Liver Disorders

Kia Saeian • Reza Shaker

Editors

Liver Disorders

A Point of Care Clinical Guide

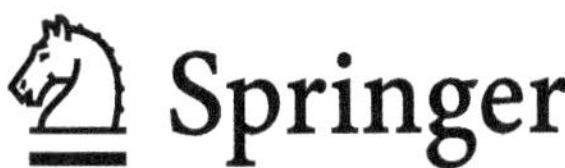 Springer

Editors
Kia Saeian
Division of Gastroenterology and Hepatology
Medical College of Wisconsin
Milwaukee, WI, USA

Reza Shaker
Division of Gastroenterology and Hepatology
Medical College of Wisconsin
Milwaukee, WI, USA

ISBN 978-3-319-30101-3   ISBN 978-3-319-30103-7   (eBook)
DOI 10.1007/978-3-319-30103-7

Library of Congress Control Number: 2016935856

Printed on acid-free paper

This Springer imprint is published by Springer Nature
The registered company is Springer International Publishing AG
The registered company address is: Gewerbestrasse 11, 6330 Cham, Switzerland

Preface

Patients with liver disease may be fearful of the diagnosis particularly since once they are told they have liver disease, they envision having cirrhosis and its associated ominous implications. Moreover, patients often receive confusing and at times contradictory responses. Beyond the typical questions of why and how they are affected by the disease, liver patients may be concerned about their long-term prognosis, whether they can drink alcohol and if so, how much, if there is truly a best approach for management moving forward, and what lifestyle changes they should undertake. The unique aspect of this handbook on liver disease is its patient-based perspective. World-class experts in the field provide cogent responses to everyday questions often posed by patients with liver disease followed by a succinct and evidence-based summary of a particular disorder. The summaries are not intended to be exhaustive but rather intended to provide the reader with a manageable and clinically relevant basis with which to care for patients with liver disease.

Disorders of the liver affect an increasingly large number of individuals, and the emergence of myriad new therapeutic options including the new direct-acting antiviral agents used in the treatment of chronic hepatitis C has changed the landscape of the management of chronic liver disease. In addition to covering the spectrum of identified liver diseases, this handbook also provides insights into appropriate testing and disease monitoring of patients, use of medications, supplements, alternative therapies and alcohol, operative risk assessment, implementation of health maintenance for patients with chronic liver disease and cirrhosis, identification and management of particular complications of cirrhosis and appropriate referral for liver transplantation, as well as management of special populations.

It is often the case that questions posed by patients are seemingly straightforward but require the provider to synthesize and distill complex and nuanced hepatology literature into a simple answer that the patient can comprehend. Each chapter will begin with patient questions followed by answers offered by the world-class experts. The answers and evidence-based summary will guide the nonhepatologist (gastroenterologists, internists, physician extenders) liver provider as well as hepatologists to easily and quickly answer common patient questions and address their medical needs. Our guiding principles have been brevity and maintenance of a very clinical focus such that the provider can derive insight into the particular disorder by reading for just a few minutes during a busy clinic day.

We are grateful to the world-class experts who kindly agreed to offer their insights and authored the chapters in this handbook and feel honored to have been able to bring together such an outstanding group.

Milwaukee, WI   Kia Saeian
Milwaukee, WI   Reza Shaker

Contents

1 What Do Abnormal Liver Tests Mean? 1
Miguel Malespin and Rebecca Tsang

2 General Care of the Liver Patient 17
Sanjay Bhandari

3 Do I Need a Liver Biopsy? 27
Kiyoko Oshima

Part I What to Do with Tumors in the Liver?

4 Incidental Hepatic Lesions 43
Syed Rizvi

5 Benign Liver Lesions 51
Syed Rizvi

6 Malignant Liver Lesions 71
Michael Loudin, Ranjan Mascarenhas, and Barry Schlansky

7 Health Maintenance in Liver Disease and Cirrhosis 89
Veronica Loy

8 Preoperative and Postoperative Care of the Liver Patient 99
Malcolm M. Wells and Thomas D. Schiano

Part II Distinct Liver Disorders

9 Viral Hepatitis: Hepatitis A and E 121
Adnan Said and Amanda DeVoss

10 Viral Hepatitis: Hepatitis B (& D) 133
Tatyana Taranukha and Venelin Kounev

11 Viral Hepatitis: Hepatitis C 143
Chalermrat Bunchorntavakul and K. Rajender Reddy

12 Viral Hepatitis: Other Viral Hepatides 165
Adnan Said and Aiman Ghufran

13 Alcoholic Liver Disease 173
Ashutosh Barve, Luis S. Marsano, Dipendra Parajuli,
Matthew Cave, and Craig J. McClain

14 Nonalcoholic Fatty Liver Disease 199
Samer Gawrieh

15 Autoimmune Liver Diseases: Autoimmune Hepatitis 217
Albert J. Czaja

16 Autoimmune Liver Diseases: Primary Biliary Cholangitits 251
Ahmad H. Ali, Elizabeth J. Carey, and Keith D. Lindor

17 Autoimmune Liver Diseases: Primary Sclerosing Cholangitis 289
José Franco

18 Autoimmune Liver Diseases: Overlap Syndromes 307
Albert J. Czaja

**19 Metabolic and Genetic Liver Diseases:
Alpha-1 Anti-trypsin Deficiency** 329
Helen S. Te

20 Metabolic and Genetic Liver Diseases: Hemochromatosis 339
Matthew J. Stotts and Bruce R. Bacon

21 Metabolic and Genetic Liver Diseases: Wilson's Disease 355
Syed Rahman and Kia Saeian

**22 Metabolic and Genetic Liver Diseases:
Glycogen Storage Diseases** 369
Grzegorz W. Telega

23 Metabolic and Genetic Liver Diseases: Urea Cycle Defects 375
Grzegorz W. Telega

24 Metabolic and Genetic Liver Diseases: Porphyrias 381
Grzegorz W. Telega

25 Drug-Induced Liver Injury 389
Raj Vuppalanchi

**26 Miscellaneous Disorders: Pregnancy-Associated Liver
Disorders, Vascular Disorders, Granulomatous Diseases,
and Amyloidosis** 405
Eric F. Martin

Part III Care of the Cirrhotic Patient

27 **Portal Hypertension** 455
Douglas A. Simonetto and Vijay H. Shah

28 **Endoscopic Management of Portal Hypertension** 469
Murad Aburajab

29 **Portosystemic Encephalopathy** 481
Jawaid Shaw and Jasmohan S. Bajaj

30 **Ascites** 507
Adam J. Schiro

31 **Spontaneous Bacterial Peritonitis (SBP)** 519
Adam J. Schiro

32 **Hepatorenal Syndrome** 531
Michael M. Yeboah

33 **Hepatopulmonary Syndrome** 545
Rahul Sudhir Nanchal and Tessa Damm

34 **Endoscopy and the Liver Patient** 555
Abdul H. Khan

35 **Liver Resection** 583
Amir H. Fathi and T. Clark Gamblin

36 **Liver Transplantation: An Overview** 599
Joohyun Kim and Johnny C. Hong

Index 621

Contributors

Murad Aburajab, M.D. Division of Gastroenterology and Hepatology, Medical College of Wisconsin, Milwaukee, WI, USA

Ahmad H. Ali, M.B.B.S. Division of Gastroenterology and Hepatology, Mayo Clinic, Phoenix, AZ, USA

Bruce R. Bacon, M.D. Division of Gastroenterology & Hepatology, St. Louis University, Saint Louis, MO, USA

Jasmohan S. Bajaj, M.D. Division of Gastroenterology, Hepatology and Nutrition, Virginia Commonwealth University, Richmond, VA, USA

McGuire VA Medical Center, Richmond, VA, USA

Ashutosh Barve, M.D. Division of Gastroenterology, Hepatology and Nutrition, Department of Medicine, University of Louisville School of Medicine, Louisville, KY, USA

Robley Rex Louisville VAMC, Louisville, KY, USA

Sanjay Bhandari, M.D. Department of General Internal Medicine, Medical College of Wisconsin, Milwaukee, WI, USA

Chalermrat Bunchorntavakul, M.D. Division of Gastroenterology and Hepatology, Department of Medicine, Hospital of the University of Pennsylvania, Philadelphia, PA, USA

Department of Medicine, Rajavithi Hospital, College of Medicine, Rangsit University, Bangkok, Thailand

Elizabeth J. Carey, M.D. Division of Gastroenterology and Hepatology, Mayo Clinic, Phoenix, AZ, USA

Matthew Cave, M.D. Division of Gastroenterology, Hepatology and Nutrition, Department of Medicine, University of Louisville School of Medicine, Louisville, KY, USA

Robley Rex Louisville VAMC, Louisville, KY, USA

Department of Pharmacology and Toxicology, University of Louisville School of Medicine, Louisville, KY, USA

Department of Biochemistry and Molecular Biology, University of Louisville School of Medicine, Louisville, KY, USA

Albert J. Czaja, M.D. Division of Gastroenterology and Hepatology, Mayo Clinic College of Medicine, Rochester, MN, USA

Tessa Damm, M.D. Department of Critical Care Medicine, Aurora St. Luke's Medical Center, Milwaukee, WI, USA

Amanda DeVoss, M.M.S., PA-C Division of Gastroenterology and Hepatology, Department of Medicine, William S. Middleton VAMC, University of Wisconsin School of Medicine and Public Health, Madison, WI, USA

Amir H. Fathi, M.D. Division of Surgical Oncology, Medical College of Wisconsin, Milwaukee, WI, USA

José Franco, M.D. Division of Gastroenterology and Hepatology, Medical College of Wisconsin, Milwaukee, WI, USA

T. Clark Gamblin, M.D., M.S. Division of Surgical Oncology, Medical College of Wisconsin, Milwaukee, WI, USA

Samer Gawrieh, M.D. Division of Gastroenterology and Hepatology, Indiana University School of Medicine, Indianapolis, IN, USA

Aiman Ghufran, M.D. Division of Gastroenterology and Hepatology, William S. Middleton VA Medical Center, University of Wisconsin School of Medicine and Public Health, Madison, WI, USA

Johnny C. Hong, M.D., F.A.C.S. Division of Transplant Surgery, Department of Surgery, Medical College of Wisconsin, Milwaukee, WI, USA

A Joint Program of Froedtert & Medical College of Wisconsin, Children's Hospital of Wisconsin & Blood Center of Wisconsin, Milwaukee, WI, USA

Abdul H. Khan, M.D. Division of Gastroenterology, Gastroenterology and Hepatology – Froedtert, Medical College of Wisconsin, Milwaukee, WI, USA

Joohyun Kim, M.D., Ph.D. Division of Transplant Surgery, Department of Surgery, Medical College of Wisconsin, Milwaukee, WI, USA

Venelin Kounev, M.D. Division of Gastroenterology & Hepatology, Medical College of Wisconsin, Milwaukee, WI, USA

Keith D. Lindor, M.D. Division of Gastroenterology and Hepatology, Mayo Clinic, Phoenix, AZ, USA

College of Health Solutions, Arizona State University, Phoenix, AZ, USA

Michael Loudin, M.D. Division of Gastroenterology and Hepatology, Department of Medicine, Oregon Health and Science University, Portland, OR, USA

Veronica Loy, D.O. Division of Hepatology, Loyola University of College, Maywood, IL, USA

Miguel Malespin, M.D. Division of Gastroenterology and Hepatology, University of Florida Health, Jacksonville, FL, USA

Luis S. Marsano, M.D. Division of Gastroenterology, Hepatology and Nutrition, Department of Medicine, University of Louisville School of Medicine, Louisville, KY, USA

Robley Rex Louisville VAMC, Louisville, KY, USA

Eric F. Martin, M.D. Division of Hepatology, Miami University Miller School of Medicine, Miami, FL, USA

Ranjan Mascarenhas, M.D. Austin Outpatient Clinic, Central Texas Veterans Health Care System, Austin, TX, USA

Craig J. McClain, M.D. Division of Gastroenterology, Hepatology & Nutrition, Department of Medicine, University of Louisville School of Medicine, Louisville, KY, USA

Robley Rex Louisville VAMC, Louisville, KY, USA

Department of Pharmacology and Toxicology, University of Louisville School of Medicine, Louisville, KY, USA

Rahul Sudhir Nanchal, M.D. Division of Pulmonary & Critical Care, Medical College of Wisconsin, Milwaukee, WI, USA

Kiyoko Oshima, M.D., Dr.Sc. Department of Pathology, Medical College of Wisconsin, Milwaukee, WI, USA

Dipendra Parajuli, M.D. Division of Gastroenterology, Hepatology and Nutrition, Department of Medicine, University of Louisville School of Medicine, Louisville, KY, USA

Robley Rex Louisville VAMC, Louisville, KY, USA

Syed Rahman, M.D. Division of Gastroenterology & Hepatology, Division of Gastroentcrology and Hepatology, Department of Medicine, Medical College of Wisconsin, Milwaukee, WI, USA

K. Rajender Reddy, M.D. Division of Gastroenterology and Hepatology, Department of Medicine, Hospital of the University of Pennsylvania, Philadelphia, PA, USA

Syed Rizvi, M.D. Division of Gastroenterology & Hepatology, Medical College of Wisconsin, Milwaukee, WI, USA

Kia Saeian, M.D., M.Sc., Epi Division of Gastroenterology and Hepatology, Medical College of Wisconsin, Milwaukee, WI, USA

Adnan Said, M.D., M.S. Division of Gastroenterology and Hepatology, Department of Medicine, William S. Middleton VAMC, University of Wisconsin School of Medicine and Public Health, Madison, WI, USA

Thomas D. Schiano, M.D. Icahn School of Medicine at Mount Sinai, The Mount Sinai Medical Center, Recanati/Miller Transplantation Institute, New York, NY, USA

Adam J. Schiro, M.D. Division of Gastroenterology & Hepatology, Department of Medicine, Medical College of Wisconsin, Milwaukee, WI, USA

Barry Schlansky, M.D. Division of Gastroenterology and Hepatology, Department of Medicine, Oregon Health and Science University, Portland, OR, USA

Vijay H. Shah, M.D. Department of Gastroenterology and Hepatology, Mayo Clinic Hospital, Rochester, MN, USA

Jawaid Shaw, M.D. Department of Medicine, McGuire VA Medical Center, Richmond, VA, USA

Douglas A. Simonetto, M.D. Department of Gastroenterology and Hepatology, Mayo Clinic Hospital, Rochester, MN, USA

Matthew J. Stotts, M.D. Banner Health Greely, Colorado, St. Louis, MO, USA

Tatyana Taranukha, M.D. Division of Gastroenterology & Hepatology, Medical College of Wisconsin, Milwaukee, WI, USA

Helen S. Te, M.D. Center for Liver Diseases, University of Chicago Medicine, Chicago, IL, USA

Grzegorz W. Telega, M.D., M.S. Department of Pediatric Gastroenterology, Hepatology and Nutrition, Medical College of Wisconsin, Milwaukee, WI, USA

Rebecca Tsang, M.D., M.P.H. Division of Gastroenterology, Loyola University Medical Center, Maywood, IL, USA

Raj Vuppalanchi, M.D. Division of Gastroenterology and Hepatology, Indiana University School of Medicine, Indianapolis, IN, USA

Malcolm M. Wells, M.D., F.R.C.P.C. Icahn School of Medicine at Mount Sinai, The Mount Sinai Medical Center, New York, NY, USA

Michael M. Yeboah, M.B.Ch.B., Ph.D. Division of Nephrology, Medical College of Wisconsin, Milwaukee, WI, USA

Chapter 1
What Do Abnormal Liver Tests Mean?

Miguel Malespin and Rebecca Tsang

Commonly Posed Patient Questions

1. What are common causes of abnormal liver tests?

   The initial step when evaluating abnormalities in liver panel testing is to determine whether these changes reflect an acute or chronic process. An acute process is typically suspected in an individual lacking a prior history or risk factors for the development of chronic liver disease. Once chronicity has been established, a differential diagnosis can then be formulated on the basis of the pattern, degree, and rapidity of liver enzyme elevation. Common acute causes of elevated liver enzymes include drug toxicity (i.e., over-the-counter, prescribed, and herbal therapy), alcohol abuse, acute viral disease (i.e., hepatitis A and B), autoimmune diseases of the liver, benign or malignant liver tumors, thrombosis of hepatic vasculature, and global hepatic hypoperfusion.

   A chronic elevation in liver panel testing can either reflect states of persistent hepatic inflammation that occur for greater than 6 months and/or hepatic dysfunction from a cirrhotic liver's inability to carry out its basic cellular processes. Common etiologies include chronic liver disease from viral hepatitis (i.e., hepatitis B and C), alcohol abuse, nonalcoholic steatohepatitis (NASH), hereditary hemochromatosis, and chronic autoimmune diseases of the liver. The initial evaluation of both the acute and chronic liver disease involves acquisition of a thorough but focused history, physical examination,

M. Malespin, M.D. (✉)
Division of Gastroenterology and Hepatology, University of Florida Health,
Jacksonville, FL, USA

4555 Emerson St. Ste. 300, Jacksonville, FL 32207, USA
e-mail: miguel.malespin@jax.ufl.edu

R. Tsang, M.D., M.P.H.
Division of Gastroenterology, Loyola University Medical Center, Maywood, IL, USA

© Springer International Publishing Switzerland 2017
K. Sacian, R. Shaker (eds.), *Liver Disorders*,
DOI 10.1007/978-3-319-30103-7_1

serologic analysis, and liver-focused imaging with either ultrasound or computed-tomography (CT) scan. A liver biopsy may be warranted in cases where the diagnosis remains elusive.

It is important to consider that some patients may also have multiple causes of liver disease. As in the case of coexisting chronic hepatitis C (HCV) and alcohol-related liver disease, a second insult can potentiate viral replication, inflammation, and fibrosis. Given the unspecific nature of certain lab abnormalities, a practitioner should remain attuned to nonhepatic causes of elevated liver enzymes. Such examples include elevated total bilirubin levels secondary to hemolytic anemia and increased levels of circulating levels of alanine aminotransferase (ALT) and aspartate aminotransferase (AST) from skeletal muscle injury.

2. How long will it take for my AST/ALT to return to normal?

Hepatocyte inflammation is expressed serologically through an elevation in levels of the transaminases, AST and ALT. The peak of injury after the insult and time to laboratory normalization are dependent on the presence of preexisting liver disease and the etiology of hepatic insult. For example, severe injury secondary to acetaminophen toxicity typically resolves within weeks while cases of penicillin or alcohol related hepatitis could take several months to normalize. On the other hand, patients being treated with antiviral therapy for hepatitis B or C demonstrate normalization of liver enzymes upon viral suppression or clearance to undetectable levels. Treatment of NASH focuses on weight loss through dietary modifications and exercise [2]. Studies have demonstrated that approximately 10 % of weight loss can lead to improvement in hepatocyte inflammation and thus improvement in liver enzymes. The time to normalization of AST/ALT can occur early but will typically vary between individuals.

3. What does it mean if my ALT and AST is low?

When evaluating laboratory values, the reported reference range signifies the parameters that include the mean 95 % of the population. Thus, there will be a reported abnormal value for liver enzymes above and below this normal range. Low values do not represent a clinically significant abnormality and thus have no repercussions. This principle also holds true for alkaline phosphatase and bilirubin levels in a normal patient with no prior history of liver disease.

Components of a Liver Profile

The term, *liver function tests*, is often used in the medical community to describe the serologic measurements ordered to evaluate for liver disease. As part of the *liver function tests*, aminotransferases are most commonly ordered as the initial test to detect liver disease. The term *liver function tests* is a misnomer and do not necessarily reflect liver function, but more so are biochemical tests that reflect inflammation. In addition to the serum aminotransferases AST and ALT, the complete liver profile also includes total and direct bilirubin, albumin, alkaline phosphatase, and occasionally gamma glutamyl transpeptidase (GGT).

It has been found that elevated aminotransferase levels are present in 7.9 % of the population when sampling asymptomatic individuals [3]. As medical providers, it is important to know how to interpret these tests to better assess and manage these patients, as there is a mortality risk associated with acute and chronic liver diseases and their complications.

Aminotransferases

Serum aminotransferases, also known as transaminases, include AST and ALT, and are good indicators of acute hepatocellular injury. Formerly known as serum glutamic oxaloacetic transaminase (SGOT), AST is located in the cytosol and mitochondria and catalyzes the transfer of the α-amino groups of the L-aspartic acid to the α-keto group of ketoglutaric acid. Though most commonly found in the liver, this enzyme is also present in striated muscle, the kidney, brain, pancreas, lung, leukocytes, and erythrocytes. Formerly known as serum glutamic pyruvic transaminases (SGPT), ALT lies in the cytosol and catalyzes the transfer of the α-amino groups of alanine to the α-keto group of ketoglutaric acid. This enzyme is also found throughout the body, but is a more specific indicator of liver injury compared to AST because it is significantly more concentrated in the liver. In hepatocellular injury, damage to tissues rich in aminotransferases causes them to leak into the serum, resulting in increased serum levels of ALT and/or AST. The absolute value of serum levels does not necessarily reflect the degree of damage, and it cannot be assumed that the higher the serum aminotransferase level, the more severe the liver injury. These enzymes have a half-life measured in days, but AST is cleared more rapidly than ALT.

Normal Range

NHANES III criteria for upper limit reference of the normal range for aminotransferases were listed as AST >37 IU/L or ALT >40 IU/L for men and AST or ALT >31 IU/L for women [4]. However, normal values for aminotransferases in serum vary widely among laboratories due to technical issues. In addition, the normal range varies between different population groups and so there is no universal definition. Similar to most clinical laboratory tests, the normal range for a particular laboratory test is established as within two standard deviations from the mean of a healthy population, which includes 95 % of a uniformly distributed population. As mentioned earlier, serum aminotransferase level below the lower reference limit is of no clinical importance, although lower levels have been seen in hemodialysis patients thought to be partly due to B_6 deficiency. Therefore, it is only when the aminotransferase level exceeds the upper reference limit that it is considered abnormal.

Aminotransferase levels vary according to age and gender. For instance, elevated aminotransferases are more common for people between ages 30 and 40 years old, and it seems to decrease after the age of 60. In a study of 975 healthy children aged 7–18 years old, the upper reference limit of ALT was 30 IU/L for boys and 21 IU/L for girls [5], which is comparatively less than adults as evidenced by NHANES III mentioned earlier. With respect to gender differences, overall the normal range for males is higher than females [3, 5].

In addition, it has been shown that ALT levels correlated strongly with BMI, as evidenced by the Prati et al. study in which 6835 healthy blood donors were screened [2]. This could be a reflection of the increased prevalence of NAFLD in patients with a higher BMI. There is also a significant prevalence of NAFLD in overweight and obese patients with diabetes mellitus type II despite normal amino-transferases [6]. This suggests that perhaps in this population, there should be a higher index of suspicion in the lower-than-normal threshold aminotransferase level in suspecting NAFLD.

Furthermore, there are ethnic differences for normal values of aminotransferases. There are higher serum levels of aminotransferases in non-Hispanic blacks and Mexican Americans compared to non-Hispanic whites [3]. In addition, serum ami-notransferases for healthy Asians are significantly lower, as shown by the Wu et al. study in Taipei with the upper limit reference of the normal range found to be 21 IU/L for men and 17 IU/L for women [7].

Of note, there have been some studies that have shown slightly increase in AST/ALT during normal pregnancy, especially in the third trimester [8, 9]. However, the majority of studies support the presence of normal aminotransferases during uncom-plicated pregnancy [10, 11], and therefore elevated aminotransferases continue to be excellent markers for liver diseases during pregnancy.

Common Causes of Elevated Aminotransferases

As previously noted, elevated aminotransferases are suggestive of hepatocellular injury. The challenge of identifying a sole etiology was highlighted in one study, illustrating that one or more causes were determined in only 31 % of patients with elevated aminotransferases, leaving 69 % of cases unexplained [3]. Some of the most common identifiable causes include alcohol use (13.5 %), hepatitis C (7.0 %), hemo-chromatosis (3.4 %), hepatitis B (0.9 %), or a combination of causes (6.1 %). Alterations in aminotransferase levels can be classified as: *mild* (<5 times the upper limit of normal), *moderate* (5–10 times the upper limit of normal), and *marked* (>10 times the upper limit of normal). Though somewhat arbitrary, different etiologies should be considered depending on magnitude of aminotransferase alteration. Table 1.1 includes common causes of elevated aminotransferases based on the degree of elevation [12].

Table 1.1 Causes of elevated aminotransferases

Moderate-to-marked elevation in aminotransferases	Mild elevation in aminotransferases
Ischemic injury[a, b]	Nonalcoholic fatty liver disease
Toxic injury[a, b]	Alcoholic hepatitis
Acute viral hepatitis[a, c, d]	Pharmacology
Acute biliary obstruction[a, d, e]	Chronic viral hepatitis (B, C)
Alcoholic hepatitis[a, d, e]	Hereditary hemochromatosis
	Autoimmune hepatitis
	Wilson's disease
	α-1-Antitripsin deficiency
	Celiac disease
	Extrahepatic causes

[a]Aminotransferase level increase of 5–10×upper limit of normal
[b]Bilirubin increase of <5×upper reference limit
[c]Aminotransferase level increase of >10×upper limit of normal
[d]Bilirubin increase of 5–10×upper limit of normal
[e]Bilirubin increase of >10×upper limit of normal

Initial Evaluation of Elevated Aminotransferases

The work-up for abnormal aminotransferases differs according to the degree of alteration, since different etiologies are considered for mild elevations compared to moderate–severe elevations. However, as mentioned earlier, the degree of elevation does not necessarily reflect the extent of liver damage. Moderate–severe elevations are more suggestive of an acute liver injury, whereas when mild elevations in aminotransferases are encountered, chronic liver diseases should also be considered in addition to acute liver injury.

Mild alterations are commonly encountered by primary care physicians. Though some expert recommendations include repeating transaminases 6 months before initiating a work-up, the clinical scenario will likely dictate the urgency of further clinical evaluation. However, if repeat transaminases are normal, this does not entirely exclude liver diseases since aminotransferases fluctuate in liver disease. The importance of a thorough history cannot be overstated. Also, there should be a focus on identifying risk factors, family history, and possible exposures to over-the-counter medications, supplements, and alcohol. If there is clear exposure such as a medication and/or the pattern of aminotransferases is typical of alcohol use (AST:ALT >2), then it is reasonable to repeat transaminases after discontinuing the exposure. Initial testing for anti-HCV and HBsAg testing should be considered, especially in patients with IV drug use, exposure to nonsterile needles, or sexual exposure to an infected person with further consideration of anti-HCV testing in the age-based cohort of persons born between 1945 and 1965 and HBsAg testing in those of Asian descent.

Additional testing includes acquisition of ferritin, iron, and total iron-binding capacity (TIBC) to screen for hereditary hemochromatosis, and if both ferritin and transferrin saturation (iron/TIBC × 100) are increased, then it is reasonable to test for HFE gene mutation. Furthermore, it is reasonable to test for antinuclear antibodies (ANA), antismooth body antibodies (ASMA), immunoglobulin levels, and occasionally anti-LKM (liver–kidney microsomes) to rule out autoimmune hepatitis, especially in young or middle-aged women with concomitant autoimmune diseases. If the earlier tests are unrevealing, further serologic work-up to consider include alpha-1 antitrypsin levels to rule out alpha-1 antitrypsin deficiency, tissue transglutaminase antibodies to rule out celiac disease, and serum ceruloplasmin levels in patients under the age of 50 to evaluate for Wilson's disease. In the absence of serological findings and a history of alcohol abuse, one shoulder consider the presence of nonalcoholic fatty liver disease (NAFLD), particularly in patients with conditions linked to metabolic syndrome and insulin resistance (i.e., increased BMI, diabetes, hyperlipidemia, hypertension). However, lack of the above-mentioned risk factors does not exclude the possibility of NAFLD. Despite the commonality and increasing prevalence of fatty liver disease [13], the lack of disease-specific serology can make the diagnosis challenging in the absence of histology.

Moderate-to-marked elevations in aminotransferases are usually more typical of acute compared to chronic liver disease. A moderate increase in aminotransferase levels has a higher sensitivity and specificity for identifying acute injury compared to mild elevations in aminotransferases. Studies have shown a sensitivity of 91 % and specificity of 95 % with an AST ≥ 200 IU/L while ALT levels ≥ 300 IU/L offer sensitivity of 96 % and specificity of 94 % [14]. Although there are certain liver injuries that are associated with markedly elevated aminotransferases, these same etiologies should be considered in mild elevations as well.

Certain patterns of liver injury are indicative of specific disease etiologies. For example, aminotransferases levels >75 times the upper limit of normal (ULN) are indicative of ischemic or toxic liver injury [15] with a subsequent rise in bilirubin levels 3–5 days after the insult. Acute viral hepatitis usually present with a more modest elevation of aminotransferases. Patients with moderate-to-marked increases (>10–20 × ULN) in aminotransferases should be tested for IgM antibodies to hepatitis A, IgM to hepatitis B core antigen, hepatitis B surface antigen, and hepatitis C antibody. If these are negative, it is reasonable to test for HCV RNA particularly in the setting of risk factors. Other considerations include acetaminophen-induced hepatic damage as it causes 54 and 16 % of acute liver failure in the United Kingdom and United States [16].

Another etiology of moderate elevations is alcohol-induced acute hepatitis damage. This can present as both acute and acute-on-chronic liver injury. The increase in AST levels is reported to be less than six to seven times the ULN in 98 % of the patients with alcoholic liver disease, and the AST:ALT ratio >1 in 92 % and >2 in 70 % of patients [17]. After these common causes have been excluded, other less common causes such as nonhepatotropic viruses such as Epstein–Barr virus, cytomegalovirus, and herpes simplex virus, as well as other infiltrative, autoimmune, extrahepatic, and congenital causes should be considered. Imaging modalities can point to extrahepatic causes by demonstrating a dilated biliary system particularly in the setting of biliary colic and/or known gallstones (Fig. 1.1).

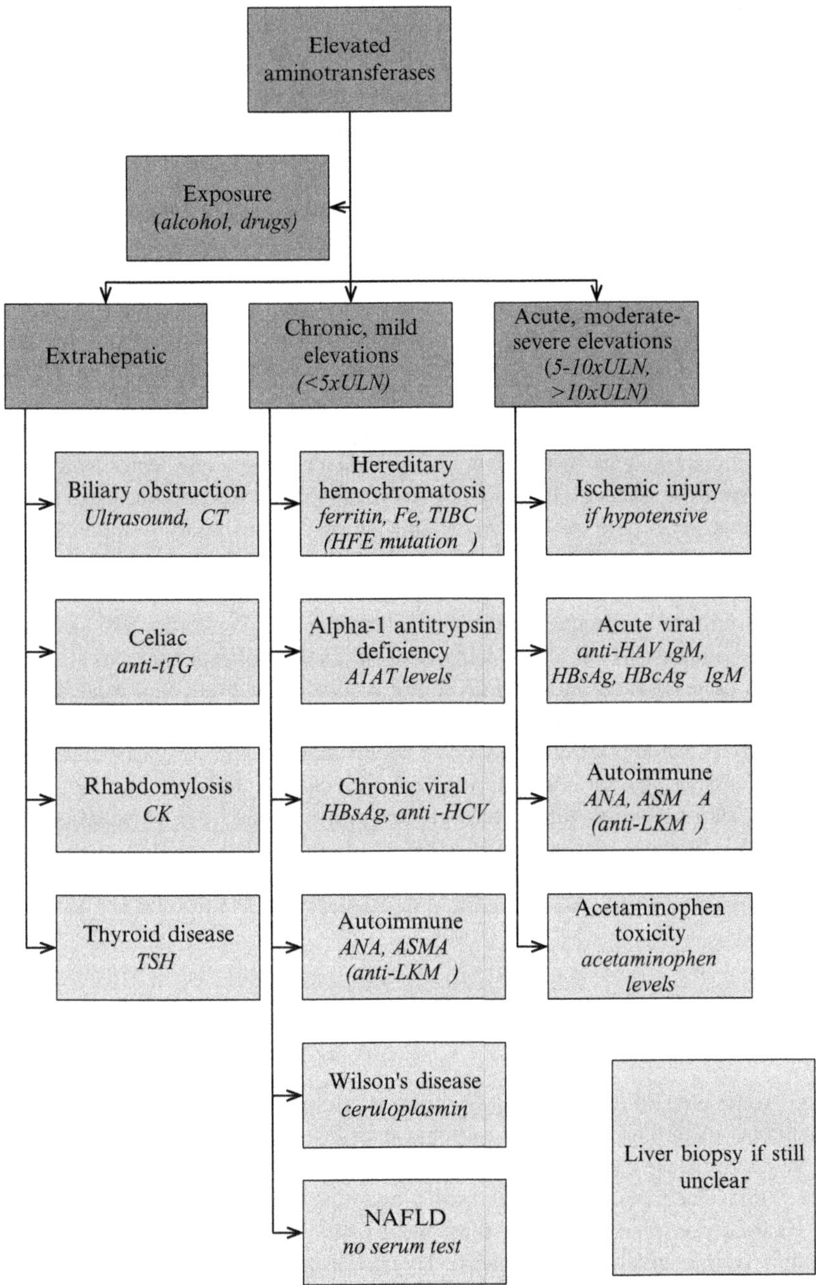

Fig. 1.1 Evaluation of transaminase elevation. *ULN* upper limit of normal, *Anti-tTG* tissue transglutaminase antibodies, *CK* creatine kinase, *Fe* iron, *TIBC* total iron binding capacity, *HBV* hepatitis B, *HCV* hepatitis C, *HBsAg* hepatitis B surface antigen, *anti-HCV* hepatitis C antibody, *ANA* antinuclear antibodies, *ASMA* antismooth body antibodies, *anti-LKM* antibodies to liver–kidney microsomes, *NAFLD* nonalcoholic fatty liver disease. Initially, if there is an obvious offending agent (i.e., drug or alcohol), liver function tests can be repeated after discontinuation of offending agent. If there is no offending agent or if no improvement in aminotransferases despite removal of offending agent, work-up should be initiated. Moderate–severe elevations are more suggestive of an acute process. Although mild elevations are more suggestive of a chronic process, acute etiologies should also be considered, especially if the chronicity of aminotransferase elevation is unclear

Alkaline Phosphatase and Gamma Glutamyl Transpeptide (GGT)

Despite being produced predominantly in the liver and bone, alkaline phosphatase isoenzymes can be found in renal, intestinal, placental tissue, or within leukocytes. In the liver, alkaline phosphatase is located on the canalicular membrane of hepatocytes and an increase in serum levels usually indicates osseous or hepatobiliary pathology. With a half-life of approximately 6 days, an increase in alkaline phosphatase levels occurs secondary to increased synthesis with leakage of the serum and not due to decreased clearance.

GGT is a microsomal enzyme located throughout the body, including hepatocytes and cholangiocytes in the liver, kidney, pancreas, spleen, heart, brain, and seminal vesicles. It has a high sensitivity for hepatobiliary disease but lacks specificity. Levels can become elevated in patients taking certain classes of medications, including anticonvulsants, oral contraceptives, barbiturates, antiretroviral therapy, as well as patients with comorbidities, such as chronic obstructive pulmonary disease, renal failure, and acute myocardial infarctions. GGT is clinically useful to identify the etiology of an isolated increase in alkaline phosphatase, as it is not elevated in bone disease. Elevated GGT levels also occur in alcohol-related liver disease, even in patients with normal alkaline phosphatase levels. Because of its high sensitivity, some physicians advocate acquisition of GGT levels as an indirect marker of current alcohol consumption [18]. Beyond alcohol liver disease, GGT levels may also be two to three times greater in more than 50% of patients with NAFLD [19]. Because elevated GGT levels are frequently elevated in most forms of liver disease, it is most useful when evaluating patients with an elevated alkaline phosphatase levels with otherwise normal liver enzymes and bilirubin levels.

Variations

There is some physiologic variation of serum alkaline phosphatase levels in certain populations, including certain physiologic circumstance in which the intestinal alkaline phosphatase can be proportionately elevated and result in elevated serum levels. For instance, because patients with blood type O and B have increased intestinal alkaline phosphatase after a fatty meal [20], some physicians recommend obtaining fasting alkaline phosphatase levels. Also, elevated intestinal alkaline phosphatase can be indicative of certain benign familial conditions, including familial intrahepatic cholestasis or benign recurrent intrahepatic cholestasis, which are typically characterized by elevations in the alkaline phosphatase despite a normal GGT with occasional elevations in the bilirubin level. The age of the individual also has an impact on the serum alkaline phosphatase levels with levels being twice as high in adolescents compared with adults due to increased bone growth. In addition, there is an unexplained increase in levels after age 30 years old, but the increase is greater in women compared to men [21].

Clinical Significance of Low Alkaline Phosphatase

Patients with Wilson's disease may have a low serum alkaline phosphatase, especially when the patient presents with fulminant hepatitis and hemolysis. It is thought that this is due to reduced activity of the enzyme, owing to displacement of the cofactor zinc by copper.

Common Causes of Elevated Alkaline Phosphatase

Table 1.2 lists the common causes of elevated levels [12]. When patients have an isolated elevated alkaline phosphatase or if the alkaline phosphatase is elevated out of proportion to the other liver enzymes, one should consider cholestatic disorders.

Table 1.2 Common causes of elevated alkaline phosphatase

Intrahepatic	
Drugs	Anabolic steroids, estrogens, ACE-I, antimicrobials, NSAIDS, allopurinol, antiepileptics, hydralazine, procainamide, quinidine, phenylbutazone
Primary biliary cirrhosis	Predominantly middle-aged women with median age of 50 years old, 95 % of patients have + AMA
Primary sclerosing cholangitis	Strongly associated with IBD, commonly in younger men, diagnosed by ERCP/MRCP
Granulomatous liver disease	Sarcoidosis, TB, fungal infections, brucellosis, Q fever, schistosomiasis
Viral hepatitis	EBV, CMV, Hepatitis A, B, C, E
Genetic conditions	Benign recurrent intrahepatic cholestasis type 1,2
Malignancy	HCC, metastatic disease, paraneoplastic syndrome
Infiltrative liver disease	Amyloidosis, lymphoma
Intrahepatic cholestasis of pregnancy	
Total parent nutrition	
Graft-versus-host disease	
Extrahepatic	
Intrinsic	
Immune-mediated duct injury	Autoimmune pancreatitis, primary sclerosing cholangitis
Malignancy	Ampullary cancer, cholangiocarcinoma
Infections	AIDS cholangiopathy, CMV, cryptosporidiosis, microsporidosis, parasitic infections
Extrinsic	
Malignancy	Gallbladder cancer, metastases, portal adenopathy, pancreatic cancer
Mirizzi syndrome	Compression of common hepatic duct by stone in neck of gallbladder
Pancreatitis	Also includes pancreatic pseudocyst

Initial Evaluation of Elevated Alkaline Phosphatase

If there is an elevated isolated alkaline phosphatase level in an asymptomatic patient, a cholestatic disorder should be considered if GGT levels are elevated or if there is elevated liver alkaline phosphatase when it is fractionated. This is particularly the case for patients in whom the elevated alkaline phosphatase levels are elevated out of proportion to aminotransferases. Initial evaluation with imaging of biliary tree help discern between intrahepatic and extrahepatic etiologies. Initial imaging is typically recommended with ultrasound to evaluate for biliary dilatation or mass lesions, but of course CT or MRI may be more definitive albeit at a higher cost and potential risk. When dilated ducts are seen on imaging, this is suggestive of an extrahepatic cause of the cholestasis. This can occur secondary to an intrinsic or extrinsic process causing biliary obstruction. Further work-up and/or management may include magnetic resonance imaging including magnetic resonance cholangiopancreatography (MRCP), endoscopic retrograde cholangiopancreatography (ERCP), and endoscopic ultrasound. In the absence of dilated ducts, further work-up should focus on intrahepatic etiologies. Part of this includes a thorough history of medications since some medications can cause a cholestatic picture. Liver biopsy is useful for evaluating hepatic disease including primary biliary cirrhosis, drug-induced liver injury, and small duct primary sclerosing cholangitis (Fig. 1.2).

Bilirubin Metabolism

Unconjugated bilirubin represents the product of the heme breakdown within the reticuloendothelial system. This unsoluble form is then bound to albumin and transported to the liver. Once it reaches the hepatic sinusoids, the albumin complex dissociates and within hepatocytes uridine-5′-diphosphate (UDP) glycuronylransferase conjugates bilirubin to glucuronic acid. The now conjugated bilirubin is then excreted into bile and travels to the distal ileum and colon where bacteria hydrolyze conjugated bilirubin to the unconjugated form. This is further reduced by bacteria to colorless urobilinogen, which is excreted or absorbed by the intestine into the portal system as urobilinogen. A minority of urobilinogen is excreted into urine while the remainder enters the enterohepatic circulation, in which the liver reexcretes it.

Laboratory Assays for Bilirubin

The laboratory tests, direct and indirect bilirubin, are the components of total bilirubin and provide rough measurements of conjugated and unconjugated bilirubin levels. This is determined by the van den Bergh reaction in which bilirubin reacts with diazotized sulfanilic acid. The conjugated fraction reacts immediately, or "directly," and can be measured within 30–60 s. The total bilirubin is measured 30–60 min

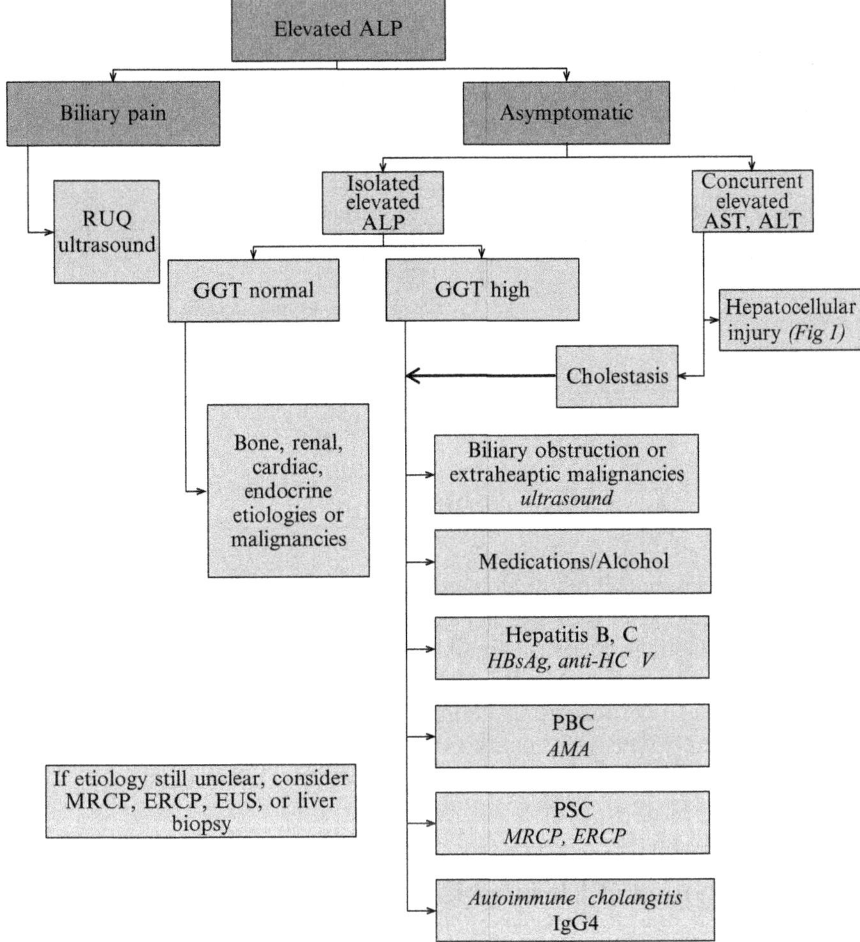

Fig. 1.2 Evaluation of alkaline phosphatase elevation. *ALP* alkaline phosphatase, *GGT* gamma glutamyl transpeptide, *HBsAg* hepatitis B surface antigen, *anti-HCV* hepatitis C antibody, *PBC* primary biliary cirrhosis, *AMA* antimitochondrial antibody, *PSC* primary sclerosing cholangitis, *MRCP* magnetic resonance cholangiopancreatography, *ERCP* endoscopic retrograde cholangiopancreatography

after adding an accelerant. Subsequently, the unconjugated, or indirect, bilirubin is the result of subtracting the direct bilirubin from the total bilirubin.

Normal Range

The normal range for total and indirect bilirubin falls between 1.0 to 1.5 and 0.8 to 1.2 mg/dL, respectively [22].

Table 1.3 Common causes of elevated bilirubin

Type	Cause
Unconjugated hyperbilirubinemia	Hemolysis
	Gilbert's syndrome
	Hematoma reabsorption
	Ineffective erythropoiesis
Conjugated hyperbilirubinemia	Bile duct obstruction
	Hepatitis
	Cirrhosis
	Autoimmune cholestatic diseases (PBC, PSC)
	Total parenteral nutrition
	Drug toxins
	Vanishing bile duct syndrome

Common Causes of Elevated Bilirubin

Findings of an elevated bilirubin can be very nonspecific and must be evaluated in the context of the other liver tests. When an elevation in bilirubin is associated with an elevation in aminotransferases and/or alkaline phosphatase, the work-up for hepatocellular injury and/or cholestatic diseases should be performed. Findings of isolated hyperbilirubinemia can reflect conditions associated with conjugated or unconjugated bilirubinemia. The most common causes of unconjugated hyperbilirubinemia are hemolysis and Gilbert's syndrome. Other causes are listed in Table 1.3.

Initial Evaluation of Elevated Bilirubin

As noted earlier, it is important to first determine whether the hyperbilirubinemia occurs in conjunction with other liver test abnormalities (i.e. aminotransferases, alkaline phosphatase). If this is the case, the evaluation should focus on investigation of common hepatocellular (Table 1.1) or cholestatic diseases (Table 1.2). However, in patients with isolated elevated bilirubin, it is important to fractionate and determine if there is a predominance of conjugated or unconjugated bilirubin. Findings of <15 % conjugated bilirubin suggest a hemolytic process, an inability to conjugate heme, or an impairment of hepatic uptake. Medications should also be reviewed to investigate for drug reactions leading to impairment of hepatocellular bilirubin uptake. If none are identified, then genetic deficiencies that impair conjugation of bilirubin should be considered, which include Gilbert's syndrome and Crigler–Najjar syndrome. Gilbert's syndrome has a reported incidence of 6–12 % in the population and occurs when due to a mutation of the UDP glycuronyl transferase gene, resulting in reduction in enzyme activity thus limiting conjugation. Gilbert's syndrome is benign,

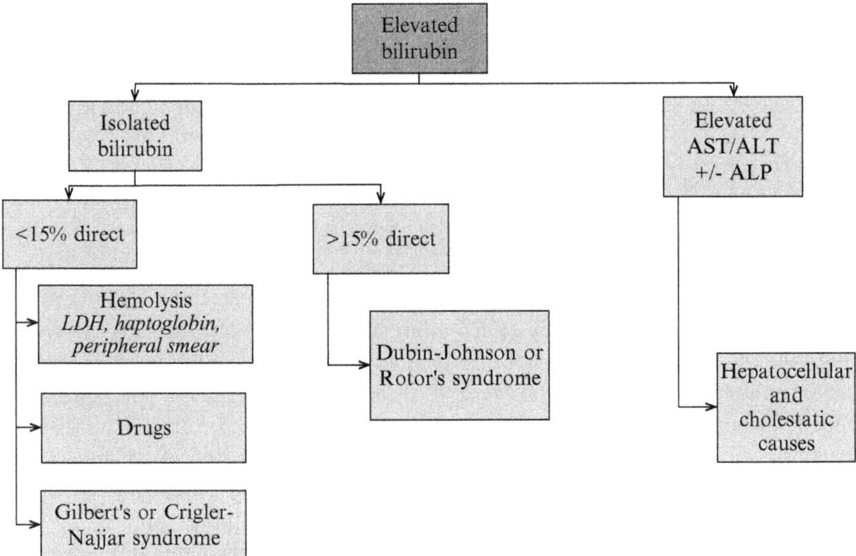

Fig. 1.3 Evaluation of bilirubin elevation. *LDH* lactate dehydrogenase. When the bilirubin is elevated in conjunction with elevated transaminases and/or alkaline phosphatase, work-up for hepatocellular and/or cholestatic etiologies should be considered (Figs. 1.1 and 1.2). For isolated bilirubin, different causes are considered depending on the fractionation of the bilirubin

unlike Crigler–Najjar syndrome which is a rare disorder related to a mutation resulting in reduced UDP glucuronyl transferase activity (<10 % in type II and absence of activity in type I). Crigler–Najjar patients are at risk for neurotoxicity secondary to hyperbilirubinemia, known as kernicterus.

Patients with isolated conjugated hyperbilirubinemia may have Dubin–Johnson syndrome or Rotor's syndrome, both uncommon, which is related to impaired excretion of conjugated bilirubin across the bile canalicular membrane. Both of these syndromes are not associated with adverse clinic outcomes (Fig. 1.3).

Albumin

Albumin is a plasma protein that is exclusively made by in the liver and accounts for 75 % of the plasma colloid pressure. The average adult procedure approximately 15 g/day and the half-life is 14–21 days [23]. This long half-life limits its reliability in acute liver injury, but is clinically helpful in chronic liver disease since hepatic synthesis of albumin is impaired in patients with advanced liver disease. However, this is not specific to liver diseases, and low serum levels can be seen in patients with nephrotic syndrome, malabsorption, protein-losing enteropathy, chronic systemic inflammatory conditions, hormonal imbalances, or malnutrition. Therefore, it is not necessarily a good screening test. It is important to interpret low albumin in the clinical context and look for other markers of liver disease. Even in patients with liver disease, if they are overloaded, the low serum albumin can be a reflection of the increased volume of distribution instead of impaired hepatic synthetic function.

Prothrombin Time

Prothrombin time is a measurement of the rate at which prothrombin is converted to thrombin, the extrinsic pathway of coagulation and depends on the activity of clotting factors II, V, VII, and X—all of which are synthesized in the liver. Therefore, prothrombin time is a reflection of liver dysfunction. Of note, factor V is sometimes checked when trying to decide if abnormal prothrombin time is due to liver disease. In chronic liver diseases, prolonged prothrombin time is a sign of advanced liver disease. In acute liver diseases, it is a more reliable indicator of immediate synthetic function since the half-life of the clotting factors are much shorter (approximately a day). International normalized ratio (INR) standardizes prothrombin time measurements based on the thromboplastin reagent used in the laboratory. It is used in a similar fashion to prothrombin time. Other etiologies of prolonged prothrombin time may be warfarin, deficiency in vitamin K, disseminated intravascular coagulopathy. Of note, obstructive jaundice can decrease absorption of vitamin K and may prolong prothrombin time but will respond to parental supplementation.

Conclusion

Interpretation of laboratory values in patients with abnormalities in liver panel testing is critical to developing a differential diagnosis and initiation an adequate work-up. The initial step when evaluating a patient with abnormalities in hepatic transaminases is to first determine whether the clinical scenario represents an acute, chronic, or acute-on-chronic process. Establishing disease chronicity is reliant on a combination of laboratory, radiologic, physical exam, and histologic findings.

Clues suggesting the presence of advanced liver disease and/or cirrhosis include the presence of hypoalbuminemia, elevation in prothrombin time, or elevated bilirubin levels. Thrombocytopenia can be used as an indirect marker of portal hypertension, particularly in the presence of splenomegaly, ascites, and portal hypertension. Other typical physical exam findings encountered in cirrhotic patients include spider angiomata, palmar erythema, gynecomastia, testicular atrophy, asterixis, and fetor hepaticus.

Acquisition of histology can be used to confirm a suspected diagnosis, rule out hepatic disease, and stage the degree of fibrosis. This procedure can be performed percutaneously with ultrasound guidance or through a transvenous approach where access to the hepatic parenchyma is obtained by introduction of a cannula through the jugular vein and into a hepatic venous system. The transvenous approach offers an added benefit of assessing for the presence of portal hypertension.

Upon establishment of chronicity, the role of the practitioner is to establish the severity of hepatic dysfunction, potential for reversibility, and the need for escalation of care. Noncirrhotic patients without a preexisting history of liver disease who develop severe hepatic injury in conjunction with encephalopathy and an elevation in INR $\geq$ 1.5 are classified as having acute liver failure. Given the increase in mortality associated with acute liver failure, transfer to a liver transplant center and intensive care unit management is recommended upon diagnosis [24].

Acknowledgements *Miguel Malespin:* Has served as a consultant for Gilead Pharmaceuticals

Conflict of interest: None of the authors have a conflict of interest.

Financial support/funding: None

References

1. Gines A, Escorsell A, Gines P, Salo J, Jimenez W, Inglada L, et al. Incidence, predictive factors, and prognosis of the hepatorenal syndrome in cirrhosis with ascites. Gastroenterology. 1993;105(1):229–36.
2. Petersen KF, Dufour S, Befroy D, Lehrke M, Hendler RE, Shulman GI. Reversal of nonalcoholic hepatic steatosis, hepatic insulin resistance, and hyperglycemia by moderate weight reduction in patients with type 2 diabetes. Diabetes. 2005;54(3):603–8.
3. Clark JM, Brancati FL, Diehl AM. The prevalence and etiology of elevated aminotransferase levels in the United States. Am J Gastroenterol. 2003;98(5):960–7.
4. Liangpunsakul S, Chalasani N. Unexplained elevations in alanine aminotransferase in individuals with the metabolic syndrome: results from the third national health and nutrition survey (NHANES III). Am J Med Sci [Internet]. 2005;329(3). http://journals.lww.com/amjmedsci/Fulltext/2005/03000/Unexplained_Elevations_in_Alanine_Aminotransferase.1.aspx.
5. Poustchi H, George J, Esmaili S, Esna-Ashari F, Ardalan G, Sepanlou SG, et al. Gender Differences in healthy ranges for serum alanine aminotransferase levels in adolescence. In: Nizami Q, editor. PLoS One. 2011;6(6):e21178.
6. Portillo Sanchez P, Bril F, Maximos M, Lomonaco R, Biernacki D, Orsak B, et al. High Prevalence of nonalcoholic fatty liver disease in patients with type 2 diabetes mellitus and normal plasma aminotransferase levels. J Clin Endocrinol Metabol. 2014;jc.2014–2739.
7. Wu W-C, Wu C-Y, Wang Y-J, Hung H-H, Yang H-I, Kao W-Y, et al. Updated thresholds for serum alanine aminotransferase level in a large-scale population study composed of 34 346 subjects. Aliment Pharmacol Ther. 2012;36(6):560–8.
8. Knopp R, Bergelin R, Wahl P, Walden C, Chapman M. Clinical chemistry alterations in pregnancy and oral contraceptive use. Obstet Gynecol. 1985;66(5):682–90.
9. Elliot JR, O'Kell RT. Normal clinical chemical values for pregnant women at term. Clin Chem. 1971;17(3):156–7.
10. Moniz CF, Nicolaides KH, Bamforth FJ, Rodeck CH. Normal reference ranges for biochemical substances relating to renal, hepatic, and bone function in fetal and maternal plasma throughout pregnancy. J Clin Pathol. 1985;38(4):468–72.
11. Carter J. Liver function in normal pregnancy. Aust N Z J Obstet Gynaecol. 1990;30(4):296–302.
12. Giannini EG, Testa R, Savarino V. Liver enzyme alteration: a guide for clinicians. Can Med Assoc J. 2005;172(3):367–79.
13. Harrison SA, Kadakia S, Lang KA, Schenker S. Nonalcoholic steatohepatitis: what we know in the new millennium. Am J Gastroenterol. 2002;97(11):2714–24.
14. Rozen P, Korn R, Zimmerman H. Computer analysis of liver function tests and their interrelationships in 347 cases of viral hepatitis. Isr J Med Sci. 1970;6(1):67–79.

15. Dufour D, Lott J, Nolte F, Gretch D. Diagnosis and monitoring of hepatic injury. I. Performance characteristics of laboratory tests. Clin Chem. 2000;46(12):2027–49.
16. O'Grady J. Acute live failure. In: O'Grady JG, Lake JR, Howelle PD, editors. Comprehensive clnical hepatology. London: Mosby; 2000. p. 16.1–16.13.
17. Cohen J, Kaplan M. The SGOT/SGPT ratio—an indicator of alcoholic liver disease. Dig Dis Sci. 1979;24(11):835–8.
18. Moussavian S, Becker R, Piepmeyer J, Mezey E, Bozian R. Serum gamma-glutamyl transpeptidase and chronic alcoholism. Influence of alcohol ingestion and liver disease. Dig Dis Sci. 1985;30(3):211–4.
19. McCullough A. Update on nonalcoholic fatty liver disease. J Clin Gastroenterol. 2002;34(3):255–62.
20. Bamford K, Harris H, Luffman J, Robson E, Cleghorn T. Serum-alkaline phosphatase and the ABO blood-groups. Lancet. 1965;1(7384):530–1.
21. Wolf P. Clinical significance of an increased or decreased seruma alkaline phosphatase level. Arch Pathol Lab Med. 1978;102:497–501.
22. Bloomer JR, Berk PD, Howe RB, Berlin NI. Interpretation of plasma on studies with. JAMA. 1971;218(2):216–20.
23. Rothschild M. Serum albumin. Hepatology. 1988;8(2):385–401.
24. Ostapowicz G, Fontana RJ, Schiødt FV, et al. Results of a prospective study of acute liver failure at 17 tertiary care centers in the United States. Ann Intern Med. 2002;137(12):947.

Chapter 2
General Care of the Liver Patient

Sanjay Bhandari

What Things Should I Avoid If I Have Liver Disease?

The liver is an important organ of metabolism. Liver carries out various essential functions, including detoxification of harmful substances present in the body and production of different vital nutrients. In the setting of underlying liver disease, it is important to avoid things which might cause further damage to the liver. These include some medications (hepatotoxic drugs) like over-the-counter acetaminophen (when used in excess) and ibuprofen or alcohol. In cirrhotics with more advanced liver disease, avoiding medications which have sedative properties and avoiding sodium intake beyond 2000 mg per day (88 mmol per day) may also be appropriate.

Hepatotoxic Drugs. There is a growing list of medications and herbal products that have been implicated as hepatotoxic [1, 2]. An online, free, and easily accessible database called LiverTox maintained by the National Institutes of Health (NIH) provides a comprehensive resource regarding up-to-date information on various hepatotoxic medications, herbals, and dietary supplements (http://www. livertox.nih.gov/). Acetaminophen overdose has been found to be the most common drug implicated in acute liver failure in the United States [3] although doses up to 2000 mg daily are generally believed to be safe even in the setting of established liver disease. Some of the other commonly used but potentially hepatotoxic medications include Nonsteroidal Anti-Inflammatory Drugs (e.g., ibuprofen, diclofenac sodium), antihypertensives (e.g., methyldopa, captopril, irbesartan), antidiabetic agents (e.g., gliclazide, glimepiride, acarbose), anticonvulsants (e.g., phenytoin, valproic acid, lamotrigine), lipid-lowering agents (e.g., simvastatin, pravastatin), psychotropic drugs (e.g., chlorpromazine, haloperidol, clozapine,

S. Bhandari, M.D. (✉)
Department of General Internal Medicine, Medical College of Wisconsin,
Milwaukee, WI 53226, USA
e-mail: sbhandari@mcw.edu

© Springer International Publishing Switzerland 2017
K. Saeian, R. Shaker (eds.), *Liver Disorders*,
DOI 10.1007/978-3-319-30103-7_2

risperidone), and antidepressants (e.g., fluoxetine) [4]. In some cases, such as the use of lipid-lowering drugs (statins), those with advanced liver disease may be at the same or slightly elevated risk of hepatotoxicity but the problem is that if the untoward hepatotoxic event occurs, then it increases the risk of hepatic decompensation in patients with established cirrhosis [5]. Nonetheless, some vital medications cannot be withheld from those who truly need them and extra caution including vigilant monitoring of liver enzymes should be employed in treating people with underlying liver disease because of the amplified risk for serious consequences [6].

Alcohol. Chronic and acute alcohol consumption can result in liver damage but the extent depends on the amount and duration of consumption. Alcohol-related liver disease or alcoholic liver disease (ALD) encompasses a spectrum of diseases falling under three categories: alcoholic fatty liver disease, alcoholic hepatitis, and alcoholic cirrhosis. The risk of cirrhosis increases proportionally with consumption of more than 30 g of alcohol per day, the highest risk being more than 120 g per day [7]. The threshold is higher in men (~40 g/day) and lower in women (~20 g/day) in general. Abstinence is the most important therapeutic intervention for people with ALD [8]. Nonabstinence from alcohol is an independent predictor for increased mortality in patients with established alcoholic cirrhosis [9]. It has been shown that abstinence improves the outcome and histological features of hepatic injury, reduces portal pressure and decreases progression to cirrhosis, and improves survival in patients with ALD [8, 10–12]. Since alcohol has a strong addictive potential, abstinence can be difficult [13]. For people with heavy alcohol use, effective support interventions should be implemented, which include referral to Alcoholics Anonymous, inpatient and outpatient rehabilitation programs, individual counseling, and pharmacological interventions to prevent relapses [14]. Complete abstinence of alcohol may not be required in those without ALD and data including a study conducted in Japan showed that light-to-moderate alcohol consumption rather has a favorable effect on incidence of nonalcoholic fatty liver [15].

Excess Intake of Sodium and Fluid. Since sodium helps retain body fluid, excess sodium may be counterproductive to cirrhotics who have increased body fluid evidenced by ascites and/or lower extremity edema. Patients with cirrhosis and ascites should be educated about restricting their daily dietary sodium restriction to 2000 mg per day (88 mmol per day) [16]. High sodium containing foods include table salt, bacon, sausage, deli meats, canned vegetables, frozen items, potato chips, pretzels certain preprepared soups, among other foods. More stringent dietary sodium restriction is not recommended because it is leads to food being unpalatable and may contribute to further worsening malnutrition that is frequently encountered in this patient population [17]. Unlike patients with volume overload due to congestive heart failure, fluid restriction is not necessary unless hyponatremia with serum sodium is <120–125 mmol/L is an issue [17].

What Steps Should I Take to Help with My Liver Disease?

In addition to the avoidance of the things mentioned earlier, there are various things that can be undertaken by a person with underlying liver disease to prevent further damage to the liver. These may include, but not limited to, vaccinations against hepatitis A and B, adjustment to various medications, maintaining a healthy diet, living an active lifestyle, screening for liver cancer (hepatocellular carcinoma) and esophageal varices, and treatment of hepatitis if present.

Vaccinations. Vaccination against hepatitis A and B for those who are not already immune can help prevent superimposed insults to the liver. Patients with chronic liver disease with superimposed infection with HAV or HBV are more likely to experience serious complications due to these infections than persons without liver disease [18]. The CDC recommends hepatitis A vaccination for all susceptible patients with chronic liver disease or those who are either awaiting or have received liver transplants [19]. However, the CDC does not recommend routine vaccination against hepatitis A for patients who have chronic HBV or HCV infection without evidence of chronic liver disease [19]. The CDC also states that anyone with chronic hepatitis C who is at risk for HBV infection should be immunized against hepatitis B [20]. Some experts recommend routine vaccination against hepatitis B for all patients with chronic liver disease in particular because of the low response rate to the vaccine if cirrhosis develops and in the setting of liver transplantation [21].

Medication adjustments. Patients with cirrhosis are at increased risk of adverse events with many medications because of impaired hepatic metabolism or renal excretion. Many medications require dose adjustments or should be avoided entirely.

Nutrition. The European Society for Clinical Nutrition and Metabolism (ESPEN) issued guidelines in 2006 may be used to guide nutritional intervention in patients with chronic liver disease [22]. The guidelines recommended use of simple bedside methods such as the Subjective Global Assessment (SGA) or anthropometry to identify patients at risk of undernutrition. Patients with cirrhosis should consume 35–40 kcal/kg body weight per day of energy and 1.2–1.5 g/kg body weight per day of protein. Supplementary enteral feeding should be initiated when oral intake is inadequate. The branched chain amino acid (BCAA)-enriched formulae may be considered in patients with hepatic encephalopathy arising during enteral nutrition. Acquisition and the palatability particularly the bitter taste of BCAA may be problematic in their use.

Lifestyle Interventions. Weight loss is recommended for people with evidence of nonalcoholic steatohepatitis (NASH) [23]. Weight loss generally reduces hepatic steatosis, achieved either by a hypocaloric diet alone or in conjunction with increased physical activity [23]. A trial that randomized 31 obese persons with NASH to intensive lifestyle changes (diet, behavior modification, and 200 min a week of moderate physical activity for 48 weeks) versus structured basic education

Table 2.1 Groups for whom HCC surveillance is recommended[a]

Population group	Incidence of HCC
Surveillance recommended	
Asian male hepatitis B carriers > age 40	0.4–0.6 %/year
Asian female hepatitis B carriers > age 50	0.3–0.6 %/year
Hepatitis B carrier with family history of HCC	Incidence higher than without family history
African/North American blacks with hepatitis B	HCC occurs at a younger age
Cirrhotic hepatitis B carriers	3–8 %/year
Hepatitis C cirrhosis	3–5 %/year
Stage 4 primary biliary cirrhosis	3–5 %/year
Genetic hemochromatosis and cirrhosis	Unknown, but probably >1.5 %/year
Alpha 1-antitrypsin deficiency and cirrhosis	Unknown, but probably >1.5 %/year
Other cirrhosis	Unknown
Surveillance benefit uncertain	
Hepatitis B carriers <40 (males) or <50 (females)	<0.2 %/year
Hepatitis C and stage 3 fibrosis	<1.5 %/year
Noncirrhotic NAFLD	<1.5 %/year

NAFLD nonalcoholic fatty liver disease

[a]Adapted from: Bruix J, Sherman M. Management of Hepatocellular Carcinoma: An Update [25]

alone found that the intensive arm had significant weight loss (9.3 % versus 0.2 % in control arm) accompanied by histological improvement [24].

Screening for Hepatocellular Carcinoma (HCC). Practice guidelines from the American Association of the Study of Liver Diseases (AASLD) have recommended HCC surveillance for patients at high risk of developing HCC [25] (Table 2.1). Liver ultrasound is recommended as the primary surveillance modality for HCC and the recommended interval between HCC surveillance tests is 6 months [25]. While no longer specifically recommended by the AASLD, measurement of the serum alpha-fetoprotein every 6 months is still practiced by many practitioners and may once again be recommended by the AASLD in the near future.

Screening for esophageal varices. Patients with cirrhosis should be screened for the presence of esophageal varices by upper endoscopy, so that prophylactic therapy such as nonselective beta blocker (i.e., propranolol, nadolol) or carvedilol can be started in those with varices that are at increased risk for bleeding [26]. In those intolerant of beta blocker therapy, prophylactic band ligation of esophageal varices should also be considered. Identifying and treating patients with high-risk varices leads to improved clinical outcomes, including reduced risk of hemorrhage and decreased mortality [26].

Treatment of Underlying Liver Disease/Hepatitis. Elimination of the underlying cause of ongoing inflammation can result in significant improvement in liver function and potentially avoidance of long-term complications. Anyone diagnosed with active chronic Hepatitis B (HBsAg positive, HBeAg positive, or HBeAg negative) should be evaluated for the treatment with antiviral medication [27]. The rationale for treatment in patients with chronic HBV is to reduce the risk of progressive chronic liver disease and hepatocellular carcinoma. The full recommendations of the American Association for the Study of Liver Diseases (AASLD) updated in 2009 regarding the treatment of chronic hepatitis B virus infection are available online (http://www.aasld.org/sites/default/files/guideline_documents/Chronic HepatitisB2009.pdf). Similarly, those with chronic hepatitis C virus (HCV) infection should be considered for treatment in order to eradicate HCV RNA as indicated by attainment of a sustained virologic response (SVR) indicating negative viral load at either 12 weeks (SVR12) or 24 weeks after cessation of therapy. The recent guidelines released jointly by the American Association for the Study of Liver Diseases (AASLD) and the Infectious Diseases Society of America (IDSA) regarding the diagnosis and management of HCV infection are available online (http:// www.hcvguidelines.org/). Sustained viral response has been associated with regression of fibrosis and cirrhosis, a reduced rate of hepatic decompensation, a reduced risk for hepatocellular carcinoma, and reduced liver-related mortality [28]. Treatment of underlying autoimmune hepatitis has similarly resulted in enhanced outcomes including fibrosis as well as in those with nonalcoholic steatohepatitis with fibrosis who have undergone bariatric surgery with concomitant weight loss.

How Do I Know How Severe My Liver Disease Is?

Severity of liver disease can be determined by different modalities, like physical examination findings, various blood tests, imaging, portal pressure measurement, liver biopsy, and use of different prognostic models.

Signs/Symptoms. Physical changes such as development of spider nevi (swollen blood vessels looking like spider's web), palmar erythema (reddening of the skin on the palmar aspect of the hands), gynecomastia (enlargement of breasts), caput medusa (distended veins, which are seen radiating from the umbilicus), Dupuytren's contractures (hand deformity where fingers are bent and cannot be fully straightened), and testicular atrophy (shrunken testes) are usually indicative of advanced liver disease and are typically not present in the absence of cirrhosis and even those with early cirrhosis. Physical signs/symptoms can help in differentiating compensated from decompensated cirrhosis. Decompensated cirrhosis is defined by the presence of complications particularly development of ascites, variceal bleeding, and/or hepatic encephalopathy (mental changes from liver disease like confused thinking). Hepatocellular carcinoma, another complication of cirrhosis, can occur in the presence or absence of decompensation. Prognosis and survival is markedly worse in decompensated cirrhosis than that in compensated cirrhosis. Thus, any patient with decompensated cirrhosis should be evaluated urgently by a hepatologist and if appropriate, referred for transplant consideration.

Laboratory Tests. There is a battery of blood tests for assessment of liver disease like serum alanine aminotransferase (ALT), aspartate aminotransferase (AST), alkaline phosphatase, direct and indirect bilirubin, serum albumin, and prothrombin time (PT). Although high elevations of aminotransferases (AST and ALT) usually over 1000 IU/L generally implement extensive hepatocellular injury, they can often be normal in patients with chronic liver disease or cirrhosis. Thus, serum aminotransferases and alkaline phosphatase do not reliably reflect disease severity but more likely reflect liver injury. On the other hand, serum bilirubin and prothrombin time, and serum albumin more so reflect liver function and the former two along with serum creatinine, are components of MELD Score, a tool used to assess the severity of liver disease and predict outcomes of interventions in patients with liver disease and to prioritize patients awaiting the liver transplant.

Imaging. Different imaging modalities are available including abdominal ultrasound, computed tomography scan, and magnetic resonance imaging. Abdominal ultrasound is typically the first radiologic study as it is widely available, less expensive, and does not expose patients to radiation or contrast hazards. Shrunken, coarsened, irregular, and nodular appearance and increased echogenicity of liver on ultrasound suggest advanced liver disease or cirrhosis. Milder changes such as fatty infiltration may also be identified. Abdominal ultrasound may reveal cirrhosis-related complications like ascites, varices, splenomegaly, and portal vein thrombosis. Ultrasound is also a screening modality for detection of hepatocellular carcinoma but CT and MRI scans are more sensitive for detection of lesions albeit at a higher monetary cost and potential complications.

Portal Pressure Measurement. Portal vein is the large vessel that carries blood from the digestive organs to the liver. In cirrhosis, resistance to the portal blood flow develops inside the liver, resulting in portal hypertension. The hepatic venous pressure gradient (HVPG) is measured to calculate the gradient (difference) in pressure between the portal vein and the inferior vena cava (large vein carrying blood from lower part of the body to the heart for purification). Portal hypertension is present if the HVPG is ≥ 6 mmHg. The risk of complications from cirrhosis and mortality rates increases as HVPG value increases. For example, with HVPG is ≥ 12 mmHg, people are at risk for variceal bleeding and the development of ascites (fluid collection in the abdomen).

Liver Biopsy. Liver biopsy remains an important tool of diagnosing some liver diseases which are otherwise not obvious from physical examination, laboratory data, and imaging. Since it is invasive, it is usually the last resort for diagnosing and assessing liver disease. Nevertheless, liver biopsy is the most accurate means of assessing severity of inflammation (grade) and degree of fibrosis (grade) of liver damage.

Prognostic Models. There are different prognostic models available for estimating disease severity and survival in patients with liver disease. Several prognostic models are currently used which are disease specific, such as the models for predicting survival in patients with primary biliary cirrhosis, primary sclerosing cholangitis, and alcoholic liver disease [29–32]. There are two models that are used commonly in the care of patients with cirrhosis in general. They are the Child–Turcotte–Pugh

(CTP) score and the Model for End-stage Liver Disease (MELD) score. Similarly King's College Hospital criteria are commonly used model for assessing prognosis in patients with acute liver failure [33].

Child–Turcotte–Pugh (CTP) Score: First developed in 1973, the Child–Pugh score was originally used to stratify the risk of portacaval shunt surgery in patients with cirrhosis, but the score has since been modified, and become a widely used tool to assess prognosis in patients with chronic liver disease and cirrhosis [34, 35]. Moreover, it was previously prior to implementation of the MELD in order to determine priority for liver transplantation. CTP Score incorporates five variables, namely the serum albumin, serum bilirubin, ascites, encephalopathy, and prothrombin time. The score ranges from 5 to 15. Depending on the score, patients can be categorized into Child–Pugh class A (5–6 points), class B (7–9 points), or class C (10–15 points). The higher the score, the more severe the liver disease is. CTP Score is a reliable predictor of survival in many liver diseases and also predicts major complications such as bleeding from varices.

Model for End-stage Liver Disease (MELD) score: Another model to predict prognosis in patients with cirrhosis is the Model for End-Stage Liver Disease (MELD) score. MELD was originally developed at the Mayo Clinic. It was originally developed to predict 3-month mortality in patients undergoing transjugular intrahepatic portosystemic shunt (TIPS) placement [36]. The MELD Score is a reliable measure of mortality risk in patients with end-stage liver disease. Different modifications have been done since its inception to accommodate different types of liver conditions or other conditions and can be easily accessed through the Mayo Clinic website (http://www.mayoclinic.org/medical-professionals/model-end-stage-liver-disease). The MELD Score has been found to be useful in determining prognosis and prioritizing for patents for receipt of a liver transplant. MELD was adopted by the United Network for Organ Sharing (UNOS) in 2002 for deceased donor liver allocation for adults with cirrhosis awaiting liver transplantation in the Unites States. The tool for calculating the MELD score as maintained by US Department of Health and Services can be easily assessed online (http://optn.transplant.hrsa.gov/converge/resources/MeldPeldCalculator.asp?index=98). The score incorporates patient's serum bilirubin, serum creatinine, and the international normalized ratio (INR) and is calculated as follows:

$$\text{MELD Score} = 3.8 \times \log_e\left(\text{serum bilirubin}[\text{mg / dL}]\right) + 11.2 \times \log_e\left(\text{INR}\right)$$
$$+ 9.6 \times \log_e\left(\text{serum creatinine}[\text{mg / dL}]\right) + 6.4$$

King's College Hospital criteria: The most widely applied prognostic system in case of acute liver failure (ALF) is the King's College Hospital criteria [33] (Table 2.2). The criteria are often employed in determining which patients are likely to succumb to their liver disease such that they should be considered urgently/emergently for liver transplantation.

Table 2.2 King's College Hospital criteria for liver transplantation in acute liver failure[a]

Acetaminophen-induced disease
Arterial pH <7.3
OR
INR >6.5, serum creatinine >3.4 mg/dl, and grade III–IV encephalopathy
All other causes of acute liver failure
INR >6.5
OR
Any three of the following variables (irrespective of the grade of encephalopathy)
1. Age <10 years or >40 years
2. Etiology: non-A, non-B hepatitis, or idiosyncratic drug reactions
3. Duration of jaundice before encephalopathy >7 days
4. INR >3.5
5. Serum bilirubin >17.5 mg/dl

[a]Data adapted from: O'Grady JG, Alexander GJ, Hayllar KM, Williams R. Early indicators of prognosis in fulminant hepatic failure [33]

References

1. Stirnimann G, Kessebohm K, Lauterburg B. Liver injury caused by drugs: an update. Swiss Med Wkly. 2010;140:w13080.
2. Bunchorntavakul C, Reddy KR. Review article: herbal and dietary supplement hepatotoxicity. Aliment Pharmacol Ther. 2013;37(1):3–17.
3. Ostapowicz G et al. Results of a prospective study of acute liver failure at 17 tertiary care centers in the United States. Ann Intern Med. 2002;137(12):947–54.
4. Chitturi S, George J. Hepatotoxicity of commonly used drugs: nonsteroidal anti-inflammatory drugs, antihypertensives, antidiabetic agents, anticonvulsants, lipid-lowering agents, psychotropic drugs. Semin Liver Dis. 2002;22(2):169–83.
5. Schenker S, Martin RR, Hoyumpa AM. Antecedent liver disease and drug toxicity. J Hepatol. 1999;31(6):1098–105.
6. Lee WM. Drug-induced hepatotoxicity. N Engl J Med. 2003;349(5):474–85.
7. Bellentani S et al. Drinking habits as cofactors of risk for alcohol induced liver damage. The Dionysos Study Group. Gut. 1997;41(6):845–50.
8. Pessione F et al. Five-year survival predictive factors in patients with excessive alcohol intake and cirrhosis. Effect of alcoholic hepatitis, smoking and abstinence. Liver Int. 2003;23(1):45–53.
9. Senanayake SM et al. Survival of patients with alcoholic and cryptogenic cirrhosis without liver transplantation: a single center retrospective study. BMC Res Notes. 2012;5:663.
10. Borowsky SA, Strome S, Lott E. Continued heavy drinking and survival in alcoholic cirrhotics. Gastroenterology. 1981;80(6):1405–9.
11. Brunt PW et al. Studies in alcoholic liver disease in Britain. I. Clinical and pathological patterns related to natural history. Gut. 1974;15(1):52–8.
12. Luca A et al. Effects of ethanol consumption on hepatic hemodynamics in patients with alcoholic cirrhosis. Gastroenterology. 1997;112(4):1284–9.
13. Riley TR, Smith JP. Preventive care in chronic liver disease. J Gen Intern Med. 1999;14(11):699–704.
14. O'Connor PG, Schottenfeld RS. Patients with alcohol problems. N Engl J Med. 1998;338(9):592–602.

15. Hamaguchi M et al. Protective effect of alcohol consumption for fatty liver but not metabolic syndrome. World J Gastroenterol. 2012;18(2):156–67.
16. Runyon BA. Care of patients with ascites. N Engl J Med. 1994;330(5):337–42.
17. Runyon BA. Management of adult patients with ascites due to cirrhosis: an update. Hepatology. 2009;49(6):2087–107.
18. Bockhold K, Riely CA, Jeffreys C. Overcoming obstacles to immunization in patients with chronic liver disease. Am J Med. 2005;118(Suppl 10A):40s–5.
19. Centers for Disease Control and Prevention. Prevention of hepatitis A through active or passive immunization: recommendations of the Advisory Committee on Immunization Practices (ACIP). Morb Mortal Wkly Rep. 1999;48(RR-12):1–37.
20. Centers for Disease Control and Prevention. Medical management of chronic hepatitis B and chronic hepatitis C. 2002. http://www.cdc.gov/idu/hepatitis/manage_chronich_hep_b-c.pdf. Accessed 11 June 2015.
21. Horlander JC et al. Vaccination against hepatitis B in patients with chronic liver disease awaiting liver transplantation. Am J Med Sci. 1999;318(5):304–7.
22. Plauth M et al. ESPEN guidelines on enteral nutrition: liver disease. Clin Nutr. 2006;25(2):285–94.
23. Chalasani N et al. The diagnosis and management of non-alcoholic fatty liver disease: practice guideline by the American Gastroenterological Association, American Association for the Study of Liver Diseases, and American College of Gastroenterology. Gastroenterology. 2012;142(7):1592–609.
24. Promrat K et al. Randomized controlled trial testing the effects of weight loss on nonalcoholic steatohepatitis. Hepatology. 2010;51(1):121–9.
25. Bruix J, Sherman M. Management of hepatocellular carcinoma: an update. Hepatology. 2011;53(3):1020–2.
26. Garcia-Tsao G et al. Prevention and management of gastroesophageal varices and variceal hemorrhage in cirrhosis. Am J Gastroenterol. 2007;102(9):2086–102.
27. Lok AS, McMahon BJ. Chronic hepatitis B: update 2009. Hepatology. 2009;50(3):661–2.
28. Ng V, Saab S. Effects of a sustained virologic response on outcomes of patients with chronic hepatitis C. Clin Gastroenterol Hepatol. 2011;9(11):923–30.
29. Dickson ER et al. Prognosis in primary biliary cirrhosis: model for decision making. Hepatology. 1989;10(1):1–7.
30. Grambsch PM et al. Extramural cross-validation of the Mayo primary biliary cirrhosis survival model establishes its generalizability. Hepatology. 1989;10(5):846–50.
31. Kim WR et al. A revised natural history model for primary sclerosing cholangitis. Mayo Clin Proc. 2000;75(7):688–94.
32. Maddrey WC et al. Corticosteroid therapy of alcoholic hepatitis. Gastroenterology. 1978;75(2):193–9.
33. O'Grady JG et al. Early indicators of prognosis in fulminant hepatic failure. Gastroenterology. 1989;97(2):439–45.
34. Pugh RN et al. Transection of the oesophagus for bleeding oesophageal varices. Br J Surg. 1973;60(8):646–9.
35. Child CG, Turcotte JG. The liver and portal hypertension. Philadelphia: WB Saunders Co.; 1964.
36. Malinchoc M et al. A model to predict poor survival in patients undergoing transjugular intrahepatic portosystemic shunts. Hepatology. 2000;31(4):864–71.

Chapter 3
Do I Need a Liver Biopsy?

Kiyoko Oshima

Abbreviations

AIH	Autoimmune hepatitis
DILI	Drug-induced liver injury
HCC	Hepatocellular carcinoma
MRI	Magnetic resonance imaging
NAFLD	Non-alcoholic fatty liver disease
PBC	Primary biliary cirrhosis
PSC	Primary sclerosing cholangitis

Patients' Questions

1. I have elevated liver enzymes found during a health checkup. Do I need a liver biopsy?

   Clinical and/or blood-based tests are sufficient to confirm many liver diseases such as hepatitis B and C. However, the liver biopsy plays an important role for patients with elevated liver enzymes of undetermined etiology to confirm diagnosis. In one study, 354 patients with abnormal liver chemistries underwent liver biopsy in the absence of diagnostic serology, and histology was investigated. Sixty-six percent had non-alcoholic fatty liver disease (NAFLD), and 19 % had treatable diseases, such as alcohol-related liver injury, autoimmune hepatitis (AIH), primary biliary cirrhosis (PBC), and hemochromatosis. Only 6 % of patients had a normal liver biopsy. Patient management was altered

K. Oshima, M.D., Dr.Sc. (✉)
Department of Pathology, Medical College of Wisconsin, Milwaukee, WI, USA
e-mail: koshima@mcw.edu

© Springer International Publishing Switzerland 2017
K. Saeian, R. Shaker (eds.), *Liver Disorders*,
DOI 10.1007/978-3-319-30103-7_3

in 18 % owing to liver biopsy findings [1]. As this study indicates, histological analysis is helpful in the setting of abnormal liver enzymes in the absence of a serological diagnosis. However, the liver biopsy has limitations as well. The liver biopsy is an essentially safe procedure, but complications including pain and bleeding may arise. Sampling error can occur because of the small size of the specimen or the variability of the disease process in the liver in certain disorders, such as primary sclerosing cholangitis (PSC). Therefore, performance of a biopsy must be individually decided based on the risks and benefits and interpreted in context [2].

2. I have hepatitis C. Do I need a liver biopsy?

The diagnosis of most cases of viral hepatitis, including hepatitis C, is confirmed by serology, and a liver biopsy is not required. The liver biopsy has been regarded as the gold standard to assess the current status of the liver injury, to predict progression, and to provide a prognosis. Grading and staging define the activity of the disease and the degree of scarring respectively. Grading is a measure of the severity of the necroinflammatory process, the activity of the ongoing disease, and the potential responsiveness to therapy. Staging refers to the degree of fibrosis, parenchymal or vascular remodeling subsequent to the necroinflammatory process [3]. However, in the era of successful new antiviral therapies, the importance of assessment for grade and stage is diminished, because cure rates are similar for all except the patients with advanced fibrosis. Non-invasive measures such as transient elastography may also mitigate the need for a liver biopsy. A liver biopsy should be considered if the patient and health care provider require information on the fibrosis stage for prognostic purposes or to make a decision regarding treatment [4]. It is still the best tool to assess concurrent disease such as fatty liver diseases of alcohol-related and non-alcoholic etiologies, AIH or iron overload. A liver biopsy is recommended when concurrent disease is suspected or when cirrhosis is suspected, but not confirmed by other means, because the presence of cirrhosis in chronic hepatitis C warrants continued surveillance for hepatocellular carcinoma (HCC) and varices, even after eradication of the virus.

3. I have AIH. Do I need a liver biopsy?

Liver biopsy examination at presentation is recommended to establish the diagnosis and to guide the treatment decisions [5]. Some patients exhibit features of both AIH and other disorders, such as PBC, PSC, or autoimmune cholangitis. A liver biopsy is the best tool to confirm such overlap syndromes. After treatment is initiated, a liver biopsy is recommended before termination of immunosuppressive therapy and relapse, because the incidence of relapse is high in residual interface hepatitis [6], which may not always be reflected by liver enzymes and/or immunoglobulin G (IgG) levels.

4. I have a tumor found on an imaging study. Do I need a liver biopsy?

The patient most likely has one of the abnormalities listed in Table 3.1, and whether the liver biopsy is needed or not depends on each specific condition. The most common hypervascular lesions found in patients without underlying liver disease are focal nodular hyperplasia and hemangioma. These lesions do not

Table 3.1 Hepatic mass lesions

Benign
Cysts (e.g., simple cyst, biliary cyst, ciliated foregut cyst, hydatid disease)
Adenoma (e.g., hepatic adenoma, biliary adenoma, biliary cyst adenoma)
Biliary hamartoma
Focal nodular hyperplasia
Hemangioma
Rare primary liver neoplasms (e.g., angiomyolipoma)
Malignant
Hepatocellular carcinoma
Cholangiocarcinoma
Metastatic
Rare primary liver neoplasm (e.g., angiosarcoma, leiomyosarcoma)
Rare primary bile duct neoplasm (e.g., biliary cyst adenocarcinoma)

need treatment if asymptomatic. The biopsy is indicated only if the imaging study is inconclusive. Hepatic adenoma is sometime hard to distinguish from well-differentiated HCC, focal nodular hyperplasia, or infrequently from metastatic carcinoma, particularly if it is multifocal. In such cases, a biopsy may be advisable. Apparent metastatic lesions without an obvious primary site should be biopsied under image guidance to confirm the diagnosis. Pathologists can narrow the possible primary sites down by utilization of immunohistochemical stains. Metastatic lesions in the setting of a previous history of malignancy should also be biopsied to confirm the diagnosis.

In patients with underlying liver disease, particularly cirrhosis, HCC and cholangiocarcinoma are more frequent and more concerning. If the radiological findings are compatible with HCC, especially if there is a market elevation in the alpha-fetoprotein level, biopsy is unnecessary [2]. When multiphase computed tomography or dynamic contrast-enhanced magnetic resonance imaging (MRI) shows arterial hypervascularity and venous or delayed phase washout in masses 2 cm or larger, particularly in the setting of cirrhosis, a diagnosis of HCC is confirmed and the biopsy is not required.

Cholangiocarcinoma often presents as a solitary lesion involving the biliary hilum or within the hepatic parenchyma. The management of cholangiocarcinoma is surgical resection, if technically feasible. The decision to liver biopsy is governed by whether or not surgical resection is considered [2]. If the possibility of transplantation arises (limited to smaller lesions often confined to the hilum and only at specialized centers), the liver biopsy should be performed under imaging guidance.

Indications for Liver Biopsy

The liver biopsy plays three major roles: diagnosis, assessment of prognosis, and therapeutic management. Indications for liver biopsy based on each role are summarized in Table 3.2 [2, 7]. Also, the diseases in which liver biopsy is indicated are listed in Table 3.3 [2, 7].

Table 3.2 Indications for liver biopsy

Diagnosis
Abnormal liver tests of unknown etiology
Hepatosplenomegaly of unknown etiology
Focal or diffuse abnormalities on imaging studies
Fever of unknown etiology
Prognosis
Staging of known parenchymal liver disease
Management
Evaluation of the efficacy or the adverse effects of treatment regimens
Evaluation of the status of the liver after transplantation or of the donor liver before transplantation

Table 3.3 Diseases for which liver biopsy is indicated

	Diagnosis	Staging/prognosis	Treatment
Viral hepatitis (HCV, HBV)	–	+++	++
Autoimmune hepatitis	+++	+++	+++
Primary biliary cirrhosis	++	+++	+
Primary sclerosing cholangitis	++	+++	+
Overlap syndrome	+++	+++	++
Alcoholic	+	+++	
NAFLD/NASH	+++	+++	+
Drug-related liver injury	++	+	+
Hemochromatosis	+	+++	+
Wilson's disease	+++	+++	–
A1AT deficiency	+	++	–
Acute liver failure	+++	+++	–
Hepatocellular carcinoma	++	–	–
Hepatocellular adenoma	+++	–	+++
Metastasis	+++	–	–

Irrelevant, + occasionally irrelevant, ++ usually irrelevant, +++ highly relevant
HCV hepatitis C virus, *HBV* hepatitis B virus, *NAFLD* non-alcoholic fatty liver disease, *NASH* non-alcoholic steatohepatitis, *A1AT* alpha-1 anti-trypsin

Diagnosis

Despite improvements in serological testing and imaging techniques, the liver biopsy remains an important diagnostic tool for diagnosing diffuse hepatic disease and hepatic lesions. For instance, liver biopsy can confirm specific disorders, leading to specific therapy in a setting of acute liver failure due to acute fatty liver of pregnancy, herpes virus infection, AIH, or Wilson's disease [8]. The liver biopsy is helpful in identifying the presence of concurrent diseases, something frequently encountered in the setting of viral hepatitis. One study reveals that 20.5 % of viral hepatitis patients had other concurrent processes (e.g., NAFLD, drug-induced liver injury (DILI), Wilson's disease, iron overload, PBC) that could potentially modify disease progression and/or alter the management strategy [9]. The liver biopsy not only confirms diagnosis, but may also determine which process is the dominant factor injuring the liver. Liver biopsy can solve the diagnostic dilemma of assessing patients with atypical features, such as anti-mitochondrial antibody-negative PBC or small bile duct PSC. Liver biopsy can distinguish between AIH and steatohepatitis for the obese patient with elevated alanine aminotransferase, IgG, and/or autoimmune markers [2]. Perhaps in no other setting is liver biopsy more essential than in evaluating allograft dysfunction after liver transplantation. It is critical to know the specific diagnosis for management, especially considering the broad potential differential diagnosis comprising acute and chronic cellular rejection, preservation injury, recurrence of the original disease, DILI, ischemic injury, or biliary obstruction. In the patient exposed to supplements or herbal medicines in whom harmful effects are suspected, liver biopsy is instrumental in making and/or confirming the diagnosis of drug-/toxin-related liver injury [10]. Please see question 4 above for the role of liver biopsy in a liver mass lesion, but do keep in mind that these biopsies typically need to be guided by imaging.

Staging

Another important role of liver biopsy is to assess the degree of fibrosis to predict liver-related morbidity and mortality. The stage reflects the degree of fibrosis and may not only guide subsequent treatment, but also help to decide whether the patient is at risk for potential complications, including portal hypertensive bleeding and HCC screening, which would be warranted in all patients with advanced fibrosis. Non-invasive methods, such as transient elastography and magnetic resonance elastography, are emerging. For example, FibroScan® (transient elastography) was approved by the FDA in 2013 for the non-invasive assessment of hepatic fibrosis and is now used in a number of clinics to monitor patients and at times even to justify proceeding with a liver biopsy. Although in the future these tests may replace liver biopsy in staging [11], validation has not been performed in all disease entities and the liver biopsy still remains the gold standard.

Treatment

A liver biopsy can be used to develop a treatment plan. For example, immunosuppression levels can be adjusted for patients with AIH or liver transplantation based on histological findings. By assessing the efficacy and the toxicity of a new medication, the liver biopsy remains the gold standard.

Preparation for Liver Biopsy

A liver biopsy is generally undertaken as an outpatient. Before liver biopsy, patients must be informed of the alternatives, risks, benefits, and limitations. Practical points, such as by whom and where the biopsy is to be performed, what kind of sedation, if any, will be used, what degree of pain is anticipated, when the patient may return to their usual level of activity, when the result will be known, and by what means this information is communicated should be discussed in advance. A written informed consent form, including the risks, benefits, and alternatives, should be obtained before the procedure [2].

Pre-biopsy Testing

Measurement of the complete blood count, including platelet count, prothorombin time, and international normalized ratio (INR), is required. Most practitioners avoid percutaneous biopsy with platelet counts less than 60,000 or an INR greater than 1.5. Patients with previously known abnormalities in laboratory tests require repeat testing before the procedure. Imaging reports should be reviewed to check that there are no abnormal findings that might be contraindications to percutaneous and nonguided biopsy, such as hemangioma, significant ascites, or biliary obstruction [2].

Management of Medication

Antiplatelet medications (i.e., aspirin, ticlodipine, clopidogrel, IIb/IIIa receptor antagonists, nonsteroidal anti-inflammatory drugs) should be discontinued typically 7 days before the biopsy. Warfarin should be discontinued at least 5 days beforehand. Depending on the indication for antiplatelet or anticoagulant therapy, the above can be modified on a case-by-case basis, but if antiplatelet/anticoagulant therapy cannot be maintained, performing the biopsy should be reconsidered and certainly consideration given to performing the biopsy via the transvenous route.

The risk of discontinuing anticoagulant medication must be weighed against the risk of bleeding during/after the liver biopsy. Antiplatelet therapy may be restarted 72–96 h after the liver biopsy, and warfarin may be restarted the day following the procedure and slowly titrated back up to therapeutic levels [2].

Liver Biopsy Methods

There are three main approaches to liver biopsy, including percutaneous biopsy, transvenous (transjugular or transfemoral) biopsy, and surgical/laparoscopic biopsy. Percutaneous biopsy can be undertaken guided by palpation/percussion, imaging, and real-time imaging. The surgical/laparoscopic approach is usually utilized by surgeons during an operation and is often performed because the liver incidentally appeared to be abnormal at the time of the operation [12].

Contraindications

Contraindications to percutaneous biopsy are listed in Table 3.4. Percutaneous biopsy is appropriate only in cooperative patients. In patients with clinically evident coagulopathy, a transvenous approach is recommended. Ascites, massive obesity, suspected vascular tumor, amyloidosis, or hydatid disease are relative contraindications to percutaneous biopsy and thus indications for considering tranvenous biopsy.

Table 3.4 Contraindications to percutaneous liver biopsy

Absolute
Uncooperative patient
Tendency to bleed
PT-INR > 1.5 s
Platelet count <50,000/mm^3
Use of a non-steroidal anti-inflammatory drug within the previous 7–10 days
Blood for transfusion unavailable
Infection of the hepatic bed
Relative
Ascites
Morbid obesity
Possible vascular lesion
Amyloidosis
Hydatid disease
Extrahepatic biliary obstruction

Complications

Because of its invasive nature, liver biopsy regardless of route may be associated with complications and this truly is the major limitation of the procedure.

Percutaneous Liver Biopsy

Complications associated with percutaneous liver biopsy are rare. Minor complications include transient localized discomfort at the biopsy site, which may radiate to the right shoulder owing to the innervation of the liver, pain, and transient hypotension. The pain is usually dull and mild. Severe pain in the abdomen should alert the physician to the possibility of a more severe complication, such as bleeding or peritonitis. Some 60 % of complications occur within 2 h and 96 % within 24 h. Although it is very rare, significant intraperitoneal hemorrhage is the most serious bleeding complication. It usually becomes apparent within the first 2–3 h after the procedure. Risk factors for hemorrhage after biopsies include older age, more than three passes with the biopsy needle, and the presence of cirrhosis or liver cancer. Other rare complications include pneumothorax, hemothorax, biliary ascites, bile pleuritis, bile peritonitis, and infection (bacteremia, abscess, sepsis). The mortality rate among those undergoing liver biopsy is approximately 0.01 %. Mortality is highest among patients who undergo biopsies of malignant lesions [8]. One study shows a very low complication rate for physicians performing more than 50 biopsies per year [13]. Specific training to carry out liver biopsy is essential and at least 50 biopsies are required to become adequately trained, although previous accreditation approved those with as few as 20 biopsies. Those educating others in the technique of liver biopsy should have completed more than several hundred live biopsies [2].

Transjugular Liver Biopsy

In this procedure, typically performed by interventional radiologists (at least in the USA) the right internal jugular vein is punctured, and a guidewire followed by a sheath is introduced into the superior vena cava, the right atrium, the inferior vena cava, and into the hepatic vein with the use of fluoroscopy. The liver tissue is obtained from within the vascular system, which minimizes the risk of bleeding. The quality of transjugular biopsy used to be questioned for smaller and more fragmented specimens compared with percutaneous biopsy. It has recently been improved by an 18- or 19-G Tru-Cut needle with at least three passes. The success rate of obtaining sufficient tissue for diagnosis is 96.8 %. Minor and major complications occur in 6.5 and 0.56 % of cases respectively [14]. During the procedure, close cardiac monitoring, including continuous electrocardiographic monitoring, is required to detect arrhythmias, which may be induced by the passage of the catheter through the heart. Complications include abdominal pain, neck hematoma, transient Horner's syndrome, transient dysphonia, cardiac arrhythmias, pneumothorax, fistula formation from the hepatic artery to the portal vein or the biliary tree, and perforation of the liver capsule. Mortality rate ranges from 0.1 to 0.5 %.

Laparoscopic Liver Biopsy

The complications include those caused by general anesthesia and local abdominal wall or intraperitoneal trauma, such as laceration of the spleen, bleeding, and prolonged abdominal pain [2, 11].

Liver Sampling and Adequacy

It is essential that the liver biopsy is adequate for the pathologists to interpret. The ideal specimen for assessing the pattern of injury, grade of inflammation, and stage of fibrosis is at least 2.5 cm long and 1.4 mm wide for visualization of ten portal tracts. Smaller specimens are often problematic and may lead to the understaging of the degree of fibrosis. This is particularly problematic because the specimen may be separated into multiple pieces, particularly in the setting of advanced fibrosis. A length of at least 1.5 cm is required to assess the underlying liver disease. Even an adequate sized liver biopsy represents approximately 1: 50,000 of the entire liver. Although a 1.5-cm biopsy specimen may be adequate for assessing many liver diseases, a short specimen less than 2.5 cm may result in a failure to recognize cirrhosis in up to 20 % [12].

One of the limitations of liver biopsy is related to the variability of the disease process in the liver itself. Although chronic liver disease is typically a diffuse process, it can have variable degrees of pathological process based upon the location. A classic example of this is PSC, which, depending on the location and degree of biliary stenosis, may show areas of variable fibrosis. Another example to keep in mind is that subcapsular liver tissue is more fibrotic, and not an ideal location for the evaluation of fibrosis.

Tissue Processing

Tissue should be fixed in 10 % neutral buffered formalin, which allows the full range of histochemical stains (hematoxylin and eosin and special stains) and immunohistochemical stains. Masson trichrome stain is most often used for the

Table 3.5 Special stains commonly used in liver biopsy

Stain	Indications
Masson's trichrome	Collagen fiber
Reticulin	Cord and acinar architecture
Prussian blue	Iron deposition
Rhodamine	Copper deposition for Wilson's disease or chronic cholestasis
Periodic acid-Schiff-diastase (PAS-d)	Globules of A1AD disease
Oil red O	Confirmation of microvesicular steatosis for fatty liver of pregnancy and Reye syndrome
Congo red	Amyloid
AFB	Acid-fast bacilli in granuloma
GMS	Fungi in granuloma
Orcein	HBV surface antigen, copper binding protein in chronic cholestasis
Vierhoff van Geisen	Elastic fiber in vessel walls
Imunohistochemical stain	Characterization of tumor, HBsAg, HBcAg

HBsAG surface antigen of the HBV, *HBcAG* hepatitis B core antigen

evaluation of fibrosis. Table 3.5 shows commonly used stains and indications [15]. Molecular studies, flow cytometry for lymphoma work-up, oil red O stain for lipids (when suspecting acute fatty liver of pregnancy), and enzyme assay for glycogen storage disease require fresh tissue. A small piece of the biopsy may need to be sent to the pathology department as separate fresh tissue. Culture can be performed, but should be stored in a sterilized container.

If Wilson's disease or iron overload is suspected, care must be taken to send a sample in a metal-free container and to specifically request copper and/or iron quantitation of the liver tissue.

Experience of a Liver Pathologist

The experience of the pathologist is an important factor in the accurate interpretation of the liver biopsy specimen. The importance of this type of experience is emphasized by a report in which re-examination of the biopsy initially read by a nonspecialist pathologist by an academic pathologist resulted in changes in diagnosis that had a significant effect on the management of 35.2 % of cases [16]. Second opinions from experienced pathologists should be liberally sought on behalf of the patient [17].

Specimen Interpretation

There are multiple systems available for assessing disease activity in chronic hepatitis and steatohepatitis. The goal of systems is to ensure that the same lesions are being evaluated and given similar diagnostic weight regardless of the observers. For chronic hepatitis, Kendoll histological activity index score (HAI), Ishak modified HAI score, Scheuer system, Metavir system, and Battss and Ludwig are available [18–22]. Batts–Ludwig system is shown in Figs. 3.1 and 3.2. All assessments are based on portal inflammation, interface activity, and lobular necroinflammatory and fibrosis. For steatohepatitis, the Brunt system and the NASH Clinical Research Network (CNR) scoring system are often used. Both systems assess grading based on the degree of steatosis, hepatocytes ballooning, and lobular inflammation [23, 24].

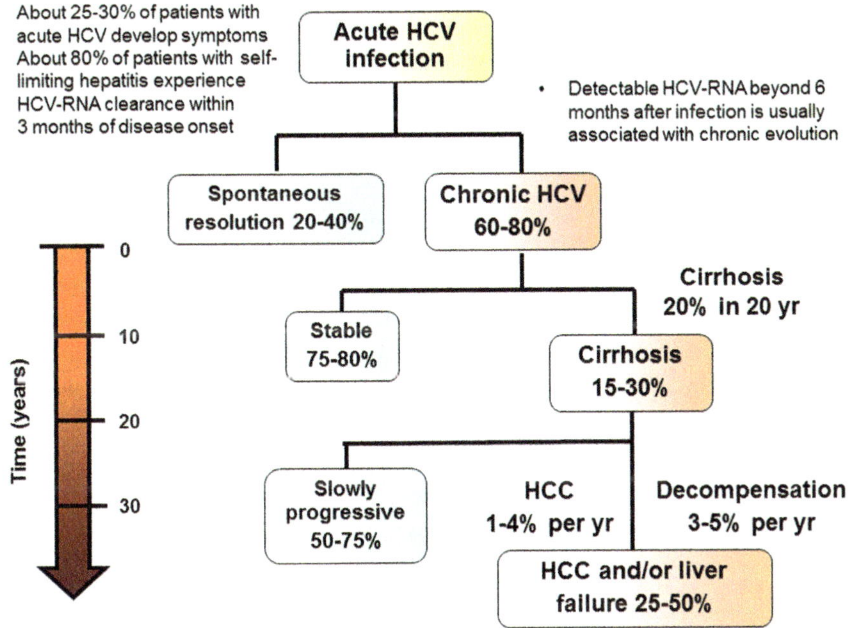

Fig. 3.1 Batts–Ludwig grading of chronic hepatitis: grade 1 (minimal activity) shows minimal portal inflammation, minimal patchy interface activity, and minimal lobular inflammation; grade 2 (mild activity) shows mild portal inflammation involving some or all portal tracts, and mild lobular activity with little hepatocellular damage; grade 3 (moderate activity) shows moderate portal inflammation involving all portal tracts and moderate lobular inflammation with noticeable hepatocellular damage; grade 4 (severe activity) shows severe portal inflammation, severe interface activity, and severe lobular inflammation with diffuse hepatocellular damage

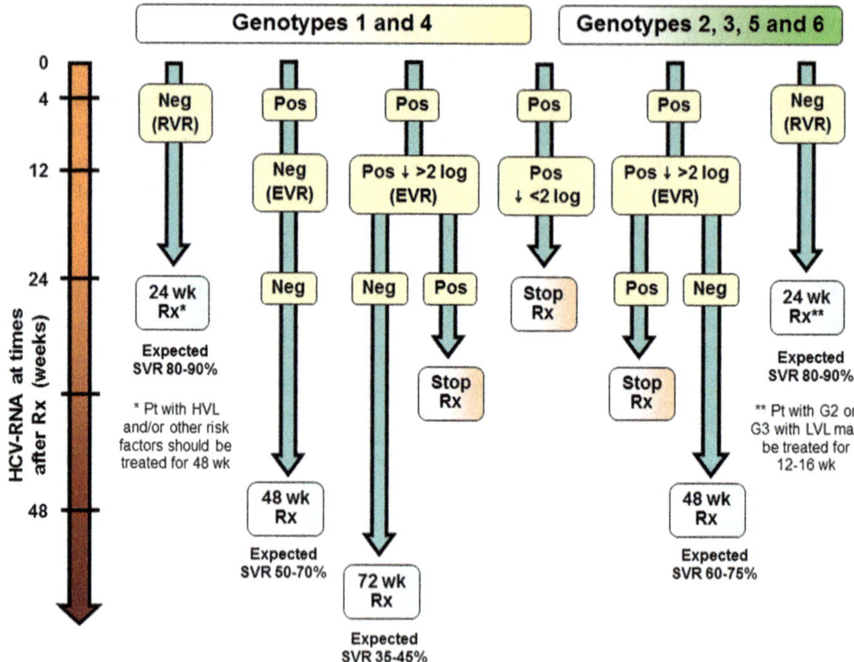

Fig. 3.2 (**a, b**) Batts–Ludwig staging of chronic hepatitis: stage 1 shows enlarged portal tracts (portal fibrosis); stage 2 shows periportal fibrosis; stage 3 shows bridging (septal) fibrosis; stage 4 shows cirrhosis

Conclusion

With adequate biopsy sampling, along with incorporation of clinical and laboratory information and close communication between the clinician and pathologist, a liver biopsy often provides not only helpful information in making a diagnosis, but also critical information for therapeutic management decisions and offering patients a reliable prognosis.

References

1. Skelly MM, James PD, Ryder SD. Findings on liver biopsy to investigate abnormal liver function tests in the absence of diagnostic serology. J Hepatol. 2001;35(2):195–9.
2. Rockey DC, Caldwell SH, Goodman ZD, Nelson RC, Smith AD, American Association for the Study of Liver D. Liver biopsy. Hepatology. 2009;49(3):1017–44.
3. Brunt EM. Grading and staging the histopathological lesions of chronic hepatitis: the Knodell histology activity index and beyond. Hepatology. 2000;31(1):241–6.
4. Ghany MG, Strader DB, Thomas DL, Seeff LB, American Association for the Study of Liver Diseases. Diagnosis, management, and treatment of hepatitis C: an update. Hepatology. 2009;49(4):1335–74.

 5. Manns MP, Czaja AJ, Gorham JD, Krawitt EL, Mieli-Vergani G, Vergani D, et al. Diagnosis and management of autoimmune hepatitis. Hepatology. 2010;51(6):2193–213.
 6. Verma S, Gunuwan B, Mendler M, Govindrajan S, Redeker A. Factors predicting relapse and poor outcome in type I autoimmune hepatitis: role of cirrhosis development, patterns of transaminases during remission and plasma cell activity in the liver biopsy. Am J Gastroenterol. 2004;99(8):1510–6.
 7. Tannapfel A, Dienes HP, Lohse AW. The indications for liver biopsy. Dtsch Arztebl Int. 2012;109(27–28):477–83.
 8. Polson J, Lee WM, American Association for the Study of Liver D. AASLD position paper: the management of acute liver failure. Hepatology. 2005;41(5):1179–97.
 9. Nair V, Fischer SE, Adeyi OA. Non-viral-related pathologic findings in liver needle biopsy specimens from patients with chronic viral hepatitis. Am J Clin Pathol. 2010;133(1):127–32.
10. Kleiner DE, Chalasani NP, Lee WM, Fontana RJ, Bonkovsky HL, Watkins PB, et al. Hepatic histological findings in suspected drug-induced liver injury: systematic evaluation and clinical associations. Hepatology. 2014;59(2):661–70.
11. Tapper EB, Castera L, Afdhal NH. FibroScan (vibration-controlled transient elastography): where does it stand in the United States practice. Clin Gastroenterol Hepatol. 2015;13(1): 27–36.
12. Bravo AA, Sheth SG, Chopra S. Liver biopsy. N Engl J Med. 2001;344(7):495–500.
13. Froehlich F, Lamy O, Fried M, Gonvers JJ. Practice and complications of liver biopsy. Results of a nationwide survey in Switzerland. Dig Dis Sci. 1993;38(8):1480–4.
14. Kalambokis G, Manousou P, Vibhakorn S, Marelli L, Cholongitas E, Senzolo M, et al. Transjugular liver biopsy – indications, adequacy, quality of specimens, and complications – a systematic review. J Hepatol. 2007;47(2):284–94.
15. Brunt EM. Liver biopsy interpretation for the gastroenterologist. Curr Gastroenterol Rep. 2000;2(1):27–32.
16. Hahm GK, Niemann TH, Lucas JG, Frankel WL. The value of second opinion in gastrointestinal and liver pathology. Arch Pathol Lab Med. 2001;125(6):736–9.
17. Bejarano PA, Koehler A, Sherman KE. Second opinion pathology in liver biopsy interpretation. Am J Gastroenterol. 2001;96(11):3158–64.
18. Knodell RG, Ishak KG, Black WC, Chen TS, Craig R, Kaplowitz N, et al. Formulation and application of a numerical scoring system for assessing histological activity in asymptomatic chronic active hepatitis. Hepatology. 1981;1(5):431–5.
19. Ishak KG. Chronic hepatitis: morphology and nomenclature. Mod Pathol. 1994;7(6): 690–713.
20. Scheuer PJ. Classification of chronic viral hepatitis: a need for reassessment. J Hepatol. 1991;13(3):372–4.
21. The French METAVIR Cooperative Study Group. Intraobserver and interobserver variations in liver biopsy interpretation in patients with chronic hepatitis C. Hepatology. 1994;20(1 Pt 1):15–20.
22. Batts KP, Ludwig J. Chronic hepatitis. An update on terminology and reporting. Am J Surg Pathol. 1995;19(12):1409–17.
23. Brunt EM, Janney CG, Di Bisceglie AM, Neuschwander-Tetri BA, Bacon BR. Nonalcoholic steatohepatitis: a proposal for grading and staging the histological lesions. Am J Gastroenterol. 1999;94(9):2467–74.
24. Kleiner DE, Brunt EM, Van Natta M, Behling C, Contos MJ, Cummings OW, et al. Design and validation of a histological scoring system for nonalcoholic fatty liver disease. Hepatology. 2005;41(6):1313–21.

What to Do with Tumors in the Liver?

Chapter 4
Incidental Hepatic Lesions

Syed Rizvi

Patients' Questions

I had a CT scan of the chest for my cough and the report says that there is a mass in the liver. What should I do?

Patient level answer: Most spots in the liver found incidentally in an otherwise healthy person are benign and can usually be quickly identified by a CT scan or MRI of the liver. Your individual risks for type of a lesion depend on age, sex, use of oral contraceptives, history of chronic liver, and recent travel. The best approach is to start with your primary care physician who can order a "triple-phase" CT scan or MRI done specifically to correctly identify this spot.

I had a CT scan of the abdomen for suspected diverticulitis on which a lesion was seen in the liver. The radiologist states that the lesion is indeterminate and advises biopsy. Is a liver biopsy necessary?

Patient level answer: Lesions in the liver are broadly divided into the category of the cysts, which are fluid-filled or solid and contain various cells and blood vessels. To correctly determine what type of lesion it is, a "triple-phase" CT scan or MRI with contrast medium can identify the type of lesion more than 90 % of the time and eliminate the need for a liver biopsy. As a biopsy not only involves risks of complications, such as bleeding, but may also not eliminate the cancer if very small, it should be reserved for when CT or MRI is not able to correctly identify the spot and/or if it is growing in size.

S. Rizvi, M.D. (⊠)
Division of Gastroenterology & Hepatology, Medical College of Wisconsin,
Milwaukee, WI, USA
e-mail: srizvi@mcw.edu

© Springer International Publishing Switzerland 2017
K. Sacian, R. Shaker (eds.), *Liver Disorders*,
DOI 10.1007/978-3-319-30103-7_4

Investigation of Incidental Hepatic Lesions

The use of imaging studies for various reasons can often lead to the finding of incidental lesions in the liver. As the utilization of imaging studies has increased over time, more of these incidental lesions are being found. Such findings may lead to anxiety on the part of the patient and to an unnecessarily exhaustive and time-consuming workup. A systemic approach to such a finding not only simplifies but also expedites the diagnostic workup and enhances patient outcomes.

A hepatic lesion may be encountered in one of three scenarios.

(a) An imaging study ordered for an unrelated reason – (e.g., CT performed to assess a pulmonary embolism shows an incidental liver lesion in abdominal sections).
(b) An abdominal scan ordered for nonspecific abdominal pain shows a small hepatic lesion unrelated to the pain.
(c) An imaging study ordered for other purposes in a patient who happens to have chronic liver disease, such as chronic hepatitis B or C.

Irrespective of which scenario is involved, the physician must include the specific characteristics of the lesion and the specific lesion that the patient has.

This systematic approach begins with a detailed history, physical examination, and laboratory testing, which inform the provider as to the appropriate subsequent imaging test if required. This approach precludes the need for a biopsy of the lesion in most cases. It may well be the case that the lesion cannot be fully characterized by the initial imaging modality and a further imaging study may indeed be required.

The Need for a Subsequent Imaging Study

Ultrasound is a safe modality that is able to detect hepatic lesions, is less costly than CT or MRI, and is often able to differentiate between a solid and a cystic lesion. Unfortunately, it cannot provide further information on the salient features or specific characteristics of the lesion needed to confidently identify it. Hence, a dynamic study, called a "liver protocol," often using CT or MRI, is of great value, because these modalities provide detailed information regarding such characteristics. As the liver receives most of its blood supply from the portal vein (approximately 70 %) and partly from the hepatic artery, the timing of uptake of contrast medium in individual phases of the blood supply may often help to identify a lesion. Hence, a triple-phase CT, which includes an early arterial phase, portal venous phase, and delayed portal venous phase can obviate the need for a liver biopsy in most cases.

With improvements in CT and MRI techniques, a biopsy of the hepatic lesion is often not required. Moreover, in the case of hypervascular lesions such as adenoma, hemangioma or hepatocellular carcinoma (HCC), a liver biopsy should be avoided because of the risk of bleeding and seeding of the cancer along the needle tract. It is also important to note that a needle biopsy of a lesion with potentially malignant features may miss the malignant cells, giving the patient and provider a false sense of security, potentially resulting in a lack of the appropriate follow-up or intervention. Hence, in most situations follow-up scans at periodic intervals may be the best approach for indeterminate lesions. Nevertheless, on rare occasions, if a lesion remains indeterminate on follow-up CT and MRI, a biopsy may be of use. A core biopsy should be ordered rather than needle aspiration, given the higher diagnostic yield.

The Systematic Approach to Incidental Hepatic Lesions

Now that we have discussed individual aspects of the diagnostic work-up for liver lesions, let us approach a lesion in a systematic manner.

History and Physical Examination

After receiving a radiology report of an ultrasound or abdominal CT or MRI, the workup should begin by determining whether or not the patient has underlying liver disease. The history should investigate the presence of risk factors such as a history of alcohol consumption, drug abuse, blood transfusions or a family history of liver disease or tumors. A history of oral contraceptives should be obtained, as this can easily give a clue with regard to hepatic adenoma. A history of cirrhosis or risk factors for cirrhosis, such as significant alcohol abuse, may point toward underlying cirrhosis, a known risk factor for HCC, and should raise the suspicion of malignancy. Similarly, a patient who is an immigrant from a country with a high prevalence of hepatitis B is at risk of HCC, even in the absence of cirrhosis. A cystic lesion found in a patient from sheep-grazing areas may have an underlying Echinococcus granulosus infection. A history of previous malignancy should raise the suspicion of metastatic disease.

Laboratory Evaluation

A liver panel should be the first test to be ordered to establish the presence or absence of underlying liver disease. Leukocytosis in the complete blood count may be found with a hepatic abscess and thrombocytopenia may point toward portal hypertension due to cirrhosis. Eosinophilia is not an often noted feature of amoebic liver disease [1]. Viral serologies should be ordered to rule out hepatitis A, B, and C. We do order tumor markers as part of the workup for solid hepatic lesions, including alpha fetoprotein (AFP), carbohydrate antigen 19-9 (CA 19-9), and carcinoembryonic antigen (CEA).

Imaging Studies

Based on imaging characteristics a liver lesion can be divided into cystic or solid. The first question to answer after an imaging study is whether or not the patient has an underlying liver disease, including cirrhosis. If the patient does have cirrhosis or an underlying liver disease considered to be at a high risk for malignancy (e.g., chronic hepatitis B) and the reported lesion is solid, then the mass should be considered an HCC until proven otherwise. If the initial study was ultrasound or nonliver protocol CT or MRI, then a dedicated triple-phase CT scan (or dedicated liver MRI if CT is not feasible) should be ordered with tumor markers (AFP, CA19-9, and CEA) to confirm the diagnosis. A finding of typical washout during the portal venous phase confirms the diagnosis of HCC, especially if the lesion measures 1 cm or more in size. AFP is a supplementary test and elevated levels, particularly those of more than 200 ng/ml or a significant rise from baseline, are highly suggestive of HCC in the presence of a solid lesion. However, it is worth noting that AFP may be normal in up to 40 % of small HCCs [2]. A suspicious lesion less than 1 cm in size needs surveillance with ultrasound every 3 months [3] and if growing, needs referral to a transplant facility. If the lesion is stable, continued surveillance is recommended. This approach avoids the need to biopsy a lesion and decreases the risks (e.g., bleeding, seeding of the needle track, false-negative diagnosis) posed by the biopsy.

A solid lesion in a noncirrhotic liver should also be approached by liver protocol CT or MRI. The most common benign lesion, hepatic hemangioma, shows peripheral nodular enhancement in the arterial phase and centripetal filling in the portal venous phase. Focal nodular hyperplasia (FNH) shows enhancement on the arterial phase with a characteristic "central scar" on CT or MRI. A hepatic adenoma shows somewhat intense enhancement in the arterial phase and becomes less intense in the delayed phase. MRI is considered more sensitive in differentiating between FNH and hepatic adenoma and may further characterize the type of adenoma, which can help in management (see next section).

Metastatic lesions in the liver are typically less vascular than HCCs, may be multiple, may have peripheral rim enhancement, and should particularly be suspected in those who have a known pre-existing extrahepatic malignancy.

A cystic lesion in the liver should be investigated by a CT or MRI to clarify whether it is a simple cyst or has suspicious features such as a thickened wall or nodularity, septations or a daughter cyst, as seen in an echinococcal cyst.

Choice of Contrast Agents for MRI of the Liver

Two types of commercially available contrast media are useful when imaging the liver: extracellular agents and hepatobiliary agents. The extracellular agents have the ability to visualize vascular perfusion and can be used to detect and characterize focal liver lesions. However, these agents only have 5 % hepatobiliary uptake.

They include gadobutrol (Gadavist™ [USA], Gadovist® [EU]; Bayer) and gadoversetamide (Optimark™, Covidien; Mallinckrodt).

Hepatobiliary agents, on the other hand, are not only taken up in vascular and extravascular spaces, but also have a 50 % [4, 5] hepatobiliary uptake. These agents are taken up from the sinusoidal side of the hepatocyte and excreted via the canalicular membrane. Hence, these agents perform extremely well in distinguishing lesions that do not contain hepatocytes (e.g., metastatic lesions) from the adjacent hepatic parenchyma. Of these agents, the ones approved by the FDA for liver imaging are Eovist and Optimark. Eovist (Gd-EOB-DTPA) is widely available in the USA after being approved by the FDA in 2008 [6, 7]. Similar to conventional MR contrast media, with the use of Eovist, first an arterial phase, then a venous phase, and finally, 20–30 min afterward, hepatobiliary phase imaging is performed.

Malignant Lesions

In malignant lesions such as HCCs (less functional hepatocytes) or metastatic disease, which contains no hepatocytes, low signal intensity foci are detected against the enhancing high signal parenchyma in the hepatobiliary phase, thus improving tumor detection. This feature is particularly useful in clearly identifying HCCs less than 2 cm in size in which MRI sensitivity is only 62 % [8]. This is because small HCCs, early in their growth, still obtain their blood supply from the portal vein compared with larger ones, which obtain their vascular supply from the hepatic artery. Hence, the low signal intensity in the hepatobiliary phase in these smaller HCCs can help to differentiate them from dysplastic nodules.

Benign Lesions

When imaging a hemangioma with MRI, whether using conventional extracellular contrast medium or hepatobiliary contrast medium, the hemangioma appears the same as its surroundings in the arterial phase. But, in the portal venous and hepatobiliary phases, with the use of hepatobiliary agents such as Eovist, a hemangioma appears iso- or hypointense compared with the adjacent parenchyma, as the hepatocytes of the surrounding normal liver appear bright compared with the hemangioma.

The use of Eovist is particularly helpful in identifying the typical characteristics of FNH. As the FNH consists of hepatocytes with abnormal canaliculi not connected to the adjacent biliary system, in the hepatocyte phase of the Eovist, the lesion appears iso- or hyperintense relative to the surrounding liver parenchyma, showing a classic "pop"-like enhancement pattern. This happens because of the accumulation of Eovist in the hepatobiliary phase. Because the characteristic central scar contains malformed vascular structures, it will be hypointense on the hepatocyte phase images using Eovist.

After injection of Eovist, hepatic adenomas frequently enhance in the arterial phase, with a washout in later phases. On hepatocyte phase images, adenomas typically appear hypointense because of the lack of biliary canaliculi, a feature that can distinguish hepatic adenoma from FNH.

Conclusion

In summary, in the appropriate setting, the use of new MRI contrast imaging techniques can more confidently classify indeterminate lesions, often obviating the need for biopsy and allowing the patient to avoid further invasive testing. The flow diagram in Fig. 4.1 gives a brief overview of the abovementioned workup, which may help to reach the diagnosis.

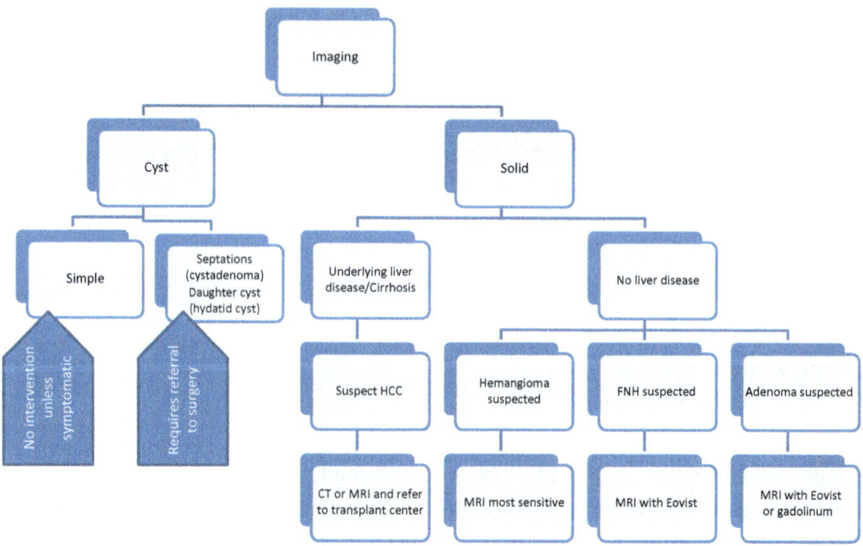

Fig. 4.1 Differential diagnosis of incidental hepatic lesions based on imaging

References

1. Reed SL. Amebiasis: An update. Clin Inf Dis. 1992;14:385–91.
2. Chen DS, Sung JL, Sheu JC, Lai MY, How SW, Hsu HC, et al. Serum alpha-fetoprotein in the early stage of human hepatocellular carcinoma. Gastroenterology. 1984;86(6):1404.
3. Briux et al. Management of hepatocellular carcinoma: an Update, Hepatology, 2011; 53:1020–1022.
4. Holzapfel K, Breitwieser C, Prinz C, et al. Contrast-enhanced magnetic resonance cholangiography using gadolinium-EOB-DTPA: preliminary experience and clinical applications [in German]. Radiologe. 2007;47:536–44.
5. Zizka J, Klzo L, Ferda J, et al. Dynamic and delayed contrast enhancement in upper abdominal MRI studies: comparison of gadoxetic acid and gadobutrol. Eur J Radiol. 2007;62:186–91.
6. Hammerstingl R, Huppertz A, Breuer J, et al. Diagnostic efficacy of gadoxetic acid (Primovist)-enhanced MRI and spiral CT for a therapeutic strategy: comparison with intraoperative and histopathologic findings in focal liver lesions. Eur Radiol. 2008;18:457–67.
7. Zech CJ, Herrmann KA, Reiser MF, et al. MR imaging in patients with suspected liver metastases: value of liver-specific contrast agent Gd-EOBDTPA. Magn Reson Med Sci. 2007;6:43–52.
8. Forner A, Vilana R, Ayuso C, Bianchi L, Sole M, Ayuso JR, et al. Diagnosis of hepatic nodules 20 mm or smaller in cirrhosis: prospective validation of the noninvasive diagnostic criteria for hepatocellular carcinoma. Hepatology. 2008;47:97–104.

Chapter 5
Benign Liver Lesions

Syed Rizvi

Patients' Questions

Question 1: My doctor told me that I have a hemangioma. Does it need to be removed?

Patient level answer: Hemangiomas are benign tumors that are noncancerous and are found in 5–10 % of the general population, who have no previous knowledge of them. Only large ones measuring more than 5 cm may occasionally cause symptoms. Hence, unless they cause pain and discomfort you do not need surgery.

Question 2: I have been diagnosed with an adenoma and I heard that it can cause problems during pregnancy. Can I get pregnant?

Patient level answer: Adenomas in the liver can grow owing to high levels of pregnancy hormones. However, the rupture of an adenoma is rare, unless it is large in size or is located on or near the surface of the liver. Hence, it is generally recommended that if it measures more than 5 cm you should see a surgeon to consider removal before pregnancy. If a decision is made not to operate, surveillance for growth in size can be performed with ultrasound during pregnancy.

Question 3: I recently had a CT scan of my chest for trouble with breathing and the emergency room physician told me that they also saw a 10-cm "simple cyst" in the liver. I don't have any pain; does it need to be taken out?

Patient level answer: Simple cysts that are small in size rarely cause symptoms and as they carry no risk of malignancy they do not need to be removed. They may cause pain and discomfort only if they are larger than 4–5 cm. Simple cysts measuring

S. Rizvi, M.D. (✉)
Division of Gastroenterology & Hepatology, Medical College of Wisconsin,
Milwaukee, WI, USA
e-mail: srizvi@mcw.edu

© Springer International Publishing Switzerland 2017
K. Saeian, R. Shaker (eds.), *Liver Disorders*,
DOI 10.1007/978-3-319-30103-7_5

more than 4–5 cm need monitoring for growth by ultrasound every 6–12 months for 2–3 years and if no growth is noted, they pose no risk. If a cyst is growing or causing symptoms, then you may need to see a surgeon.

Question 4: A 35-year-old female patient presents to your clinic with her husband. They have been married 5 years. They have been seen in the fertility clinic and are planning to undergo in vitro fertilization. The gynecologist told her that she has a 1-cm hemangioma that should probably be taken out, because it may grow and be dangerous during pregnancy. She was diagnosed with irritable bowel syndrome at age 25 and has sporadic abdominal pain on the right side that improves after a bowel movement. Is the hemangioma really causing her right-sided abdominal pain? Is this enough of a danger with regard to her large dose of hormonal therapy and anticipated pregnancy to warrant intervention?

Patient level answer: Your situation raises two questions, is a 1-cm hemangioma the cause of the pain in your abdomen and can a hemangioma pose a threat to your pregnancy?

The liver is very accommodating to small spots; hence, a hemangioma has to measure at least 5 cm to cause pain. With a spot in the liver measuring 1 cm, your physician should look for other reasons for the abdominal pain. Although a hemangioma in the liver may grow during pregnancy or with hormonal therapy, this connection is weak. In one study, 27 pregnancies in women with hepatic hemangiomas of sizes ranging 2.4–61 cm, 12 hemangiomas grew and only 1 case reported a rupture that was very large (10 cm) [1]. Hence, based on expert guidelines, there is no contraindication to proceeding with pregnancy unless it is very large [2].

Hepatic Hemangioma

This is the most common benign hepatic lesion. Although it may occur at any age, the majority are found between the ages of 30 and 50 years, with a female predominance by a ratio of 3:1 [1, 2]. This gender predominance may be explained by the growth of hemangioma observed during pregnancy and regression after withdrawal of hormonal therapy [3, 4]. However, there is no definitive effect of hormonal therapy on the development of hemangioma, as noted in a well-performed case–control study [5].

Clinical Presentation

Hemangiomas are largely asymptomatic, irrespective of size. To cause symptoms, a hemangioma should typically measure more than 4–5 cm. Most common symptoms are abdominal pain or right upper quadrant fullness. In addition, acute abdominal pain can be observed in cases of thrombosis or bleeding. In rare cases, giant hemangiomas may cause consumptive coagulopathy, known as Kasabach–Merritt syndrome, which manifests as thrombocytopenia, disseminated intravascular coagulation, and systemic bleeding [6].

Diagnosis

Ultrasound, CT, and MRI, in increasing order of sensitivity and specificity, are helpful in accurately diagnosing the hepatic hemangioma.

Ultrasound

Hemangioma on ultrasound appears as a homogeneous, hyperechoic mass. However, in the case of fatty liver, it can appear to be hypoechoic because of the bright signals from the surrounding parenchyma.

Computed Tomography

In the case of unenhanced CT, a hemangioma may appear as a homogeneous hypodense mass. However, similar to ultrasound in patients with fatty liver, it may appear hyperdense.

The addition of IV contrast medium shows a typical peripheral nodular pattern in the early contrast phase with "filling in" toward the center of the lesion in the delayed venous phase of the study, which can be diagnostic.

MRI

Magnetic resonance imaging is probably the most sensitive and specific test [7, 8]. In our practice, an MRI is the study of choice for a suspected hemangioma. It shows a smooth, well-demarcated, homogeneous mass that has low signal intensity on T1-weighted images and is hyperintense (light bulb sign) on T2-weighted images. Scintigraphy with technetium labeled RBC delayed scan is an obsolete study in the age of MRI.

Needle Biopsy

Because of the vascular nature of hemangioma, a biopsy is considered high risk. As most cases are diagnosed correctly on imaging, the role of biopsy is almost nil in current practice.

Management

As hemangiomas rarely grow, an incidentally found hepatic hemangioma requires no intervention. Those that tend to bleed are larger, hence, for hemangiomas >10 cm, or for smaller ones in patients for whom other competing etiologies of abdominal discomfort have been ruled out, surgical intervention may be considered [9, 10].

Follow up imaging of classic hemangioma is not required. For hemangiomas measuring more than 5 cm, which rarely have the potential to grow, a repeat imaging study after 6–12 months can be carried out. If no change in size is noted, no further follow-up imaging is warranted.

> **Hemangioma Summary**
> - Hemangiomas have no malignant potential.
> - A large hemangioma may even be asymptomatic.
> - The best confirmatory test is a liver MRI protocol.
> - Liver biopsy is not required to confirm the diagnosis.
> - Surgery is only considered if symptomatic.

Hepatic Adenoma

Hepatic adenoma is a benign epithelial tumor that arises de novo in the liver and has a causal relationship with hormonal abnormality or with metabolic syndrome. It is often noted in women at a young age and is mostly asymptomatic.

Risk Factors

Although they can be found without risk factors, there is a clear and established link between hormonal abnormalities and hepatic adenomas. Several studies have shown a marked increase in adenomas with the use of oral contraceptives (OCPs). In one study the incidence of hepatic adenoma was 1–1.3 per million in women not on OCPs compared with 34 per one million in women who were on OCPs [11]. Also, regression has been noted in patients who stopped using OCPs, further confirming a causal relationship. Just as they are linked with female hormones, there is evidence of increased association of hepatic adenoma with the use of androgens. Discontinuation of androgens may also result in regression [12, 13].

Other risk factors associated with hepatic adenomas include glycogen storage disease Ia and III. In such patients there is a male to female ratio of 2:1 in developing hepatic adenomas and they are typically found at a much younger age.

Several studies have proposed metabolic syndrome as a risk factor for the development of hepatic adenomas [14, 15] with the use of OCPs, with the risk of hepatic adenoma increasing further in patients who are obese. Although the chance of developing adenomas is higher in women, the risk of the malignant transformation of an existing hepatic adenoma is 10 times higher in obese men than in obese women [16].

Complications

Risk Factors for Malignant Transformation

Malignant transformation has been linked to a size >5 cm, beta catenin mutation, and the presence of glycogen storage disease.

Hemorrhage

Large adenomas can bleed ; with the use of OCPs, pregnancy or if sub-capsular in location, the risk of bleeding is increased.

Clinical Presentation

Hepatic adenomas are often asymptomatic, but if symptoms are present, the most common presentation is epigastric or right upper quadrant abdominal pain. Large adenomas may present with bleeding and shock. Approximately 11–29 % of hepatic adenomas may develop spontaneous hemorrhage due to rupture, with nearly all instances occurring in lesions measuring >5 cm [17–19].

Diagnosis

Ultrasound

Adenomas are well demarcated and hyperechoic on ultrasound

CT

Well-demarcated with peripheral enhancement during the early phase with centripetal flow during the portal venous phase, a characteristic of adenoma [20]. In the delayed venous phase, the lesion becomes isodense or hypodense.

MRI

On MRI most adenomas are hyperintense on T1-weighted images and on T2-weighted images. An advantage of MRI over CT is that not only can it help to differentiate from other lesions, it can also determine the subtype of hepatic adenoma, obviating the need for a biopsy (Table 5.1).

Table 5.1 Types of hepatic adenoma

Type of adenoma	Prevalence	Malignant transformation	MRI characteristics
Inflammatory HCAs	30–50 %	5–10 %	Plain MRI: hyperintense on T2WI; hypointense on T1WI
HNF-1 α -mutated HCAs	30–35 %	Minimal	Heterogeneous hypointense areas on T1 out-phased sequences with significant signal drops (sensitivity 85 %, specificity 100 %) On T2WI iso- or hypointense nodule, without significant restriction on DWI
β -Catenin-mutated HCAs	10–15 %	20–30 %	

HNF hepatocyte nuclear factor, *HCA* hepatocellular adenoma, *T2WI* T2-weighted imaging, *T1WI* T1-weighted imaging, *DWI* diffusion-weighted imaging

Biopsy of Hepatic Adenoma

Because of the risk of a beta-catenin type of hepatic adenoma transforming into a hepatocellular carcinoma (HCC), a biopsy of the hepatic adenoma can be helpful in determining the subtype; however, owing to the vascular nature of the lesion, there is an increased risk of bleeding. As MRI with contrast medium can help to determine the subtype, liver biopsy is seldom required and should be reserved for cases in which the diagnosis is in question.

Management

Incidental Diagnosis, <5-cm Adenoma with No Symptoms

The first step in the management of the lesion should be to stop taking OCPs if they are involved. Then, 6 months after this, repeat imaging should be performed to document regression or stability in size. Surveillance should be carried out every 6 months for 2 years, and, if stable, annual imaging should be performed [21].

Symptomatic, >5-cm Adenomas

Lesions larger than 5 cm should be considered for resection because of their risk of malignant transformation, spontaneous hemorrhage, and symptoms. Nonsurgical management such as embolization is an alternative for high-operative-risk patients. Because of the higher risk of "beta-catenin" (a phenotypic expression)-type adenoma with regard to malignant transformation, patients should be referred for surgical resection irrespective of the size.

Women Contemplating Pregnancy or Who Are Pregnant

Hepatic adenomas are known to grow during pregnancy and hence there is a risk of acute rupture. However, owing to the rare nature of this disease, clear guidelines on managing these lesions in patients planning to be pregnant are not available. However, in general, lesions <5 cm can be observed with no intervention is required [22].

Hepatic Adenomas in Glycogen Storage Disease

Hepatic adenoma in these patients does pose a risk for malignant transformation. Management is slightly different. Nocturnal tube feeding intended to control the disease has been shown to decrease the size of the adenoma [23]. Given the risk for malignant transformation, resection can be offered. Liver transplantation in patients who develop HCC is curative for both HCC and glycogen storage disease.

Liver Adenomatosis

Liver adenomatosis is the condition where >3 to >10 adenomas are present [24, 25]. Nature and disease behavior are the same and hence similar management criteria apply in this subtype.

> **Adenomas Summary**
> - Adenomas can grow with the use of OCPs.
> - They are mostly asymptomatic.
> - They may grow in size in women on hormonal therapy or during pregnancy.
> - Pregnancy is not contraindicated; however, adenomas measuring more than 5 cm should be addressed surgically before pregnancy.
> - Adenomas have malignant potential for HCC.

Focal Nodular Hyperplasia

Focal nodular hyperplasia is the second most commonly found hepatic lesion in the liver, with a reported prevalence rate of 0.03–0.3 % in autopsy series [26, 27]. FNH is proposed to be due to the arteriovenous malformation resulting in a response from the hepatic stellate cells, resulting in a "central scar" appearance on imaging.

Focal nodular hyperplasia is most frequently diagnosed incidentally, but can be symptomatic in 20–40 % of cases [28, 29]. It has a female preponderance and is proposed to be present at birth and likely to grow under the effect of female hormones. This is slightly different than hepatic adenoma, which may develop de novo under the influence of hormonal stimulation. However, similar to hemangioma, no clear link is found between the discontinuation of OCPs and a reduction in the size of FNH.

Diagnosis

Diagnosis is usually made by identifying the characteristic features on imaging. Liver enzymes as a rule are normal and tumor markers are not elevated. Differential diagnosis includes hepatic hemangiomas or hepatic adenomas. Caution should be observed as the central scar characteristic of FNH can also be seen in the fibrolamellar type of HCC

Imaging

Most of the lesions are solitary; however, multiple FNHs have been reported in 7–20 % of cases. A diagnosis of FNH can be confidently made by identifying the central scar on imaging.

Ultrasound

Focal nodular hyperplasia can be hyper-, hypo- or isoechoic on ultrasound and a central scar can only be identified in 20 % of the cases.

CT with Intravenous Contrast Medium

An appropriately timed liver CT protocol. The lesion is hyperdense in the arterial phase and either hypodense or isodense with a central scar in the portal venous phase.

MRI

On MRI, the FNH can be isointense or hypointense. A central scar can be seen on the delayed phase. In the T2 phase it is slightly hyperintense or isointense. MRI is the definitive imaging modality for FNH.

Management

Focal nodular hyperplasia usually remains stable and rarely causes symptoms. Unlike hepatic adenoma, it does not have the potential for malignant transformation. Thus, intervention with operative removal is only warranted when symptoms are clearly associated or there is diagnostic uncertainty.

FNH and OCPs

Although there may be a hormonal influence, discontinuation of OCPs is not absolutely recommended. However, in women who wish to continue taking OCPs, an annual ultrasound focusing on the change in size can be performed for 2–3 years. In women who discontinue OCPs, follow-up imaging is not required.

> **FNH Summary**
> - FNHs are benign lesions in the liver.
> - They are identified by a central scar on imaging.
> - They rarely grow.
> - There is no risk of malignancy.

Nodular Regenerative Hyperplasia

Nodular regenerative hyperplasia (NRH) is a benign transformation of hepatic parenchyma into nodular form. This is described as a consequence of changes in blood flow through the hepatic parenchyma. This, in turn, leads to hyperplasia of the hepatic architecture to compensate for atrophic hepatocytes in ischemic zones, resulting in a nodular appearance. NRH is associated with immunological and hematological disorders, cardiac or pulmonary disorders, and certain drugs and toxins have been implicated in NRH (Table 5.3).

Diagnosis

There are no classic imaging characteristics of NRH on imaging, although patients are often mistakenly diagnosed as having cirrhosis (Table 5.2).

Clinical features

Although itself a painless condition, NRH may cause a pre-sinusoidal type of portal hypertension, leading to ascites, splenomegaly, and varices. Hence, the diagnosis of NRH is based on:

- Exclusion of cirrhosis using imaging and serological markers for chronic liver disease.
- Exclusion of noncirrhotic etiologies of portal hypertension; namely, congenital hepatic fibrosis, alcoholic hepatitis, sarcoidosis, schistosomiasis, and portal vein thrombosis.
- Drugs and toxin history (see Table 5.3).
- Liver biopsy, which is compatible and shows the absence of cirrhosis with reticulin staining, is helpful in accentuating the nodularity.

Table 5.2 Imaging characteristics of benign lesions

	Ultrasound	CE ultrasound	CT	MRI
HCA	Heterogeneous; hyperechoic if steatotic, but anechoic center if hemorrhagic	Arterial phase; hyperenhancement; hypoenhancement in portal phase and no enhancement in late phase	Well-demarcated with peripheral enhancement; homogeneous more often than heterogeneous; hypodense if steatotic, hyperdense if hemorrhagic	HNF-1α: signal lost on chemical shift: moderate arterial enhancement without persistent enhancement during delayed phase IHCA: markedly hyperintense on T2WI with stronger signal peripherally: persistent enhancement in delayed phase B-catenin: inflammatory subtype has same appearance as IHCA; noninflammatory is heterogeneous with no signal dropout on chemical shift, isointense on T1WI and T2WI with strong arterial enhancement and delayed washout
THCA	Variable appearance	Subcapsular feeding arteries with mixed or centripetal fitting: arterial phase shows hyperenhancement with hypoenhancement and no enhancement in the portal and late phases respectively	Hypo- to isoattenuating	T1WI: heterogeneous and well-defined iso-to hyperintense mass Strongly hyperintense with persistent contrast enhancement in delayed phase
FNH	Generally isoechoic	Arterial phase: hyperenhancement; portal and late phases: isoenhancement	Central scar. Arterial phase shows homogenous hyperdense lesion; returns to precontrast density during portal phase, which is hypo- or isodense	T1WI: isointense or slightly hypointense. Gadolinium produces early enhancement with central scar enhancement during delayed phase T2WI: slightly hyperintense or isointense

NRH	Isoechoic/hyperechoic	Isoenhancement during arterial, portal, and late phases	Unenhancing nodules, sometimes hypodense, with variable sizes (most sub-centimeter)	T1WI: hyperintense T2WI: varied intensity (hypo-/iso-/hyperintense)
Hemangioma	Hyperechoic with well-defined rim and with few intranodular vessels	Arterial phase: discontinuous peripheral nodular enhancement: progressive and centripetal fill in the portal and late phases	Discontinuous peripheral nodular enhancement isoattenuating to aorta with progressive centripetal fill-in	T1WI: hypointense: discontinuous peripheral enhancement T2WI: hyperintense relative to spleen
SHC	Homogeneous anechoic fluid-filled space without clear walls and with posterior acoustic enhancement	No enhancement during arterial, portal, or late phases. Lack of enhancement because of avascularity	Isodense to water (because of lack of vascularity): well-demarcated	T1WI: hypointense (no enhancement with gadolinium) T2WI: hyperintense to spleen and isointense relative to simple fluid
HBCA	Anechoic with irregular walls and internal septations	Arterial phase: hyperenhancement of cystic wall, internal septations, and intracystic solid portion: enhancement washes out progressively: hypoenhancement during portal and late phases	Isodense lesion with well-defined thick wall, mural nodules, and internal septations	T1WI: multilocular mass with homogeneous hyperintensity

IHCA inflammatory hepatocellular adenoma, *THCA* telangiectatic hepatocellular adenoma, *FNH* focal nodular hyperplasia, *NRH* nodular regenerative hyperplasia, *SHC* sarcomatoid hepatocellular carcinoma, *HBCA* hepatobiliary cystadenomas

Table 5.3 Diseases associated with nodular regenerative hyperplasia

Immunological	Hematological	Drugs and toxins	Cardiac and pulmonary disorders	Other
Autoimmune	Myeloproliferative neoplasms	Chemotherapeutic agents	Cardiac	Neoplasia
Polyarteritis nodosa	Chronic myelogenous leukemia	6-thioguanine	Congenital heart	Massive hepatic
Rheumatoid arthritis	Primary myelofibrosis (myeloid	Busulfan and 6-thioguanine	disease	metastasis
Felty's syndrome	metaplasia)	Doxyrubicin	Congestive heart	Hepatocellular
Systemic lupus erythematosus	Polycythemia vera	Cyclophosphamide	failure	carcinoma
Progressive systemic sclerosis	Essential thrombocytosis	Chlorambucil	Myocardial	Carcinoid syndrome
Antiphospholipid syndrome Primary	Lymphoproliferative neoplasms	Cytosine arabinoside	infarction	Organ transplantation
biliary cirrhosis	Chronic lymphocytic leukemia	Bleomycin	Endocardial cushion	Bone marrow
Celiac disease	Hodgkin's lymphoma	Carmustine	defect	transplantation
CREST syndrome	Non-Hodgkin's lymphoma	Oxaliplatin	Infections,	Renal transplantation
Primary Sjögren's syndrome	Waldenström's	Azathioprine	endocarditis	Liver transplantation
Polymyalgia rheumatic	macroglobulinemia	HIV drugs	Pulmonary	Miscellaneous
Lymphocytic thyroiditis Schnitzler	Other	Nevirapine	Pulmonary	Portal vein agenesis
syndrome	Thrombotic thrombocytopenic	Didanosine	emphysema	Diabetes mellitus
Immunodeficiency	purpura	IL-2 therapy	Bronchial asthma	Budd–Chiari syndrome
Hypogammaglobulinemia	Sickle cell anemia	Other	Interstitial	Age greater than 80
Common variable immunodeficiency	Mastocytosis	Toxic oil syndrome	pneumonia	years
Hyper IgM syndrome	Aplastic anemia	Anabolic androgenic	Pulmonary	Amyloidosis
Bruton syndrome		steroids	hypertension	Visceral leishmaniasis
HIV patients		6-mercaptopurine	Tuberculosis	Familial idiopathic
Acquired protein S deficiency				pulmonary fibrosis
Thrombophilia				Chronic renal disease

CREST calcinosis, Raynaud's phenomenon, esophageal dysmotility, sclerodactyly, and telangiectasia

Biopsy samples obtained via a percutaneous or transvenous route may not be sufficiently large and thus laparoscopic sampling may be required to demonstrate the nodular pattern. The nodular pattern can be differentiated from that of cirrhosis by the presence of surrounding atrophic parenchyma, the lack of fibrous septa, and curvilinear compression of the central lobule. Unlike cirrhosis, NRH is not known to increase the risk of HCC.

Management

The management of NRH is twofold. First is the management of complications, such as ascites and esophageal varices. Second, the underlying cause of NRH should be sought (see list of risk factors, Table 5.3) and if necessary addressed.

NRH Summary
- NRH has a pseudotumor appearance in the liver.
- It is often a manifestation of some other disease.
- It may cause portal hypertension.
- Patients need endoscopy to screen for esophageal varices.
- Ascites may develop.

Hepatic Cysts

Hepatic cysts are a group of heterogeneous, fluid-filled spaces originating in either the hepatic parenchyma or the biliary tree.

Hepatic cysts can be broadly divided into three types:

1. Simple cysts, including polycystic liver disease (PCLD).
2. An infective type, such as hydatid cysts.
3. Cystadenomas and cystadenocarcinomas.

In general, hepatic cysts are rarely symptomatic and are almost always discovered incidentally.

Simple Cysts

Simple cysts are usually small, measuring up to 5 cm. By definition, there should be less than 3 of them and if there are more, this raises the possibility of PCLD [30]. They are rarely symptomatic and have no malignant potential.

A simple cyst can be easily differentiated from other types of cysts on ultrasound, CT or MRI. On ultrasound, it is anechoic, homogeneous, and fluid-filled with smooth margins. On CT, it is a well-demarcated, water-attenuated, smooth lesion with no septations or wall thickening. On MRI, it is recognized as a homogeneous lesion with no contrast enhancement. On T1-weighted images, it is hypointense, and on T2 imaging it is hyperintense. Liver enzymes are normal.

Simple cysts have a benign course and require no further follow-up [31]. Rarely, those cysts that are large, symptomatic, and show interval growth require further intervention and should be referred for surgery.

Polycystic Liver Disease

Polycystic liver disease is identified by the presence of numerous cysts. It usually presents in association with autosomal dominant polycystic kidney disease (ADPKD) [32, 33] but can be present as isolated disease [34]. It is usually discovered in adulthood and is largely asymptomatic. However, symptoms may occur in 10–15 % of patients, mostly women. Symptoms range from abdominal fullness, pain, to bleeding into a cyst. Patients may present with jaundice because of the extrinsic compression of the bile duct. Rarely, patients may develop portal hypertension with ascites owing to compression of hepatic veins or associated congenital hepatic fibrosis.

Diagnosis

Liver enzymes are normal. On ultrasound, CT or MRI, multiple hepatic cysts, with similar characteristics to simple cysts, are seen.

Management

The management of PCLD is dependent on the patient's symptoms. De-roofing, fenestration with or without sclerosants, or resection are all options, but unfortunately recurrences are frequent. In severe forms, liver transplantation with or without kidney transplantation may be required.

Biliary cystadenomas and biliary cystadenocarcinomas

Biliary cystadenomas are best described as congenitally derived, aberrant bile duct remnants. Despite their origin, they have no communication with the bile ducts. Structurally, the biliary cystadenoma has septations, giving it a loculated appearance on imaging, and it is filled with mucinous fluid.

Diagnosis

The presence of septations and irregular walls on ultrasound are consistent with biliary cystadenomas. With these findings on ultrasound, a CT or MRI should be performed to better delineate the characteristics, namely, a thickened wall, septations, papillary formation, and to confirm the diagnosis. On MRI, the cysts are usually hyperintense on T2-weighted imaging. Aspiration and biopsy should not be attempted.

Management

Given the risk of malignancy, a patient with a biliary cystadenoma or biliary cystadenocarcinoma should be referred to a hepatobiliary surgeon for surgical excision [35–38].

Hydatid Cysts

Hydatid cysts are formed as a result of an infestation of *Echinococcosis granulosus* in patients from sheep-grazing areas such as South America, Australia, East Africa, or the Mediterranean, where humans act as accidental hosts. The eggs hatch in the intestine and embryos migrate to the liver and lungs via the vasculature, eventually resulting in hydatid cysts. Mostly, they are small (<5 cm) and asymptomatic; however, larger cysts may cause abdominal discomfort.

Diagnosis

Eosinophilia may be found in approximately 30 % of patients. On ultrasound, hydatid cysts may be unilocular or multilocular with thickened walls and hypo-/hyperechoic content. Daughter cysts may be seen at the periphery. On CT, a hypodense lesion with a hypervascular wall due to calcification may be noted. Loculations and daughter cysts can be seen at the periphery of the mother cyst. On MRI, hydatid cysts are hypointense on T1- and hyperintense on T2-weighted images. Daughter cysts are seen at the periphery of the mother cyst.

Management

The management of hydatid cysts includes the use of anthelminthic drugs, such as albendazole and mebendazole, percutaneous drainage, or surgical removal. No clear guideline is available about the timing and modality of treatment. Anthelminthics alone are not indicated for symptomatic cysts, as efficacy is not 100 %, treatment is long term, and there is a risk of recurrence; however, they can be used as an adjunct to other interventions. Cyst drainage by puncture, aspiration, injection, and re-aspiration (PAIR) is used as an alternative to surgery where a sclerosant such as 95 % ethanol or hypertonic saline is injected and aspirated. PAIR should not be used if there is a connection to the bile duct because of the risk of sclerosing cholangitis. Surgery, including de-roofing or radical pericystectomy, can be performed in patients who can tolerate surgery (Table 5.4).

Table 5.4 Management strategies for benign solid and cystic hepatic tumors

	Associated complications (rate if known)	Malignant potential (rate if known)	OCP use	Pregnancy	Biopsy (yes or no)	Follow-up	Management
HCA	Hemorrhage and spontaneous rupture (11–29 %)	Yes (5–10 %), almost exclusively of β-catenin subtype	Discontinue	Generally contradicted, but can be individualized if carefully managed	Generally no. In select cases if diagnosis is uncertain and histological, genetic, and molecular markers to be used	Confirm diagnosis and monitor if treatment is conservative	Conservative treatment if <5 cm and asymptomatic for HNF-1α, and IHCA subtypes. Resect if asymptomatic and/or ≥5 cm, or if β-catenin subtype
LA	Hemorrhage and rupture	Yes	Discontinue	Generally contraindicated, but can be individualized if carefully managed	Same as for HCA	Monitor	Variable; resection of largest lesions combined with RFA is suggested when possible
THCA	Hemorrhage and rupture	Unknown	Discontinue	Generally contraindicated, but can be individualized if carefully managed	Same as for HCA	Investigate treatment options	Resect or ablate tumor
FNH	Association with other vascular anomalies; spontaneous rupture is extremely rare	Rare if any	Not absolutely contraindicated	Not contraindicated	No	Classic features require no follow-up; atypical lesions should be monitored	Conservative. Surgical intervention required for severely symptomatic tumors, or tumors without a firm diagnosis

NRH	Portal hypertension: ascites; esophageal varices	No	Not contraindicated	Not contraindicated	Yes	Determine underlying disease	Treat underlying condition and manage portal hypertension
Hemangioma	Rare: obstructive jaundice; consumptive coagulopathy	No	Not absolutely contraindicated	Not contraindicated	No	Classic features require no follow-up	Conservative
SHC	Rare: obstructive jaundice; portal hypertension; hemorrhage; rupture; infection	No	Not contraindicated	Not contraindicated	No	Monitor	Conservative
PCLD	Hemorrhage; rupture; infection; portal hypertension; biliary obstruction	Rare	Not contraindicated	Not contraindicated	No	Monitor closely with imaging	Conservative management of asymptomatic cysts. Symptomatic cysts can be managed surgically
HBCA		Yes (as high as 26 %)	Not contraindicated	Not contraindicated	No	Investigate surgical options	Complete resection of the tumor whenever possible

OCP oral contraceptive, *LA* liver adenomatosis, *RFA* radiofrequency ablation, *PCLD* polycystic liver disease

Conclusion

Benign liver lesions are often found incidentally. Radiologically they can be differentiated as cystic or solid lesions.

With relevant history including that of medications such as OCPs in the case of adenomas, physical exam as well as labs to look for clues of underlying liver disease, benign liver lesions can be diagnosed with a good certainty with the help of cross sectional imaging. Biopsy is often not needed. It should be also be remembered that in cases of adenomas or in hemangiomas biopsy carries a risk of catastrophic bleed and is not of additional value to the radiographic diagnosis. Although majority of the benign lesions do not warrant surgical intervention only those with symptoms or those with risk of potential growth or malignant transformation such as hepatic adenomas or biliary cystadenomas may need intervention. Nodular regenerative hyperplasia gives pseudotumor appearance on imaging. It is a manifestation of another underlying medical problem or exposure to drugs or toxins which warrant further investigation.

References

1. Farges O, Daradkeh S, Bismuth H. Cavernous hemangiomas of the liver: are there any indications for resection? World J Surg. 1995;19(1):19–24.
2. Gandolfi L et al. Natural history of hepatic haemangiomas: clinical and ultrasound study. Gut. 1991;32(6):677–80.
3. DuPre CT, Fincher RM. Case report: cavernous hemangioma of the liver. Am J Med Sci. 1992;303(4):241–4.
4. Saegusa T et al. Enlargement of multiple cavernous hemangioma of the liver in association with pregnancy. Intern Med. 1995;34(3):207–11.
5. Gemer O et al. Oral contraceptives and liver hemangioma: a case-control study. Acta Obstet Gynecol Scand. 2004;83(12):1199–201.
6. Kasabach H, Merritt K. Capillary hemangioma with extensive purpura: report of a case. Am J Dis Child. 1940;59:1063–70.
7. Lee MG et al. The diagnostic accuracy/efficacy of MRI in differentiating hepatic hemangiomas from metastatic colorectal/breast carcinoma: a multiple reader ROC analysis using a jack-knife technique. J Comput Assist Tomogr. 1996;20(6):905–13.
8. McFarland EG et al. Hepatic hemangiomas and malignant tumors: improved differentiation with heavily T2-weighted conventional spin-echo MR imaging. Radiology. 1994;193(1):43–7.
9. Ehrl D et al. "Incidentaloma" of the liver: management of a diagnostic and therapeutic dilemma. HPB Surg. 2012;2012:891787.
10. Shaked O, et al. Biologic and clinical features of benign solid and cystic lesions of the liver. Clin Gastroenterol Hepatol. 2012; 9(7): 547–62 e1–4.
11. Rooks JB et al. Epidemiology of hepatocellular adenoma. The role of oral contraceptive use. JAMA. 1979;242(7):644–8.
12. Carrasco D et al. Multiple hepatic adenomas after long-term therapy with testosterone enanthate. Review of the literature. J Hepatol. 1985;1(6):573–8.
13. Resnick MB, Kozakewich HP, Perez-Atayde AR. Hepatic adenoma in the pediatric age group. Clinicopathological observations and assessment of cell proliferative activity. Am J Surg Pathol. 1995;19(10):1181–90.

14. Bioulac-Sage P, et al. Hepatocellular adenoma subtypes: the impact of overweight and obesity. Liver Int. 2012;32(8):1217–21.
15. Bunchorntavakul C, et al. Clinical features and natural history of hepatocellular adenomas: the impact of obesity. Aliment Pharmacol Ther. 2011;34(6):664–74.
16. Farges O, et al. Changing trends in malignant transformation of hepatocellular adenoma. Gut. 2011;60(1):85–9.
17. Cho SW et al. Surgical management of hepatocellular adenoma: take it or leave it? Ann Surg Oncol. 2008;15(10):2795–803.
18. Deneve JL et al. Liver cell adenoma: a multicenter analysis of risk factors for rupture and malignancy. Ann Surg Oncol. 2009;16(3):640–8.
19. Ribeiro Junior MA et al. Surgical management of spontaneous ruptured hepatocellular adenoma. Clinics (Sao Paulo). 2009;64(8):775–9.
20. Grazioli L et al. Hepatic adenomas: imaging and pathologic findings. Radiographics. 2001;21(4):877–92. discussion 892–4.
21. Leese T, Farges O, Bismuth H. Liver cell adenomas. A 12-year surgical experience from a specialist hepato-biliary unit. Ann Surg. 1988;208(5):558–64.
22. Broker ME et al. The management of pregnancy in women with hepatocellular adenoma: a plea for an individualized approach. Int J Hepatol. 2012;2012:725735.
23. Parker P et al. Regression of hepatic adenomas in type Ia glycogen storage disease with dietary therapy. Gastroenterology. 1981;81(3):534–6.
24. Flejou JF et al. Liver adenomatosis. An entity distinct from liver adenoma? Gastroenterology. 1985;89(5):1132–8.
25. Ribeiro A et al. Management of liver adenomatosis: results with a conservative surgical approach. Liver Transpl Surg. 1998;4(5):388–98.
26. Craig JR, et al. Tumor of the liver and intrahepatic bile ducts. Armed Forces Institute of Pathology, Washington DC: Atlas of Tumor Pathology: 1989. p. 280.
27. Karhunen PJ. Benign hepatic tumours and tumour like conditions in men. J Clin Pathol. 1986;39(2):183–8.
28. Cherqui D et al. Management of focal nodular hyperplasia and hepatocellular adenoma in young women: a series of 41 patients with clinical, radiological, and pathological correlations. Hepatology. 1995;22(6):1674–81.
29. Luciani A et al. Focal nodular hyperplasia of the liver in men: is presentation the same in men and women? Gut. 2002;50(6):877–80.
30. Cowles RA, Mulholland MW. Solitary hepatic cysts. J Am Coll Surg. 2000;191(3):311–21.
31. Doty JE, Tompkins RK. Management of cystic disease of the liver. Surg Clin North Am. 1989;69(2):285–95.
32. D'Agata ID et al. Combined cystic disease of the liver and kidney. Semin Liver Dis. 1994;14(3):215–28.
33. Summerfield JA et al. Hepatobiliary fibropolycystic diseases. A clinical and histological review of 51 patients. J Hepatol. 1986;2(2):141–56.
34. Karhunen PJ, Tenhu M. Adult polycystic liver and kidney diseases are separate entities. Clin Genet. 1986;30(1):29–37.
35. Hansman MF et al. Management and long-term follow-up of hepatic cysts. Am J Surg. 2001;181(5):404–10.
36. Lee JH et al. Biliary cystadenoma and cystadenocarcinoma of the liver: 10 cases of a single center experience. Hepatogastroenterology. 2009;56(91–92):844–9.
37. Sanchez H et al. Surgical management of nonparasitic cystic liver disease. Am J Surg. 1991;161(1):113–8. discussion 118–9.
38. Vogt DP, Henderson JM, Chmielewski E. Cystadenoma and cystadenocarcinoma of the liver: a single center experience. J Am Coll Surg. 2005;200(5):727–33.

Chapter 6
Malignant Liver Lesions

Liver Disorders: A Point-of-Care Clinical Guide

Michael Loudin, Ranjan Mascarenhas, and Barry Schlansky

Abbreviations

AFP	Alpha-fetoprotein
BCLC	Barcelona clinic liver cancer
CCA	Cholangiocarcinoma
CEA	Carcinoembryonic antigen
CT	Computerized tomography
EHE	Epithelioid hemangioendothelioma
HB	Hepatoblastoma
HBV	Hepatitis B
HCC	Hepatocellular carcinoma
HCV	Hepatitis C
HIV	Human immunodeficiency virus
HSTCL	Hepatosplenic T-cell lymphoma
MRI	Magnetic resonance imaging

M. Loudin, M.D. • B. Schlansky, M.D., M.P.H. (✉)
Division of Gastroenterology and Hepatology, Department of Medicine,
Oregon Health and Science University, 3181 SW Sam Jackson Park Road, L-461,
Portland, OR 97239, USA
e-mail: loudin@ohsu.edu; schlansk@ohsu.edu

R. Mascarenhas, M.D.
Austin Outpatient Clinic, Central Texas Veterans Health Care System,
7901 Metropolis Drive, Austin, TX 78744, USA
e-mail: Ranjan.Mascarenhas@va.gov

© Springer International Publishing Switzerland 2017
K. Saeian, R. Shaker (eds.), *Liver Disorders*,
DOI 10.1007/978-3-319-30103-7_6

Patient Questions

Is My Liver Mass a Cancer?

Liver masses are either benign (noncancerous) or malignant (cancerous). Malignant liver masses either originate in the liver itself (primary liver cancer) or move to the liver from another organ (metastatic cancer to the liver). Benign masses are generally confined to the liver. Rarely, certain benign liver masses (hepatocellular adenomas) harbor the potential to change into a liver cancer, particularly if they are larger in size. The most common type of malignant liver mass is a liver metastasis. Metastases from a cancer in another organ most frequently come from the lungs, breasts, colon, or pancreas. The two most common types of cancer that arise from liver cells (primary liver cancer) are hepatocellular carcinoma (HCC) and cholangiocarcinoma (CCA).

HCC is the most common form of primary liver cancer and is usually diagnosed by imaging studies. In some cases, HCC cannot be diagnosed with imaging, and a biopsy is required. In contrast, CCA and other more rare forms of liver cancer almost always require a biopsy for diagnosis. Certain blood tests called tumor markers may be elevated in liver cancer. Although these tests may be used to monitor a response to treatment after liver cancer is diagnosed, the tumor markers by themselves are not enough to establish the initial cancer diagnosis.

What Are the Treatment Options for My Liver Cancer?

The treatment options for liver cancer depend on the cancer type, the extent of the cancer (the stage), and whether scarring (fibrosis or cirrhosis) is present in the liver. Conceptually, treatments for primary liver cancer are separated between those that have the possibility of curing the cancer, and those therapies that are intended to improve survival with a low likelihood of cure (palliate the cancer). Treatments which have the ability to cure liver cancer include surgical removal of the cancer (resection), chemical destruction of the cancer with 100% ethanol (percutaneous ethanol injection), heat destruction of the cancer (radiofrequency ablation), and liver transplantation (replacement of the liver with a donor organ). The choice of therapy is complex and based on the type, size, location, and number of tumors in the liver, spread of the tumor outside the liver or into blood vessels, and underlying liver health. Statistically, less than 15% of all liver cancers are diagnosed early enough for curative therapies to help. Palliative therapies are broken down into liver-directed therapies and systemic therapies (therapies that affect the whole body). The selection of an appropriate therapy is again complex and depends on the type size, location, and number of tumors in the liver, spread outside the liver or into blood vessels, and underlying liver health. Liver-directed therapies are a group of treatments that directly target the cancer inside the liver, whereas systemic therapies are regimens that introduce treatments either orally or directly into the blood supply (intravenous) and affect all organ systems. Liver-directed therapies attack the cancer through direct injection of substances into the artery feeding the tumor or through external beam radiation. Substances which are injected into the tumor include ones that block the artery feeding the cancer (embolizing agents), direct injection of chemotherapy with or without an embolizing agent, and the direct injection of radioactive beads. Currently, only one systemic chemotherapy agent is approved for the treatment of HCC (sorafenib); this is an oral drug taken twice per day.

The primary treatment for early CCA is surgical resection or rarely liver transplantation. CCA tends to be an aggressive type of liver cancer and often recurs after resection. In CCA that comes back after surgery, or in CCA detected at an advanced stage, chemotherapy is the preferred treatment, and prolongs life, but does not offer the prospect of a cure.

Rare liver cancers, including epithelioid hemangioendothelioma, hepatic angiosarcoma, and hepatoblastoma are treated with surgical resection, liver transplantation (except angiosarcoma), or burning the tumor (percutaneous ablation) if they are detected at an early stage. As with HCC and CCA, chemotherapy is typically used for recurrent or advanced cancers.

What Is the Likely Course of My Cancer?

Prognosis is the medical term for the course of a disease. The prognosis of liver cancer is affected by several factors. The type of cancer, the cancer stage, the presence of underlying liver disease, and the presence of other medical conditions all interact to determine the availability of various treatments and the prognosis. In general, fewer curative options are available for cancers that are more advanced, when the background liver function is poor, or when other health issues such as lung or heart disease make certain treatment options unsafe.

The prognosis of HCC depends on the stage at diagnosis. Five-year survival with very early stage HCC treated with surgical resection or percutaneous ablation is theoretically over 90 %. Early stage HCC treated with nonsurgical therapy offers a 5-year survival rate of 50–75 %. Intermediate stage HCC confined to the liver treated with transarterial chemoembolization is associated with a 3-year survival of about 50 %. Finally, the average survival of advanced HCC that is treated with chemotherapy is about 11 months.

Due to frequent cancer recurrence, the 5-year survival of CCA is only 25–50 %, even when it is diagnosed early and treated with surgical resection. Liver transplantation may offer better long-term survival for a small subgroup of patients with early CCA located at the base of the liver who respond well to chemotherapy and radiation. The 5-year survival for more advanced CCA treated with chemotherapy is about 10 %. The prognosis for the rare types of liver cancer strongly depends on the cancer type and how widespread it is at diagnosis. In general, hepatoblastoma carries the best prognosis, followed by epithelioid hemangiosarcoma and then angiosarcoma.

Malignant Liver Lesions

Introduction

The incidence of primary liver cancer has been rising over the past decade in the United States, with an estimated 35,660 new cases expected in 2015. Primary liver cancer has a high fatality rate, with the number of annual deaths approaching the cancer incidence (24,550 deaths) [1]. The initial evaluation of a potentially malignant liver lesion includes a detailed history, physical exam, imaging and laboratory studies, and sometimes a tumor biopsy [2]. This chapter summarizes the epidemiology, risk factors, and approach to the diagnosis and management of malignant liver lesions.

Hepatocellular Carcinoma

Epidemiology

Hepatocellular carcinoma is the most common primary liver cancer (Fig. 6.1) [3]. Worldwide, HCC is the sixth most common cancer (5th most common in men, 9th in women) and the second most common cause of cancer deaths [4]. In the United States (U.S.), HCC is the 14th most common cancer and the fastest rising cause of cancer deaths [1]. Most HCC (80 %) occurs in patients with underlying cirrhosis [1, 5]. The annual risk of developing HCC in cirrhotic patients ranges from 0.5 to 8 %, depending on the underlying cause of liver disease (Table 6.1) [6, 7].

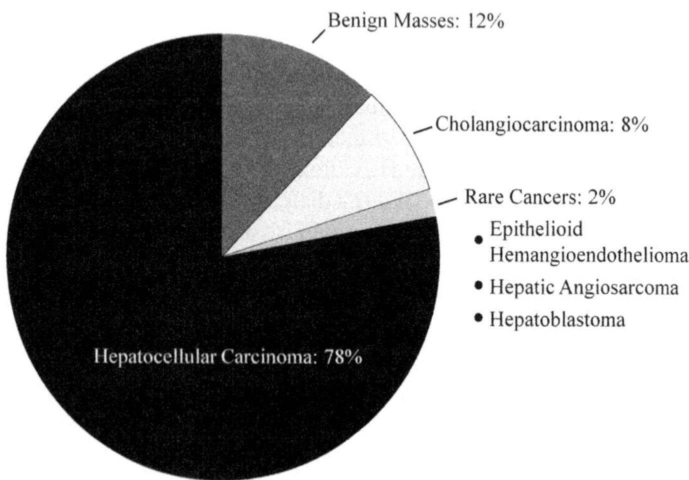

Fig. 6.1 Relative frequency of primary liver masses. Adapted from: Goodman ZD. Neoplasms of the liver. *Mod Pathol* 2007 Feb;20 Suppl 1:S49–60

Table 6.1 Annual incidence of hepatocellular carcinoma in cirrhosis by etiology of liver disease

Liver disease etiology	Annual incidence of hepatocellular carcinoma
Hepatitis C	3–5%
Hepatitis B	3–8%
Hemochromatosis	4%
Stage 4 primary biliary cirrhosis	3–5%
Non-alcoholic steatohepatitis	0.5–3%
α-1-antitrypsin deficiency	1.5%
Autoimmune	1.1%
Alcohol	Unknown
Cryptogenic	Unknown

Adapted from (Bruix and Sherman. American Association for the Study of Liver Diseases. Management of hepatocellular carcinoma: an update. Hepatology 2011;53(3):1020–1022)

Some conditions confer a risk for HCC without concurrent cirrhosis. These include chronic hepatitis B, with an annual incidence of HCC in noncirrhotic patients of approximately 0.5% per year, and nonalcoholic fatty liver disease, with an annual incidence of HCC in noncirrhotic patients of approximately 1.5% per year [7]. Additionally, while most benign liver masses (focal nodular hyperplasia, hemangiomas, and simple cysts) do not harbor a risk of malignant transformation to hepatocellular carcinoma, hepatocellular adenomas are the exception. The overall risk of malignant transformation of hepatocellular adenomas is low (4.2%). Risk factors for transformation of a hepatocellular adenoma include larger diameter ($\geq$5-cm), anabolic steroid use, male sex, and glycogen storage diseases [8].

Risk Factors

Chronic hepatitis C (HCV) infection is the most common cause of cirrhosis in the U.S. and the most common HCC risk factor [7]. Other risk factors, concomitant with HCV infection, further increase HCC risk, including older age at the time of HCV infection, male sex, coinfection with human immunodeficiency virus (HIV) or hepatitis B (HBV), alcohol or tobacco abuse, and possibly diabetes and obesity [6, 9].

Chronic HBV infection is a strong promoter of hepatocarcinogenesis and the leading risk factor for HCC in Asia and Africa [7, 10]. Unlike most other HCC risk factors, HCC frequently occurs in HBV-infected patients without cirrhosis [7]. As with HCV, several risk factors interact with HBV infection to increase HCC risk, including male sex, older age, duration of HBV infection, high HBV replication, family history of HCC, aflatoxin exposure, coinfection with HCV, HIV, or hepatitis D, alcohol or tobacco abuse, and infection with HBV genotype C [6, 9]. Predictive models are available to estimate the risk of developing HCC with chronic HBV infection [11, 12].

Factors that protect against the development of HCC have also been identified. Viral suppression of HBV and cure of HCV reduce but do not completely abrogate HCC risk [7]. Smoking and alcohol cessation may reduce HCC risk, even after cirrhosis has already developed [13, 14]. Additionally, population-level studies have shown a lower HCC incidence with high coffee consumption in both cirrhotic and noncirrhotic patients [15].

Diagnosis

The diagnosis of HCC is typically made using cross-sectional imaging studies, without the need for tumor biopsy. Dynamic computerized tomography (CT) or magnetic resonance imaging (MRI) with imaging acquisition in the arterial, portal venous, and delayed phases has a high sensitivity, specificity, and accuracy for HCC diagnosis [6, 7]. HCC enhances more than the background liver in the arterial phase and enhances less (washes out) in the portal venous and delayed phases because its principal blood supply derives from the hepatic artery, while blood supply to the background liver primarily derives from the portal vein [7]. In tumors over 2-cm in diameter, the diagnosis of HCC can usually be made when a solid liver mass exhibits arterial enhancement and portal venous and delayed phase washout on dynamic CT or MRI (Fig. 6.2). The presence of an enhancing ring around the periphery of the mass, a pseudocapsule, also supports a HCC diagnosis, particularly when the mass is between 1 and 2 cm. However, imaging-based diagnosis is less accurate for tumors smaller than 2-cm in diameter or when cirrhosis is not present [6].

If a suspected HCC does not possess characteristic imaging findings or occurs in a noncirrhotic liver, a biopsy may be necessary to establish the diagnosis [2]. The risk of tumor seeding the needle track with biopsy is low (2.7 %) and should not discourage its use when an imaging-based diagnosis is not possible [16]. The serum alpha-fetoprotein (AFP) level may be elevated in HCC, but it may also be elevated in other liver conditions, including CCA, metastatic colon cancer, and chronic viral hepatitis, making the use of AFP in the diagnosis of HCC controversial [7]. Additionally, the AFP level is normal in approximately 40 % of HCC patients, even when the cancer is advanced. However, the trajectory of the AFP level is useful as a marker of treatment response in patients with AFP-producing tumors [7].

Staging

Accurate staging of HCC is a crucial determinant for treatment selection and prognostication. Multiple staging systems have been proposed, including the American Joint Committee on Cancer Tumor-Node-Metastasis system, the Okuda classification, the Barcelona Clinic Liver Cancer (BCLC) staging system, and others. The BCLC system is most frequently used because it unifies the cancer stage, liver function, and comorbid illnesses into a clinically practical approach that facilitates the selection of HCC treatment [7]. BCLC staging incorporates tumor size,

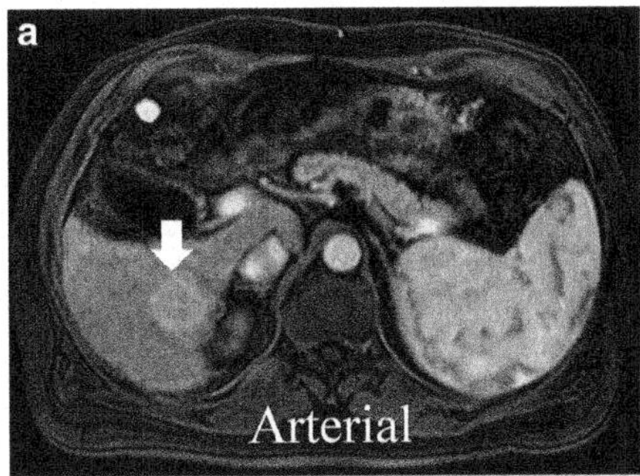

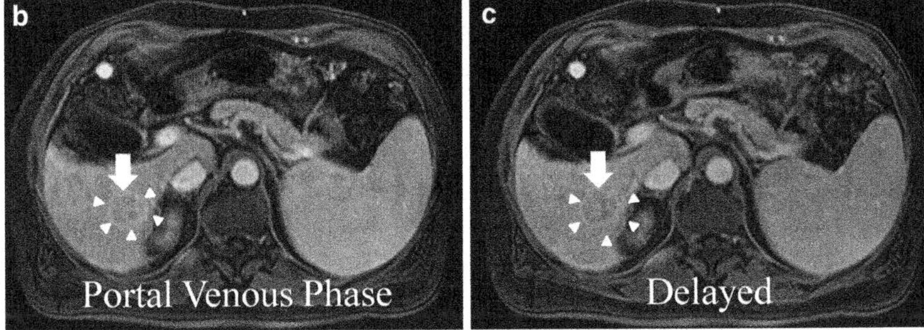

Fig. 6.2 Multiphase contrast-enhanced magnetic resonance imaging demonstrating the typical radiographic features of hepatocellular carcinoma. The liver mass (*arrow* in all panels) prominently enhances in the arterial phase (panel **a**) and is hypoenhancing to the surrounding liver parenchyma (washes out) in the portal venous (panel **b**) and delayed phases (panel **c**). A ring of enhancement (pseudocapsule) encircles the periphery of the mass (*arrowheads* in panels **b** and **c**). Images provided by Alice Fung, MD

number, extent, liver function (represented by the Child–Pugh score), and comorbid illnesses (represented by the performance status) to stage patients as stage 0 (very early HCC), stage A (early HCC), stage B (intermediate HCC), stage C (invasive or metastatic HCC), and stage D (end-stage HCC) (Fig. 6.3). Each BCLC stage is linked to a suggested treatment and prognosis.

Management

Optimal management of HCC requires a multidisciplinary approach with the involvement of gastroenterologists/hepatologists, hepatobiliary and transplant surgeons, diagnostic and interventional radiologists, and medical and radiation oncologists. Patients with very early HCC (BCLC stage 0), who have single tumors less than 2-cm in diameter with excellent liver function and performance status, may be treated with surgical resection or percutaneous ablation. Resection is the treatment of choice, though only 5 % of patients in Western countries are candidates due to surgical contraindications such as portal hypertension, poor liver function, or non-liver-related comorbidities [7]. In cirrhotic patients, resection may induce hepatic

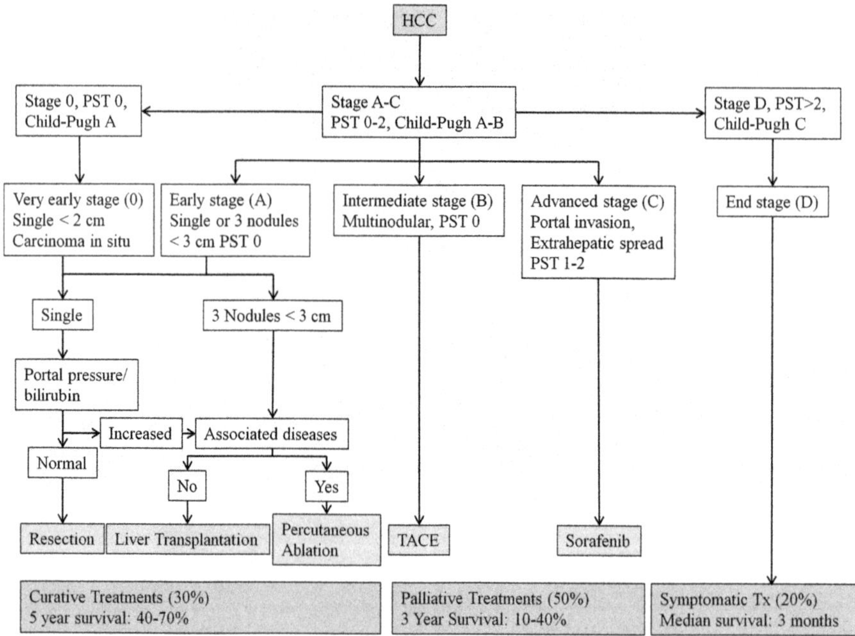

Fig. 6.3 The Barcelona clinic liver cancer staging system for hepatocellular carcinoma. *HCC* hepatocellular carcinoma, *PST* performance status, *TACE* transarterial chemoembolization. Adapted from: Bruix J, Llovet JM. Major achievements in hepatocellular carcinoma. *Lancet* 2009;373: 614–616

decompensation, and careful preoperative patient selection may prevent this potentially deadly complication. The 5-year overall survival after resection of very early HCC is theoretically over 90%, but recurrence is common, occurring in approximately 70% of patients within 5 years [6, 7].

Early stage HCC (BCLC stage A) may be treated with surgical resection if only 1 tumor is present with preserved liver function and good performance status. Therapeutic options for nonresectable BCLC stage A HCC include percutaneous ablation, transarterial chemoembolization, transarterial radioembolization, and radiation therapy, with liver transplantation available as an adjunctive treatment in selected patients. Percutaneous ablation includes percutaneous ethanol injection, radiofrequency ablation, cryoablation, microwave ablation, and irreversible electroporation [7]. Percutaneous ethanol injection is an effective treatment for small tumors (<2-cm), achieving a necrosis rate of 90–100%, but it is less effective for larger tumors (only 50% tumor necrosis is achieved for tumors greater than 3-cm) and it requires multiple procedures [6, 7]. Radiofrequency ablation involves the insertion of electrodes into the tumor that deliver directed heat to induce tumor necrosis [7]. The efficacy of radiofrequency ablation is similar to ethanol injection for tumors less than 2-cm, generally requires fewer repeat procedures, and is much more effective than ethanol injection for larger tumors up to 5-cm in diameter [17,

18]. Both ethanol injection and radiofrequency ablation are associated with a small risk of needle-track tumor seeding [19, 20].

Candidacy for liver transplantation depends on the extent of the tumor and the presence of medical and psychosocial comorbidities (including substance abuse). Most liver transplant centers in the U.S. employ the Milan criteria as the upper limit of cancer size and number to permit transplantation [21]. These criteria require a single tumor less than 5-cm in diameter or up to 3 tumors, all less than 3-cm in diameter, and predict a 4-year posttransplant survival of over 70 %. A small number of U.S. transplant centers utilize less restrictive selection criteria for the transplantation of HCC, including the University of California San Francisco criteria, which allow tumors up to 6.5-cm in diameter, or transplantation only after cancer treatment has reduced the size and number of tumors to within the Milan criteria ("downstaging") [22, 23].

HCC that initially meets criteria for transplantation may later grow to exceed transplant criteria, leading to deactivation on the liver transplant wait-list. The rate of wait-list exclusion secondary to cancer progression is up to 25 % when the waiting time is greater than 1 year [24]. To reduce waiting time for transplantation, patients with HCC are given additional priority for liver transplantation (termed "MELD exceptions") [7]. Enactment of MELD exceptions for HCC greatly increased the proportion of HCC patients receiving liver transplantation [25].

Patients with intermediate stage HCC (BCLC stage B) are primarily treated with transarterial chemoembolization or radioembolization, and are not candidates for surgical resection or liver transplantation. Transarterial chemoembolization involves catheterization of the femoral artery, followed by injection of chemotherapeutic agents and embolization of the branch of the hepatic artery feeding the tumor [7]. Careful patient selection is necessary because transarterial chemoembolization may induce liver failure in patients with decompensated liver disease (Child–Pugh class B or C) [7]. A self-limited postembolization syndrome characterized by fever, abdominal pain, nausea, and/or ileus occurs in 50 % of patients. Transarterial chemoembolization is not curative, but it has been shown to delay tumor progression and prolong survival (20–60 % at 2 years) [26, 27]. Transarterial radioembolization is a newer approach that is best suited for the treatment of larger, infiltrative tumors and involves the catheter-based delivery of a radioactive isotope (yttrium-90) bound to glass microspheres into the hepatic artery branch feeding the tumor [28]. No randomized trials comparing transarterial chemoembolization with radioembolization have been performed, although observational studies suggest similar efficacy. Radioembolization has been associated with shorter hospitalization after treatment and better short-term quality of life [29, 30].

In patients with advanced HCC with preserved liver function and performance status (BCLC stage C) or in patients who failed liver-directed treatments, chemotherapy with sorafenib, an oral multikinase inhibitor, improves survival. In two randomized controlled trials, the median survival with sorafenib ranged from 6.5 to 10.7 months, compared to 4.2–7.9 months with placebo [31, 32]. Sorafenib may cause adverse effects including diarrhea, nausea, fatigue, weight loss, and a rash involving the palms and soles of the hands and feet (hand-foot syndrome) [32].

Patients with end-stage HCC (BCLC stage D) are not candidates for HCC therapy due to severe comorbidities, advanced liver disease, or poor performance status, regardless of the extent of their HCC. The prognosis of BCLC stage D HCC is poor (3-month median survival), and none of the therapies discussed earlier improve survival or quality of life [7]. The primary treatment for BCLC stage D HCC includes symptomatic/palliative care approaches, and early referral to hospice is advised.

Fibrolamellar Carcinoma

Fibrolamellar carcinoma is a rare variant of HCC, making up 0.85 % of primary liver cancers [33]. Unlike typical HCC, fibrolamellar carcinoma generally occurs in noncirrhotic patients without a male predominance and is also more frequent in younger patients of white race [33, 34]. Like HCC, the diagnosis can usually be made solely with dynamic CT or MRI, and only rarely requires tumor biopsy [34]. Compared to typical HCC, fibrolamellar carcinoma is more often amenable to surgical resection. Despite this advantage, fibrolamellar carcinoma has a prognosis similar to that of HCC in noncirrhotic patients [34, 35]. When resection is not an option, liver transplantation is sometimes possible [36]. Because fibrolamellar carcinoma is rare, scant data are available for the use of liver-directed treatments and systemic chemotherapy [35].

Cholangiocarcinoma

Epidemiology

Accounting for 8 % of primary liver cancers, cholangiocarcinoma (CCA) is the second most common primary liver cancer after HCC [3]. CCA is classified according to its location within the biliary tree: intrahepatic (5–10 %), perihilar (60–70 %), or extrahepatic (20–30 %) [37]. CCA treatment varies by the location of involvement.

Risk Factors

The strongest risk factor for CCA is primary sclerosing cholangitis [38]. Cirrhosis is also a strong risk factor for intrahepatic CCA. Other, weaker risk factors for CCA largely involve inflammatory disorders, toxic exposures, and congenital malformations of the biliary tract. These include tobacco or alcohol abuse, older age, liver fluke infection, Caroli's disease, choledochal cysts, bile duct adenomas, chronic intrahepatic biliary stones, vinyl chloride exposure (an intermediate product in plastics manufacturing), and Thorotrast exposure (a commonly used radiocontrast agent in the 1930–1940s) [39, 40]. However, a large proportion of CCA occurs in patients without known risk factors [3].

Diagnosis

Unlike HCC, the diagnosis of CCA cannot be established with imaging alone and requires tumor biopsy. In patients with tumors that are considered to be technically resectable based on the extent of liver and bile duct involvement and the absence of medical comorbidities or major liver dysfunction, surgical resection is the initial diagnostic and treatment modality of choice [41]. In patients who are not candidates for liver resection, needle core biopsy is required [2]. Dynamic CT and MRI supplement biopsy for cancer staging and treatment planning, allowing the evaluation of vascular invasion, metastatic spread, and in surgical candidates, the size of the potential liver remnant [2, 40]. The tumor marker CA 19-9 is elevated in some CCA patients but has a sensitivity and specificity of only 62 and 63 % for CCA diagnosis [42]. AFP and carcinoembryonic antigen (CEA) levels may also be elevated in CCA but are nonspecific [7, 41].

Management

The 1-year mortality of untreated CCA is high (50–70 %), and aggressive treatment is warranted when possible [43]. Surgical resection is the only curative treatment for CCA. Unfortunately, recurrence following resection occurs in most patients within 2 years, and the median survival after resection is 36 months [44]. Surgical candidacy requires the absence of nodal or distant metastases or vascular invasion [45]. Patients who are not candidates for surgical resection are treated with chemotherapy (gemcitabine and cisplatin), which achieves a median survival of 11.7 months, compared to 8.1 months for gemcitabine alone [46].

Historically, cholangiocarcinoma has been a contraindication for liver transplantation. However, recent studies have shown that carefully selected patients with early stage perihilar CCA may be treated with liver transplantation with good posttransplant survival (53 % at 5 years) [47]. The restrictive protocol for transplantation of perihilar HCC requires an unresectable early stage perihilar CCA with a good tumor response to external beam radiation therapy and chemotherapy, followed by diagnostic laparoscopy showing no metastatic disease. A quarter of patients with potentially transplantable CCA drop off the transplant waiting list due to tumor progression or inability to complete pretransplant chemoradiation [43].

Rare Primary Liver Tumors

Epithelioid Hemangioendothelioma

Epithelioid hemangioendothelioma (EHE) is an uncommon vascular tumor with moderate malignant potential. According to the most recent World Health Organization classification, EHE is considered a malignant vascular tumor similar to angiosarcoma, though with a better prognosis [48]. The incidence of EHE is less than 1/1,000,000 [49]. EHE risk factors are largely unknown given its low incidence, but it is most commonly diagnosed in young to middle-aged women [49]. Oral contraceptive pills, vinyl chloride, and Thorotrast exposures have also been implicated as potential EHE risk factors [50]. EHE is usually multifocal (81 %) and mimics metastatic disease on imaging studies, necessitating tumor biopsy for diagnosis [49]. Because of its multifocality, resection is frequently not possible and liver transplantation is required for cure [51]. The 1-year and 5-year survival rates of EHE without treatment are 39.3 and 4.5 %, respectively, but improve to 96 and 54.5 % with liver transplantation, and 100 and 75 % with surgical resection [49]. In patients who are not candidates for resection or transplantation, chemotherapy and radiation regimens similar to those for angiosarcoma are recommended, typically including celecoxib, paclitaxel, and antiangiogenic drugs. The 1-year and 5-year survival rates with combination chemotherapy and radiation are 73.3 and 30 %, respectively [49].

Hepatic Angiosarcoma

Hepatic angiosarcoma is a rare primary liver cancer, representing 0.5–2 % of primary liver cancers. Less than 5 % of all angiosarcomas arise from the liver [52]. Angiosarcoma risk factors are largely environmental, with exposure to vinyl chloride the most common (25 % of cases) [53, 54]. Arsenic and Thorotrast exposures have also been implicated in hepatic angiosarcoma [53]. Finally, sparse data suggest that long-term anabolic steroid exposure may also increase hepatic angiosarcoma risk [52]. Hepatic angiosarcoma can mimic HCC, EHE, and hepatic adenomas on imaging, mandating tissue evaluation for diagnosis [55]. The utility of needle core biopsy is compromised by frequent false negative results, and surgical biopsy or resection is often necessary. Treatment for angiosarcoma includes a combination of surgical resection, chemotherapy, and/or radiation therapy. Without treatment, the median survival for hepatic angiosarcoma is 5 months, but the median survival increases to 17 months when these treatments are employed [53]. Hepatic angiosarcoma may be complicated by spontaneous or biopsy-related tumor hemorrhage, and transarterial embolization may be used to effectively prevent or treat this complication [53]. Hepatic angiosarcoma is a contraindication to liver transplantation due to frequent posttransplant cancer recurrence [56, 57].

Hepatoblastoma

Hepatoblastoma (HB) is the most common primary liver cancer in children (80 %), with a peak incidence in the first 3 years of life, but it is nevertheless rare, representing only 1 % of all pediatric cancers [58]. Approximately forty cases of HB have been reported in adults [59]. Premature birth, low birth weight, and male sex are possible risk factors [58]. Tumor biopsy is required for diagnosis, but dynamic CT or MRI may be used to assess vascular involvement, which determines candidacy for resection [58, 60]. Historically, early stage HB was treated with neoadjuvant chemotherapy and surgical resection; however, primary resection with adjuvant chemotherapy has more recently been shown to confer longer survival in selected patients [58]. Liver transplantation is the recommended treatment for HB with extensive liver involvement and yields similar survival to early stage HB treated with resection (75 % 5-year survival) [58, 60].

Metastatic Lesions and Lymphoma

Metastatic Liver Lesions

Metastatic lesions are by far the most common type of liver cancer, occurring about 30 times more often than primary liver cancer in noncirrhotic patients. In contrast, primary liver cancers outnumber metastases by about three to one in patients with cirrhosis [3]. Liver metastases occur at a lower absolute frequency in cirrhotic compared to noncirrhotic patients, implying that fibrosis may make the liver less hospitable to metastatic deposition [61]. The most common primary cancer sites for liver metastases are the lung, breast, colon, and pancreas, but metastases may originate from almost anywhere in the body. Liver metastases from head and neck cancers and sarcomas are distinctly uncommon [3].

Treatment of liver metastases greatly depends on the site of origin and may include chemotherapy, radiation, liver-directed therapy, resection, and in rare cases, liver transplantation. Good surgical candidates with isolated liver metastases from colorectal cancer are frequently treated with hepatic resection, though up to two-thirds of patients will experience cancer recurrence within 5 years [62]. Radio-frequency ablation, transarterial chemoembolization, and radiation therapy are alternative approaches in nonsurgical candidates with a low burden of disease in the liver, with higher reported rates of recurrence [62, 63]. Patients with neuroendocrine tumors, often of pancreatic origin, frequently experience liver metastases (40–75 %), which may be treated with surgical resection or liver transplantation, depending on the burden of hepatic disease and surgical candidacy [62, 64]. The 5-year survival after resection of metastatic neuroendocrine tumors is good (60–75 %), but recurrence is common (85–100 %) [62, 63]. Liver transplantation is an option in selected patients with large hepatic tumor burdens, with 5-year survival rates of 49 % [65].

As with colorectal cancer metastases, liver-directed therapies and radiation can be applied in nonsurgical candidates. Metastases to the liver from primary sites other than colorectal and neuroendocrine cancers are not treated with resection due to a high risk of cancer recurrence (61–80%) [66].

Hepatic Lymphoma

Lymphomas are a heterogeneous group of hematologic malignancies with a primary origin in any organ that contains lymphocytes, frequently involving the lymph nodes but sometimes only extranodal sites, including the liver. Lymphomas are classified as Hodgkin's disease and non-Hodgkin lymphoma [67]. Non-Hodgkin lymphoma frequently involves the liver (26–40%), presenting as diffuse infiltration or focal liver masses [68]. The cornerstone of treatment for hepatic lymphoma is chemotherapy. Antiviral treatment for HCV should also be considered with HCV-associated lymphoma subtypes, although it is unknown whether a HCV cure impacts lymphoma progression or recurrence [69].

Hepatosplenic T-cell lymphoma (HSTCL) is a uniformly fatal, rare lymphoma (3% of T-cell lymphomas) that occurs most often in young men [70, 71]. About one-third of HSTCLs are associated with immunosuppressed states, especially inflammatory bowel disease treatment regimens that include azathioprine [72]. Treatment of HSTCL includes chemotherapy or bone marrow transplantation, but survival remains poor (8-month median survival) [71, 73].

Conclusion

The diagnosis and management of liver cancer is challenging and requires a multidisciplinary approach. The future burden of primary liver cancer in the U.S., the majority of which is HCC, will be shaped by changes in the prevalence of risk factors for cirrhosis, such as nonalcoholic steatohepatitis and HCV. Population-level studies using the Surveillance, Epidemiology, and End Results cancer registry suggest that HCC incidence may be nearing its peak in the U.S., and the increasing application of newly available direct-acting HCV therapies promises to further reduce the incidence of HCV-related cirrhosis and HCC over the next decade [74–77]. On the other hand, the rising incidence of diabetes, obesity, and metabolic syndrome have fueled an epidemic of nonalcoholic steatohepatitis, the most common liver disease in Western countries and an emerging, common risk factor for cirrhosis [78, 79]. As the epidemic of HCV infection recedes, a continued reduction in HCC incidence will require that attention be turned to the development of effective strategies to stem the tide of nonalcoholic fatty liver disease.

Acknowledgements *Financial Support/Disclosure:* No external funding was used for this study. No authors report conflicts of interest.

References

1. American Cancer Society. Cancer facts and figures. http://seer.cancer.gov/statfacts/html/livibd.html. Accessed 3 Feb 2015.
2. Marrero JA, Ahn J, Rajender Reddy K, American College of Gastroenterology. ACG clinical guideline: the diagnosis and management of focal liver lesions. Am J Gastroenterol. 2014;109(9):1328–47. quiz 1348.
3. Goodman ZD. Neoplasms of the liver. Mod Pathol. 2007;20 Suppl 1:S49–60.
4. Ferlay J, Soerjomataram I, Ervik M, Dikshit R, Eser S, Mathers C, Rebelo M, Parkin DM, Forman D, Bray F. GLOBOCAN 2012 v1.0, Cancer incidence and mortality worldwide: IARC Cancer Base No. 11. http://globocan.iarc.fr. Accessed 16 Feb 2015.
5. Fattovich G, Stroffolini T, Zagni I, Donato F. Hepatocellular carcinoma in cirrhosis: incidence and risk factors. Gastroenterology. 2004;127(5 Suppl 1):S35–50.
6. El-Serag HB. Hepatocellular carcinoma. N Engl J Med. 2011;365(12):1118–27.
7. Bruix J, Sherman M, American Association for the Study of Liver Diseases. Management of hepatocellular carcinoma: an update. Hepatology. 2011;53(3):1020–2.
8. Stoot JH, Coelen RJ, De Jong MC, Dejong CH. Malignant transformation of hepatocellular adenomas into hepatocellular carcinomas: a systematic review including more than 1600 adenoma cases. HPB (Oxford). 2010;12(8):509–22.
9. Donato F, Tagger A, Gelatti U, Parrinello G, Boffetta P, Albertini A, et al. Alcohol and hepatocellular carcinoma: the effect of lifetime intake and hepatitis virus infections in men and women. Am J Epidemiol. 2002;155(4):323–31.
10. Bosch FX, Ribes J, Borras J. Epidemiology of primary liver cancer. Semin Liver Dis. 1999;19(3):271–85.
11. Yang HI, Sherman M, Su J, Chen PJ, Liaw YF, Iloeje UH, et al. Nomograms for risk of hepatocellular carcinoma in patients with chronic hepatitis B virus infection. J Clin Oncol. 2010;28(14):2437–44.
12. Yuen MF, Tanaka Y, Fong DY, Fung J, Wong DK, Yuen JC, et al. Independent risk factors and predictive score for the development of hepatocellular carcinoma in chronic hepatitis B. J Hepatol. 2009;50(1):80–8.
13. Shih WL, Chang HC, Liaw YF, Lin SM, Lee SD, Chen PJ, et al. Influences of tobacco and alcohol use on hepatocellular carcinoma survival. Int J Cancer. 2012;131(11):2612–21.
14. Marrero JA, Fontana RJ, Fu S, Conjeevaram HS, Su GL, Lok AS. Alcohol, tobacco and obesity are synergistic risk factors for hepatocellular carcinoma. J Hepatol. 2005;42(2):218–24.
15. Sang LX, Chang B, Li XH, Jiang M. Consumption of coffee associated with reduced risk of liver cancer: a meta-analysis. BMC Gastroenterol. 2013;13:34-230X-13-34.
16. Silva MA, Hegab B, Hyde C, Guo B, Buckels JA, Mirza DF. Needle track seeding following biopsy of liver lesions in the diagnosis of hepatocellular cancer: a systematic review and meta-analysis. Gut. 2008;57(11):1592–6.
17. Livraghi T, Goldberg SN, Lazzaroni S, Meloni F, Solbiati L, Gazelle GS. Small hepatocellular carcinoma: treatment with radio-frequency ablation versus ethanol injection. Radiology. 1999;210(3):655–61.
18. Lencioni RA, Allgaier HP, Cioni D, Olschewski M, Deibert P, Crocetti L, et al. Small hepatocellular carcinoma in cirrhosis: randomized comparison of radio-frequency thermal ablation versus percutaneous ethanol injection. Radiology. 2003;228(1):235–40.
19. Llovet JM, Vilana R, Bru C, Bianchi L, Salmeron JM, Boix L, et al. Increased risk of tumor seeding after percutaneous radiofrequency ablation for single hepatocellular carcinoma. Hepatology. 2001;33(5):1124–9.
20. Livraghi T, Solbiati L, Meloni MF, Gazelle GS, Halpern EF, Goldberg SN. Treatment of focal liver tumors with percutaneous radio-frequency ablation: complications encountered in a multicenter study. Radiology. 2003;226(2):441–51.

21. Mazzaferro V, Regalia E, Doci R, Andreola S, Pulvirenti A, Bozzetti F, et al. Liver transplantation for the treatment of small hepatocellular carcinomas in patients with cirrhosis. N Engl J Med. 1996;334(11):693–9.
22. Patel SS, Arrington AK, McKenzie S, Mailey B, Ding M, Lee W, et al. Milan criteria and UCSF criteria: a preliminary comparative study of liver transplantation outcomes in the United States. Int J Hepatol. 2012;2012:253517.
23. Yao FY, Ferrell L, Bass NM, Bacchetti P, Ascher NL, Roberts JP. Liver transplantation for hepatocellular carcinoma: comparison of the proposed UCSF criteria with the Milan criteria and the Pittsburgh modified TNM criteria. Liver Transpl. 2002;8(9):765–74.
24. Yao FY, Bass NM, Nikolai B, Davern TJ, Kerlan R, Wu V, et al. Liver transplantation for hepatocellular carcinoma: analysis of survival according to the intention-to-treat principle and dropout from the waiting list. Liver Transpl. 2002;8(10):873–83.
25. Ioannou GN, Perkins JD, Carithers Jr RL. Liver transplantation for hepatocellular carcinoma: impact of the MELD allocation system and predictors of survival. Gastroenterology. 2008;134(5):1342–51.
26. Bruix J, Sala M, Llovet JM. Chemoembolization for hepatocellular carcinoma. Gastroenterology. 2004;127(5 Suppl 1):S179–88.
27. Llovet JM, Bruix J. Systematic review of randomized trials for unresectable hepatocellular carcinoma: chemoembolization improves survival. Hepatology. 2003;37(2):429–42.
28. Mahnken AH, Spreafico C, Maleux G, Helmberger T, Jakobs TF. Standards of practice in transarterial radioembolization. Cardiovasc Intervent Radiol. 2013;36(3):613–22.
29. Moreno-Luna LE, Yang JD, Sanchez W, Paz-Fumagalli R, Harnois DM, Mettler TA, et al. Efficacy and safety of transarterial radioembolization versus chemoembolization in patients with hepatocellular carcinoma. Cardiovasc Intervent Radiol. 2013;36(3):714–23.
30. Salem R, Gilbertsen M, Butt Z, Memon K, Vouche M, Hickey R, et al. Increased quality of life among hepatocellular carcinoma patients treated with radioembolization, compared with chemoembolization. Clin Gastroenterol Hepatol. 2013;11(10):1358–1365.e1.
31. Cheng AL, Kang YK, Chen Z, Tsao CJ, Qin S, Kim JS, et al. Efficacy and safety of sorafenib in patients in the Asia-Pacific region with advanced hepatocellular carcinoma: a phase III randomised, double-blind, placebo-controlled trial. Lancet Oncol. 2009;10(1):25–34.
32. Llovet JM, Ricci S, Mazzaferro V, Hilgard P, Gane E, Blanc JF, et al. Sorafenib in advanced hepatocellular carcinoma. N Engl J Med. 2008;359(4):378–90.
33. El-Serag HB, Davila JA. Is fibrolamellar carcinoma different from hepatocellular carcinoma? A US population-based study. Hepatology. 2004;39(3):798–803.
34. Njei B, Konjeti VR, Ditah I. Prognosis of patients with fibrolamellar hepatocellular carcinoma versus conventional hepatocellular carcinoma: a systematic review and meta-analysis. Gastrointest Cancer Res. 2014;7(2):49–54.
35. Mavros MN, Mayo SC, Hyder O, Pawlik TM. A systematic review: treatment and prognosis of patients with fibrolamellar hepatocellular carcinoma. J Am Coll Surg. 2012;215(6):820–30.
36. Grossman EJ, Millis JM. Liver transplantation for non-hepatocellular carcinoma malignancy: indications, limitations, and analysis of the current literature. Liver Transpl. 2010;16(8):930–42.
37. Maddrey WC, Sorrell MF, Schiff ER, Schiff L, Schiff ER. Schiff's diseases of the liver. Schiff's diseases of the liver 11e; Diseases of the liver 2012.
38. Razumilava N, Gores GJ, Lindor KD. Cancer surveillance in patients with primary sclerosing cholangitis. Hepatology. 2011;54(5):1842–52.
39. Rimola J, Forner A, Reig M, Vilana R, de Lope CR, Ayuso C, et al. Cholangiocarcinoma in cirrhosis: absence of contrast washout in delayed phases by magnetic resonance imaging avoids misdiagnosis of hepatocellular carcinoma. Hepatology. 2009;50(3):791–8.
40. Khan SA, Thomas HC, Davidson BR, Taylor-Robinson SD. Cholangiocarcinoma. Lancet. 2005;366(9493):1303–14.
41. Khan SA, Davidson BR, Goldin RD, Heaton N, Karani J, Pereira SP, et al. Guidelines for the diagnosis and treatment of cholangiocarcinoma: an update. Gut. 2012;61(12):1657–69.

42. Blechacz B, Komuta M, Roskams T, Gores GJ. Clinical diagnosis and staging of cholangio-carcinoma. Nat Rev Gastroenterol Hepatol. 2011;8(9):512–22.
43. Rosen CB, Heimbach JK, Gores GJ. Surgery for cholangiocarcinoma: the role of liver transplantation. HPB (Oxford). 2008;10(3):186–9.
44. Endo I, Gonen M, Yopp AC, Dalal KM, Zhou Q, Klimstra D, et al. Intrahepatic cholangiocarcinoma: rising frequency, improved survival, and determinants of outcome after resection. Ann Surg. 2008;248(1):84–96.
45. Rajagopalan V, Daines WP, Grossbard ML, Kozuch P. Gallbladder and biliary tract carcinoma: a comprehensive update, part 1. Oncology (Williston Park). 2004;18(7):889–96.
46. Valle J, Wasan H, Palmer DH, Cunningham D, Anthoney A, Maraveyas A, et al. Cisplatin plus gemcitabine versus gemcitabine for biliary tract cancer. N Engl J Med. 2010;362(14):1273–81.
47. Darwish Murad S, Kim WR, Harnois DM, Douglas DD, Burton J, Kulik LM, et al. Efficacy of neoadjuvant chemoradiation, followed by liver transplantation, for perihilar cholangiocarcinoma at 12 US centers. Gastroenterology. 2012;143(1):88–98.e3. quiz e14.
48. Fletcher CD. The evolving classification of soft tissue tumours—an update based on the new 2013 WHO classification. Histopathology. 2014;64(1):2–11.
49. Mehrabi A, Kashfi A, Fonouni H, Schemmer P, Schmied BM, Hallscheidt P, et al. Primary malignant hepatic epithelioid hemangioendothelioma: a comprehensive review of the literature with emphasis on the surgical therapy. Cancer. 2006;107(9):2108–21.
50. Woodall CE, Scoggins CR, Lewis AM, McMasters KM, Martin RC. Hepatic malignant epithelioid hemangioendothelioma: a case report and review of the literature. Am Surg. 2008;74(1):64–8.
51. Remiszewski P, Szczerba E, Kalinowski P, Gierej B, Dudek K, Grodzicki M, et al. Epithelioid hemangioendothelioma of the liver as a rare indication for liver transplantation. World J Gastroenterol. 2014;20(32):11333–9.
52. Poggi Machuca L, Ibarra Chirinos O, Lopez Del Aguila J, Villanueva Pflucker M, Camacho Zacarias F, Tagle Arrospide M, et al. Hepatic angiosarcoma: case report and review of literature. Rev Gastroenterol Peru. 2012;32(3):317–22.
53. Zheng YW, Zhang XW, Zhang JL, Hui ZZ, Du WJ, Li RM, et al. Primary hepatic angiosarcoma and potential treatment options. J Gastroenterol Hepatol. 2014;29(5):906–11.
54. Huang NC, Wann SR, Chang HT, Lin SL, Wang JS, Guo HR. Arsenic, vinyl chloride, viral hepatitis, and hepatic angiosarcoma: a hospital-based study and review of literature in Taiwan. BMC Gastroenterol. 2011;11:142-230X-11-142.
55. Koyama T, Fletcher JG, Johnson CD, Kuo MS, Notohara K, Burgart LJ. Primary hepatic angiosarcoma: findings at CT and MR imaging. Radiology. 2002;222(3):667–73.
56. Orlando G, Adam R, Mirza D, Soderdahl G, Porte RJ, Paul A, et al. Hepatic hemangiosarcoma: an absolute contraindication to liver transplantation—the European Liver Transplant Registry experience. Transplantation. 2013;95(6):872–7.
57. Maluf D, Cotterell A, Clark B, Stravitz T, Kauffman HM, Fisher RA. Hepatic angiosarcoma and liver transplantation: case report and literature review. Transplant Proc. 2005;37(5):2195–9.
58. Czauderna P, Lopez-Terrada D, Hiyama E, Haberle B, Malogolowkin MH, Meyers RL. Hepatoblastoma state of the art: pathology, genetics, risk stratification, and chemotherapy. Curr Opin Pediatr. 2014;26(1):19–28.
59. Zheng MH, Zhang L, Gu DN, Shi HQ, Zeng QQ, Chen YP. Hepatoblastoma in adult: review of the literature. J Clin Med Res. 2009;1(1):13–6.
60. Otte JB. Progress in the surgical treatment of malignant liver tumors in children. Cancer Treat Rev. 2010;36(4):360–71.
61. Melato M, Laurino L, Mucli E, Valente M, Okuda K. Relationship between cirrhosis, liver cancer, and hepatic metastases. An autopsy study. Cancer. 1989;64(2):455–9.
62. Johnston FM, Mavros MN, Herman JM, Pawlik TM. Local therapies for hepatic metastases. J Natl Compr Canc Netw. 2013;11(2):153–60.
63. Mayo SC, Pawlik TM. Thermal ablative therapies for secondary hepatic malignancies. Cancer J. 2010;16(2):111–7.

64. Reddy SK, Clary BM. Neuroendocrine liver metastases. Surg Clin North Am. 2010;90(4):853–61.
65. Gedaly R, Daily MF, Davenport D, McHugh PP, Koch A, Angulo P, et al. Liver transplantation for the treatment of liver metastases from neuroendocrine tumors: an analysis of the UNOS database. Arch Surg. 2011;146(8):953–8.
66. Groeschl RT, Nachmany I, Steel JL, Reddy SK, Glazer ES, de Jong MC, et al. Hepatectomy for noncolorectal non-neuroendocrine metastatic cancer: a multi-institutional analysis. J Am Coll Surg. 2012;214(5):769–77.
67. Eichenauer DA, Engert A, Dreyling M, ESMO Guidelines Working Group. Hodgkin's lymphoma: ESMO clinical practice guidelines for diagnosis, treatment and follow-up. Ann Oncol. 2011;22 Suppl 6:vi55–8.
68. Gobbi PG, Ferreri AJ, Ponzoni M, Levis A. Hodgkin lymphoma. Crit Rev Oncol Hematol. 2013;85(2):216–37.
69. Hartridge-Lambert SK, Stein EM, Markowitz AJ, Portlock CS. Hepatitis C and non-Hodgkin lymphoma: the clinical perspective. Hepatology. 2012;55(2):634–41.
70. Weidmann E. Hepatosplenic T cell lymphoma. A review on 45 cases since the first report describing the disease as a distinct lymphoma entity in 1990. Leukemia. 2000;14(6):991–7.
71. Visnyei K, Grossbard ML, Shapira I. Hepatosplenic gammadelta T-cell lymphoma: an overview. Clin Lymphoma Myeloma Leuk. 2013;13(4):360–9.
72. Kotlyar DS, Osterman MT, Diamond RH, Porter D, Blonski WC, Wasik M, et al. A systematic review of factors that contribute to hepatosplenic T-cell lymphoma in patients with inflammatory bowel disease. Clin Gastroenterol Hepatol. 2011;9(1):36–41.e1.
73. Subramaniam K, Yeung D, Grimpen F, Joseph J, Fay K, Buckland M, et al. Hepatosplenic T-cell lymphoma, immunosuppressive agents and biologicals: what are the risks? Intern Med J. 2014;44(3):287–90.
74. Morgan RL, Baack B, Smith BD, Yartel A, Pitasi M, Falck-Ytter Y. Eradication of hepatitis C virus infection and the development of hepatocellular carcinoma: a meta-analysis of observational studies. Ann Intern Med. 2013;158(5 Pt 1):329–37.
75. van der Meer AJ, Veldt BJ, Feld JJ, Wedemeyer H, Dufour JF, Lammert F, et al. Association between sustained virological response and all-cause mortality among patients with chronic hepatitis C and advanced hepatic fibrosis. JAMA. 2012;308(24):2584–93.
76. Altekruse SF, Henley SJ, Cucinelli JE, McGlynn KA. Changing hepatocellular carcinoma incidence and liver cancer mortality rates in the United States. Am J Gastroenterol. 2014;109(4):542–53.
77. Njei B, Rotman Y, Ditah I, Lim JK. Emerging trends in hepatocellular carcinoma incidence and mortality. Hepatology. 2015;61(1):191–9.
78. Michelotti GA, Machado MV, Diehl AM. NAFLD, NASH and liver cancer. Nat Rev Gastroenterol Hepatol. 2013;10(11):656–65.
79. White DL, Kanwal F, El-Serag HB. Association between nonalcoholic fatty liver disease and risk for hepatocellular cancer, based on systematic review. Clin Gastroenterol Hepatol. 2012;10(12):1342–1359.e2.

Chapter 7
Health Maintenance in Liver Disease and Cirrhosis

Veronica Loy

Patient Questions

1. Should I receive vaccinations if I have liver disease?
2. Should I be evaluated for bone disease if I have liver disease?
3. Can I drink coffee?
4. What can I take for pain if I have liver disease?

Question One: Should I Receive Vaccinations If I Have Liver Disease?

Answer: Patients with liver disease are at an increased risk of worsening of their underlying liver disease or developing acute hepatitis by contracting viral hepatitis and should be vaccinated for hepatitis A and B. Patients with cirrhosis in particular also have an increased risk of worsening liver function from influenza or pneumococcal infection and thus should be vaccinated. Cirrhotics should avoid live vaccines if feasible due to the potential risk of developing infection.

V. Loy, D.O. (✉)
Division of Hepatology, Loyola University of Chicago,
2160 S First Avenue, Maywood, IL 60153, USA
e-mail: veronica.loy@luhs.org

© Springer International Publishing Switzerland 2017
K. Saeian, R. Shaker (eds.), *Liver Disorders*,
DOI 10.1007/978-3-319-30103-7_7

Table 7.1 Recommended vaccinations for cirrhotic patients

Vaccinations	Brand names	Dose	Schedule
Hepatitis A	Havrix Vaqta	1440 EL.U in 1 mL IM 50 U in 1 mL IM	0, 6–12 months
Hepatitis B	Engerix-B Recombivax HB	20 mig in 1 mL IM 10 mig in 1 mL IM	0, 1, 6 months
Hepatitis A/B	Twinrix (Havrix and Engerix-B)	720 EL.U HAV and 20 mig HBsAG in 1 mL IM	0, 1, 6 months
H. influenza	Fluarix FluLaval	0.5 mL IM	Annual
Pneumococcal	PCV13 (Prevnar 13) PPSV23 (Pneumovax)	0.5 mL IM 0.5 mL IM	PCV13 followed by PPSV23 in 8 weeks PPSV23 every 3–5 years
TdaP	Daptacel Infanrix	0.5 mL IM 0.5 mL IM	10 Years

Hepatitis A Vaccination

Acute hepatitis A virus (HAV) infection in patients with chronic liver disease has been shown to have a higher risk for fulminant hepatic failure or hepatic decompensation. Between 1983 and 1988, 115,551 cases of HAV were reported to the CDC. While the overall fatality rate in these cases was only 0.33 % in patients who were HBsAG carriers, the calculated rate was 11.7 % or a 50-fold higher risk of death in a hepatitis B carrier. These effects appear more pronounced in older patients with histological evidence of chronic hepatitis or frank cirrhosis [1]. Similarly, patients with chronic hepatitis C virus (HCV) infection who are then infected with HAV have a significant increase in morbidity and mortality. One study showed that of 432 HCV patients, 3.9 % developed acute HAV. Of those who were infected with HAV, 41 % developed fulminant hepatitis; this rate is dramatically higher than the rate in the general population (<1 %) [2]. These rates have not been confirmed in other studies. Reports of fulminant HAV infection in patients with cryptogenic cirrhosis or alcohol-related liver disease support the conclusion that patients with chronic liver disease are at risk for poor outcomes with acute HAV infection.

A protective vaccination for hepatitis A exists. All patients with chronic liver disease, who are not immigrants from an endemic area such as India, should be tested for immunity against hepatitis A. Patients from endemic areas are thought to have nearly 100 % immunity [3]. Since prevalence in the USA of HAV immunity ranges from 30 to 65 %, targeted vaccination strategies have been found to be the most cost effective [4]. Patients should have hepatitis A virus IgG serology evaluation prior to vaccination administration. If patients do not exhibit IgG antibody to HAV, they should be offered vaccination with two formalin-inactivated hepatitis A virus vaccinations at 0 and 6 months (Table 7.1).

The vaccine is only slightly less immunogenic in patients with chronic liver disease than the general population, with seroconversion rate of 93% [5]. In patients with decompensated cirrhosis conversion rate is 20–50% compared to 99% in immunocompetent hosts [6]. One series illustrated that predictors of non-response were the presence of an alcoholic component of liver disease and a worse stage of liver failure [7]. Evidence supports as disease worsens response to HAV vaccine worsens; therefore, vaccination should be given as early as possible in the disease course of chronic liver disease when the patient has a better chance of achieving seroconversion. To document response, anti-HAV IgG may be assessed 3 months after final vaccination.

Hepatitis B Vaccination

Much like hepatitis A, acute hepatitis B virus (HBV) has been implicated in fulminant hepatitis in patients with chronic liver disease such as those with hepatitis C [8]. Additionally, patients with chronic HBV and HCV co-infection have worse outcomes than patients with either infection alone [9]. One study shows significantly high rates of cirrhosis (95% vs. 48%) and hepatocellular carcinoma (63% vs. 15%).

Similar to the case of HAV, the CDC also recommends vaccination of all patients with chronic liver disease against hepatitis B (Table 7.1). Because the prevalence of previous infection is more than 30% in patients with chronic liver disease, it is cost effective to screen patients prior to vaccination [10]. Patients should be tested for immunity and if negative should be given three doses at 0, 1, and 6 months. Immunogenicity is diminished in cirrhotic patients. The proportion of antibody response is 40–70% in cirrhotic patients and 30–50% in decompensated cirrhotics; this again suggests that vaccination early in the disease course is preferred [11]. Antibody response should be verified 2–3 months after completion of vaccination. For those without a response, a second series will result in immunity in 60% of patients [12]. If patients are over 18 years of age a combined vaccination for hepatitis A and B is available called Twinrix. This may be used if both vaccinations are indicated.

Influenza Vaccination

Patients with cirrhosis are at high risk for complications of influenza. While influenza is not more common in cirrhotic patients than the general population, it may increase the risk of decompensation by producing TNF alpha, and IL-1 and IL-6 cytokines [13]. One study illustrated that the influenza vaccine reduced the risk of decompensation in cirrhotic patients [14]. The CDC recommends annual influenza vaccination for patients with cirrhosis as soon as the flu season begins in September. While the CDC does not have guidelines about cirrhotic patients receiving live vaccinations, typically the inactivated vaccination is preferred in these patients.

Pneumococcal Vaccination

Patients with chronic liver disease are at higher risk for pneumococcal infection [15]. Patients with cirrhosis have higher rates of mortality during a pneumococcal infection than non-cirrhotic patients. Patients with cirrhosis are more likely to have bacteremia during a pneumococcal infection [16]. For this reason, pneumococcal vaccination is recommended in all cirrhotic patients. In 2010 the CDC guidelines recommended adults who had not previously received PCV13 pneumococcal conjugate vaccine (PCV13) or pneumococcal polysaccharide vaccine (PPSV23) should receive a dose of PCV13 first, and followed by a dose of PPSV23 at least 8 weeks later. A second PPSV23 dose is recommended 5 years after the first PPSV23 dose. Patients who previously have received ≥ 1 doses of PPSV23 should be given a PCV13 dose ≥ 1 year after the last PPSV23 dose was received.

Question Two: Should I Be Evaluated for Bone Disease If I Have Liver Disease?

Answer: The majority of patients with liver disease should be evaluated with bone densitometry for low bone density. There is a high prevalence of bone disease in patients with liver disease. This is particularly true in cholestatic liver disease such as primary biliary cirrhosis, alcohol-related liver disease, or cirrhosis of any etiology. Additionally, fat-soluble vitamin levels such as vitamin D are often low, which can contribute to osteopenia and osteoporosis.

Vitamin D Deficiency

The prevalence of vitamin D deficiency is 60 % in cirrhotic patients and as high as 96 % at the time of liver transplantation [17]. Despite the high prevalence of vitamin deficiency, osteomalacia (defective bone mineralization with subsequent softening of the bones) is rare but osteoporosis and osteopenia are not uncommon. Low vitamin D has been associated with low bone mineral density, hip fracture, and high bone turnover and contributes to osteoporosis in patients with chronic liver disease. A recent study by Venu et al. showed insufficient vitamin D in 83 % of cirrhotic patients [18]. Osteopenia or osteoporosis was noted in 45 and 18 % of cirrhotic patients, respectively; of those patients with osteoporosis, 100 % had vitamin D deficiency. Etiology of liver disease (including cholestatic etiology versus other) was not predictive of who developed vitamin D deficiency.

Low Bone Density

Patients with chronic liver disease exhibit many risk factors for low bone density and osteoporosis. Known risk factors include poor nutrition, steroid use, alcohol intake, and hypogonadism [17]. Cirrhotic patients are not the only patients with liver disease at risk for low bone density. One study showed that alcohol intake was inversely related to bone mineral density in men. Additionally, in 76 men who drank 216 g/day or more for 24 years, 30 % had vertebral fractures regardless of stage of fibrosis on histology [19]. Non-cirrhotic patients with hemochromatosis also have high rates of osteoporosis which seem to correlate with the degree of hepatic iron level.

Patients with non-cirrhotic biliary disease have been examined for increased rates of osteopenia and osteoporosis. The incidence of osteoporosis in primary sclerosing cholangitis (PSC) is between 3 and 32 %. It does not appear that treatment with urso-deoxycholic acid improves bone density in this patient population [20]. According to the American Association for the Study of Liver Disease (AASLD) practice guidelines, bone density should be evaluated with any new PSC diagnosis and at subsequent 2–3-year intervals [21]. The AASLD guidelines also recommend calcium and additional vitamin D to promote calcium absorption in patients with proven osteopenia [21]. Patients with end-stage primary biliary cirrhosis (PBC) have significantly greater risk of osteopenia and osteoporosis than do age-matched and sex-matched controls, although this has been subject to controversy. Recent studies show that PBC patients have a fourfold increased risk of osteoporosis [22]. The American Gastroenterological Association (AGA) guidelines suggest that bone mineral density evaluation should be considered in all patients with PBC at diagnosis, whereas other recommendations limit bone mineral density evaluation to patients with bilirubin greater than three times the upper limit of normal [23, 24]. The AASLD recommends baseline and regular screening every 2–3 years using bone mineral density testing [25]. The AASLD also recommends measuring annual vitamin D levels in patients with advanced disease. In PBC patients with osteoporosis, alendronate has been shown in a randomized controlled trial to significantly improve bone density when compared to placebo. Therefore, AASLD recommends alendronate for osteoporosis, but only if the patient has no known varices or reflux [25].

Cirrhotic patients of all etiologies are at an increased risk for osteoporosis. Prevalence of osteoporosis varies in studies but ranges from 12 to 55 % [26, 27]. Rates of osteoporosis increase with worsening hepatic function reflected by a higher Child's score and do not seem to correlate with degree of cholestasis. AASLD suggests screening densitometry in all cirrhotic patients and all patients undergoing transplant evaluation [28].

Low bone density and osteoporosis are particularly concerning in liver transplant recipients. In the first 3 months following liver transplantation, bone density falls dramatically [29]. This is a time when patients are limited in their mobility and typically receiving high-dose corticosteroids to prevent rejection. Fracture rates of 15–35 % have been reported, with most fractures occurring within the first 2 years of transplantation. A recent study showed that 25 % of patients have new fracture

Table 7.2 Benefits of coffee in liver disease

Decrease in ALT and GGT
Decrease in fibrosis progression in HCV, NASH, and other causes of liver disease
Higher SVR in patients treated for HCV with IFN+RBV
Decreased risk of NAFLD
Decreased risk of HCC in cirrhotic patients
Decreased mortality in alcoholic cirrhosis
All-cause decrease in mortality

IFN interferon, *RBV* ribavirin

within the first 6 months after liver transplantation. Another study showed that bone density decreases in the first 6 months and remains low in the femoral neck, but improves to exceed pretransplantation density in the lumbar spine by 2 years [29]. The role of calcineurin inhibitors in bone turnover following transplantation remains controversial. However, long-term steroid use increases the risk for decreased bone mineral density.

Question Three: What Effect Does Coffee Have on My Liver

Answer: Coffee has been shown to be beneficial in many types of liver disease. Increased coffee consumption reduces mortality, decreases progression of nonalcoholic fatty liver disease (NAFLD), decreases the rate of scarring in the liver and progression to cirrhosis, decreases rate of liver cancer development, and increases treatment response to hepatitis C antiviral interferon-based therapy (Table 7.2).

Coffee has been shown to decrease the risk of all-cause mortality and be beneficial in many medical conditions. Numerous studies between 1996 and 2010 have shown an inverse relationship between coffee consumption and liver enzymes including GGT and ALT. A large study of over 12,000 patients completed in Japan showed a strong inverse relationship between coffee consumption and GGT in male alcohol drinkers ($P<0.0001$) [30]. The third National Health and Nutrition Examination Survey (NHANES) also found that coffee consumption and caffeine were associated with decrease in ALT in patients who were at high risk for liver disease [31].

Several studies also show decreased risk of fibrosis progression in patients with chronic liver disease who are coffee drinkers. One notable study completed by Modi et al. demonstrated that those who drank >2 cups of coffee a day was associated with lower rates of fibrosis (OR 0.3 95 % CI 0.14–0.8 $P=0.015$) [32]. Long-term follow-up of 19 years showed that patients who drank more than two cups of coffee a day had less than half the rate of chronic liver disease. Interestingly, this effect was not seen with non-coffee caffeine sources [33].

Coffee has been shown to decrease the mortality risk in both alcoholic and nonalcoholic cirrhosis, with RR 0.77 per cup per day [34]. Long-term studies show a dose-dependent decrease in risk of cirrhosis [35]. Coffee use in patients with hepatitis C has been shown to decrease fibrosis progression. In the well-known HALT-C trial, coffee drinkers had decreased rates of fibrosis progression [36]. Hepatitis C virus patients who drank coffee while on interferon/ribavirin antiviral therapy had a higher rate of sustained virologic response (SVR), which in part may be due to a higher tolerance of interferon-associated side effects (60 % vs. 50 %) [37].

NAFLD is perhaps the most well-studied patient population in respect to the effect of coffee on liver disease. NHANES illustrated that caffeine intake was associated with decreased risk of NAFLD [38]. Cross-sectional studies show that coffee consumption was associated with decreased risk in fibrosis in nonalcoholic steatohepatitis (NASH) patients [38]. Molloy et al. studied 306 patients' coffee consumption and evaluated the stage of fibrosis showing that an increase in coffee consumption inversely correlated with fibrosis stage with RR −0.7 [38].

Finally, coffee appears to be protective against the development of hepatocellular carcinoma (HCC). Several case-controlled studies illustrate that increase in coffee intake was associated with a dose-dependent decrease in HCC risk. Montella et al. found a dose-effect relationship between coffee intake and risk of HCC for people who consumed four or more cups daily (OR 0.4, 95 % CI 0.2–1.1) [39]. Several studies analyzing the Japan Collaborative Cohort Study demonstrate decreased risk of HCC and death with increased coffee consumption [40–42].

Question Four: What Can I Take for My Pain?

Answer: Most medications utilize the liver for clearance, detoxification, and excretion. Pain medications must be used with caution. Pain management is particularly challenging in cirrhotic patients. In general nonsteroidal anti-inflammatory drugs (NSAIDs) and opioids should be avoided. Acetaminophen at doses less than 2–3 g/day or tramadol is a more appropriate choice for pain management.

Acetaminophen

Acetaminophen is an excellent analgesic that is safe in proper doses. It can cause acute liver damage and fulminant liver failure when not dosed properly. In patients with cirrhosis lower doses should be used. One study showed that up to 4 g/day was safe in patients with chronic liver disease. Another study showed that up to 2 g/day in cirrhotic patients was safe in those not actively drinking alcohol. The threshold for safety is lower for those actively drinking alcohol and the malnourished.

NSAIDs

NSAIDs should be avoided in patients with cirrhosis. Cirrhotic patients have altered coagulation and risk for bleeding. NSAIDs cause impairment in platelet function which may propagate bleeding. Additionally cirrhotic patients are at risk for renal insufficiency. NSAIDs decrease renal blood flow and may also lead to renal failure. For these reason, NSAIDs should be avoided in cirrhotic patients.

Tramadol

Tramadol is a centrally acting synthetic analgesic that is not an opiate. It has good analgesic properties and short half-life of 6 h. There have been no prospective controlled trials in cirrhotic patients; however, it is commonly used for pain management.

Opioids

Patients with cirrhosis have a decreased creatinine clearance. Opioids can accumulate and cause severe respiratory depression. There is a risk of increased accumulation with repeat dosing. Opioids have also been implicated in causation of hepatic encephalopathy directly and also secondarily through worsening constipation. If opioids are used in cirrhotic patients they should be given at the lowest possible dose with the longest possible interval between doses.

Acknowledgements This review did not receive financial support from a funding agency or institution, and Veronica Loy, DO, has no conflict of interests to declare.

References

1. Keeffe EB. Is hepatitis A more severe in patients with chronic hepatitis B and other chronic liver diseases? Am J Gastroenterol. 1995;90(2):201–5.
2. Vento S et al. Fulminant hepatitis associated with hepatitis A virus superinfection in patients with chronic hepatitis C. N Engl J Med. 1998;338(5):286–90.
3. Xavier S, Anish K. Is hepatitis A vaccination necessary in Indian patients with cirrhosis of liver? Indian J Gastroenterol. 2003;22(2):54–5.
4. Jacobs RJ, Koff RS, Meyerhoff AS. The cost-effectiveness of vaccinating chronic hepatitis C patients against hepatitis A. Am J Gastroenterol. 2002;97(2):427–34.
5. Lee SD et al. Safety and immunogenicity of inactivated hepatitis A vaccine in patients with chronic liver disease. J Med Virol. 1997;52(2):215–8.
6. Arguedas MR, McGuire BM, Fallon MB. Implementation of vaccination in patients with cirrhosis. Dig Dis Sci. 2002;47(2):384–7.

7. Smallwood GA et al. Can patients awaiting liver transplantation elicit an immune response to the hepatitis A vaccine? Transplant Proc. 2002;34(8):3289–90.
8. Feray C et al. Hepatitis C virus RNA and hepatitis B virus DNA in serum and liver of patients with fulminant hepatitis. Gastroenterology. 1993;104(2):549–55.
9. Benvegnu L et al. Specificity and patterns of antibodies to hepatitis C virus in hepatocellular carcinoma. Hepatology. 1991;14(5):959.
10. Lemon SM, Thomas DL. Vaccines to prevent viral hepatitis. N Engl J Med. 1997;336(3): 196–204.
11. Jacobs RJ, Meyerhoff AS, Saab S. Immunization needs of chronic liver disease patients seen in primary care versus specialist settings. Dig Dis Sci. 2005;50(8):1525–31.
12. Poland GA. Hepatitis B immunization in health care workers. Dealing with vaccine nonresponse. Am J Prev Med. 1998;15(1):73–7.
13. Duchini A et al. Hepatic decompensation in patients with cirrhosis during infection with influenza A. Arch Intern Med. 2000;160(1):113–5.
14. Song JY et al. Clinical impact of influenza immunization in patients with liver cirrhosis. J Clin Virol. 2007;39(3):159–63.
15. Kyaw MH et al. The influence of chronic illnesses on the incidence of invasive pneumococcal disease in adults. J Infect Dis. 2005;192(3):377–86.
16. Bouza E et al. Nosocomial bloodstream infections caused by Streptococcus pneumoniae. Clin Microbiol Infect. 2005;11(11):919–24.
17. Collier J. Bone disorders in chronic liver disease. Hepatology. 2007;46(4):1271–8.
18. Venu M et al. High prevalence of vitamin A deficiency and vitamin D deficiency in patients evaluated for liver transplantation. Liver Transpl. 2013;19(6):627–33.
19. Peris P et al. Vertebral fractures and osteopenia in chronic alcoholic patients. Calcif Tissue Int. 1995;57(2):111–4.
20. Lindor KD et al. Bone disease in primary biliary cirrhosis: does ursodeoxycholic acid make a difference? Hepatology. 1995;21(2):389–92.
21. Chapman R et al. Diagnosis and management of primary sclerosing cholangitis. Hepatology. 2010;51(2):660–78.
22. Solaymani-Dodaran M et al. Fracture risk in people with primary biliary cirrhosis: a population-based cohort study. Gastroenterology. 2006;131(6):1752–7.
23. Collier JD, Ninkovic M, Compston JE. Guidelines on the management of osteoporosis associated with chronic liver disease. Gut. 2002;50 Suppl 1:i1–9.
24. Leslie WD, Bernstein CN, Leboff MS. AGA technical review on osteoporosis in hepatic disorders. Gastroenterology. 2003;125(3):941–66.
25. Lindor KD et al. Primary biliary cirrhosis. Hepatology. 2009;50(1):291–308.
26. Guichelaar MM et al. Bone mineral density before and after OLT: long-term follow-up and predictive factors. Liver Transpl. 2006;12(9):1390–402.
27. Sokhi RP et al. Bone mineral density among cirrhotic patients awaiting liver transplantation. Liver Transpl. 2004;10(5):648–53.
28. Martin P, et al. Evaluation for liver transplantation in adults: 2013 practice guideline by the AASLD and the American Society of Transplantation. 2013; http://www.aasld.org/sites/default/files/guideline_documents/evaluationadultltenhanced.pdf.
29. Ninkovic M et al. Incidence of vertebral fractures in the first three months after orthotopic liver transplantation. Eur J Gastroenterol Hepatol. 2000;12(8):931–5.
30. Tanaka K et al. Coffee consumption and decreased serum gamma-glutamyltransferase and aminotransferase activities among male alcohol drinkers. Int J Epidemiol. 1998;27(3):438–43.
31. Ruhl CE, Everhart JE. Coffee and caffeine consumption reduce the risk of elevated serum alanine aminotransferase activity in the United States. Gastroenterology. 2005;128(1):24–32.
32. Modi AA et al. Increased caffeine consumption is associated with reduced hepatic fibrosis. Hepatology. 2010;51(1):201–9.
33. Ruhl CE, Everhart JE. Coffee and tea consumption are associated with a lower incidence of chronic liver disease in the United States. Gastroenterology. 2005;129(6):1928–36.

34. Klatsky AL, Armstrong MA, Friedman GD. Coffee, tea, and mortality. Ann Epidemiol. 1993;3(4):375–81.
35. Klatsky AL et al. Coffee, cirrhosis, and transaminase enzymes. Arch Intern Med. 2006;166(11):1190–5.
36. Freedman ND et al. Coffee intake is associated with lower rates of liver disease progression in chronic hepatitis C. Hepatology. 2009;50(5):1360–9.
37. Freedman ND et al. Coffee consumption is associated with response to peginterferon and ribavirin therapy in patients with chronic hepatitis C. Gastroenterology. 2011;140(7):1961–9.
38. Birerdinc A et al. Caffeine is protective in patients with non-alcoholic fatty liver disease. Aliment Pharmacol Ther. 2012;35(1):76–82.
39. Montella M et al. Coffee and tea consumption and risk of hepatocellular carcinoma in Italy. Int J Cancer. 2007;120(7):1555–9.
40. Kurozawa Y et al. Dietary habits and risk of death due to hepatocellular carcinoma in a large scale cohort study in Japan. Univariate analysis of JACC study data. Kurume Med J. 2004; 51(2):141–9.
41. Kurozawa Y et al. Coffee and risk of death from hepatocellular carcinoma in a large cohort study in Japan. Br J Cancer. 2005;93(5):607–10.
42. Wakai K et al. Liver cancer risk, coffee, and hepatitis C virus infection: a nested case-control study in Japan. Br J Cancer. 2007;97(3):426–8.

Chapter 8
Preoperative and Postoperative Care of the Liver Patient

Malcolm M. Wells and Thomas D. Schiano

Introduction

Patients with cirrhosis undergoing surgery are at increased risk of morbidity and mortality. Advances in surgery, anesthesiology, intensive care medicine, hematology, and liver transplantation medicine have decreased overall mortality rates; however, cirrhotic patients still remain high surgical risk candidates. Absolute contraindications for surgery include acute viral hepatitis, alcoholic hepatitis and fulminant liver failure. Otherwise, surgical risk in patients with cirrhosis can be assessed using the Child–Turcotte–Pugh (CTP) classification (see Table 8.1) and the Model for End Stage Liver Disease (MELD) score. The invasiveness (laparoscopic vs. open) and the acuity (emergent vs. elective) of the surgery have an appreciable impact on a patient's morbidity and mortality as well.

Prior to surgery, the condition of patients with decompensated cirrhosis should be optimized as much as possible in order to minimize complications. A tool such as the Preoperative Liver Assessment (POLA) checklist (see Table 8.2) provides a simple to use, yet comprehensive approach, in optimizing patients with decompensated cirrhosis. In the following chapter, we will review and discuss the assessment of surgical risk and the management of perioperative complications in patients with cirrhosis who are undergoing surgery.

M.M. Wells, M.D., F.R.C.P.C. • T.D. Schiano, M.D. (✉)
Icahn School of Medicine at Mount Sinai, The Mount Sinai Medical Center,
Recanati/Miller Transplantation Institute, One Gustave Levy Place,
Box 1104, New York, NY 10029-6574, USA
e-mail: thomas.schiano@mountsinai.org

© Springer International Publishing Switzerland 2017
K. Saeian, R. Shaker (eds.), *Liver Disorders*,
DOI 10.1007/978-3-319-30103-7_8

Table 8.1 Child–Turcotte–Pugh classification

	1 Point	2 Points	3 Points
Bilirubin (mg/dL)	<2	2–3	>3
Albumin (g/dL)	>3.5	2.8–3.5	<2.8
PT prolong (sec)	<4	4–6	>6
Ascites	None	Easily controlled	Poorly controlled
Encephalopathy	None	Grade 1–2	Grade 3–4

A total Child–Turcotte–Pugh score of 5–6 is considered class A (well-compensated disease); 7–9 is class B (significant functional compromise); and 10–15 is class C (decompensated disease). Adapted from Pugh et al. [90]

Table 8.2 Preoperative liver assessment (POLA) checklist

- **Emergent or elective**
  - If surgery is potentially life-saving, proceed with surgery with adequate informed consent, but also consider nonsurgical alternatives like such as ongoing medical therapy or interventional radiologic procedures or palliative care as appropriate
- **Characterize liver disease**
  - Determine cause and chronicity of liver disease
    - o If acute viral or alcoholic hepatitis or severe drug-induced injury, postpone surgery for at least 3 months
    - o If chronic but mild liver disease, proceed with surgery
    - o If there is evidence of cirrhosis or non-cirrhotic portal hypertension, continue with liver assessment
- **Identify significant comorbid conditions**
  - Focus on presence of diabetes, chronic kidney disease, and cardiovascular disease
  - If moderate or severe nutritional deficiency is present, optimize nutrition by oral, enteral, or even parenteral means before surgery
- **Perform liver imaging**
  - MRI or CT are preferred to evaluate for liver appearance, vessel patency, hepatocellular carcinoma, and evidence of portal hypertension (e.g., Intra-abdominal varices, spleen size)
  - Ultrasound with Doppler is sufficient if there are contraindications to CT or MRI such as acute liver injury
- **Obtain history of prior hepatic decompensation**
  - Ascites: if yes, consider future impact on wound healing with postoperative recurrence
  - Encephalopathy: if yes, adjust planned sedation and analgesia, and monitor for regular bowel movements
    - o Do not restrict dietary protein (give 1.2–1.5 g/kg protein daily)
  - Variceal bleeding: if yes, perform upper endoscopy and initiate variceal hemorrhage prophylaxis
- **Evaluate for current hepatic decompensation**
  - Ascites: if yes, perform diagnostic paracentesis to evaluate for SBP
    - o If moderate or severe, perform LVP before surgery
    - o Consider preoperative TIPS if diuretic resistant and MELD < 15, but not typically for emergent cases
      - □ Give 2 g sodium diet, 35–45 kcal/g daily

(continued)

Table 8.2 (continued)

– Encephalopathy: if yes, optimize lactulose to achieve 2–4 bowel movements/day (even by NGT) and give rifaximin
o Do not restrict dietary protein (give 1.2–1.5 g/kg protein daily)
o Order aspiration precautions
– Variceal bleeding: if yes, perform upper endoscopy and initiate variceal hemorrhage prophylaxis
– Hypoxemia or CHF: if yes, consider hepatopulmonary syndrome or portopulmonary hypertension
o Perform ABG, contrast-enhanced echocardiography
• **Estimate liver function and likelihood of portal hypertension**
– Check serum total bilirubin, albumin, INR, creatinine, platelets, hepatic venous pressure gradient, if available
• **Calculate CTP, MELD, and modified MELD for surgery at several time points**
– Calculator for postoperative mortality risk in patients with cirrhosis found at http://www.mayoclinic.org/meld/mayomodel9.html
o Compensated cirrhosis is ASA stage III
o Decompensated cirrhosis is ASA stage IV
– If Child C or MELD >12 or high risk, consider alternatives to surgery or transfer to liver transplant center
– If Child C or MELD >12 or high risk, consider completing liver transplant evaluation before surgery
• **Evaluate coagulopathy and anemia**
– Give subcutaneous vitamin K supplementation leading up to surgery
– Give DDAVP/desmopressin if renal insufficiency present
– Consider use of recombinant factor VIIa for refractory hemorrhage
– In the absence of hemorrhage, do not transfuse platelets if count $>50 \times 10^3/\mu L$ or cryoprecipitate if fibrinogen > 50 mg/dL
– Avoid overtransfusion to correct anemia (use hemoglobin goal of 7 g/dL) to avoid increasing portal pressures
• **Review medications**
– Avoid hepatotoxic medications like herbal supplementations and acetaminophen >2 g per day
– Avoid nephrotoxic medications like NSAIDs (i.e., ketorolac, ibuprofen) or aminoglycosides (i.e., gentamicin)
– Avoid all benzodiazepines for anxiety/insomnia and narcotics or administer those with short half-lives
– Monitor and correct for electrolyte and acid–base disturbances that may precipitate encephalopathy
– Avoid prophylactic antibiotics with greater risks of drug-induced liver injury like amoxicillin-clavulanate (Augmentin), nitrofurantoin, TMP/SMX (Bactrim), ciprofloxacin, and levofloxacin

Ref. [10]

Assessing Surgical Risk

Doctor, The Out-Pouching in My Belly Button Is Bothering Me. I Have Also Been Told I Am Suffering from Alcoholic Hepatitis. Given My Liver Condition, Can I Have This Umbilical Hernia Fixed?

There are a number of settings in which elective surgery is contraindicated, as the perioperative mortality is unacceptably high. Patients with acute hepatitis (whether secondary to viral infection, toxic insults, alcohol, ischemia, or drugs) have increased perioperative mortality and morbidity. Studies have shown that patients with acute viral hepatitis have a 10 % perioperative mortality and an additional 11 % morbidity [2, 3]. Patients with acute alcoholic hepatitis who underwent open surgical liver biopsy had a fivefold increase in mortality compared with closed biopsy [4], Mortality rates as high as 100 % in patients with acute alcoholic hepatitis undergoing open liver biopsy [4, 5], portosystemic shunt surgery [5–8], or exploratory laparotomy [5, 9] have been reported. Patients with acute alcoholic hepatitis should not undergo surgery for at least 12 weeks or until their condition has improved and the hepatitis and clinical symptoms have resolved. Acute liver failure (ALF), characterized by acute liver injury, hepatic encephalopathy, and coagulopathy, is treated with supportive care and liver transplantation. Elective surgery is contraindicated in patients with ALF.

Doctor, Does It Make a Difference What Type of Anesthesia I Receive, and What Are the Effects of Anesthesia on My Liver?

General anesthesia with neuromuscular blocking agents and volatile anesthetics reduce hepatic blood flow which can lead to liver decompensation. Aside from halothane which is rarely used anymore, commonly used anesthetics do not have associated direct hepatotoxicity [10]. Thus, the type of general anesthesia administered does not really matter. Monitored sedation with propofol, which is typically used during endoscopic procedures, does not alter hepatic blood flow appreciably and does not require any dose modifications in the setting of liver dysfunction. Spinal or epidural anesthetics may reduce mean arterial pressure and impose significant bleeding risks in cirrhotic patients having coagulopathy [10].

When I Went for My Preoperative Testing the Anesthesiologist Wrote That I Was ASA Class 3: What Does That Mean?

The American Society of Anesthesiologists (ASA) physical status classification system (see Table 8.3) is a general predictor of postoperative mortality [11, 12]. It was initially created in 1941 to assess the degree of a patient's "sickness" or "physical state" prior to selecting the anesthetic or prior to performing surgery [11].

Table 8.3 American Society of Anaesthesiologists' (ASA) classification of physical health

I	Patient is a completely healthy fit patient
II	Patient has mild systemic disease
III	Patient has severe systemic disease that is not incapacitating
IV	Patient has incapacitating disease that is a constant threat to life
V	A moribund patient who is not expected to live 24 h with or without surgery

Adapted from Ref. [91]

A large prospective study validating the ASA Physical Status classification system found that intraoperative blood loss, postoperative morbidity and postoperative mortality increased with increasing ASA class [13]. Thirty-day mortality was 0.1, 0.7, 3.5, and 18.3 % for Class I, II, III, and IV, respectively [13]. ASA class III and IV had risk odds ratios for 30-day mortality of 2.2 and 4.2, respectively [13]. Most patients having cirrhosis are ASA Class 3 (see Table 8.3).

During My Workup for the Liver Transplant, The Heart Doctor Did an Echocardiogram and Told Me That I Have High Lung Pressures That will Make Any Future Surgery Dangerous. Is This Related to My Liver Condition?

Portopulmonary hypertension (PPHTN) occurs in upwards of 0.61–0.73 % of cirrhotic patients [14]. All cirrhotic patients should be screened for PPHTN with echocardiography prior to undergoing any type of surgical procedure. Perioperative mortality rates are prohibitively high in the presence of severe pulmonary hypertension, whether it is related to underlying liver disease or not. Thus, timely diagnosis and treatment are necessary before any elective surgical procedure [15–18]. Prior to undergoing surgery, patients with chronic liver disease should receive clearance from a hepatologist, as well as receive clearance from an internist in order to optimize any preexisting medical comorbidities, such as diabetes and other cardiac risk factors [15–18].

I Have Early Cirrhosis That Doesn't Require a Liver Transplant and I Need Colon Surgery. Does the Severity of My Liver Disease Impact the Risks Surrounding This Surgery?

In patients without an absolute contraindication to surgery, a preoperative evaluation is performed. This includes assessment of the severity of the patient's liver disease, the nature of the operation, the presence of other comorbidities, as well as the urgency of the surgery.

In the setting of chronic hepatitis, there is limited data on patients with milder forms of liver disease undergoing surgery. The CPT classification (see Table 8.1) and MELD score have been studied regarding the estimation of perioperative mortality. CTP classes A, B, and C have been associated with 30-day mortality rates of 10 %, 17–31 %

and 63–82%, respectively [19–21]. Patients with a MELD score of less than 10, 10–15, and greater than 15 are estimated to have a 30-day postoperative mortality of 9, 19 and 54%, respectively [19]. In another study, 30-day mortality ranged from 5.7% (MELD score<8) to more than 50% (MELD score >20) [22]. In the same study, the median survival among all patients with digestive, orthopedic or cardiovascular surgery was 4.8 years for MELD scores of 0–7 ($n=351$), 3.4 years for scores of 8–11 ($n=257$), 1.6 years for scores of 12–15 ($n=106$), 64 days for scores of 16–20 ($n=35$), 23 days for scores of 21–25 ($n=13$), and 14 days for a MELD score of 26 or greater ($n=10$) [22].

In a retrospective study of 140 cirrhotic patients undergoing surgery, the MELD score was the only statistically significant predictor of 30-day mortality, with an approximate 1% increase in mortality risk for each 1-point increase in the MELD score from 5 to 20, and a 2% increase in mortality risk for each 1-point increase in the MELD score when >20 [23]. Thus, patients who are CTP Class C or have a MELD score greater than 15 should if at all possible not undergo elective surgery. Patients who have CTP Class B cirrhosis or a MELD of 10–15 still have significant risk of perioperative mortality and elective surgery is a relative contraindication.

I Was Recently Admitted to the Hospital with a Gallbladder Attack. Is It Better If I Have My Gall Bladder Removed Laparoscopically or Through the Traditional Way?

Although data are limited, the manner in which the surgery is performed impacts upon outcome. In one study, the outcomes of patients with cirrhosis undergoing emergent or elective cholecystectomy, umbilical herniorrhaphy, or colectomy [24] were evaluated. Most surgeries were completed laparoscopically, with some requiring conversion to an open procedure. The authors reported a 30-day postoperative mortality of 2% for patients who were CTP A, and 12% for both CTP B and CTP C groups (see Fig. 8.1) [24]. A similar trend was observed when patients were compared using their MELD scores. Thirty-day postoperative mortality was 3, 8, 29, and 0% in patients with a MELD score of less than 10, 10–14, 15–25, and greater than 25, respectively (see Fig. 8.2) [24]. Morbidity remained high in cirrhotic patients undergoing laparoscopic surgeries, with rates comparable to studies in which open surgeries were performed. Cirrhotic patients had increasing rates of morbidity with increasing CTP class or MELD score. Thirty-day postoperative morbidity was 20% for patients who were CTP A, 58% for CTP B and 80% for CTP C [24]. Thirty-day postoperative morbidity rates were 35, 50, 60, and 100% in patients with a MELD score of less than 10, 10–14, 15–25, and greater than 25, respectively [24]. Major morbidities included wound complications (infections, hematomas, leakage of ascites), liver decompensation, ileus or obstruction, respiratory failure, sepsis, variceal bleeding, and anastomotic leakage [24]. Thirty-day mortality was markedly lower in this study [24] compared to other studies in which open surgeries were performed [19–21]. Albeit studies are very limited with no direct comparison between laparoscopic and open techniques, it would appear laparoscopic as opposed to open, may be a safer surgical approach in cirrhotic patients.

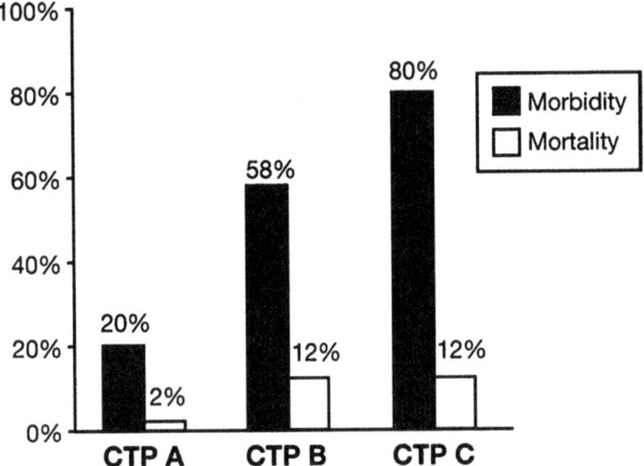

Fig. 8.1 Thirty-day morbidity and mortality in cirrhotic patients undergoing surgery by CTP score [24]

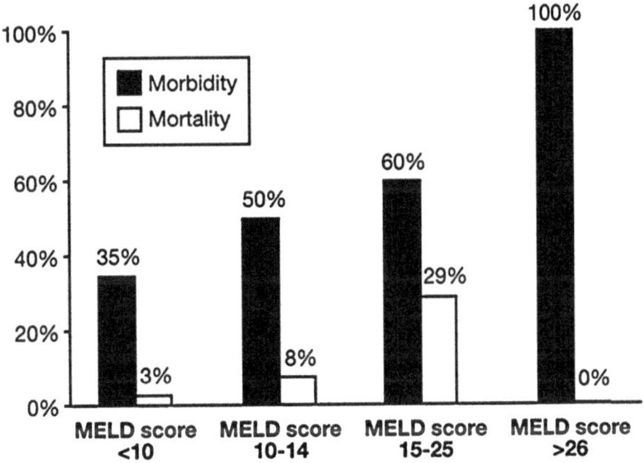

Fig. 8.2 Thirty-day morbidity and mortality in cirrhotic patients undergoing surgery by MELD [24]

Timing of Surgery: Emergency Surgery, Elective Surgery, and Deferring Surgery

My Mother Requires Emergency Surgery for a Bowel Obstruction. Does Having Emergency Surgery Increase the Risk, Given Her Cirrhosis?

The acuity of surgery impacts on the morbidity, mortality and need for liver transplantation in patients having cirrhosis. In seven studies comparing elective vs. emergent surgery in cirrhotic patients, mortality ranged from 6 to 18 % for elective surgery and 19–86 % for emergent surgery, a 1.1- to 8.6-fold increase in mortality [19–21, 24–27]. This is not an unexpected result as emergent surgery is precipitated by life-threatening presentations. Increased morbidity and mortality is also seen with emergent vs. elective surgery in non-cirrhotic patients [28–30].

If My Heart Surgery will Be Risky, Can the Surgery Be Done at the Same Time as My Liver Transplant?

There is limited experience of elective surgery performed concurrently with liver transplantation. There are a handful of case reports and a case series of successful simultaneous combined liver transplantation and coronary artery bypass grafting procedures (CABG) [31–36]. Although successful cases have been reported, simultaneous cardiac surgery and OLT remains technically difficult and should be limited to very specialized centers.

Optimizing Patients Medically

My Father Has Cirrhosis and May Need Lung Surgery. Can Anything Be Done to Make His Liver Better Before Surgery?

Preoperative checklists can be used to reduce morbidity and mortality in cirrhotic patients [37, 38]. Similarly, the Preoperative Liver Assessment (POLA) checklist (Table 8.2) has been proposed to simplify the process of assessing and optimizing surgical risk in patients having chronic liver disease [10].

My Wife Has End Stage Liver Disease and She Is Often Foggy Mentally. Can Anything Be Done Prior to Surgery to Reduce the Risk Postoperatively?

Hepatic encephalopathy is a debilitating complication of decompensated cirrhosis, leading to significant morbidity and mortality. In patients with cirrhosis, HE contributes to functional decline and consumption of appreciable health care resources [39]. In evaluating patients prior to surgery, potential signs and symptoms of HE should be explored. HE manifests in a broad array of neurologic and psychiatric symptoms ranging from minimal hepatic encephalopathy (MHE) to overt hepatic encephalopathy (OHE). Patients with MHE have minimal or subclinical symptoms and the diagnosis is made via psychometric testing [40–43]. Patients with OHE have a wide range of presentations including day-night wake reversal, agitation, somnolence, stupor, and finally coma [44, 45].

There is some evidence for the benefit of prophylaxis of OHE in certain settings. Acute variceal bleeding occurs in 25–30 % of patients with cirrhosis and is an important precipitant of OHE, leading to increased morbidity and mortality [46, 47]. In the setting of acute variceal bleeding, lactulose vs. placebo prophylaxis in one study resulted in significantly less OHE (14 % vs. 40 %) and trended towards less mortality (8.5 % vs. 17 %) [48]. In a second study, rifaximin and lactulose appear to be equally effective for primary prophylaxis in the setting of an acute variceal bleeding, with no significant difference in development of HE (10/60 vs. 9/60; $p = 1.0$) and mortality (8/60 vs. 9/60; $p = 1.0$) [49]. There is also evidence for the benefit of secondary prophylaxis of OHE in cirrhotic patients. Lactulose, rifaximin and probiotics are effective at preventing subsequent episodes of OHE in patients with cirrhosis who had a previous episode of OHE [50–52].

Identification and treatment of precipitating factors are the primary therapeutic option for patients with OHE [53]. Gastrointestinal bleeding, infection (including spontaneous bacterial peritonitis), hypokalemia and/or metabolic alkalosis, renal failure, hypovolemia, hypoxia, sedative or tranquilizer use, hypoglycemia, constipation, and hepatocellular carcinoma and/or vascular occlusion (hepatic vein or portal vein thrombosis) can all precipitate OHE [53]. In addition to the optimization and treatment of these precipitating factors, medical management is the cornerstone of treatment. Two meta-analyses demonstrated that both oral non-absorbable disaccharides (lactulose or lactitol) and rifaximin are equally effective in the management of OHE with rifaximin being better tolerated [54, 55].

Lactulose or lactitol are effective in patients with MHE, with trials demonstrating improvement in psychometric testing [56, 57], reduced progression to OHE [56], reduced ammonia levels [56, 57] and improved health-related quality of life [56]. Adverse events were not serious and all were related to the gastrointestinal tract (diarrhea, flatulence, abdominal pain, and nausea) [57].

Limiting opiate analgesics for pain may help prevent the development of hepatic encephalopathy postoperatively, especially in patients also taking iron and calcium supplements, all of which contribute to constipation [58]. Concurrent lactulose use may contribute to the development of ileus or small bowel obstruction, as well as dehydration leading to hypovolemia. For analgesia, acetaminophen up to 2 g total daily is safe to use and is preferred over NSAIDs (i.e., ketorolac), which may predispose to renal dysfunction

My Husband Has Liver Disease. He Bruises Easily and Often Has Persistent Nosebleeds. Can Anything Be Done to Decrease His Risk of Bleeding During Surgery?

Patients with cirrhosis commonly have accompanying coagulopathy. It is recommended to supplement with vitamin K 10 mg subcutaneously daily for 3 days in order to correct any nutritional deficiency that may raise a patient's International Normalized Ratio (INR) and calculated MELD score. Overtransfusion of blood products is to be avoided so as to not increase portal pressures and precipitate variceal bleeding. A restrictive Packed Red Blood Cell (PRBC) transfusion strategy is advised, with a threshold serum hemoglobin of 7–8 g/dL. Fresh frozen plasma (FFP) is given if a patient's INR is greater than 1.5 preoperatively despite administration of vitamin K. Platelets are transfused for serum platelet levels below $50 \times 10^3/\mu L$ preoperatively. Cryoprecipitate is transfused to increase fibrinogen concentration to above 50–100 mg/dL in nonsurgical settings and to approximately 100–200 mg/dL for surgical prophylaxis [59, 60]. DDAVP can be used in patients having renal dysfunction to correct qualitative platelet dysfunction. DDAVP nasal spray may be used instead of blood products in cirrhotic patients undergoing dental extractions who have a modest degree of coagulopathy [61]

I Have Abdominal Distension with Ascites Fluid. How Can This Be Controlled Prior to Surgery and will It Be a Problem Afterwards?

For patients with cirrhosis, a low-sodium diet (<2 g daily) is advised. Patients with ascites should undergo a diagnostic paracentesis preoperatively to exclude spontaneous bacterial peritonitis (SBP). If there is no SBP, patients with moderate to severe ascites can undergo a large volume paracentesis (LVP). A Transjugular Intrahepatic Portosystemic Shunt (TIPS) can be considered preoperatively if the surgery is not emergent, if the ascites is diuretic-resistant or if the patient's MELD if not greater than 15. TIPS reduces portal hypertension by creating a communication between intrahepatic branches of the hepatic vein and portal vein [62]. It is effective for treatment of acute variceal hemorrhage and refractory ascites [62, 63]. The beneficial effects of TIPS in variceal bleeding rapidly occur but the humoral and hemodynamic changes that lead to the improvement and resolution of ascites may take upwards of 6–8 weeks or longer. Older patients and those with preexisting renal dysfunction have less of a chance to resolve their ascites after TIPS, with the associated risks of developing or worsening OHE being much greater. Contraindications to TIPS include: severe heart failure or pulmonary hypertension, portal vein thrombosis with cavernous transformation, and polycystic liver disease [62]. The MELD score was originally developed to predict the 3-month mortality of patients undergoing elective TIPS [64]. Patients with higher MELD scores, particularly MELD scores greater than 18, have a poorer prognosis, with higher 3-month mortality [65–68].

Aggressive management of ascites prior to abdominal surgery is essential to afford optimized wound closure and healing of any tissue anastomoses. Liver dysfunction precipitated by surgery can often manifest as an increase in ascites. Leakage of ascites through an abdominal incision may lead to fascial breakdown, poor wound healing, infection and the precipitation of renal failure. Diuretic use and paracentesis postoperatively may need to be utilized to prevent ascites development. A worsening of ascites may also result in the development of a hepatic hydrothorax, and its attendant morbidity [69–71].

My Primary Care Physician Says My Kidney Function Is Poor and It Is Likely Related to My Cirrhosis. What Investigations and Management Should I Have Performed Prior to Surgery

Acute kidney injury (AKI) is a common complication in all patients in the perioperative setting. Although the majority of patients with AKI have significant recovery in glomerular filtration rates, AKI may lead to chronic kidney disease (CKD) and the need for hemodialysis [72]. AKI significantly increases mortality postoperatively, with increased duration and severity of AKI increasing mortality [73]. Therefore, it is important to prevent and treat AKI in patients undergoing surgery.

Hepatorenal syndrome (HRS) accounts for 45% of renal failure in patients with cirrhosis [74]. Type 1 HRS is characterized by a rapid decline in renal function with creatinine rising from baseline to greater than 2.5 mg/dL in less than 2 weeks [75–77]. Type 2 HRS shows a steady, progressive decline in renal function [75–77]. The diagnosis of HRS is one of exclusion. Major diagnostic criteria include: cirrhosis with ascites, serum creatinine >1.5 mg/dL, no improvement with 2 days of diuretic withdrawal and volume expansion with albumin, absence of shock, no current or recent nephrotoxic medications, and no parenchymal renal disease (proteinuria < 0.5 g/day, no microscopic hematuria, and a normal renal ultrasound) [75–77]. Treatment for HRS [75, 77] includes vasoconstrictors (terlipressin, octreotide, vasopressin, or norepinephrine), with midodrine plus albumin. Worsening HRS may necessitate the consideration of hemodialysis or TIPS. Liver transplantation is the most effective treatment for HRS. Combined liver and kidney transplantation may be required for patients requiring HD for more than 8–12 weeks [78, 79], with recent data suggesting that combined transplantation may be necessary after as little as 2 weeks of HD [80].

Other causes of AKI should be investigated and treated appropriately [75–77]. A thorough review of prescription and over-the-counter medications should be performed so as to avoid nephrotoxic agents such as NSAIDs (i.e., ibuprofen, ketorolac), aminoglycoside antibiotics (for example, gentamicin) and other antimicrobials (sulfonamides, acyclovir). Infection is a common cause of AKI and should be ruled out with blood cultures, urine culture, stool analysis (culture and sensitivity, ova and parasites and Clostridium difficile toxin) and a diagnostic paracentesis. AKI may be precipitated by hypovolemia (secondary to diuretics, intra-abdominal or gastrointestinal bleeding), acute tubular necrosis, parenchymal renal diseases (diabetic nephropathy, glomerulonephritis due to hepatitis B or C, interstitial nephritis, or IgA nephropathy), obstructive uropathy, or radiocontrast [74–77].

I Have Cirrhosis and Am Scheduled for an Elective Surgery, However I Have Had Several Episodes of Black Tarry Stool Recently. Should I Be Concerned?

Variceal bleeding is a severe complication of portal hypertension and cirrhosis [46, 62, 74, 81]. Variceal bleeding is associated with high mortality and is the most lethal complication of cirrhosis [46]. Esophagogastroduodenoscopy to screen for esophageal and gastric varices is recommended at the time of diagnosis of cirrhosis [46]. Primary prophylaxis of gastroesophageal variceal hemorrhage with nonselective beta-blockers or band ligation is recommended for medium or large varices [46]. Performance of an upper endoscopy prior to surgery is important to assess whether prophylactic beta blockade is warranted. Infection, overhydration, development of portal vein thrombosis, and overtransfusion all may lead to an increase in portal pressure and hence the risk of variceal bleeding. Prophylactic acid suppression is not routinely recommended for cirrhotic patients undergoing surgery.

Since I Was Diagnosed with Cirrhosis, I Have Lost a Significant Amount of Weight and Muscle in My Shoulder Girdle. I Am Scheduled to Have a Hernia Repair. How Should My Nutrition Be Managed While I Am in the Hospital?

The European Society for Clinical Nutrition and Metabolism (ESPEN) has made recommendations for assessing and improving the nutritional status of patients with cirrhosis pre- and post-surgery [82]. Simple bedside methods such as the Subjective Global Assessment (SGA; see Table 8.4) or anthropometry should be used to identify patients at risk of malnutrition. A complete diet or enteral nutrition should be initiated within 12–24 h after surgery, including after liver transplantation. Energy intake is recommended to be 35–40 kcal/kg/day (147–168 kJ/kg/day) consisting of a protein intake of 1.2–1.5 g/kg/day. Nasogastric tubes can be considered for early enteral nutrition, but may increase the aspiration risk. Whole protein formulas are generally recommended, however, in patients with ascites, concentrated high-energy formulas are preferred. Severe muscle depletion or sarcopenia often occurs along with malnutrition. Sarcopenia is one of the most common complications in patients with cirrhosis [83, 84] and it is associated with a higher risk of mortality in these patients [84–86]. Physical activity is a valuable countermeasure to sarcopenia in its treatment and prevention [87].

Alcohol Withdrawal

My Mom's Liver Disease Is from Drinking Alcohol. When Does She Need to Stop Drinking Prior to Surgery?

Alcohol abuse is a common etiology for cirrhosis and thus cirrhotic patients undergoing surgery should be screened for alcohol use and withdrawal. Symptoms of alcohol withdrawal, include tremor, anxiety, headache, diaphoresis and seizures, and may begin within 6 h of the last alcoholic drink [88]. Hallucinations may begin within 12–48 h and delirium tremens may begin within 48–96 h [88]. Thus, the patient should stop drinking alcohol as early as possible prior to surgery and should inform their physicians of this so the requisite precautions can be taken. Patients taking methadone should not stop their typical maintenance dose prior to surgery and should alert their treatment team as to the dosing. Thiamine and multivitamin are used to prevent Wernicke's Syndrome. Clinical Institute Withdrawal Assessment for Alcohol Scale—Revised (CIWA-Ar; Table 8.5) is used to assess the severity of withdrawal [89]. Patients with a score of 8 or more should be treated with benzodiazepines to prevent more severe symptoms.

Table 8.4 Features of the subjective global assessment

(A) Patients related medical history:

1. Weight change (overall change in past 6 months)

1	2	3	4	5
No weight change or gain	Minor weight loss (<5 %)	Weight loss 5–10 %	Weight loss 10–15 %	Weight loss >15 %

2. Dietary intake

1	2	3	4	5
No change	Suboptimal solid diet	Full liquid diet or moderate overall decrease	Hypo-caloric liquid	Starvation

3. Gastrointestinal symptoms

1	2	3	4	5
No symptoms	Nausea	Vomiting or moderate GI symptoms	Diarrhea	Severe anorexia

4. Functional capacity (nutritionally related functional impairment)

1	2	3	4	5
None (improved)	Difficulty with ambulation	Difficulty with normal activity	Light activity	Bed/chair-ridden with no or little activity

5. Comorbidity

1	2	3	4	5
Dialysis <12 months and healthy otherwise	Dialysis 1–2 years or mild comorbidity	Dialysis 2–4 years or age>75 or moderate comorbidity	Dialysis >4 years or severe comorbidity	Very severe multiple comorbidity

(B) Physical exam:

1. Decreased fat stores or loss of subcutaneous fat (below eyes, triceps, biceps, chest)

1	2	3	4	5
None (no change)		Moderate		Severe

2. Signs of muscle wasting (temple, clavicle, scapula, ribs, quadriceps, knee, interosseous)

1	2	3	4	5
None (no change)		Moderate		Severe

Malnutrition score: (sum of all numbers)

The fully quantitative version of the SGA, also known as modified SGA or DMS. Five scale parameters are used, and the values are summed. A value of 7 is normal, and 35 is the most severe malnutrition. Adapted from Ref. [92]

Summary

Patients with cirrhosis undergoing surgery are at increased risk of morbidity and mortality. The Child–Turcotte–Pugh classification and the Model for End-stage Liver Disease score have been used to assess perioperative mortality. Patients with decompensated liver disease should be optimized prior to proceeding with surgery.

Table 8.5 Clinical Institute Withdrawal Assessment of Alcohol Scale, Revised (CIWA-Ar)

Patient: _________________________
Date: _________________________
Time: _________________________ (24 h clock, midnight = 00:00)
Pulse or heart rate, taken for 1 min: _________________________
Blood pressure: _________________________
Nausea and vomiting Ask: "Do you feel sick to your stomach? Have you vomited?"
0: No nausea and no vomiting
1: Mild nausea with no vomiting
2:
3:
4: Intermittent nausea with dry heaves
5:
6:
7: Constant nausea, frequent dry heaves and vomiting
Tremor arms extended and fingers spread apart
0: No tremor
1: Not visible, but can be felt fingertip to fingertip
2:
3:
4: Moderate, with patient's arms extended
5:
6:
7: Severe, even with arms not extended
Paroxysmal sweats
0: No sweat visible
1: Barely perceptible sweating, palms moist
2:
3:
4: Beads of sweat obvious on forehead
5:
6:
7: Drenching sweats
Anxiety Ask: "Do you feel nervous?"
0: No anxiety, at ease
1: Mild anxious
2:
3:
4: Moderately anxious, or guarded, so anxiety is inferred
5:
6:
7: Equivalent to acute panic states as seen in severe delirium or acute schizophrenic reactions

(continued)

Table 8.5 (continued)

Agitation
0: Normal activity
1: Somewhat more than normal activity
2:
3:
4: Moderately fidgety and restless
5:
6:
7: Paces back and forth during most of the interview, or constantly thrashes about

Tactile disturbances Ask: "Have you any itching, pins and needles sensations, any burning, any numbness, or do you feel bugs crawling on or under your skin?"

0: None
1: Very mild itching, pins and needles, burning or numbness
2: Mild itching, pins and needles, burning or numbness
3: Moderate itching, pins and needles, burning or numbness
4: Moderately severe hallucinations
5: Severe hallucinations
6: Extremely severe hallucinations
7: Continuous hallucinations

Auditory disturbances Ask: "Are you more aware of sounds around you? Are they harsh? Do they frighten you? Are you hearing anything that is disturbing to you? Are you hearing things you know are not there?"

0: Not present
1: Very mild harshness or ability to frighten
2: Mild harshness or ability to frighten
3: Moderate harshness or ability to frighten
4: Moderately severe hallucinations
5: Severe hallucinations
6: Extremely severe hallucinations
7: Continuous hallucinations

Visual disturbances Ask: "Does the light appear to be too bright? Is its color different? Does it hurt your eyes? Are you seeing anything that is disturbing to you? Are you seeing things you know are not there?"

0: Not present
1: Very mild sensitivity
2: Mild sensitivity
3: Moderate sensitivity
4: Moderately severe hallucinations
5: Severe hallucinations
6: Extremely severe hallucinations
7: Continuous hallucinations

(continued)

Table 8.5 (continued)

Headache, fullness in head Ask: "Does your head feel different? Does it feel like there is a band around your head?" Do not rate for dizziness or lightheadedness. Otherwise, rate severity

0: Not present
1: Very mild
2: Mild
3: Moderate
4: Moderately severe
5: Severe
6: Very severe
7: Extremely severe

Orientation and clouding of sensorium Ask: "What day is this? Where are you? Who am I?"

0: Oriented and can do serial additions
1: Cannot do serial additions or is uncertain about date
2: Disoriented for date by no more than 2 calendar days
3: Disoriented for date by more than 2 calendar days
4: Disoriented for place/or person

Total CIWA-Ar score ______

Rater's initials ______

Maximum possible score 67

Patients scoring less than 10 do not usually need additional medication for withdrawal

Adapted from [89]

The Preoperative Liver Assessment (POLA) checklist can be useful in assessing and optimizing patients prior to surgery.

Acknowledgements None

Disclosures

Wells: none

Schiano: none

References

1. Murray CJ, Atkinson C, Bhalla K, Birbeck G, Burstein R, Chou D, et al. The state of US health, 1990-2010: burden of diseases, injuries, and risk factors. JAMA. 2013;310(6):591–608.
2. Harville DD, Summerskill WH. Surgery in acute hepatitis. Causes and effects. JAMA. 1963;184:257–61.
3. Hardy KJHE. Laparotomy in viral hepatitis. Med J Aust. 1968;1:710–2.
4. Greenwood SM, Leffler CT, Minkowitz S. The increased mortality rate of open liver biopsy in alcoholic hepatitis. Surg Gynecol Obstet. 1972;134(4):600–4.
5. Friedman LS. The risk of surgery in patients with liver disease. Hepatology. 1999;29(6):1617–23.
6. Mikkelsen WP. Therapeutic portacaval shunt. Preliminary data on controlled trial and morbid effects of acute hyaline necrosis. Arch Surg. 1974;108(3):302–5.

7. Mikkelsen WP, Kern WH. The influence of acute hyaline necrosis on survival after emergency and elective portacaval shunt. Major Probl Clin Surg. 1974;14:233–42.
8. Mikkelsen WP, Turrill FL, Kern WH. Acute hyaline necrosis of the liver. A surgical trap. Am J Surg. 1968;116(2):266–72.
9. Powell-Jackson P, Greenway B, Williams R. Adverse effects of exploratory laparotomy in patients with unsuspected liver disease. Br J Surg. 1982;69(8):449–51.
10. Im GY, Lubezky N, Facciuto M, Schiano TD. Surgery in Patients with Portal Hypertension: A Preoperative Checklist and Strategies for Attenuating Risk. In: Herrera JL, editor. Portal hypertension. Philadelphia, PA: Elsevier; 2014. p. 477–505.
11. Saklad M. Grading of patients for surgical procedures. Anesthesiology. 1941;2:281–4.
12. Dripps D. New classification of physical status. Anesthesiology. 1963;24:111.
13. Wolters U, Wolf T, Stutzer H, Schroder T. ASA classification and perioperative variables as predictors of postoperative outcome. Br J Anaesth. 1996;77(2):217–22.
14. McDonnell PJ, Toye PA, Hutchins GM. Primary pulmonary hypertension and cirrhosis: are they related? Am Rev Respir Dis. 1983;127(4):437–41.
15. Forrest P. Anaesthesia and right ventricular failure. Anaesth Intensive Care. 2009;37(3):370–85.
16. Kaw R, Pasupuleti V, Deshpande A, Hamieh T, Walker E, Minai OA. Pulmonary hypertension: an important predictor of outcomes in patients undergoing non-cardiac surgery. Respir Med. 2011;105(4):619–24.
17. Lai HC, Lai HC, Wang KY, Lee WL, Ting CT, Liu TJ. Severe pulmonary hypertension complicates postoperative outcome of non-cardiac surgery. Br J Anaesth. 2007;99(2):184–90.
18. Rodriguez RM, Pearl RG. Pulmonary hypertension and major surgery. Anesth Analg. 1998;87(4):812–5.
19. Neeff H, Mariaskin D, Spangenberg HC, Hopt UT, Makowiec F. Perioperative mortality after non-hepatic general surgery in patients with liver cirrhosis: an analysis of 138 operations in the 2000s using child and MELD scores. J Gastrointest Surg. 2011;15(1):1–11.
20. Garrison RN, Cryer HM, Howard DA, Polk Jr HC. Clarification of risk factors for abdominal operations in patients with hepatic cirrhosis. Ann Surg. 1984;199(6):648–55.
21. Mansour A, Watson W, Shayani V, Pickleman J. Abdominal operations in patients with cirrhosis: still a major surgical challenge. Surgery. 1997;122(4):730–5. discussion 5-6.
22. Teh SH, Nagorney DM, Stevens SR, Offord KP, Therneau TM, Plevak DJ, et al. Risk factors for mortality after surgery in patients with cirrhosis. Gastroenterology. 2007;132(4):1261–9.
23. Northup PG, Wanamaker RC, Lee VD, Adams RB, Berg CL. Model for end-stage liver disease (MELD) predicts nontransplant surgical mortality in patients with cirrhosis. Ann Surg. 2005;242(2):244–51.
24. Telem DA, Schiano T, Goldstone R, Han DK, Buch KE, Chin EH, et al. Factors that predict outcome of abdominal operations in patients with advanced cirrhosis. Clin Gastroenterol Hepatol. 2010;8(5):451–7.
25. Aranha GV, Greenlee HB. Intra-abdominal surgery in patients with advanced cirrhosis. Arch Surg. 1986;121(3):275–7.
26. Doberneck RC, Sterling Jr WA, Allison DC. Morbidity and mortality after operation in non-bleeding cirrhotic patients. Am J Surg. 1983;146(3):306–9.
27. Farnsworth N, Fagan SP, Berger DH, Awad SS. Child-Turcotte-Pugh versus MELD score as a predictor of outcome after elective and emergent surgery in cirrhotic patients. Am J Surg. 2004;188(5):580–3.
28. Brittenden J, Heys SD, Eremin O. Femoral hernia: mortality and morbidity following elective and emergency surgery. J R Coll Surg Edinb. 1991;36(2):86–8.
29. Cogbill CL. Operation in the aged. Mortality related to concurrent disease, duration of anesthesia, and elective or emergency operation. Arch Surg. 1967;94(2):202–5.
30. Greenburg AG, Saik RP, Coyle JJ, Peskin GW. Mortality and gastrointestinal surgery in the aged: elective vs emergency procedures. Arch Surg. 1981;116(6):788–91.
31. Axelrod D, Koffron A, Dewolf A, Baker A, Fryer J, Baker T, et al. Safety and efficacy of combined orthotopic liver transplantation and coronary artery bypass grafting. Liver Transpl. 2004;10(11):1386–90.

32. Eckhoff DE, Frenette L, Sellers MT, McGuire BM, Contreras JL, Bynon JS, et al. Combined cardiac surgery and liver transplantation. Liver Transpl. 2001;7(1):60–1.
33. Lebbinck H, Bouchez S, Vereecke H, Vanoverbeke H, Troisi R, Reyntjens K. Sequential off-pump coronary artery bypass and liver transplantation. Transplant Int. 2006;19(5):432–4.
34. Manas DM, Roberts DR, Heaviside DW, Chaudhry S, Tocewicz K, Hudson M, et al. Sequential coronary artery bypass grafting and orthotopic liver transplantation: a case report. Clin Transplant. 1996;10(3):320–2.
35. Kniepeiss D, Iberer F, Grasser B, Schaffellner S, Tscheliessnigg KH. Combined coronary artery bypass grafting and orthotopic liver transplantation: a case report. Transplant Proc. 2003;35(2):817–8.
36. Massad MG, Benedetti E, Pollak R, Chami YG, Allen BS, DeCastro MA, et al. Combined coronary bypass and liver transplantation: technical considerations. Ann Thorac Surg. 1998;65(4):1130–2.
37. Haynes AB, Weiser TG, Berry WR, Lipsitz SR, Breizat AH, Dellinger EP, et al. A surgical safety checklist to reduce morbidity and mortality in a global population. N Engl J Med. 2009;360(5):491–9.
38. Morrow R. Perioperative quality and improvement. Anesthesiol Clin. 2012;30(3):555–63.
39. Rakoski MO, McCammon RJ, Piette JD, Iwashyna TJ, Marrero JA, Lok AS, et al. Burden of cirrhosis on older Americans and their families: analysis of the health and retirement study. Hepatology. 2012;55(1):184–91.
40. Amodio P, Montagnese S, Gatta A, Morgan MY. Characteristics of minimal hepatic encephalopathy. Metab Brain Dis. 2004;19(3-4):253–67.
41. Gitlin N, Lewis DC, Hinkley L. The diagnosis and prevalence of subclinical hepatic encephalopathy in apparently healthy, ambulant, non-shunted patients with cirrhosis. J Hepatol. 1986;3(1):75–82.
42. Lockwood AH. "What's in a name?" Improving the care of cirrhotics. J Hepatol. 2000;32(5):859–61.
43. McCrea M, Cordoba J, Vessey G, Blei AT, Randolph C. Neuropsychological characterization and detection of subclinical hepatic encephalopathy. Arch Neurol. 1996;53(8):758–63.
44. Teasdale G, Jennett B. Assessment of coma and impaired consciousness. A practical scale. Lancet. 1974;2(7872):81–4.
45. Khungar V, Poordad F. Hepatic encephalopathy. Clin Liver Dis. 2012;16(2):301–20.
46. Garcia-Tsao G, Sanyal AJ, Grace ND, Carey W, Practice Guidelines Committee of the American Association for the Study of Liver Diseases, Practice Parameters Committee of the American College of Groups. Prevention and management of gastroesophageal varices and variceal hemorrhage in cirrhosis. Hepatology. 2007;46(3):922–38.
47. Grace ND, Groszmann RJ, Garcia-Tsao G, Burroughs AK, Pagliaro L, Makuch RW, et al. Portal hypertension and variceal bleeding: an AASLD single topic symposium. Hepatology. 1998;28(3):868–80.
48. Sharma P, Agrawal A, Sharma BC, Sarin SK. Prophylaxis of hepatic encephalopathy in acute variceal bleed: a randomized controlled trial of lactulose versus no lactulose. J Gastroenterol Hepatol. 2011;26(6):996–1003.
49. Maharshi S, Sharma BC, Srivastava S, Jindal A. Randomised controlled trial of lactulose versus rifaximin for prophylaxis of hepatic encephalopathy in patients with acute variceal bleed. Gut 2015;64(8):1341–2.
50. Agrawal A, Sharma BC, Sharma P, Sarin SK. Secondary prophylaxis of hepatic encephalopathy in cirrhosis: an open-label, randomized controlled trial of lactulose, probiotics, and no therapy. Am J Gastroenterol. 2012;107(7):1043–50.
51. Sharma P, Sharma BC. Disaccharides in the treatment of hepatic encephalopathy. Metab Brain Dis. 2013;28(2):313–20.
52. Bass NM, Mullen KD, Sanyal A, Poordad F, Neff G, Leevy CB, et al. Rifaximin treatment in hepatic encephalopathy. N Engl J Med. 2010;362(12):1071–81.
53. Riordan SM, Williams R. Treatment of hepatic encephalopathy. N Engl J Med. 1997;337(7):473–9.
54. Eltawil KM, Laryea M, Peltekian K, Molinari M. Rifaximin vs. conventional oral therapy for hepatic encephalopathy: a meta-analysis. World J Gastroenterol. 2012;18(8):767–77.

55. Jiang Q, Jiang XH, Zheng MH, Jiang LM, Chen YP, Wang L. Rifaximin versus nonabsorbable disaccharides in the management of hepatic encephalopathy: a meta-analysis. Eur J Gastroenterol Hepatol. 2008;20(11):1064–70.
56. Luo M, Li L, Lu CZ, Cao WK. Clinical efficacy and safety of lactulose for minimal hepatic encephalopathy: a meta-analysis. Eur J Gastroenterol Hepatol. 2011;23(12):1250–7.
57. Als-Nielsen B, Gluud LL, Gluud C. Non-absorbable disaccharides for hepatic encephalopathy: systematic review of randomised trials. BMJ. 2004;328(7447):1046.
58. Perumalswami PV, Schiano TD. The management of hospitalized patients with cirrhosis: the Mount Sinai experience and a guide for hospitalists. Dig Dis Sci. 2011;56(5):1266–81.
59. Bornikova L, Peyvandi F, Allen G, Bernstein J, Manco-Johnson MJ. Fibrinogen replacement therapy for congenital fibrinogen deficiency. J Thromb Haemost. 2011;9(9):1687–704.
60. Mannucci PM, Duga S, Peyvandi F. Recessively inherited coagulation disorders. Blood. 2004;104(5):1243–52.
61. Stanca CM, Montazem AH, Lawal A, Zhang JX, Schiano TD. Intranasal desmopressin versus blood transfusion in cirrhotic patients with coagulopathy undergoing dental extraction: a randomized controlled trial. J Oral Maxillofac Surg. 2010;68(1):138–43.
62. Toubia N, Sanyal AJ. Portal hypertension and variceal hemorrhage. Med Clin North Am. 2008;92(3):551–74. viii.
63. Rossle M, Gerbes AL. TIPS for the treatment of refractory ascites, hepatorenal syndrome and hepatic hydrothorax: a critical update. Gut. 2010;59(7):988–1000.
64. Malinchoc M, Kamath PS, Gordon FD, Peine CJ, Rank J, Borgter PC. A model to predict poor survival in patients undergoing transjugular intrahepatic portosystemic shunts. Hepatology. 2000;31(4):864–71.
65. Ripamonti R, Ferral H, Alonzo M, Patel NH. Transjugular intrahepatic portosystemic shunt-related complications and practical solutions. Semin Intervent Rad. 2006;23(2):165–76.
66. Angermayr B, Cejna M, Karnel F, Gschwantler M, Koenig F, Pidlich J, et al. Child-Pugh versus MELD score in predicting survival in patients undergoing transjugular intrahepatic portosystemic shunt. Gut. 2003;52(6):879–85.
67. Ferral H, Gamboa P, Postoak DW, Albernaz VS, Young CR, Speeg KV, et al. Survival after elective transjugular intrahepatic portosystemic shunt creation: prediction with model for end-stage liver disease score. Radiology. 2004;231(1):231–6.
68. Salerno F, Merli M, Cazzaniga M, Valeriano V, Rossi P, Lovaria A, et al. MELD score is better than Child-Pugh score in predicting 3-month survival of patients undergoing transjugular intrahepatic portosystemic shunt. J Hepatol. 2002;36(4):494–500.
69. Mouroux J, Perrin C, Venissac N, Blaive B, Richelme H. Management of pleural effusion of cirrhotic origin. Chest. 1996;109(4):1093–6.
70. Runyon BA, Greenblatt M, Ming RH. Hepatic hydrothorax is a relative contraindication to chest tube insertion. Am J Gastroenterol. 1986;81(7):566–7.
71. Temes RT, Davis MS, Follis FM, Pett Jr SB, Wernly JA. Videothoracoscopic treatment of hepatic hydrothorax. Ann Thorac Surg. 1997;64(5):1468–9.
72. Siew ED, Deger SM. Recent advances in acute kidney injury epidemiology. Curr Opin Nephrol Hypertens. 2012;21(3):309–17.
73. Coca SG, King Jr JT, Rosenthal RA, Perkal MF, Parikh CR. The duration of postoperative acute kidney injury is an additional parameter predicting long-term survival in diabetic veterans. Kidney Int. 2010;78(9):926–33.
74. Salerno F, Cazzaniga M, Merli M, Spinzi G, Saibeni S, Salmi A, et al. Diagnosis, treatment and survival of patients with hepatorenal syndrome: a survey on daily medical practice. J Hepatol. 2011;55(6):1241–8.
75. European Association for the Study of the L. EASL clinical practice guidelines on the management of ascites, spontaneous bacterial peritonitis, and hepatorenal syndrome in cirrhosis. J Hepatol. 2010;53(3):397–417.
76. Guevara M, Arroyo V. Hepatorenal syndrome. Expert Opin Pharmacother. 2011;12(9):1405–17.
77. Ng CK, Chan MH, Tai MH, Lam CW. Hepatorenal syndrome. Clin Biochem Rev. 2007;28(1):11–7.

78. Northup PG, Argo CK, Bakhru MR, Schmitt TM, Berg CL, Rosner MH. Pretransplant predictors of recovery of renal function after liver transplantation. Liver Transpl. 2010;16(4):440–6.
79. Ruiz R, Kunitake H, Wilkinson AH, Danovitch GM, Farmer DG, Ghobrial RM, et al. Long-term analysis of combined liver and kidney transplantation at a single center. Arch Surg. 2006;141(8):735–41.
80. Wong F, Leung W, Al Beshir M, Marquez M, Renner EL. Outcomes of patients with cirrhosis and hepatorenal syndrome type 1 treated with liver transplantation. Liver Transpl. 2015;21(3):300–7.
81. Abraldes JG, Bosch J. The treatment of acute variceal bleeding. J Clin Gastroenterol. 2007;41 Suppl 3:S312–7.
82. Plauth M, Cabre E, Riggio O, Assis-Camilo M, Pirlich M, Kondrup J, et al. ESPEN guidelines on enteral nutrition: liver disease. Clin Nutr. 2006;25(2):285–94.
83. O'Brien A, Williams R. Nutrition in end-stage liver disease: principles and practice. Gastroenterology. 2008;134(6):1729–40.
84. Dasarathy S. Consilience in sarcopenia of cirrhosis. J Cachexia Sarcopenia Muscle. 2012;3(4):225–37.
85. Montano-Loza AJ, Meza-Junco J, Prado CM, Lieffers JR, Baracos VE, Bain VG, et al. Muscle wasting is associated with mortality in patients with cirrhosis. Clin Gastroenterol Hepatol. 2012;10(2):166–73. 73 e1.
86. Periyalwar P, Dasarathy S. Malnutrition in cirrhosis: contribution and consequences of sarcopenia on metabolic and clinical responses. Clin Liver Dis. 2012;16(1):95–131.
87. Pillard F, Laoudj-Chenivesse D, Carnac G, Mercier J, Rami J, Riviere D, et al. Physical activity and sarcopenia. Clin Geriatric Med. 2011;27(3):449–70.
88. Etherington JM. Emergency management of acute alcohol problems. Part 1: uncomplicated withdrawal. Can Fam Phys. 1996;42:2186–90.
89. Sullivan JT, Sykora K, Schneiderman J, Naranjo CA, Sellers EM. Assessment of alcohol withdrawal: the revised clinical institute withdrawal assessment for alcohol scale (CIWA-Ar). Br J Addict. 1989;84(11):1353–7.
90. Pugh RN, Murray-Lyon IM, Dawson JL, Pietroni MC, Williams R. Transection of the oesophagus for bleeding oesophageal varices. Br J Surg. 1973;60(8):646–9.
91. Daabiss M. American Society of Anaesthesiologists physical status classification. Indian J Anaesth. 2011;55(2):111–5.
92. Steiber AL, Kalantar-Zadeh K, Secker D, McCarthy M, Sehgal A, McCann L. Subjective Global Assessment in chronic kidney disease: a review. J Ren Nutr. 2004;14(4):191–200.

Part II
Distinct Liver Disorders

Chapter 9
Viral Hepatitis: Hepatitis A and E

Adnan Said and Amanda DeVoss

Questions from Patients

1. *How do I become infected with hepatitis A and/or hepatitis E?*

   Both hepatitis A and hepatitis E are viral illnesses. They are brought into the body through the mouth, usually by drinking unclean water. The virus then travels to the liver to multiply.

2. *What are the signs and symptoms of hepatitis A and E infection?*

   For hepatitis A, symptoms can begin around 28 days after initial ingestion. The illness typically starts suddenly with fever, fatigue, anorexia, nausea, abdominal discomfort, dark urine, and jaundice. These symptoms last less than 2 months and do not cause long-term damage. Symptoms from this disease can be linked to your age. In children less than 6 years of age, most (70 %) do not have any symptoms (asymptomatic). In older children and adults, most infections do have symptoms and more than 70 % of patients have jaundice, or yellowing of their skin and eyes. Specific treatment for hepatitis A is not present, so many of the treatments that are used are directed at symptoms. These may include intravenous fluids, anti-nausea medication and acetaminophen for fever.

   Hepatitis E can present very similar to hepatitis A. The symptoms usually start about 2–10 weeks after the initial ingestion. The first symptoms that appear are fever, lack of appetitive, nausea, vomiting, diarrhea, and abdominal pain. These typically last for a few days. As these symptoms lessen, the patient can often become jaundiced or yellow. This is self-limited and will disappear in a few weeks. Chronic disease due to hepatitis E is unlikely in the majority of patients. Treatment for hepatitis E is very similar to hepatitis A.

A. Said, M.D., M.S. (✉) • A. DeVoss, M.M.S., PA-C
Division of Gastroenterology and Hepatology, Department of Medicine, William
S. Middleton VAMC, University of Wisconsin School of Medicine and Public Health,
Madison, WI, USA
e-mail: axs@medicine.wisc.edu

© Springer International Publishing Switzerland 2017
K. Saeian, R. Shaker (eds.), *Liver Disorders*,
DOI 10.1007/978-3-319-30103-7_9

3. *Can I protect myself against getting hepatitis A and E infection?*

A vaccine against hepatitis A does exist. It is given in two doses (0 and 6 months). Nearly 100 % of people who receive both dosages of the vaccine develop immunity to hepatitis A. It is recommended in the USA that all children receive this vaccine between 12 and 23 months of age. It is also recommended for many groups of adults including those who are international travelers, men who have sex with men and persons with chronic liver disease.

Unfortunately, there currently is not an approved vaccine for hepatitis E. This infection is prevented by safe drinking water techniques, proper disposal of human feces and education about personal hygiene.

Outline of Chapter

A. Epidemiology of hepatitis A and hepatitis E

A.1 Incidence of hepatitis A and E in the USA and worldwide
A.2 Geographic distribution
A.3 Age distribution
A.4 Changing incidence over time

Hepatitis A is a reportable illness in the USA [1]. Since the initiation of the hepatitis A vaccine into the routine vaccination schedule for children, there has been a dramatic decrease in the incidence of hepatitis A. This has translated into a two-thirds decrease in admissions to hospitals and markedly lower medical expenditures between 1996 and 2004 [2]. The incidence of hepatitis A in the USA in 2011 was reported at 1398 and estimated to be at 2700 cases. As can be seen in Fig. 9.1, this is significantly lower than in the past decades [1].

Worldwide, approximately 1.5 million clinical cases of hepatitis A occur annually but the rate of infection is likely ten times higher. The incidence rate is strongly related to economics and access to clean drinking water: as mean-income rises and access to clean water improves, the incidence of hepatitis A infection decreases [2].

Distribution of hepatitis A infection worldwide is classified as areas of high, intermediate or low endemicity (see Fig. 9.2) [1, 2]. These areas are differentiated by standards of hygiene and sanitation, the age-dependent clinical expression of the disease, and lifelong immunity [3]. In highly endemic areas of the world, poor sanitation and hygiene lead to most persons being infected at a very young age, when the disease usually has no symptoms. These areas include most of Africa, Asia, and Central/South America.

In developing countries, such as Eastern Europe and other parts of Africa, Asia, and America, sanitation and hygiene is variable [2]. This allows many children to avoid infection in early childhood. Peak incidence in these countries is often in later childhood and adolescents. Infection is later childhood is associated with higher rate of symptomatology. Outbreaks in these countries are often associated with person-to-person contact and are harder to control with standard hygiene measures [2].

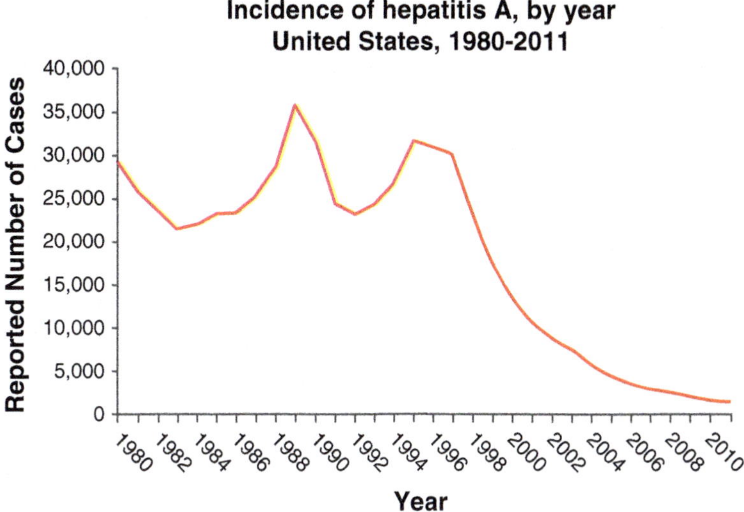

Fig. 9.1   Annual number of cases of hepatitis A in the USA according to the CDC

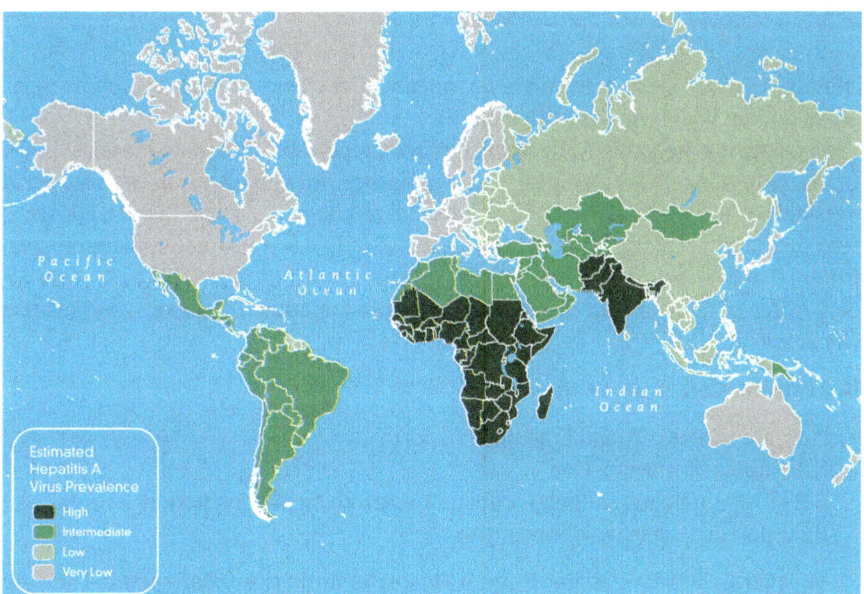

Fig. 9.2   Worldwide prevalence of hepatitis A

In more developed countries, such as North America, Western Europe, Australia, and Japan, sanitation and hygiene is better. This leads to a low incidence and infection rate of hepatitis A. Outbreaks in these countries are often seen with large person-to-person outbreaks (often single source outbreaks such as infected food handler or a contaminated food source from an endemic country) or in specific

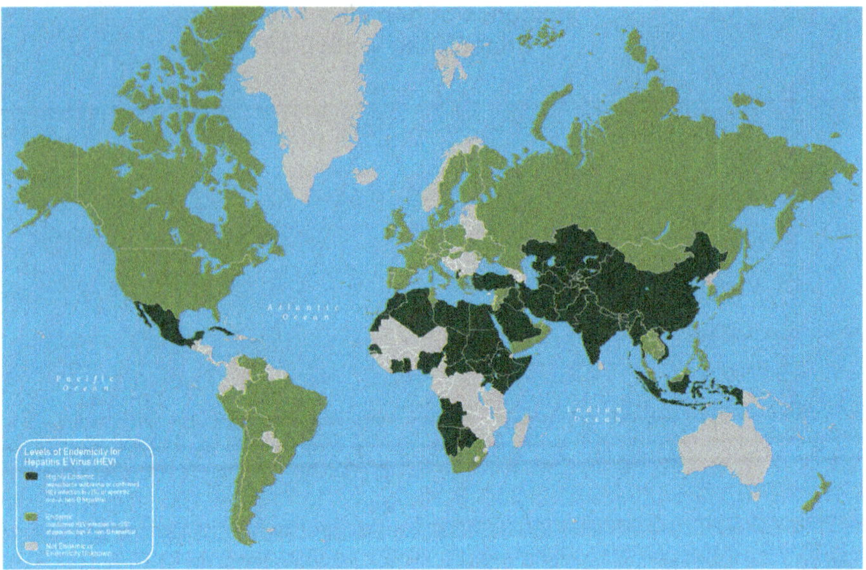

Fig. 9.3 Worldwide epidemiology of hepatitis E

adult risk groups such as travelers to endemic areas, persons who use intravenous drugs or men who have sex with men [2].

In contrast to hepatitis A, hepatitis E is not a reportable disease to the CDC in the USA, so less is known about the exact incidence. Worldwide, it is estimated that one-third of the population has been infected, although the actual disease burden is unknown [4]. Similarly to hepatitis A, hepatitis E has a distinct epidemiological pattern that is based on different rates of infection (see Fig. 9.3] [4]. These areas not only differ in numbers but in routes of transmission, affected persons, and disease characteristics [5].

B. Transmission of hepatitis A and E

How are hepatitis A and E spread?
B.1 Routes of transmission
B.2 Hosts (humans, animals), infectivity period, incubation period
B.3 Sporadic versus epidemic forms

In general, hepatitis A and E are both spread through similar routes. They are both enteric pathogens and are spread through fecal–oral route. Most commonly this is through ingestion of contaminated drinking water. This is where the similarities end, as hepatitis E has the ability to take other routes of infectivity, including different hosts [6, 7].

The incubation period of hepatitis A is roughly 28 days (range of 15–50 days).

Hepatitis A, after infection, replicates in the liver [1]. Humans are the only host for hepatitis A. During the initial period of infectivity (10–12 days), the virus is present in blood and excreted via the biliary system into the feces. It reaches peak titers about 2 weeks before the onset of symptoms. As viral replication and excretion begins to wane, symptoms begin to appear. These symptoms are often indistinguishable from other viral hepatitis'. They include a sudden onset of fever, fatigue, anorexia, nausea, abdominal discomfort, dark urine, and jaundice. Viral excretion has significantly decreased by 7–10 days after the onset of symptoms, with most infected patients no longer shedding virus in the feces by the third week of illness [7, 8].

The clinical illness associated with hepatitis A does not usually last greater than 2 months, but can develop a prolonged or relapsing state in 10–15 % of patients [1]. This can last up to 6 months, with virus being excreted during these relapses [1].

Hepatitis E can have different modes of transmission and reservoirs based on endemic locations worldwide [5]. In areas of the world that are highly endemic, such as Asia, Africa, and Central America, infection is most often transmitted through the fecal–oral route with contaminated drinking water. Water contamination is often related to heavy rainfall and floods. This can lead to large outbreaks of the disease, often affecting thousands of individuals. One to fifteen percent of the population can often be affected by these outbreaks, with young adults being most affected. Men often outnumber women, thought to be related to increased exposure to contaminated water [5].

In regions of the world with lower endemic rates, such as the USA, Western Europe, and developed countries of the Asia-Pacific, hepatitis E infection is quite infrequent [5]. Most are related to recent travel to endemic areas, but an occasional small foodborne outbreak due to locally acquired infection has occurred. Several observations, based on viral genomics, have led to the realization that zoonotic isolates (genotype 3 in the USA, genotype 4 in Asia) of hepatitis E can be spread to humans. This has been observed with ingestion of contaminated wild boar, wild deer and commercially available pig liver. This has led to sporadic outbreaks of hepatitis E in low endemic areas, which differ greatly than larger epidemic outbreaks seen in highly endemic areas [5].

Infectivity rates of hepatitis E are similar to hepatitis A. Viremia and fecal shedding of the hepatitis E virus begin 1–2 weeks prior to symptoms. Fecal shedding of virus lasts approximately 2–4 weeks after the onset of symptoms [4]. Incubation period ranges from 15 to 60 days.

C. Pathogenesis of viral hepatitis A and E including basic virology and hepatitis

Hepatitis A is a small, non-enveloped single-stranded RNA virus. Based on outbreaks and clinical presentation, it was initially thought to be an enterovirus [7]. In 1992, it was classified as a member of the Hepatovirus genus of the family Picornaviridae. This virus replicates inside the hepatocytes and interferes with liver function. This leads to an immune response, thus leading to liver inflammation [2].

Hepatitis E was also initially known as an enterically transmitted non-A, non-B hepatitis virus, which was subsequently named hepatitis E. It is classified in the genus *Hepevirus* and family *Hepeviridae* [7]. This family also includes related viruses that infect pigs, rabbits, rats, deer, and mongoose. Within the genus *Hepevirus*, at least four genotypes have been recognized; Genotype 1 and 2 are restricted to humans, while Genotype 3 and 4 have many hosts (including humans) and are zoonotic [5]. Interspecies transmission has been demonstrated, which has lead to sporadic outbreaks of hepatitis E in non-endemic areas of the world. The hepatitis E virions are small, non-enveloped single-stranded RNA, similar to hepatitis A [7]. This virus infects hepatocytes, leading to replication. It is not directly cytopathic, but instead leads to liver injury due to the host immune response [5].

D. Clinical Presentation of hepatitis A and E

What are the typical and atypical presentations of hepatitis A and E?
D.1 Signs and symptoms
D.2 Clinical spectrum from asymptomatic, to acute hepatitis, acute liver failure, relapsing and cholestatic hepatitis. Chronic hepatitis E in immunosuppressed populations.
D.3 Risk factors for severe outcome
D.4 Natural history of hepatitis A and hepatitis E self limited hepatitis

Hepatitis A and E both have clinical symptoms that are indistinguishable from other forms of acute hepatitis. Both present with nonspecific symptoms including fever, malaise, weakness, anorexia, nausea, vomiting, arthralgias, and myalgias. The prodromal symptoms tend to subside with the onset of jaundice. Jaundice is usually self-limited and lasts for a few weeks. Physical examination often will reveal jaundice, hepatomegaly, and splenomegaly. These are considered to be the typical manifestations of the disease and usually lead to a self-limited disease course [1, 2, 5].

For hepatitis A, symptomatology varies greatly with age. Around 50 % of children, under the age of 6 who become infected are asymptomatic [2]. Of those who do develop symptoms, most are mild and often not recognized to be related to hepatitis. Between 5 and 10 % of children, less than 6, who are infected develop jaundice. Beginning at age 6 and older, more than 75 % of patients develop hepatitis symptoms such as jaundice and dark urine [2].

There are also some atypical features of hepatitis A, which include relapsing hepatitis and prolonged cholestasis [8]. Relapsing hepatitis is characterized by a biphasic peak of serum aminotransferases, with a 4–7 week period in between the phases.

Prolonged cholestatic hepatitis A is characterized by prolonged jaundice often beyond 12 weeks, pruritus, fatigue, loose stools and weight loss in addition to cholestasis [8]. This manifestation can be predicted by detection of plasma hepatitis A RNA after 20 days of illness, while relapsing hepatitis cannot be predicted. Persistence of serum hepatitis A IgM antibodies in serum is also seen in cholestatic hepatitis A.

In both the relapsing and cholestatic form of hepatitis A, the clinical course is spontaneous recovery of liver function [9].

Hepatitis A infection does have the ability to cause acute liver failure and death, although this is a rare occurrence resulting in 0.2 % of cases [10]. The risk of these outcomes increases with age at infection and the presence of underlying chronic liver disease. In some studies, this outcome was thought to be due to a severe host immune response and not direct viral effect [2, 10].

The clinical presentation for hepatitis E varies greatly between high and low endemic areas. In highly endemic regions of the world the most common clinical presentation is an acute icteric hepatitis. Infection in children is often asymptomatic, so many residents may not be aware of an active infection. This form of hepatitis E is often self-limited and will improve in a few weeks [5].

Hepatitis E also has the ability to cause a super infection in those with a preexisting chronic liver disease. These patients can present with an acute-on-chronic liver disease or liver failure. They are at high risk for poor outcome [5]. Lastly, this disease has a higher disease attack rate in pregnant women [5, 11]. These women are more likely to develop fulminant hepatic failure and death with mortality rates reported up to 25 %. These risks appear to increase as the woman advances in her pregnancy [11]. Infants who develop vertically acquired hepatitis E can develop hepatitis and are at greater risk for death [12].

In areas of low disease prevalence, the clinical manifestation of the hepatitis E can look very similar to those in high endemic areas. This includes icteric hepatitis, anicteric illness with nonspecific symptoms and asymptomatic transaminase elevation [5]. Because routine serologic testing for hepatitis E is not available in the USA, this disease is mostly recognized after investigations for all other causes are exhausted. These individuals are usually older, male patients with a high frequency of underlying liver disease or alcohol use. They typically have nonspecific symptoms. Mortality in these regions appears to be higher, but may be due to older age of infection and the presence of comorbid conditions [13, 14]. Prolonged cholestasis (up to 6 months) can also occur after hepatitis E infection

While hepatitis E is overwhelmingly an acute, self-limited infection, it was recently discovered in 2008 in France that immunosuppressed patients, most often solid organ transplant recipients were found to have a chronic form of the disease. It was noted to be due to genotype 3 (often seen in animals) [15]. Chronic hepatitis E infection has also been found in patients with hematological diseases, human immunodeficiency virus infection and those receiving anticancer chemotherapy [16, 17]. Liver biopsies in these patients did confirm the presence of progressing fibrosis, leading to the possibility of the development of cirrhosis in some patients [18].

Among otherwise healthy individuals or in highly endemic areas, chronic infection has not been found in genotype 1 or 2 hepatitis E [5].

E. Diagnosis and Treatment of hepatitis A and E

What is the best way of diagnosing hepatitis A and E and is a liver biopsy necessary?

E.1 Diagnostic tests for hepatitis A and E-evolution, accuracy, sensitivity, specificity (serum, stool, antibodies and PCR)

E.2 Diagnostic tests-role of liver biopsy

E.3 Prognostic tests—how to distinguish markers of poor prognosis and acute liver failure

E.4 Treatment-supportive, role of steroids, role of antivirals, role of liver transplantation.

As previously discussed, the symptoms of both hepatitis A and E are often indistinguishable from other types of hepatitis. Because symptoms are not specific, further diagnostic testing needs to be completed in order to confirm a diagnosis. Initial laboratory testing should include serum transaminases (AST and ALT), total bilirubin, alkaline phosphatase, albumin and coagulation studies, such as PT/INR. In both infections, AST and ALT are the predominately elevated and can often reach levels in the thousands with acute hepatitis A. Alkaline phosphatase is usually only minimally elevated. Bilirubin is usually elevated to coincide with the icteric phase. Coagulopathy can occur in more severe forms of the disease [1, 2, 5–7].

Acute hepatitis A is diagnosed by testing for immunoglobulin M (IgM) antibodies to hepatitis A [1]. This test has a high sensitivity and specificity when drawn on patients with typical symptoms [6]. There is a risk of false positives when drawn on asymptomatic patients. IgM anti-hepatitis A is usually detectable once symptoms have appeared and levels slowly decline to undetectable levels by 6-months in most patients. There have been case reports of IgM anti-hepatitis A remaining positive for greater than 1 year after initial infection was reported [2].

Immunoglobulin G (IgG) anti-hepatitis A develops shortly after infection, and remains positive for a patient's lifetime. Total anti-hepatitis A antibodies can be drawn to investigate immunity but do not identify an acute infection [2]. These laboratory changes can be seen in Fig. 9.4 [18].

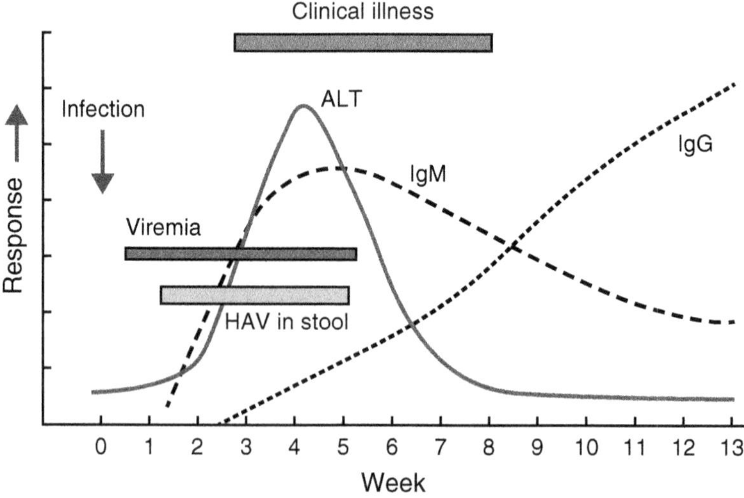

Fig. 9.4 Time course of hepatitis A

Nucleic acid amplification techniques are used primarily for research to detect hepatitis A RNA in serum and stool. Specimens can be frozen during an outbreak to later detect genotyping for epidemiologic purposes [19].

Liver biopsy is often reserved for severe forms of hepatitis A or in situations where the diagnosis is not clear. Since hepatitis A has the ability to cause acute liver failure, attention should be paid to the patient's mental status and coagulation parameters. If a patient develops mental status changes in the setting of increasing bilirubin and PT/INR, referral and transport should be arranged to a liver transplant center for further monitoring.

As hepatitis A is often self-limited, treatment is usually supportive including assuring adequate rest, hydration and nutrition. The patient should be educated to avoid hepatotoxins such as alcohol and acetaminophen [6]. No specific antiviral medication is recommended. In the case of a prolonged, cholestatic course of hepatitis A, corticosteroids have been shown to play a role in shortening the clinical course [19].

Diagnosis of hepatitis E is more difficult as there are no currently FDA approved assays for detection of anti-HEV antibodies in the USA. In highly endemic areas, detection of IgM anti-hepatitis E antibodies is used to indicate a current infection [5]. In these areas, testing is often available. In nonendemic areas, such as the USA, detection of IgM anti-hepatitis E antibodies can also be used, but testing is usually handled through research laboratories or the Center for Disease Control (CDC). Hepatitis E nucleic acid detection using amplification techniques can provide more accurate detection and allows for genotypes to be identified. Because the time course of viremia and viral shedding is brief, this mode of testing often lacks sensitivity [5]. A timeline of these serologic changes can be seen in Fig. 9.5 [5].

Similarly to hepatitis A, hepatitis E is often treated with supportive measures. In patients with suspected acute liver failure, prompt transport and referral to a liver transplant center should be initiated. Treatment with pegylated interferon alpha-2a/alpha-2b or ribavirin alone for 3–12 months has been tried in patients with chronic

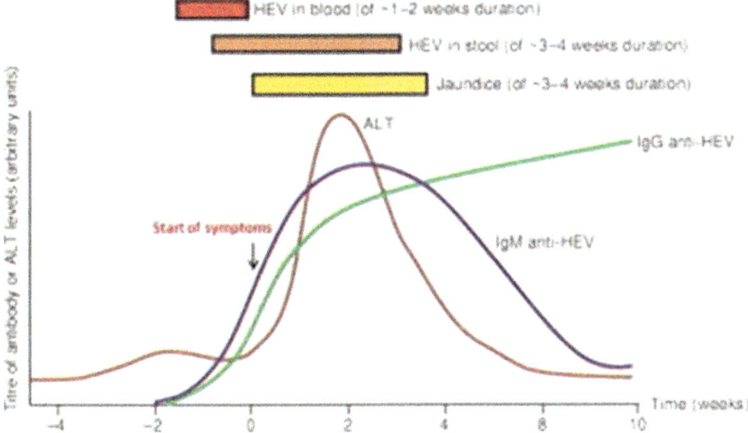

Fig. 9.5 Time course of hepatitis E

or persistent infections [20, 21]. This data was only collected in case reports, and data from controlled trials is not available. In patients with high doses of immunosuppressive medications, dose reduction should be initiated before antiviral medications are given [5]. Patients with chronic hepatitis E with progression to cirrhosis should be monitored for liver decompensation. Referral to a liver transplant center should be initiated in cases of decompensation.

F. Prevention of hepatitis A and E

What precautions should be taken for those suspected of exposure to hepatitis A or E?
F.1 Post-exposure prophylaxis
F.2 Vaccination—who should be vaccinated

Hepatitis A and E can both be prevented through the use of clean drinking water, proper disposal of human feces and education about personal hygiene. During outbreaks, boiling of water can be useful. For zoonotic infections, proper handling and cooking of pig and deer meat is recommended [1, 2, 5].

Although treatment of the patient is supportive, those individuals who are at risk of being infected with hepatitis A are eligible for post-exposure prophylaxis [3]. Immune globulin (IG) is preferred for persons older than 40 years of age, children younger than 12 months of age, immunocompromised persons, and persons with chronic liver disease. In healthy persons aged 12 months to 40 years of age, hepatitis A vaccination is the preferred method of prophylaxis. Administration of IG should be given to eligible persons within 2 weeks of exposure to prevent development or reduce the severity of the disease [3].

For hepatitis A prevention, two inactivated whole virus vaccines are available: HAVRIX (GlaxoSmithKline) and VAQTA (Merck) [3]. Both vaccines are available in pediatric and adult formulations. Both vaccines provide excellent protection against hepatitis A, with more than 95 % of adults developing protective antibody within 4 weeks of the single dose of the vaccine, and close to 100 % of persons will seroconvert after two doses. In children and teens, close to 97 % of persons will be seropositive within 4 weeks of a single dose, and all persons had seroconverted after two doses [3].

Hepatitis A vaccines were originally targeted to persons with increased risk of infection when introduced in 1995 [6]. These mainly included persons who traveled to endemic areas, men who have sex with men, and persons with chronic liver disease. Then in 2005, the Advisory Committee on Immunization Practices (ACIP) recommended that universal hepatitis A vaccination be implemented into the routine childhood vaccination schedule at age 1–2 years. The CDC later adopted this practice into their vaccine recommendations in January 2006 [6].

Unfortunately for hepatitis E, there are no commercially available vaccines or immunoglobulin. Two vaccines have undergone clinical trials that do show efficacy, but have not been brought to market for various issues [5].

References

1. Center for Disease Control. The pink book -epidemiology & prevention of vaccine-preventable diseases. http://www.cdc.gov/vaccines/pubs/pinkbook/downloads/hepa.pdf. Accessed 20 Oct 2014.
2. Franco E, Meleleo C, Serino L, Sorbara D, Zaratti L, Hepatitis A. Epidemiology and prevention in developing countries. World J Hepatol. 2012;4(3):68–73.
3. World Health Organization. Global alert and response: hepatitis A. http://www.who.int/csr/disease/hepatitis/whocdscsredc2007/en/index4.html. Accessed 20 Oct 2014.
4. World Health Organization. Hepatitis E fact sheet. http://www.who.int/mediacentre/factsheets/fs280/en/. Accessed 20 Oct 2014.
5. Aggarwal R, Jameel S. Hepatitis E. Hepatology. 2011;54:2218–26.
6. Brundage S, Fitzpatrick A. Hepatitis A. Amer Fam Phy. 2006;73:2162–8.
7. Sjogren M. Hepatitis A. In: Schiff E, Sorrell M, Maddrey W, editors. Schiff's diseases of the liver. Philadelphia: Lippincott-Raven; 1999. p. 745–56.
8. Jeong S, Lee H, Hepatitis A. Clinical manifestations and management. Intervirology. 2010;53:15–9.
9. Sagnelli E, Coppola N, et al. HAV replication in acute hepatitis with typical and atypical clinical course. J Med Vir. 2003;71:1–6.
10. Rezende G, Roque-Afonso A, Samuel D, et al. Viral and clinical factors associated with the fulminant course of hepatitis A infection. Hepatology. 2003;38:613–8.
11. Khuroo MS, Teli MR, et al. Incidence and severity of viral hepatitis in pregnancy. Am J Med. 1981;70(2):252–5.
12. Khuroo MS, Kamili S, Khuroo MS. Clinical course and duration of viremia in vertically transmitted hepatitis E (HEV) infection in babies born to HEV-infected mothers. J Viral Hep. 2009;16:519–23.
13. Borgen K, Herremans T, Duizer E, et al. Non-travel related hepatitis E virus genotype 3 infections in the Netherlands; a case series 2004-2006. BMC Infect Dis. 2008;8:61.
14. Mansuy JM, Peron JM, Abravanel F, et al. Hepatitis E in the south west of France in individuals who have never visited an endemic area. J Med Virol. 2004;74:419–24.
15. Kamar N, Selves J, Mansuy JM, et al. Hepatitis E virus and chronic hepatitis in organ-transplant recipients. N Engl J Med. 2008;358(8):811–7.
16. Tamura A, Shimizu YK, Tanaka T, et al. Persistent infection of hepatitis E virus transmitted by blood transfusion in a patient with T-cell lymphoma. Hepatol Res. 2007;37(2):113–20.
17. Dalton HR, Bendall RP, Keane FE, et al. Persistent carriage of hepatitis E virus in patients with HIV infection. N Engl J Med. 2009;361:1025–7.
18. Kumar A, Aggarwal R, Naik SR, et al. Hepatitis E virus is responsible for decompensation of chronic liver disease in an endemic region. Indian J Gastro. 2004;23(2):59–62.
19. Yoon EL, Yim HJ, Kim SY, et al. Clinical courses after administration of oral corticosteroids in patients with severely cholestatic acute hepatitis A: three cases. Korean J Hep. 2010;16:329–33.
20. Kamar N, Rostaing L, Abravanel F, et al. Pegylated interferon-alpha for treating chronic hepatitis E virus infection after liver transplantation. Clin Infect Dis. 2010;50:30–3.
21. Kamar N, Rostaing L, Abravanel F, et al. Ribavirin therapy inhibits viral replication in patients with chronic hepatitis E virus infection. Gastroenterology. 2010;139:1612–8.

Chapter 10
Viral Hepatitis: Hepatitis B (& D)

Tatyana Taranukha and Venelin Kounev

What Is the Significance of Having Both Hepatitis B Surface Antibody and Hepatitis B Surface Antigen at the Same Time?

Seroconversion of the HBs antigen and emergence of HBs antibody are associated with clearance of HBV virus and emergence of immunity. However, in approximately 3–5 % of patients with chronic hepatitis B, HBsAg persists despite development of the protective antibody [1, 2]. This is thought to be due to the rise of immune variants which have an altered anti-HBs-binding site. Thus, despite seroconversion, viral replication is able to persist due to failure of recognition by the host immune system. These individuals are at risk for progressive liver disease due to active HBV replication and chronic hepatitis [3]. Chronic infection in such individuals may also be missed if the mutated HBsAg is not detected or screened for. To avoid misdiagnosis, HBsAg, anti-HBs, and anti-HBc antibodies should be checked during routine HBV screening [3].

What Is the Risk of Reactivation?

Patients who are inactive HBsAg carriers and those who have previously recovered from HBV infection are at risk for reactivation during chemotherapy, immunosuppression following organ transplantation, and treatment with corticosteroids or

T. Taranukha, M.D.
Division of Gastroenterology & Hepatology, Medical College of Wisconsin,
Milwaukee, WI, USA
e-mail: ttaranukha@mcw.edu

V. Kounev, M.D. (✉)
Division of Gastroenterology & Hepatology, Medical College of Wisconsin,
Milwaukee, WI, USA
e-mail: vkounev@mcw.edu

© Springer International Publishing Switzerland 2017
K. Saeian, R. Shaker (eds.), *Liver Disorders*,
DOI 10.1007/978-3-319-30103-7_10

immune-modulating agents [4]. Reactivation can be severe, leading to acute liver failure or chronic hepatitis [4]. Delay of treatment until elevation of HBV DNA levels is dangerous and not recommended. Groups at high risk for reactivation include individuals being treated with B-cell-depleting agents particularly rituximab, anthracycline derivates, or 10 mg or greater of prednisone daily for 4 or more weeks. Antiviral prophylaxis for these individuals should be provided for at least 6 months following completion of the immunosuppressive therapy and at least for 12 months following B-cell-depleting agents [5]. To date, there has been insufficient evidence to guide recommendations regarding the role of anti-HBs status in prophylaxis [5].

In terms of treatment, a nucleotide or nucleoside analogue with a more favorable resistance profile than lamivudine should be initiated for the necessary duration of time [5]. Entecavir has recently been shown to be a more effective prophylactic agent in decreasing the risk of HBV reactivation and hepatitis flares when compared to lamivudine in patients undergoing chemotherapy for diffuse large B-cell lymphoma [6].

How Do You Distinguish Acute Hepatitis B Infection from Recurrence or Flare of Chronic Hepatitis B Infection?

Acute HBV infection is classified by appearance of HBsAg and anti-HBc IgM [7]. HBV infection persisting for greater than 6 months is considered chronic [7]. In addition to checking for the presence of anti-HBc IgM, distinction between acute hepatitis and flare of chronic hepatitis can be made by looking at sera from both patient groups. Patients with chronic hepatitis demonstrate higher levels of anti-HBe as well as HBeAg/anti-HBe and HBsAg/anti-HBs immune complexes compared to patients with acute hepatitis [8].

Upon resolution of HBV infection, patients demonstrate both anti-HBc and anti-HBs antibodies. Anti-HBc antibodies persist for life and do not develop in individuals who develop immunity through HBV vaccinations [7].

Should Patients with Isolated Hepatitis B Core Antibody Be Considered for Vaccination?

Isolated presence of anti-HBc is not specific and can be indicative of either the "window period" during acute hepatitis B infection, chronic carrier state where HBsAg is unable to be detected, past infection with waning immunity, or presence of a cross-reacting antibody [9, 10]. In the literature, a wide range (up to 20%) of patients have been reported to be isolated hepatitis B core antibody carriers. Vaccination for hepatitis B in such individuals can help determine the significance of the isolated anti-HBc as well as provide protection to nonimmune individuals.

In previously immune patients, administration of the HBV vaccine would generate an early, high anti-HBs response. The same result would not, however, be observed in individuals who are chronic nonimmune carriers or who have not previously received the HBV vaccine. A follow-up anti-HBs antibody should be ordered 2 weeks after the administration of the HBV vaccine to evaluate response. In individuals with a falsely positive anti-HBc, full immunity would be expected after the administration of the standard three-dose vaccine series [10].

Do I Need a Liver Biopsy If I Have Hepatitis B and My Viral Load Is Low?

A liver biopsy may be helpful in establishing the extent of liver damage in patients with chronic hepatitis who may otherwise not meet guidelines for treatment [11]. ALT is a convenient marker when assessing liver injury; however, ALT levels can exhibit great variability along the course of the HBV infection. In patients with normal liver transaminases and low HBV viral load, treatment is generally not recommended. However, when a liver biopsy was performed on HBeAg-negative patients with HBV viral loads equal to or less than 10,000 copies/mL (equivalent to 2000 IU/mL) and normal ALT levels, severe hepatic fibrosis was noted in 12 % of patients and mild-to-moderate necroinflammation in 26 % of patients [12]. In this case, a liver biopsy was able to identify individuals with progressive liver disease who should receive hepatitis B treatment. Thus, particularly in patients who are HBeAg(−) who have a borderline low viral load and ALT levels <2× the upper limits of normal, consideration should be given to a liver biopsy to help assess whether treatment should be implemented.

When Do I Need to Worry About Occult Hepatitis B?

Occult hepatitis B infection is defined as the presence of viral HBV DNA in liver tissues in individuals who test negative for HBsAg [13]. Occurrence of occult HBV is highest among hepatitis C carriers. It is a significant issue for blood banks and those involved in organ transplantation in which case HBV can be transmitted to the recipient. Though post-transfusion hepatitis remains a rare occurrence in Western countries, in case of orthotopic liver transplantation (OLT), rates of HBV transmission have been estimated to be between 17 and 94 % from HBsAg-negative/anti-HBc-positive donors [13]. Similarly, individuals with occult hepatitis B undergoing OLT may develop reinfection of their graft with concomitant complications and need for therapy. Another concern is the potential for reactivation of occult hepatitis B during periods of immunosuppression leading to acute severe hepatitis as well as acceleration of chronic liver disease and development of HCC, especially in individuals simultaneously co-infected with HCV [13]. Thus, a high level of suspicion and liberal virologic testing must be performed to detect this rare but real issue associated with hepatitis B particularly in those from endemic areas.

What If I Miss a Dose of the Hepatitis B Vaccine Series? Do I Have to Repeat all the Shots?

Primary vaccination for HBV consists of three doses of the intramuscular hepatitis B vaccine administered at 0, 1, and 6 months of age to individuals born in the USA. Typically, a protective antibody response is seen in 30–55 % of individuals less than 40 years of age after the first dose, in approximately 75 % of individuals after the second dose, and in greater than 90 % of individuals after the third dose [14]. Age, smoking, obesity, and immune suppression can contribute to decreased vaccine response [14]. No significant effect is seen on development of immunity by increasing the time between the administrations of the first two vaccine doses. The third dose acts primarily as a booster and provides maximal long-term protection. Thus, it is not necessary to repeat all the shots in a vaccination series if a single dose of the vaccine is missed. However, by increasing the time interval between the doses, there is increased risk of acquiring HBV infection in individuals who have a delayed or incomplete response to vaccination [14].

Though follow-up testing after completion of the vaccination series is not necessary, it is recommended for persons who are at high risk of infection such as healthcare workers, infants of HBsAg-positive mothers, and sexual partners of those with chronic HBV infection [11].

How Do I Prevent Transmission of Hepatitis B to My Baby If I Am Pregnant?

Infants born to HBV-positive mothers should be given hepatitis B immune globulin (HBIG) and hepatitis B vaccine within 12 h of delivery [15]. Combination of HBIG and hepatitis B vaccine has been shown to be up to 95 % effective in preventing transmission of HBV through birth [11]. Furthermore, both the European Association for the Study of Liver Disease and the Asian Pacific Association for the Study of Liver Disease recommend initiation of antiviral therapy during the third trimester for HBsAg-positive mothers with greater than five million copies/mL and ten million copies/mL of HBV DNA, respectively. Lamivudine, telbivudine, or tenofovir should be started between 28 and 32 weeks, or earlier if the viral load is greater than 10^8 copies/mL [15]. Telbivudine and tenofovir both carry the advantage of being pregnancy category B drugs [16]. Antiviral therapy should be stopped within 3 months of delivery or immediately after birth if the mother plans to breastfeed her child [15].

What Is the Risk of Passing HBV to Those I Live With?

Patients with HBV need to be informed regarding the risk of HBV transmission to others. Hepatitis B can be transmitted by close person-to-person contact through open cuts and sores, direct contact with mucosal surfaces, as well as exposure to blood and infectious body fluids such as serum, saliva, and semen [14]. It is recommended that persons with HBV cover up open wounds, clean blood stains with detergent or bleach, and not share toothbrushes or razors [14]. In fact, hepatitis B virus can remain stable at room temperatures for greater than 7 days [14]. Sexual partners also need to be vaccinated against HBV. If a sexual partner is not vaccinated then barrier protection should always be used.

Overall, the risk of developing chronic infection after exposure to HBV ranges from 25 to 30 % in infants and children under the age of five to less than 5 % in adults [11].

What Is My Risk of Liver Cancer?

Individuals who acquired hepatitis B during the perinatal period have the greatest chance of developing hepatocellular carcinoma (HCC), approximately 5 % per decade during their life [17]. Additional risk factors for development of HCC include male gender, family history of HCC, older age, cirrhosis, elevated ALT level, presence of HBeAg, prolonged elevations of HBV DNA, genotype C, and coinfection with hepatitis C [11, 17].

What Can I Do to Reduce My Risk of Cirrhosis?

Active HBV replication, older age, HBV genotype C, ongoing chronic alcohol use, and coinfection with hepatitis C all strongly contribute to development of cirrhosis. It is estimated that progression to cirrhosis occurs at an incidence of 2–6 % in patients with chronic hepatitis B [18]. To decrease the risk of progressive liver disease, patients with HBV should seek treatment if they are HBeAg positive with elevated ALT levels or HBeAg negative with presence of HBV DNA greater than 2000 IU/mL [11]. Adhering to abstinence from alcohol and other potentially hepatotoxic compounds may also further prevent progression of liver disease.

What Can I Do to Reduce My Risk of Liver Cancer?

Hepatitis B-infected patients who are at high risk for hepatocellular carcinoma (HCC) include Africans and African-Americans, Asian men over the age of 40, Asian women over the age of 50, individuals with cirrhosis, family history of HCC, and any carrier of HBV over 40 years of age with persistent or intermittent ALT elevations or HBV DNA level greater than 2000 IU/mL. Robust treatment data indicate that in hepatitis B patients with advanced fibrosis, cirrhosis, or chronic hepatitis B, reduction of HBV DNA leads to a decreased risk of developing HCC [19]. Nucleotide and nucleotide analogues have previously been shown to reduce HBV viral loads and most recently entecavir, an NA, has been demonstrated to have reduced rates of HCC compared to no treatment at 5 years of follow-up [19].

In addition, high-risk individuals should be screened with ultrasound of the liver every 6–12 months. Alpha-fetoprotein (AFP) measurement alone can be used when ultrasound is not available [11]. Periodic AFP testing can also be considered in low-risk individuals in endemic areas as it has a high negative predictive value [20]. Unfortunately, AFP measurement alone is less able to identify lesions at an earlier stage at which point a wider range of treatment options are viable.

Why and When Should HBV Be Treated?

HBV should be treated to halt progression of liver disease, and prevent liver failure and development of hepatocellular carcinoma (HCC) [16, 17]. Per guidelines published by the American Association for the Study of Live Disease (AASLD), treatment is recommended for patients with chronic hepatitis B who are HBeAg positive if they have elevated ALT levels (>2× upper limit of normal (ULN)) or moderate-to-severe hepatitis on biopsy and HBV DNA>20,000 IU/mL as well as those with icteric flares. Consideration should be given to delaying treatment for 3–6 months in those with compensated liver disease in order to determine whether spontaneous HBeAg seroconversion would take place. For patients who are HBeAg negative, there is some discrepancy between various society guidelines but in general the threshold viral load for initiation of therapy is HBV DNA $\geq$ 2000 IU/mL for those with ALT levels >2× ULN [11]. HBeAg(−) patients with HBV DNA $\geq$ 2000 IU/mL but lesser elevations in liver enzymes may benefit from a liver biopsy in deciding whether to initiate treatment if there is moderate-to-severe inflammation or significant fibrosis. Patients with chronic hepatitis B who do not meet the above criteria particularly based on a lower than threshold HBV DNA level but have advanced fibrosis or cirrhosis should also be considered for treatment [21].

What Are the Treatment Options and for How Long Should HBV Be Treated?

In the USA, there are seven medications that are currently approved for treatment of adults with chronic hepatitis B. They are classified either as interferons (interferon-α, pegylated interferon-α), nucleoside analogues (lamivudine, entecavir, and telbivudine), or nucleotide analogues (adefovir, tenofovir) [17, 22]. While all treatments are effective at decreasing HBV DNA levels, nucleoside and nucleotide analogues offer more convenient administration and improved safety profile compared to interferon therapy [17, 21]. Tenofovir and entecavir are currently recommended as first-line oral antiviral agents because of their favorable resistance and efficacy profiles [23].

Duration of treatment depends upon the agent used. Interferons which are typically used with the intent of cure or a sustained virologic response (negative HBV DNA 6 months after cessation of therapy) are given for a defined course of 16–48 weeks. Due to the more limited subgroup of patients likely to respond to and tolerate interferons (HBeAg(+) with higher inflammatory activity, lower viral load, compensated liver disease, and particularly genotype A infection), treatment with this regimen is typically limited to younger and healthier patients particularly those who do not want to remain on long-term therapy.

Nucleoside and nucleotide analogues (NAs) are typically much better tolerated than interferons due to their better side effect profile but the length of therapy is dependent on a number of factors including the patient's baseline characteristics as well as treatment response. They can be used in a wider range of patients than interferons not only due to their much lesser side effect profile but also proven efficacy in a broader group of patients including those who are HBeAg(−) and those with advanced liver disease including those with decompensated liver disease. While resistance is not an issue with interferons, it has been a significant problem with the NAs. Perhaps the main reason entecavir and tenofovir are considered first-line agents is their resistance profile. Entecavir therapy has been reported to have a very low resistance profile in treatment-naïve patients (approximately 1 % after 5 years on therapy) [24]. Documented resistance to tenofovir in the hepatitis B population has not been documented to date. An option available particularly in the HIV population is to use the approved HIV combination medication comprised of tenofovir and emtricitabine since the latter medication also has activity against hepatitis B.

Unfortunately, the required length of therapy with these agents is significantly longer and dictated both by the HBeAg status and the presence or absence of cirrhosis as well as response to therapy. Loss of HBsAg, reduction of HBV DNA level to undetectable levels, seroconversion in HBeAg-positive patients, ALT level normalization, and improvement in liver histology have all been studied as end points to HBV treatment with NAs [7, 17, 21]. The best therapeutic marker, however, appears to be loss of HBsAg as it signifies clearance of the virus as well as development of immunity to hepatitis B. Most patients with chronic hepatitis B who are undergoing treatment with NAs will require 4–5 years of treatment while some patients may need to be treated indefinitely [16].

In a slight oversimplification, most experts essentially do not stop treatment in those with cirrhosis due to concerns about flares and further decompensation with cessation of therapy. In the non-cirrhotic HBeAg(+) population, cessation of treatment can be considered if there is an undetectable viral load and HBeAg seroconversion (development of anti-HBe antibodies). Typically an extended 12 months of consolidation therapy follows the seroconversion before cessation is undertaken. In those who are HBeAg(+) and without cirrhosis, we often counsel the patient that an almost indefinite length of therapy may be warranted. The only subgroup in this population that treatment cessation is considered are those who demonstrate consistent negative HBV DNA viral loads and HBsAg loss (this may or may not be accompanied by development of anti-HBs antibodies). Some experts do extend a consolidation interval of additional treatment for 6–12 months before cessation of the medication.

What Are the Side Effects of HBV Medications?

Both interferon therapy and nucleoside and nucleotide analogues (NAs) are associated with individual side effects. Interferons require subcutaneous injections and are known to cause headaches, nausea, depression, flulike symptoms, as well as anemia and neutropenia. They are also contraindicated in decompensated cirrhosis due to potential for life-threatening side effects [4]. Alternatively, nucleoside and nucleotide analogues can be used during all stages of disease. They are given orally while side effects can include renal and mitochondrial toxicity [16, 17]. Adefovir and tenofovir have both been associated with significant renal dysfunction with prolonged treatment when used at higher doses [4, 16]. Patients taking these NAs should have their creatinine levels monitored regularly and therapy should be modified or discontinued at first sign of renal toxicity. Tenofovir has also been associated with bone loss and reduced bone mineral density while telbivudine has been associated with myopathy [4, 21].

Can My Medications Ever Be Stopped?

Interferons are given for 16–48 weeks [17]. Nucleoside and nucleotide analogues (NAs) are continued until desired therapeutic effect is achieved. Premature discontinuation of NAs can lead to increase in HBV DNA levels and reactivation of hepatitis leading to potential for decompensated liver failure [16, 17]. Most patients undergoing treatment with NAs will require treatment for 4–5 years while some patients particularly those with cirrhosis will likely need to be treated indefinitely [16]. Please see details above.

Should I Be Treated with More Than One Medication to Prevent Resistance?

Combination therapy is used primary in individuals who have developed resistance to the initial treatment of HBV [21]. Though various combination therapies have been investigated, none of the combinations have yet been shown to be superior to monotherapy when the more potent of the two agents is used alone [4]. There was also no increase in long-term response when peginterferon was used in combination with lamivudine in treatment of HBV [4]. Given favorable efficacy and resistance profiles, tenofovir monotherapy remains an excellent choice for patients who have previously developed resistance to other nucleoside or nucleotide analogues [21]. The use of nucleotide and nucleoside combination therapy is promising for those with previously established resistance but cannot be routinely advocated at this time.

What Is the Risk of Resistance?

Treatment of HBV with nucleoside and nucleotide analogues (NAs) can lead to antiviral resistance defined as increase of circulating HBV DNA with decreased efficacy against the antiviral agent [4]. NAs can be classified as L-nucleosides (lamivudine, telbivudine, clevudine), acyclic phosphonates (adefovir, tenofovir), and cyclopentenes (entecavir). It has been shown that development of resistance to lamivudine makes other drugs in the same class ineffective [4]. Risk of drug resistance increases with duration of therapy, persistently elevated HBV levels, patient nonadherence to therapy, previous treatment with nucleotide or nucleoside analogues, and incomplete viral suppression during the first 6 months of therapy [22].

Lamivudine has the highest rate of resistance, estimated to be 70 % after 4 years of continuous treatment. Adefovir, though it has been shown to be effective against both naïve and lamivudine-resistant HBV, also carries a resistance rate of approximately 29 % by year five of treatment [22]. The rate of resistance of entecavir, which requires mutations in multiple locations to reduce its efficacy, is increased from less than 1 % when used in treatment-naïve patients to 43 % after 5 years of therapy in patients with lamivudine-resistant mutants [22]. Tenofovir, the most recently introduced nucleotide analogue, has the best resistance profile to date. As of yet, there has been no noted resistance up to 5 years of therapy [21, 22]. Similarly, there is also no risk of drug-induced resistance associated with the use of interferons [22].

References

1. Lada O, Benhamou Y, Poynard T, Thibault V. Coexistance of hepatitis B surface antigen (HBs Ag) and anti-HBs antibodies in chronic hepatitis B virus carriers: influence of "a" determinant variants. J Virol. 2006;80(6):2968–75.
2. Galati G, Vincentis A, Vespasiani-Gentilucci U, Gallo P, Vincenti D, Solmone M, et al. Coexistance of HBsAg and HBsAb in a difficult-to-treat chronic hepatitis B: loss of HBsAg with entecavir plus tenofovir combination. BMC Gastroenterol. 2014;14(94):1–4.
3. Colson P, Borentain P, Motte A, Henry M, Moal V, Botta-Fridlund D, et al. Clinical and virological significance of the co-existance of HBsAg and anti-HBs antibodies in hepatitis B chronic carriers. Virology. 2007;367:30–40.
4. Hoofnagle J, Doo E, Liang J, Fleischer R, Lok A. Management of hepatitis B; summary of clinical research workshop. Hepatology. 2007;45(4):1056–75.
5. Reddy K, Beavers K, Hammond S, Lim J, Falck-Ytter Y. American Gastroenterological Association Institute Guideline on the prevention and treatment of hepatitis B virus reactivation during immunosuppresive drug therapy. Gastroenterology. 2015;148(1):215–9.

6. Huang H, Li X, Zhu J, Ye S, Zhang H, Wang W, et al. Entecavir vs lamivudine for prevention of hepatitis B virus reactivation among patients with untreated diffuse large B-cell lymphoma receiving R-CHOP chemotherapy: a randomized clinical trial. JAMA. 2014;312(23):2521–30.

7. LeFevre M. Screening for hepatitis B virus infection in nonpregnant adolescents and adults: U.S. Preventative Services Task Force Recommendation Statement. Ann Intern Med. 2014;161(1):58–67.

8. Maruyama T, Schodel F, Iino S, Koike K, Yasuda K, Peterson D, et al. Distinguishing between acute and symptomatic chronic hepatitis B virus infection. Hepatology. 1988;8(4):766–70.

9. Draelos M, Morgan T, Schifman R, Sampliner R. Significance of isolated antibody to hepatits B core antigen determined by immune response to hepatitis B vaccination. JAMA. 1987;258(9):1193–5.

10. Al-Mekhaizeem K, Miriello M, Sherker A. The frequency and significance of isolated hepatitis B core antibody and the suggested management of patients. Can Med Assoc J. 2001;165(8):1063–4.

11. Lok A, McMahon J. AASLD practice guidelines: chronic hepatitis B. Hepatology. 2007;45(2):507–39.

12. Al-Mahtab M, Rahman S, Akbar S, Kamal M, Khan M. Clinical use of liver biopsy for the diagnosis and management of inactive and aymptomatic hepatitis B virus carriers in Bangladesh. J Med Virol. 2010;82:1350–4.

13. Raimondo G, Pollicino T, Cacciola I, Squadrito G. Occult hepatitis B virus infection. J Hepatol. 2007;46:160–70.

14. Mast E, Weinbaum C, Fiore A, Alter M, Bell B, Finelli L, et al. A comprehensive immunization strategy to eliminate transmission of hepatitis B virus infection in the United States. Recommendations of the Advisory Committee on Immunization Practices (ACIP) part II: immunization of adults. MMWR. 2006;54(RR16):1–23.

15. Sarkar M, Terrault N. Ending vertical transmission of hepatitis B: the third trimester intervention. Hepatology. 2014;60(2):448–51.

16. Reddy K, Pavri T. Long-term safety of HBV therapies and when to stop therapy. Crit Issues HBV. 2014;1(1):17–9.

17. Sorrell M, Belongia E, Costa J, Gareen I, Grem J, Inadomi J, et al. National Institutes of Health Consensus Development Conference Statement: management of hepatitis B. Ann Intern Med. 2009;150(2):104–10.

18. Chu C, Liaw Y. Hepatitis B virus-related cirrhosis: natural history and treatment. Semin Liver Dis. 2006;26(2):142–52.

19. Hosaka T, Suzuki F, Kobayashi M, Seko Y, Kawamura Y, Sezaki H, et al. Long-term entecavir treatment reduces hepatocellular carcinoma incidence in patients with hepatitis B virus infection. Hepatology. 2013;58(1):98–107.

20. Keefe E, Dieterich D, Han S, Jacobson I, Martin P, Schiff E, et al. A treatment algoright for the management of chronic hepatitis B virus infection in the United States. Clin Gastroenterol Hepatol. 2004;2(2):87–106.

21. Wong R, Gish R. Implementing best practices when initiating hepatitis B virus therapy. Crit Issues HBV. 2014;1(1):5–10.

22. Lau D, Javaid A. Evaluating underlying causes of HBV treatment failure. Crit Issues HBV. 2014;1(1):13–5.

23. Lok A, McMajon B. Chronic hepatitis B: update 2009. Hepatology. 2009;50(3):661–2.

24. Heo NY, Lim YS, Lee HC, Chung YH, Lee YS, Suh DJ. Lamivudine plus adefovir or entecavir for patients with chronic hepatitis B resistant to lamivudine and adefovir. J Hepatol. 2010; 53(3):449.

Chapter 11
Viral Hepatitis: Hepatitis C

Chalermrat Bunchorntavakul and K. Rajender Reddy

Questions

What Are the Risk Factors for HCV Infection and What Are the Clinical Features of Acute Hepatitis C?

Acute hepatitis C (AHC) has a spectrum of clinical presentation and course, and its diagnosis can be challenging in a significant proportion of patients. Risk factors of HCV infection and persons for whom HCV screening is recommended are summarized in Table 11.1 [1]. However, it should be noted that these risk factors may not be present in up to one-third of patients, especially among Asians [2–4]. The prompt diagnosis of AHC is crucial in order to allow close monitoring and early treatment, which effectively prevent disease transmission and consequences of liver disease. Nowadays, AHC is often encountered among intravenous drug users, men who have sex with men, and in the health care associated settings [3–5].

Clinical presentation of AHC ranges from asymptomatic alanine aminotransferase (ALT) elevation to acute icteric hepatitis with symptoms of nausea, vomiting, and abdominal pain [3–5]. The most frequently used individual criteria for defining

C. Bunchorntavakul, M.D.
Division of Gastroenterology and Hepatology, Department of Medicine, Hospital of the University of Pennsylvania, 2 Dulles, 3400 Spruce Street, Philadelphia, PA 19104, USA

Department of Medicine, Rajavithi Hospital, College of Medicine, Rangsit University, Rajavithi Road, Ratchathewi, Bangkok 10400, Thailand
e-mail: dr.chalermrat@gmail.com

K.R. Reddy, M.D. (⊠)
Division of Gastroenterology and Hepatology, Department of Medicine, Hospital of the University of Pennsylvania, 2 Dulles, 3400 Spruce Street, Philadelphia, PA 19104, USA
e-mail: rajender.reddy@uphs.upenn.edu

© Springer International Publishing Switzerland 2017
K. Saeian, R. Shaker (eds.), *Liver Disorders*,
DOI 10.1007/978-3-319-30103-7_11

"

Table 11.1 Risk factors for HCV infection and the recommendation for HCV testing

Persons born between 1945 and 1965
Persons with risk behaviors, exposures, and conditions associated with an increased risk of HCV infection
• Risk behaviors
– Injection-drug use (current or ever)
– Intranasal illicit drug use
• Risk exposures
– Long-term dialysis
– Getting a tattoo or body piercing in unregulated setting
– Healthcare, emergency medical and public safety workers after needle sticks, sharps, or mucosal exposure to HCV-related blood
– Children born to HCV-infected women
– Prior recipients of transfusions or organ transplantation before 1992
– Persons who were ever incarcerated
• Other medical conditions
– HIV infection
– Unexplained chronic liver disease and chronic hepatitis
– Medical conditions that may causality related to HCV infection, such as mixed cryoglobulinemia and membranoproliferative glomerulonephritis

a case includes anti-HCV seroconversion, acute ALT elevation, and HCV-RNA detection [6]. Testing for anti-HCV alone cannot be used to diagnose AHC in the early phase, since it generally is detected after 4–12 weeks after HCV inoculation [3–5]. Substantial changes in HCV-RNA and ALT activity are commonly seen in patients with AHC, whereas intermittent and transient HCV-RNA negativity and ALT normalization can also be observed [4, 5, 7]. Thus, patients with acute hepatitis C warrant careful monitoring with repeated testing of HCV-RNA, ALT and serology, as well as exclusion of other causes of acute hepatitis.

The majority (60–80 %) of individuals exposed to HCV evolve on to chronic infection [3]. Several host and viral factors, including younger age, female gender, presence of symptoms and/or jaundice, antiviral broadly specific, durable and polyfunctional T cell response, immunogenetic polymorphisms such as IL28B, human immune-deficiency virus (HIV) infection, low dose HCV inoculum, and high initial HCV-RNA, have been known to favorably impact spontaneous resolution of acute hepatitis C [3–5, 8, 9]. Approximately 80 % of patients with self-limiting hepatitis C experience HCV-RNA clearance within 3 months of onset of infection. Persistent viremia beyond 6 months of infection is usually associated with evolution to chronic infection [10–12].

The *European Association for the Study of the Liver* (EASL) guidelines suggest following HCV-RNA every 4 weeks, and that only those who remain positive at 12 weeks from onset be treated [13–15]. Treatment of AHC had traditionally been with pegylated interferon (PEG-IFN) monotherapy for 12–24 weeks, with expected successful rate around 90 % [12–17]. Initiation of treatment before or at week 12 after onset of AHC results in higher sustained virological response (SVR) rates than initiation beyond week 20 [15, 18]. The combination of PEG-IFN plus ribavirin (RBV) and direct acting antivirals (DAA)-based regimens are also likely to be effective in AHC, but these need large clinical trials to confirm [1, 14]. Also, the use of DAAs alone is likely to be influenced by their availability in resource constrained regions of the World.

What Are the Natural History and the Consequences of Chronic HCV Infection?

Persistent viremia beyond 6 months of infection indicates chronic infection [10–12]. Once chronic infection is established, spontaneous clearance of HCV is very rare. Published estimates of fibrosis progression and time to cirrhosis are dependent on study design and the patient population, while one large systematic review of 111 studies estimated prevalence of cirrhosis at 20 years after the infection to be 14–19 % [19] (Fig. 11.1). Fibrosis progression in chronic hepatitis C is variable and depends on numerous host, viral, and environmental factors, such as age at acquisition of infection, sex, race, genetic factors, alcohol consumption, insulin resistance, and coinfection with other viruses [20] (Table 11.2). Identification of these factors is important because modifiable factors can be altered and high-risk patients should be treated promptly. For example, insulin resistance, obesity, and/or hepatic steatosis

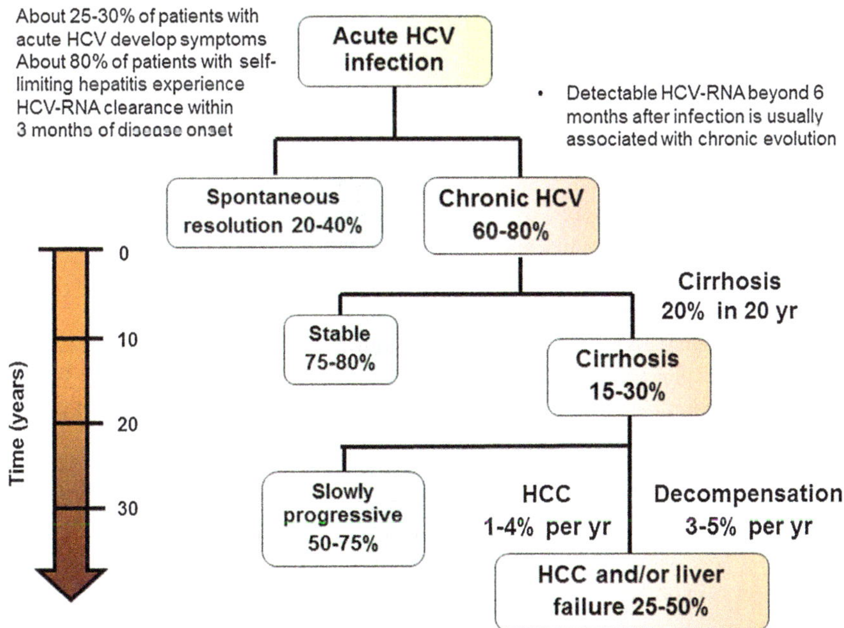

Fig. 11.1 Natural history of hepatitis C. *HCV* hepatitis C virus, *HCC* hepatocellular carcinoma

Table 11.2 Factors associated with HCV disease progression

Established factors	Possible factors
• Age at infection >40 years	• Male gender
• Caucasians	• HCV genotype 3
• Obesity[a]	• Cigarette smoking[a]
• Fatty liver[a]	• Increased hepatic iron concentration
• Metabolic syndrome/insulin resistance[a]	• High level of serum transaminases
• Alcohol consumption >20 g/day[a]	
• Daily use of marijuana[a]	
• Immunosuppressed state[a]	
• Schistosomiasis	
• HIV coinfection	
• Hepatitis B coinfection	

[a]Modifiable risk factors

have shown to accelerate progression of fibrosis and possibly increase risk of HCC in patients with HCV [21]. Weight reduction is associated with decrease in hepatic steatosis and the rate of fibrosis progression [21].

It should be noted that serum ALT level has high visit-to-visit variability and is not a good indicator of liver disease activity or fibrosis in HCV patients [22]. Prospective data from community-based cohort of 1,235 HCV-infected persons found that ALT levels were persistently normal in 42 %, persistently elevated in 15 %, and intermittently elevated in 43 % [22]. Patients with persistently normal serum ALT levels tend to have significantly lower scores for inflammation and fibrosis, compared with patients with elevated serum ALT levels; however advanced fibrosis/cirrhosis and portal inflammation can be observed histologically in 12 and 26 % of those with persistently normal and abnormal ALT, respectively [23]. Traditionally, the gold standard for the assessment of the stage of fibrosis in HCV has been to perform percutaneous liver biopsy and then staging by METAVIR, Ishak, or Knodell scoring systems. However, in real-life practice, liver biopsy may be limited by patient's acceptance, pain, risk of bleeding, and the possibility for sampling error. Therefore, noninvasive methods to assess liver injury and fibrosis (e.g., transient elastography, serum direct and indirect fibrotic markers) have been evaluated and are becoming increasingly available and used. Although no single noninvasive test or combination of tests developed to date can parallel the information obtained from actual histology, noninvasive methods, particularly when used in combination, can reliably differentiate between minimal and significant fibrosis or cirrhosis, and thereby avoid liver biopsy in a significant percentage of patients [24].

Among patients with HCV-induced cirrhosis, manifestations of liver failure (e.g., ascites, variceal bleeding, encephalopathy, and hepatorenal syndrome) develop in 3–5 % per year, and HCC develops in 1–4 % per year [25–27]. Once decompensation has developed, survival rate is about 50 % at 5 years and LT is the only effective therapy [25–27] (Fig. 11.1).

HCV infection can be associated with other extrahepatic conditions, such as impaired quality of life, insulin resistance, mental impairment, depression, lymphoproliferative (e.g., essential mixed cryoglobulinemia and lymphoma) and autoimmune disorders [28, 29]. Further, HCV generates a major financial burden to society. In 1997, the total cost of HCV-related illness in the USA was estimated to be $5.46 billion ($1.80 billion direct costs and $3.66 billion indirect costs) [30]. The projected annual direct medical care cost of HCV treatment from 2010 to 2019 is $6.5–$13.6 billion, with indirect costs expected to reach $75.5 billion [31].

Do I Require Treatment for Chronic Hepatitis C?

Antiviral therapy should be considered for all patients with chronic HCV infection. In most circumstances, the decision of whether or not to proceed with treatment is based on the patient's desire and the need for therapy. The degree of the need is a subjective assessment that is made upon considering the stage of liver disease, presence or absence of favorable factors for treatment response, safety and efficacy of the available treatment options, age and comorbid conditions.

The primary goal of treatment of HCV infection is eradication or "cure" of the virus. Sustained virologic response (SVR, undetectable HCV-RNA by sensitive assay after 12–24 weeks after completion of therapy) is known to be an excellent surrogate marker for the cure of HCV. In an extensive review of 44 long-term follow studies after treatment-induced SVR, HCV-RNA was noted to have remained undetectable in 97 % of a combined total of >4,000 HCV patients, many of whom were immunosuppressed, during their follow-up periods (range from 2 to >10 years) [32, 33]. Several studies have clearly demonstrated that SVR is associated with a substantial reduction in hepatic inflammation, reversal of fibrosis and even of cirrhosis, as well as improvement in health-related quality of life [34–38]. Hence, the risk of liver failure, at least over the short term, is virtually eliminated in patients with cirrhosis who achieve an SVR [36–38]. Notably, the risk of HCC after SVR in patients with cirrhosis is reduced by more than one half; however the risk is not eliminated and surveillance for HCC in cirrhotics must continue [37, 38]. Additional cirrhosis care, in those who achieved SVR, such as surveillance for varices is necessary although we currently do not know if the frequency of surveillance should remain the same as for those without viral clearance or those with other etiologies for cirrhosis. Successful treatment of HCV has been associated with a decrease in liver related mortality, need for liver transplantation, and also with a decrease in all-cause mortality [39].

How Effective Has Interferon-Based Regimen Been and What Have the Challenges Been?

Interferon-based regimen, mainly with PEG-IFN plus ribavirin (RBV), had been the standard of care of HCV therapy for more than a decade [14, 40]. Two forms of PEG-IFN are available (PEG-IFN alfa-2a and alfa-2b), and RBV should be administered according to the body weight of the patient. Although smaller trials from Europe have suggested slightly higher SVR rates with PEG-IFN alfa-2a [41, 42], a large US multicenter study did not detect any significant difference in SVR between the two PEG-IFNs plus RBV [43]. While IFN-based therapies have almost been completely replaced by IFN-free DAA-based therapies in the USA, a combination of PEG-IFN/RBV will be still widely utilized in the developing countries for quite some time because access to new drugs are restricted and delayed by policies, limited resources, and economic barriers.

PEG-IFN/RBV treatment is administered for either 48 weeks (for HCV genotypes 1, 4, 5, and 6) or for 24 weeks (for HCV genotypes 2 and 3), inducing SVR rates of 40–50 % in those with genotype 1, 50–60 % in those with genotype 4, 60–90 % in those with genotype 6, and >70–85 % in those with genotypes 2 and 3 infection [14, 40, 44]. Several host (e.g., age, race, IL-28 B genotype, obesity, metabolic, comorbidities and presence of advanced fibrosis and cirrhosis), viral (e.g., viral load and genotype), environmental (e.g., substance and alcohol abuse), and treatment-related factors (e.g., side effects, adherent to therapy) have been shown to influence the SVR rates following IFN-based therapy. It should be noted that HCV treatment outcome with PEG-IFN/RBV in Asians seems to be superior to that of non-Asian populations, and this may be due to several factors that include a favorable IL28B genotype [2, 44]. Host genetic polymorphisms located on chromosome 19 near the region coding for IL28B (or IFN lambda-3) is associated with SVR following treatment with PEG-IFN/RBV in HCV genotype 1, but also to a lesser extent for genotype 2 and 3 [45, 46]. IL28B testing is useful to predict virologic response at week 4 as a predictive marker for the success of treatment with PEG-IFN/RBV, but its role in protease inhibitor-based triple therapy is less significant, and is insignificant in IFN-free treatment regimen [45, 46]. Improvement of SVR rates with IFN-based therapy can be achievable by correction of modifiable risk factors, treatment adherence and response-guided adjustment of the treatment duration (response-guided therapy, RGT) [14] (Fig. 11.2).

One of the challenges in utilizing PEG-IFN/RBV therapy is management of the treatment-related side effects. The common side effects of PEG-IFN include influenza-like syndrome (fever, headache, malaise, and myalgia), cytopenia, sleep disturbance, hair loss and psychiatric effects, whereas the unusual and severe side effects include seizure, psychosis, severe depression, autoimmune reactions, bacterial infections, and thyroid dysfunction. The major side effects of RBV are hemolytic anemia, cough, rash, and teratogenicity. These side effects are generally manageable by pretreatment advice, proper clinical and laboratory monitoring, symptomatic treatment, and appropriate dose reduction of the related drugs. In cases with significant RBV-induced anemia (hemoglobin <10 g/dL), a stepwise RBV dose decrement is suggested to maintain RBV exposure during treatment in order to minimize virologic relapse [14, 47]. This strategy has been proven not to compromise the SVR rate, and erythropoiesis-stimulating agents may also be useful in select patients with difficulty in management of anemia especially in those with cirrhosis and/or multiple comorbidities [47, 48].

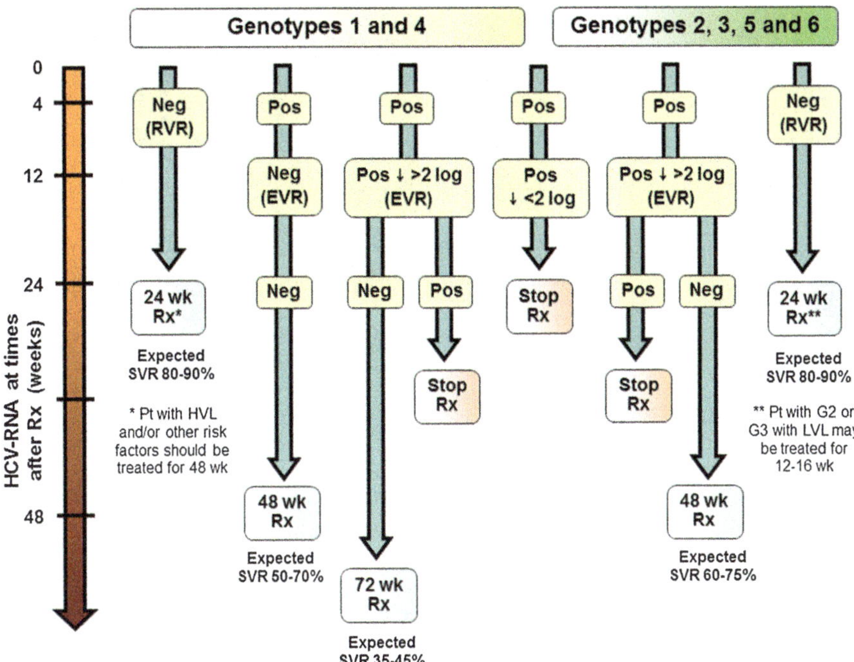

Fig. 11.2 Recommendations for response-guided therapy with pegylated interferon plus ribavirin and the expected sustained virological response rates. *SVR* sustained virological response, *RVR* rapid virological response, *EVR* early virological response, *HVL* high viral load, *LVL* low viral load, *Pt* patients, *G* genotype

What Are the Current Treatment Options?

Therapies for chronic HCV have been evolving rapidly over the past few years, mainly due the development of new DAA targeting NS3/4A, NS5A, and NS5B HCV proteins (Table 11.3) [1, 13, 49, 50]. Accordingly, treatment-induced SVR rates have been consistently improving, and now IFN-free DAA combination regimen with short duration of treatment (<3 months), single or few pills per day, and >95 % SVR rates have become widely available. Currently, some of these all-oral combinations (such as sofosbuvir/ledipasvir with or without RBV, sofosbuvir plus simeprevir, paritaprevir/ritonavir/ombitasvir plus dasabuvir with or without RBV) have already been approved in the USA and some countries in Europe. Most recently, daclatasvir in combination with sofosbuvir with or without RBV has also been approved for use in the USA, and previously in Europe and in Japan and provides a viable option particularly for those with genotype 3 infection. At this evolving stage of HCV management, it is suggested to continuously update the most recent recommendations for HCV treatment via the American Association for the Study of Liver Disease (AASLD), and EASL websites [1, 13]. The recent Infectious

Table 11.3 Pharmacologic properties and potential for drug–drug interactions of anti-HCV medications

Drugs	Metabolism/excretion route	Interaction with CYP and substrate transporters	Dosage adjustment in patients with renal impairment (RI)	Dosage adjustment in patients with liver impairment
Pegylated interferons (PEG-IFN)				
PEG-IFN alfa-2a	Renal (main) and hepatic (minor)	No	135 µg/week (25–45 % reduction) for severe RI/ESRD	Not recommended for CTP class B/C
PEG-IFN alfa-2b	Renal	No	1.125 µg/kg/week (25 % reduction) for moderate RI; 0.75 µg/kg/week (50 % reduction) for severe RI/ESRD	Not recommended for CTP class B/C
Ribavirin				
Ribavirin	Renal	No	200–400 mg/day for moderate RI; 200 mg/day for severe RI/ESRD	No dose adjustment is required for cirrhosis (with careful monitoring)
NS3/4A protease inhibitors				
Telaprevir	Hepatic (CYP3A)	Strong CYP3A inhibitor, moderate P-gp inhibitor	No dose adjustment is required for any degree of RI (clinical data is limited)	No dose adjustment is required in compensated cirrhosis; not recommended for CTP class B/C
Boceprevir	Hepatic (CYP3A, aldoketo-reductase)	Moderate CYP3A inhibitor, weak P-gp inhibitor	No dose adjustment is required for any degree of RI (clinical data is limited)	No dose adjustment is required in compensated cirrhosis; not recommended for CTP class B/C
Simeprevir	Hepatic (CYP3A)	Mild CYP1A2 and CYP3A inhibitor, inhibitor of OATP1B1 and MRP2	No dose adjustment is required for mild-severe RI; no data in ESRD	No dose adjustment is required in compensated cirrhosis; not recommended for CTP class C
Paritaprevir (ABT-450)/ritonavir	Hepatic (CYP3A)	Strong CYP3A inhibitor (ritonavir), inhibitor of OATP1B1, substrate of P-gp and BCRP	No dose adjustment is required for mild-moderate RI; no data in severe RI/ESRD	No dose adjustment is required in compensated cirrhosis; not recommended for CTP class C

Asunaprevir	Hepatic (CYP3A)	Weak CYP3A4 inducer, moderate CYP2D6 inhibitor, inhibitor of P-gp and OATP1B1	No dose adjustment is required for any degree of RI (clinical data is limited)	No dose adjustment is required in compensated cirrhosis; not recommended for CTP class B/C
NS5A replication complex inhibitors				
Daclatasvir	Hepatic (CYP3A)	Not a CYP3A inducer/inhibitor, moderate inhibitor of P-gp and OATP1B1	No dose adjustment is required for any degree of RI (clinical data is limited)	No dose adjustment is required in compensated cirrhosis; not recommended for CTP class C
Ledipasvir	Feces (major); hepatic and renal (minor)	Not a CYP inducer/inhibitor, weak inhibitor of P-gp and OATP1B1	No dose adjustment is required for mild-moderate RI; no data in severe RI/ESRD	No dose adjustment is required for any degree of liver impairment
Ombitasvir (ABT-267)	Amide hydrolysis and oxidative metabolism	Not a CYP inducer/inhibitor, substrate of P-gp and BCRP	No dose adjustment is required for mild-moderate RI; no data in severe RI/ESRD	No dose adjustment is required in compensated cirrhosis; not recommended for CTP class C
NS5B nucleotide polymerase inhibitors				
Sofosbuvir	Renal	Not a CYP inducer/inhibitor, substrate of P-gp	No dose adjustment is required for mild-moderate RI; no data in severe RI/ESRD	No dose adjustment is required for any degree of liver impairment
NS5B non-nucleoside polymerase inhibitors				
Dasabuvir (ABT-333)	Hepatic (CYP2C8 60 %, CYP3A4 30 % and CYP2D6 10 %)	Not a CYP inducer/inhibitor, substrate of P-gp and BCRP	No dose adjustment is required for mild-moderate RI; no data in severe RI/ESRD	No dose adjustment is required in compensated cirrhosis; not recommended for CTP class C

Adapted from Tischer S, Fontana RJ. J Hepatol 2014;60:872–84 and Bunchorntavakul C, Tanwandee T. Gastroenterol Clin North Am 2015; in press
CYP cytochrome P450, *P-gp* P-glycoprotein, *BCRP* breast cancer resistance protein, *MRP* multiple drug resistance protein, *OATP* organic anion transporting polypeptide, *RI* renal impairment, *ESRD* end-stage renal disease, *CTP* Child–Turcotte–Pugh

Diseases Society of America (IDSA)/AASLD guidance is summarized in Table 11.4, and with these regimens, the expected SVR rates are over 90% for non-cirrhotic and cirrhotic patients with any of the HCV genotypes [1]. However, in real-life practice, treatment regimen for HCV may not be generalizable due to many reasons such as patient's comorbidities, physician's preference, availability and cost of DAA in each country, as well as the reimbursement policy. Therefore, the appropriate HCV treatment regimens should be tailored based on the risk of progressive liver disease in an individual patient, associated comorbidities, local or regional treatment guidelines and cost-effectiveness analyses.

What Are the Challenges, If Any, in Treating Special Populations Such as Those With, Renal Failure, Decompensated Liver Disease, Liver Transplantation, and HIV Infection?

The management of HCV in special populations is challenging, particularly when treating with IFN-based therapy, due to reduced efficacy of treatment, increased treatment-related side effects, altered pharmacokinetics, as well as the potential for drug–drug interactions. Important pharmacokinetic and metabolic properties of PEG-IFN, RBV and selected DAA are summarized in Table 11.3 [49, 50]. New generation DAA-based therapy, especially the IFN-free/RBV-free regimens, are preferred. The efficacy and safety data of the currently approved all-oral DAA combinations is compelling for use is special HCV populations, as recently been recommended by the AASLD/IDSA guidance (Table 11.5).

HCV Infection in Patients with End-Stage Renal Disease (ESRD) (Fig. 11.3)

HCV infection in patients with ESRD is associated with more rapid liver disease progression, more liver-related mortality and reduced renal graft and patient survival following kidney transplantation [51–55]. It should also be noted that serum ALT levels in patients with ESRD are lower than in the general population, and there is a weak correlation between ALT levels and liver disease activity in this population [53, 56]. The pharmacokinetics of IFN, RBV and some DAA, such as sofosbuvir, are altered in patients with ESRD. With dose adjustment and careful monitoring, treatment with PEG-IFN plus RBV in HCV patients with ESRD can be associated with SVR rates nearly comparable to those with normal renal function [53, 56, 57]. In patients with severe renal impairment (creatinine clearance, CrCl <30 mL/min) or ESRD on dialysis, the dose recommendations are 135 µg/week for PEG-IFN alfa-2A, and 1 µg/kg/week or 50% reduction for PEG-IFN alfa-2B), and 200 mg/day for ribavirin [1]. Based on the

Table 11.4 AASLD/IDSA guidance for the treatment of chronic HCV infection

	Treatment-naïve patients	Patients whom prior PEG-IFN plus RBV treatment has failed
HCV genotype 1a	• SOF-LDV for 12 weeks • PTV-RTV-OMV + DSV + RBV for 12 weeks (no cirrhosis) or 24 weeks (cirrhosis) • SOF + SMV, ±RBV for 12 weeks (no cirrhosis) or 24 weeks (cirrhosis) • DCV + SOF for 12 weeks (no cirrhosis) or DCV + SOF ± RBV for 24 weeks (cirrhosis)	• Same as treatment-naïve • Patients in whom PEG-IFN + RBV ± PI has failed: SOF-LDV for 12 weeks (no cirrhosis) or SOF-LDV + RBV for 12 weeks (cirrhosis) or SOF-LDV 24 week (cirrhosis)
HCV genotype 1b	• SOF-LDV for 12 weeks • PTV-RTV-OMV + DSV for 12 weeks • SOF + SMV ± RBV for 12 weeks (no cirrhosis) or 24 weeks (cirrhosis) • DCV + SOF for 12 weeks (no cirrhosis) or DCV + SOF ± RBV for 24 weeks (cirrhosis)	• Same as treatment-naïve • Patients in whom PEG-IFN + RBV ± PI has failed: SOF-LDV for 12 weeks (no cirrhosis) or SOF-LDV + RBV for 12 weeks (cirrhosis) or SOF-LDV 24 week (cirrhosis)
HCV genotype 2	• SOF + RBV for 12 weeks (no cirrhosis) or 16 weeks (cirrhosis) • DCV + SOF for 12 weeks (no cirrhosis) or for 16 weeks (cirrhosis) in RBV-intolerant	• SOF + RBV for 16–24 weeks • SOF + RBV + PEG-IFN[a] for 12 weeks • DCV + SOF ± RBV[a] for 24 weeks if IFN-ineligible
HCV genotype 3	• DCV + SOF for 12 weeks (no cirrhosis) or DCV + SOF ± RBV for 24 weeks (cirrhosis) • SOF + RBV + PEG-IFN for 12 weeks if IFN-eligible • SOF + RBV[a] for 24 weeks	• Same as treatment naïve
HCV genotype 4	• SOF-LDV for 12 weeks • PTV-RTV-OMV + DSV + RBV for 12 weeks • SOF + RBV for 24 weeks • SOF + RBV + PEG-IFN[a] for 12 weeks	• Same as treatment-naïve • SOF + RBV + PEG-IFN for 12 weeks
HCV genotype 5	• SOF-LDV for 12 weeks • SOF + RBV + PEG-IFN[a] for 12 weeks	• Same as treatment-naïve
HCV genotype 6	• SOF-LDV for 12 weeks • SOF + RBV + PEG-IFN[a] for 12 weeks	• Same as treatment-naïve

SOF sofosbuvir, *LDV* ledipasvir, *SMV* simeprevir, *PTV* paritaprevir, *RTV* ritonavir, *OMV* ombitasvir, *DSV* dasabuvir, *PEG-IFN* pegylated interferon, *RBV* ribavirin, *DCV* daclatasvir, *PI* protease inhibitors
[a]Alternative regimens

Table 11.5 Summary of AASLD/IDSA guidance for the treatment of chronic HCV infection in special populations

Decompensated cirrhosis	
HCV genotype 1 or 4	• SOF-LDV + RBV (initial dose of 600 mg, increased as tolerate) for 12 weeks (consider 24 weeks for prior sofosbuvir failure) • DCV + SOF + RBV (initial dose of 600 mg, increased as tolerate) for 12 weeks • DCV + SOF for 24 weeks (if RBV intolerant or ineligible)
HCV genotype 2 or 3	• DCV + SOF + RBV (initial dose of 600 mg, increased as tolerate) for 12 weeks • SOF + RBV for up to 48 weeks
Recurrent HCV post liver transplantation	
HCV genotype 1	• SOF-LDV + RBV for 12 weeks (including compensated cirrhosis) • DCV + SOF + RBV (initial dose of 600 mg, increased as tolerate) for 12 weeks (including compensated cirrhosis) • SOF-LDV[a] for 24 weeks (including compensated cirrhosis) • DCV + SOF[a] for 24 weeks (including compensated cirrhosis) • PTV-RTV-OMV + DSV + RBV[a] for 24 weeks (for early recurrence: fibrosis stage 0–2) • SOF[a] + SMV ± RBV for 12 weeks
HCV genotype 2	• DCV + SOF + RBV (initial dose of 600 mg, increased as tolerate) for 12 weeks • SOF + RBV for 24 weeks • DCV[a] + SOF for 24 weeks
HCV genotype 3	• DCV + SOF + RBV (initial dose of 600 mg, increased as tolerate) for 12 weeks • SOF + RBV for 24 weeks • DCV[a] + SOF for 24 weeks
HCV genotype 4	• SOF-LDV + RBV for 12 weeks • DCV + SOF + RBV (initial dose of 600 mg, increased as tolerate) for 12 weeks • SOF-LDV[a] for 24 weeks • DCV[a] + SOF for 24 weeks
HIV-HCV coinfection	
DCV	• DCV requires dose adjustment with ritonavir-boosted atazanavir (a decrease to 30 mg daily) and efavirenz or etravirine (an increase to 90 mg daily)
SOF-LDV	• Because LDV increases tenofovir levels, concomitant use of LDV with tenofovir disoproxil fumarate mandates consideration of CrCl rate and should be avoided in those with CrCl below 60 mL/min • Because potentiation of this effect is expected when tenofovir is used with RTV-boosted HIV protease inhibitors, LDV should be avoided with this combination (pending further data) unless ARV cannot be changed and the urgency of treatment is high

(continued)

Table 11.5 (continued)

PTV-RTV-OMV+DSV	• PTV-RTV-OMV+DSV should be used with ARV with which it does not have substantial interactions: raltegravir, dolutegravir, enfuvirtide, tenofovir, emtricitabine, lamivudine, and atazanavir
	• The dose of RTV used for boosting of HIV protease inhibitors may need to be adjusted (or held) when administered with PTV-RTV-OMV+DSV and then restored when HCV treatment is completed
	• HIV protease inhibitor should be administered at the same time as the fixed-dose HCV combination
SMV	• SMV should only be used with ARV with which it does not have clinically significant interactions: raltegravir (and probably dolutegravir), rilpivirine, maraviroc, enfuvirtide, tenofovir, emtricitabine, lamivudine, and abacavir

SOF sofosbuvir, *LDV* ledipasvir, *SMV* simeprevir, *PTV* paritaprevir, *RTV* ritonavir, *OMV* ombitasvir, *DSV* dasabuvir, *PEG-IFN* pegylated interferon, *RBV* ribavirin, *DCV* daclatasvir, *PI* protease inhibitors

[a]Alternative regimens

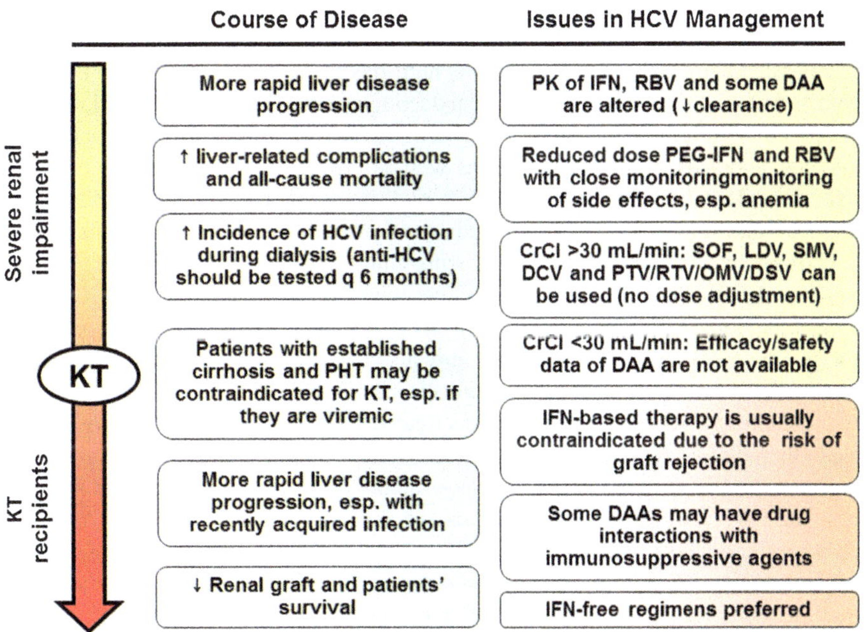

Fig. 11.3 Natural history and management of hepatitis C in patients with severe renal impairment and kidney transplantation. *HCV* hepatitis C virus, *KT* kidney transplantation, *PHT* portal hypertension, *PEG IFN* pegylated interferon, *RBV* ribavirin, *PK* pharmacokinetics, *DAA* direct acting antivirals, *SOF* sofosbuvir, *LDV* ledipasvir, *DCV* daclatasvir, *SMV* simeprevir, *PTV* paritaprevir, *RTV* ritonavir, *OMV* ombitasvir, *DSV* dasabuvir, *CrCl* creatinine clearance

available data, the AASLD/IDSA guidance advised that no dose reduction is needed when using sofosbuvir in HCV patients with mild to moderate renal impairment (CrCl ≥30 mL/min). However, sofosbuvir is not recommended in patients with severe renal impairment/ESRD (CrCl <30 mL/min) or those who require dialysis until more data becomes available [1]. For DAA with primarily hepatic metabolism (e.g., boceprevir, simeprevir, daclatasvir), no dosage adjustment is required for patients with mild/moderate to severe renal impairment although these agents have not been adequately studied in patients with ESRD, including those requiring dialysis [1]. For patients with mild to moderate renal impairment (CrCl >30 mL/min), no dose adjustment is required when using sofosbuvir, simeprevir, fixed-dose combination of sofosbuvir/ledipasvir, or fixed-dose combination of paritaprevir/ritonavir/ombitasvir plus dasabuvir [1]. However, the safety and efficacy data of all-oral DAA regimens are limited in those with CrCl <30 mL/min [1].

HCV Infection in Patients with Decompensated Cirrhosis (Fig. 11.4)

Treatment of HCV is strongly recommended for patients with advanced fibrosis and compensated cirrhosis as an SVR in this high-risk group is associated with a significant decrease of the incidence of clinical decompensation and HCC [38, 39]. Further, successful viral eradication may then facilitate delay, or, in a small proportion of patients, avoid liver transplantation, as well as prevent HCV recurrence following liver transplantation. However, the SVR rates are generally lower with IFN-based therapies and side effects occur more commonly in patients with advanced fibrosis or cirrhosis when compared to patients with mild to moderate fibrosis [38, 39, 58]. Treatment with PEG-IFN/RBV in patients with decompensated cirrhosis is somewhat disappointing due to low efficacy (SVR 7–30 % for genotype 1, and 44–57 % for genotype 2/3) and high rates of treatment-related side effects (led to dose reduction in 40–70 % and treatment discontinuation in 13–40 %) [59, 60]. A French cohort (CUPIC Study Group) of HCV cirrhosis treated with boceprevir- or telaprevir-based triple therapy ($N=674$) reported a high incidence of serious adverse events, including death, in those with platelet count <100,000/mm^3 and/or albumin <3.5 g/L at baseline [61]. Further the real-world experience (HCV-TARGET study ($N=2084$; 38 % had cirrhosis) revealed that triple therapy was associated with high rate of adverse events (12 % had serious adverse events) and involved frequent treatment modifications [62]. Therefore, these triple therapies have no role in patients with decompensated liver disease, and newer generation DAA, preferably IFN-free regimens, are required in this population. The pharmacokinetics of sofosbuvir, ledipasvir and daclatasvir do not appear to change significantly in patients with moderate or severe liver impairment. A fixed-dose combination of paritaprevir/ritonavir/ombitasvir plus dasabuvir and RBV appear to be safe in patients with compensated cirrhosis, but should not be used in decompensated patients. Similarly, simeprevir is not recommended in Child Class B and C cirrhosis. The AASLD/IDSA guideline recommends that patients with decompensated cirrhosis can be treated with all-oral DAA

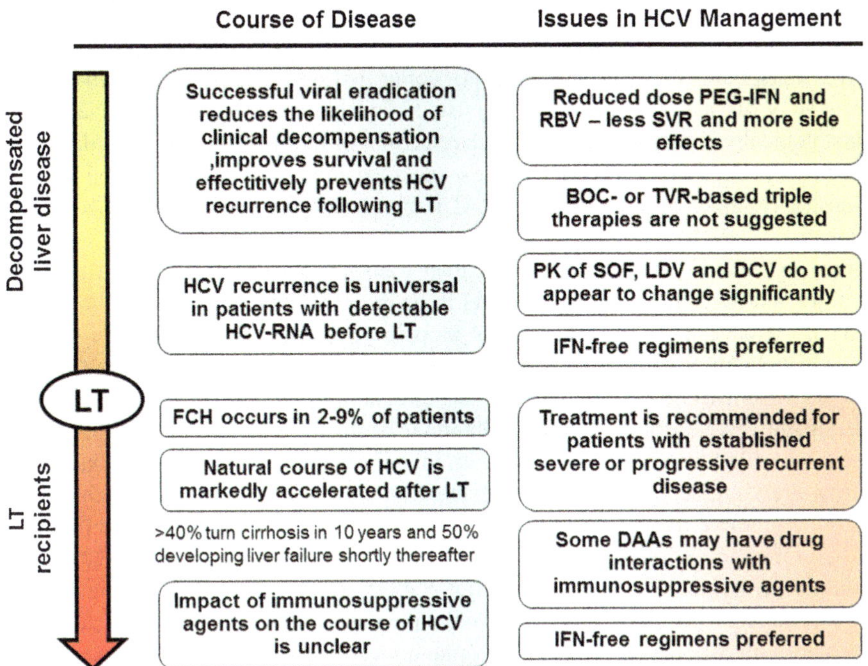

Fig. 11.4 Natural history and management of hepatitis C in patients with decompensated liver disease and liver transplantation. *HCV* hepatitis C virus, *LT* liver transplantation, *FCH* fibrosing cholestatic hepatitis, *SVR* sustained virological response, *PEG-IFN* pegylated interferon, *RBV* ribavirin, *DAA* direct acting antivirals, *PK* pharmacokinetics, *BOC* boceprevir, *TVR* telaprevir, *SOF* sofosbuvir, *LDV* ledipasvir, *DCV* daclatasvir

regimens containing sofosbuvir, ledipasvir, and RBV, according to the HCV genotypes (Table 11.5). These recommended all-oral combination regimens are generally associated with SVR rates nearly similar to that of patients without decompensated cirrhosis [1]. The majority of patients with decompensated cirrhosis will improve their liver function following SVR, which may sometimes facilitate the avoidance of liver transplantation; however liver disease progression can be observed in some patients, particularly those with pretreatment MELD >15 [63]. The antiviral treatment should be started at least 3 months before anticipated surgery with a goal of undetectable HCV-RNA for at least 30 days [63].

HCV Infection in Liver Transplant Recipients (Fig. 11.4)

Liver transplantation in HCV patients is associated with suboptimal graft survival which is attributable to universal recurrence of HCV in the graft [59, 64, 65]. The natural course of HCV is accelerated in liver transplant recipients, with more than

40% progressing to cirrhosis within 10 years and approximately 50% developing liver failure shortly thereafter [59, 64, 65]. The recommended standard of care for liver transplant recipients is treatment of confirmed significant or progressive recurrent HCV disease, based either on persistent, unexplained elevated ALT levels or on histologically confirmed fibrosis once rejection, biliary obstruction, vascular complication, and other causes have been excluded [59, 64, 65]. Due to the lack of sensitivity and specificity of serum ALT in determining the severity of recurrent hepatitis C, HCV recipients ideally should undergo protocol liver biopsies starting from around 6–12 months following liver transplantation [59, 64, 65]. The availability and high success rate of DAAs in treating this patient population may ultimately obviate the need for protocol biopsies. Treatment with PEG-IFN/RBV is associated with SVR rates of 24–40% in LT recipients, but adverse effects are common (two-thirds of patients required dose reductions and one-fourth discontinued treatment early). Boceprevir- and telaprevir-based triple therapy has been associated with higher rates of SVR, but with higher rates of side effects, and has major drug–drug interaction issues in which the immunosuppressive regimens needs to be closely monitored and preemptively adjusted during the treatment period [59, 66]. Therefore, these triple therapies are not recommended by the recent AASLD/IDSA and EASL guidelines. The AASLD/IDSA guidance recommend that patients with recurrent HCV post-liver transplant, including those with compensated cirrhosis, be treated with all-oral DAA regimens containing sofosbuvir, ledipasvir, simeprevir, daclatasvir, and RBV, according to the genotypes. Tacrolimus or cyclosporine dose adjustments are not needed when treating with these combinations. However, careful monitoring is recommended because of the lack of safety data in this group of patients (Table 11.5). The fixed-dose combination of paritaprevir/ritonavir/ombitasvir plus dasabuvir and RBV for 24 weeks can be an alternative regimen for patients with genotype 1 in the allograft, without cirrhosis [1]. Notably, ritonavir is a strong CYP3A inhibitor, and therefore the dose of calcineurin inhibitors should be adjusted and closely monitored during the treatment. The benefit of immunosuppressive strategy on the natural history HCV recurrence has not been well elucidated, although there has been evidence suggesting a neutral or small beneficial effect of cyclosporine A, mycophenolate mofetil, and sirolimus [59, 64, 65].

HCV Infection in Patients With Human Immunodeficiency Virus (HIV) Infection

In developed countries, approximately 15–25% of HIV-infected persons are chronically infected with HCV [67–69]. The prevalence of HIV/HCV coinfection varies markedly depending on the route of HIV acquisition, being lower among persons reporting high-risk sexual exposure (8–15%) and higher in those reporting injection drug use (50–90%) [68, 69]. HIV infection adversely affects the natural history of HCV, leading to increased viral persistence after acute infection, higher levels of viremia, accelerated progression to cirrhosis and ESLD, and increased risk of liver-related death [68–70]. Successful HCV eradication in HIV-infected patients not only prevents liver disease progression, but is also associated with a reduction in the risk of antiretroviral (ARV)-induced hepatotoxicity, HIV disease progression and non–liver-related mortality [68, 69, 71, 72].

Prompt treatment for HCV should be considered in all patients with HIV/HCV coinfection; however, in patients with CD4+ cell count <200 cells/mm^3, it may be preferable to improve the CD4+ cell count by starting ARV before HCV treatment [1, 13, 14]. In the interferon era, HCV treatment in HIV-infected patients was limited due to historically low response rates, patient comorbidities, physician perception, adverse effects associated with IFN-based therapy and drug–drug interactions [1]. Treatment with PEG-IFN plus RBV, can eradicate HCV in 14–29 % of HIV-infected patients coinfected with HCV genotype 1 and 44–73 % of patients coinfected with HCV genotype 2 or 3) [73] With the availability of HCV DAAs, SVR rates have markedly improved, but treatment requires awareness of complex drug interactions between DAAs and ARV therapy (Table 11.3). The AASLD//IDSA guidance has recommended that HIV/HCV coinfected patients be treated and retreated the same as non-HIV patients, after recognizing and managing interactions with ARV (Tables 11.4 and 11.5). These recommended all-oral combination regimens are generally associated with SVR rates of >90 % and similar to that of non-HIV patients. Sofosbuvir generally has no/minimal interaction with ARV, but it is not recommended for use with tipranavir because of the potential of this drug to induce P-gp [1]. Ledipasvir can increase the concentration of tenofovir that is in ARV regimen and present risk of nephrotoxicity. Simeprevir concentration are significantly decreased when dosed with efavirenz and increased when dosed with darunavir/ritonavir [1]. Because 100 mg of ritonavir is coformulated with paritaprevir and ombitasvir, the total dose of ritonavir must be carefully considered and adjusted when using ritonavir-boosted regimen [1, 74]. The combined use of RBV and didanosine is contraindicated due to the potential for dangerous interactions resulting in mitochondrial toxicity causing hepatic steatosis, liver failure, peripheral neuropathy, pancreatitis, and lactic acidosis [75]. The combined use of RBV and zidovudine should also be avoided due to increased rate of anemia [76].

Acknowledgements *Conflict of Interest:* KRR: Advisory Board: Abbvie, Merck, Gilead, BMS, and Janssen. Grant support paid to the University of Pennsylvania: Abbvie, Merck, Gilead, BMS, and Janssen. CB: Nothing to disclose.

References

1. American Association for the Study of Liver Diseases and Infectious Diseases Society of America. Recommendations for testing, managing, and treating hepatitis C. http://www.hcvguidelines.org/full-report-view.
2. Nguyen LH, Nguyen MH. Systematic review: Asian patients with chronic hepatitis C infection. Aliment Pharmacol Ther. 2013;37(10):921–36.
3. Kamal SM. Acute hepatitis C: a systematic review. Am J Gastroenterol. 2008;103(5):1283–97. quiz 98.

4. Wang CC, Krantz E, Klarquist J, Krows M, McBride L, Scott EP, et al. Acute hepatitis C in a contemporary US cohort: modes of acquisition and factors influencing viral clearance. J Infect Dis. 2007;196(10):1474–82.
5. Bunchorntavakul C, Jones LM, Kikuchi M, Valiga ME, Kaplan DE, Nunes FA, et al. Distinct features in natural history and outcomes of acute hepatitis C. J Clin Gastroenterol. 2015;49(4):e31–40.
6. Hajarizadeh B, Grebely J, Dore GJ. Case definitions for acute hepatitis C virus infection: a systematic review. J Hepatol. 2012;57(6):1349–60.
7. Loomba R, Rivera MM, McBurney R, Park Y, Haynes-Williams V, Rehermann B, et al. The natural history of acute hepatitis C: clinical presentation, laboratory findings and treatment outcomes. Aliment Pharmacol Ther. 2011;33(5):559–65.
8. Liu L, Fisher BE, Thomas DL, Cox AL, Ray SC. Spontaneous clearance of primary acute hepatitis C virus infection correlated with high initial viral RNA level and rapid HVR1 evolution. Hepatology. 2012;55(6):1684–91.
9. Tillmann HL, Thompson AJ, Patel K, Wiese M, Tenckhoff H, Nischalke HD, et al. A polymorphism near IL28B is associated with spontaneous clearance of acute hepatitis C virus and jaundice. Gastroenterology. 2010;139(5):1586–92. 92 e1.
10. Gerlach JT, Diepolder HM, Zachoval R, Gruener NH, Jung MC, Ulsenheimer A, et al. Acute hepatitis C: high rate of both spontaneous and treatment-induced viral clearance. Gastroenterology. 2003;125(1):80–8.
11. Santantonio T, Medda E, Ferrari C, Fabris P, Cariti G, Massari M, et al. Risk factors and outcome among a large patient cohort with community-acquired acute hepatitis C in Italy. Clin Infect Dis. 2006;43(9):1154–9.
12. Kamal SM, Moustafa KN, Chen J, Fehr J, Abdel Moneim A, Khalifa KE, et al. Duration of peginterferon therapy in acute hepatitis C: a randomized trial. Hepatology. 2006;43(5):923–31.
13. European Association for the Study of the Liver Recommendations on Treatment of Hepatitis C.http://www.easl.eu/_newsroom/latest-news/easl-recommendations-on-treatment-of-hepatitis-c-2014.
14. EASL. Clinical Practice Guidelines: management of hepatitis C virus infection. J Hepatol. 2011;55(2):245–64.
15. Kamal SM, Fouly AE, Kamel RR, Hockenjos B, Al Tawil A, Khalifa KE, et al. Peginterferon alfa-2b therapy in acute hepatitis C: impact of onset of therapy on sustained virologic response. Gastroenterology. 2006;130(3):632–8.
16. Santantonio T, Fasano M, Sagnelli E, Tundo P, Babudieri S, Fabris P, et al. Acute hepatitis C: a 24-week course of pegylated interferon alpha-2b versus a 12-week course of pegylated interferon alpha-2b alone or with ribavirin. Hepatology. 2014;59(6):2101–9.
17. Wiegand J, Buggisch P, Boecher W, Zeuzem S, Gelbmann CM, Berg T, et al. Early monotherapy with pegylated interferon alpha-2b for acute hepatitis C infection: the HEP-NET acute-HCV-II study. Hepatology. 2006;43(2):250–6.
18. Corey KE, Mendez-Navarro J, Gorospe EC, Zheng H, Chung RT. Early treatment improves outcomes in acute hepatitis C virus infection: a meta-analysis. J Viral Hepat. 2010;17(3):201–7.
19. Thein HH, Yi Q, Dore GJ, Krahn MD. Estimation of stage-specific fibrosis progression rates in chronic hepatitis C virus infection: a meta-analysis and meta-regression. Hepatology. 2008;48(2):418–31.
20. Missiha SB, Ostrowski M, Heathcote EJ. Disease progression in chronic hepatitis C: modifiable and nonmodifiable factors. Gastroenterology. 2008;134(6):1699–714.
21. Goossens N, Negro F. The impact of obesity and metabolic syndrome on chronic hepatitis C. Clin Liver Dis. 2014;18(1):147–56.
22. Inglesby TV, Rai R, Astemborski J, Gruskin L, Nelson KE, Vlahov D, et al. A prospective, community-based evaluation of liver enzymes in individuals with hepatitis C after drug use. Hepatology. 1999;29(2):590–6.

23. Shiffman ML, Stewart CA, Hofmann CM, Contos MJ, Luketic VA, Sterling RK, et al. Chronic infection with hepatitis C virus in patients with elevated or persistently normal serum alanine aminotransferase levels: comparison of hepatic histology and response to interferon therapy. J Infect Dis. 2000;182(6):1595–601.

24. Smith JO, Sterling RK. Systematic review: non-invasive methods of fibrosis analysis in chronic hepatitis C. Aliment Pharmacol Ther. 2009;30(6):557–76.

25. Alberti A, Vario A, Ferrari A, Pistis R. Review article: chronic hepatitis C—natural history and cofactors. Aliment Pharmacol Ther. 2005;22 Suppl 2:74–8.

26. Seeff LB. Natural history of chronic hepatitis C. Hepatology. 2002;36(5 Suppl 1):S35–46.

27. Afdhal NH. The natural history of hepatitis C. Semin Liver Dis. 2004;24 Suppl 2:3–8.

28. Jacobson IM, Cacoub P, Dal Maso L, Harrison SA, Younossi ZM. Manifestations of chronic hepatitis C virus infection beyond the liver. Clin Gastroenterol Hepatol. 2010;8(12):1017–29.

29. Zignego AL, Ferri C, Pileri SA, Caini P, Bianchi FB. Extrahepatic manifestations of hepatitis C Virus infection: a general overview and guidelines for a clinical approach. Dig Liver Dis. 2007;39(1):2–17.

30. Leigh JP, Bowlus CL, Leistikow BN, Schenker M. Costs of hepatitis C. Arch Intern Med. 2001;161(18):2231–7.

31. Wong JB, McQuillan GM, McHutchison JG, Poynard T. Estimating future hepatitis C morbidity, mortality, and costs in the United States. Am J Public Health. 2000;90(10):1562–9.

32. Seeff LB. Sustained virologic response: is this equivalent to cure of chronic hepatitis C? Hepatology. 2013;57(2):438–40.

33. Welker MW, Zeuzem S. Occult hepatitis C: how convincing are the current data? Hepatology. 2009;49(2):665–75.

34. Poynard T, Moussalli J, Munteanu M, Thabut D, Lebray P, Rudler M, et al. Slow regression of liver fibrosis presumed by repeated biomarkers after virological cure in patients with chronic hepatitis C. J Hepatol. 2013;59(4):675–83.

35. John-Baptiste AA, Tomlinson G, Hsu PC, Krajden M, Heathcote EJ, Laporte A, et al. Sustained responders have better quality of life and productivity compared with treatment failures long after antiviral therapy for hepatitis C. Am J Gastroenterol. 2009;104(10):2439–48.

36. Maylin S, Martinot-Peignoux M, Moucari R, Boyer N, Ripault MP, Cazals-Hatem D, et al. Eradication of hepatitis C virus in patients successfully treated for chronic hepatitis C. Gastroenterology. 2008;135(3):821–9.

37. George SL, Bacon BR, Brunt EM, Mihindukulasuriya KL, Hoffmann J, Di Bisceglie AM. Clinical, virologic, histologic, and biochemical outcomes after successful HCV therapy: a 5-year follow-up of 150 patients. Hepatology. 2009;49(3):729–38.

38. Singal AG, Volk ML, Jensen D, Di Bisceglie AM, Schoenfeld PS. A sustained viral response is associated with reduced liver-related morbidity and mortality in patients with hepatitis C virus. Clin Gastroenterol Hepatol. 2010;8(3):280–8. 8 e1.

39. van der Meer AJ, Veldt BJ, Feld JJ, Wedemeyer H, Dufour JF, Lammert F, et al. Association between sustained virological response and all-cause mortality among patients with chronic hepatitis C and advanced hepatic fibrosis. JAMA. 2012;308(24):2584–93.

40. Ghany MG, Strader DB, Thomas DL, Seeff LB. Diagnosis, management, and treatment of hepatitis C: an update. Hepatology. 2009;49(4):1335–74.

41. Ascione A, De Luca M, Tartaglione MT, Lampasi F, Di Costanzo GG, Lanza AG, et al. Peginterferon alfa-2a plus ribavirin is more effective than peginterferon alfa-2b plus ribavirin for treating chronic hepatitis C virus infection. Gastroenterology. 2010;138(1):116–22.

42. Rumi MG, Aghemo A, Prati GM, D'Ambrosio R, Donato MF, Soffredini R, et al. Randomized study of peginterferon-alpha2a plus ribavirin vs peginterferon-alpha2b plus ribavirin in chronic hepatitis C. Gastroenterology. 2010;138(1):108–15.

43. McHutchison JG, Lawitz EJ, Shiffman ML, Muir AJ, Galler GW, McCone J, et al. Peginterferon alfa-2b or alfa-2a with ribavirin for treatment of hepatitis C infection. N Engl J Med. 2009;361(6):580–93.

44. Bunchorntavakul C, Chavalitdhamrong D, Tanwandee T. Hepatitis C genotype 6: a concise review and response-guided therapy proposal. World J Hepatol. 2013;5(9):496–504.

45. Balagopal A, Thomas DL, Thio CL. IL28B and the control of hepatitis C virus infection. Gastroenterology. 2010;139(6):1865–76.
46. Ge D, Fellay J, Thompson AJ, Simon JS, Shianna KV, Urban TJ, et al. Genetic variation in IL28B predicts hepatitis C treatment-induced viral clearance. Nature. 2009;461(7262):399–401.
47. Bunchorntavakul C, Reddy KR. Ribavirin: how does it work and is it still needed? Curr Hepatitis Rep. 2011;10:168–78.
48. Sulkowski MS, Shiffman ML, Afdhal NH, Reddy KR, McCone J, Lee WM, et al. Hepatitis C virus treatment-related anemia is associated with higher sustained virologic response rate. Gastroenterology. 2010;139(5):1602–11. 11 e1.
49. Kiser JJ, Burton Jr JR, Everson GT. Drug-drug interactions during antiviral therapy for chronic hepatitis C. Nat Rev Gastroenterol Hepatol. 2013;10(10):596–606.
50. Tischer S, Fontana RJ. Drug-drug interactions with oral anti-HCV agents and idiosyncratic hepatotoxicity in the liver transplant setting. J Hepatol. 2014;60(4):872–84.
51. Okoh EJ, Bucci JR, Simon JF, Harrison SA. HCV in patients with end-stage renal disease. Am J Gastroenterol. 2008;103(8):2123–34.
52. Fabrizi F, Takkouche B, Lunghi G, Dixit V, Messa P, Martin P. The impact of hepatitis C virus infection on survival in dialysis patients: meta-analysis of observational studies. J Viral Hepat. 2007;14(10):697–703.
53. Liu CH, Kao JH. Treatment of hepatitis C virus infection in patients with end-stage renal disease. J Gastroenterol Hepatol. 2011;26(2):228–39.
54. Mahmoud IM, Elhabashi AF, Elsawy E, El-Husseini AA, Sheha GE, Sobh MA. The impact of hepatitis C virus viremia on renal graft and patient survival: a 9-year prospective study. Am J Kidney Dis. 2004;43(1):131–9.
55. Mathurin P, Mouquet C, Poynard T, Sylla C, Benalia H, Fretz C, et al. Impact of hepatitis B and C virus on kidney transplantation outcome. Hepatology. 1999;29(1):257–63.
56. Al-Freah MA, Zeino Z, Heneghan MA. Management of hepatitis C in patients with chronic kidney disease. Curr Gastroenterol Rep. 2012;14(1):78–86.
57. Berenguer M. Treatment of chronic hepatitis C in hemodialysis patients. Hepatology. 2008;48(5):1690–9.
58. Saxena V, Manos MM, Yee HS, Catalli L, Wayne E, Murphy RC, et al. Telaprevir or boceprevir triple therapy in patients with chronic hepatitis C and varying severity of cirrhosis. Aliment Pharmacol Ther. 2014;39(10):1213–24.
59. Bunchorntavakul C, Reddy KR. Management of hepatitis C before and after liver transplantation in the era of rapidly evolving therapeutic advances. J Clin Translational Hepatol. 2014;2:124–33.
60. Roche B, Samuel D. Hepatitis C virus treatment pre- and post-liver transplantation. Liver Int. 2012;32 Suppl 1:120–8.
61. Hezode C, Fontaine H, Dorival C, Larrey D, Zoulim F, Canva V, et al. Triple therapy in treatment-experienced patients with HCV-cirrhosis in a multicentre cohort of the French Early Access Programme (ANRS CO20-CUPIC) - NCT01514890. J Hepatol. 2013;59(3):434–41.
62. Gordon SC, Muir AJ, Lim JK, Pearlman B, Argo CK, Ramani A, et al. Safety profile of boceprevir and telaprevir in chronic hepatitis C: real world experience from HCV-TARGET. J Hepatol. 2015;62(2):286–93.
63. Flamm SL, Everson GT, Charlton M, Denning JM, Arterburn S, Brandt-Sarif T, Pang PS, McHutchison JG, Reddy KR, Afdhal NH, editors. Ledipasvir/sofosbuvir with ribavirin for the treatment of HCV in patients with decompensated cirrhosis: preliminary results of a prospective, multicenter study. 65th Annual Meeting of the American Association for the Study of Liver Diseases (AASLD) November 1–5, 2014; Boston, MA.
64. Gane EJ. The natural history of recurrent hepatitis C and what influences this. Liver Transpl. 2008;14 Suppl 2:S36–44.
65. Watt K, Veldt B, Charlton M. A practical guide to the management of HCV infection following liver transplantation. Am J Transplant. 2009;9(8):1707–13.

66. Coilly A, Roche B, Dumortier J, Leroy V, Botta-Fridlund D, Radenne S, et al. Safety and efficacy of protease inhibitors to treat hepatitis C after liver transplantation: a multicenter experience. J Hepatol. 2014;60(1):78–86.
67. Sherman KE, Rouster SD, Chung RT, Rajicic N. Hepatitis C Virus prevalence among patients infected with human immunodeficiency virus: a cross-sectional analysis of the US adult AIDS Clinical Trials Group. Clin Infect Dis. 2002;34(6):831–7.
68. Sulkowski MS, Thomas DL. Hepatitis C in the HIV-infected patient. Clin Liver Dis. 2003;7(1):179–94.
69. Sulkowski MS, Thomas DL. Hepatitis C in the HIV-infected person. Ann Intern Med. 2003;138(3):197–207.
70. Weber R, Sabin CA, Friis-Moller N, Reiss P, El-Sadr WM, Kirk O, et al. Liver-related deaths in persons infected with the human immunodeficiency virus: the D:A:D study. Arch Intern Med. 2006;166(15):1632–41.
71. Berenguer J, Alejos B, Hernando V, Viciana P, Salavert M, Santos I, et al. Trends in mortality according to hepatitis C virus serostatus in the era of combination antiretroviral therapy. AIDS. 2012;26(17):2241–6.
72. Labarga P, Soriano V, Vispo ME, Pinilla J, Martin-Carbonero L, Castellares C, et al. Hepatotoxicity of antiretroviral drugs is reduced after successful treatment of chronic hepatitis C in HIV-infected patients. J Infect Dis. 2007;196(5):670–6.
73. Sulkowski MS. Viral hepatitis and HIV coinfection. J Hepatol. 2008;48(2):353–67.
74. Sulkowski MS, Eron JJ, Wyles D, Trinh R, Lalezari J, Wang C, et al. Ombitasvir, paritaprevir co-dosed with ritonavir, dasabuvir, and ribavirin for hepatitis C in patients co-infected with HIV-1: a randomized trial. JAMA. 2015;313(12):1223–31.
75. Fleischer R, Boxwell D, Sherman KE. Nucleoside analogues and mitochondrial toxicity. Clin Infect Dis. 2004;38(8):e79–80.
76. Alvarez D, Dieterich DT, Brau N, Moorehead L, Ball L, Sulkowski MS. Zidovudine use but not weight-based ribavirin dosing impacts anaemia during HCV treatment in HIV-infected persons. J Viral Hepat. 2006;13(10):683–9.

Chapter 12
Viral Hepatitis: Other Viral Hepatides

Adnan Said and Aiman Ghufran

Questions from Patients

1. *How do I know I have viral hepatitis?*
   Hepatitis means inflammation of the liver. Drugs, toxins, heavy use of alcohol, reduced blood supply to the liver, and microorganisms including viruses may cause it. However, signs and symptoms of hepatitis from any virus are similar and the specific cause is often undistinguishable without blood tests. Sometimes patients have no symptoms. When patients do experience symptoms, these may include jaundice (yellowing of the eyes and skin), fatigue, lethargy, nausea, vomiting, loss of appetite, abdominal pain, and fever. In severe cases, patients may start noticing swelling of feet, abdomen, or confusion and drowsiness. If any combination of these symptoms occurs, medical care should be sought immediately.

2. *How does it occur? Is it contagious?*
   Most viral hepatitis occurs from human-to-human transmission, though animal-to-human transmission may also occur. Different viruses may be transmitted either from contaminated water and food; bodily secretions like blood, semen, and saliva (e.g., herpesviruses); or droplets when people cough or sneeze (influenza). The mechanism of transmission and its contagiousness is specific to each virus.

3. *How are these infections treated?*
   Hepatitis caused by viruses is usually treated symptomatically, meaning treating the symptoms of liver inflammation rather than the virus itself. However, some

A. Said, M.D., M.S. (✉)
Division of Gastroenterology and Hepatology, Department of Medicine, William
S. Middleton VAMC, University of Wisconsin School of Medicine and Public Health,
Madison, WI, USA
e-mail: axs@medicine.wisc.edu

A. Ghufran, M.D.
Division of Gastroenterology and Hepatology, William S. Middleton VA Medical Center,
University of Wisconsin School of Medicine and Public Health, Madison, WI, USA

© Springer International Publishing Switzerland 2017
K. Sacian, R. Shaker (eds.), *Liver Disorders*,
DOI 10.1007/978-3-319-30103-7_12

viruses may have a specific antiviral that can be used to eradicate it and prevent progression of the disease.
4. *How do I know if I am getting better?*
   Recovery after viral hepatitis typically starts with gradual resolution of nausea, vomiting, abdominal pain, and return of appetite and energy. The jaundice is usually the last to resolve.

Introduction

1. *Besides the known hepatitis viruses, which other viruses cause hepatitis?*
   The hepatotropic viruses are the most common cause of viral hepatitis worldwide, of which hepatitis B and C cause chronic hepatitis. However, non-hepatotropic viruses only cause acute hepatitis and/or acute liver failure, without causing any chronic damage to the liver. These viruses do not primarily target the liver; hence the term non-hepatotropic is used in their description. These viruses include the herpesviruses (Epstein-Barr virus (EBV), cytomegalovirus [CMV], and herpes simplex virus), parvovirus, adenovirus, influenza, and severe acute respiratory syndrome (SARS)-associated coronavirus [1].

   The risk of acquiring infection from any of the non-hepatotropic viruses is specific to each virus and is detailed below. Considerations for determining the risk of infection include sanitary conditions, prior exposure, host immune status, and duration of infection in the contact.

Human Herpesviruses

This class of viruses includes varicella zoster (VZV), EBV, CMV, and herpes simplex virus (HSV).

Herpes Simplex Virus

Approximately 90% of people worldwide have been exposed to one or both HSV viruses [2]. HSV-1 is more common, with 65% of persons in the USA being seropositive to HSV-1 [3]. It is almost universal in the developing world, usually acquired in childhood secondary to close contact with infected family members and causes oral cold sores [2]. HSV-2 on the other hand is less ubiquitous and incidence varies from 15 to 80%, depending on the population. Transmission is almost exclusively during sexual activity [2].

2. Which subgroups are at a particularly high risk for liver involvement with HSV?
   The infection in the liver with HSV is uncommon. However, when it does occur, it frequently leads to acute liver failure with a high mortality. Severe HSV

infections are typically associated with impaired cell-mediated immunity that may occur in a transplant recipient or in patients on high-dose steroids. Females in the third trimester of pregnancy are also particularly at risk for acute liver failure.

The diagnosis is often missed as skin lesions that provide clinical clues to the diagnosis are often lacking in patients with HSV-associated hepatitis. A high degree of suspicion, even in the absence of skin lesions, combined with early diagnostic modalities and early institution of appropriate therapy with parenteral acyclovir may dramatically improve survival [4].

Four mechanisms of HSV dissemination and resultant hepatitis have been hypothesized [5]: (a) a large HSV inoculant overwhelming the defense system; (b) an impairment in host macrophages, cytotoxic T lymphocytes, and delayed-type hypersensitivity reactions; (c) enhanced virulence; and (d) activation of a latent hepatovirulent strain.

HSV hepatitis is characterized by rapid development of fulminant hepatic necrosis with serum aminotransferase levels 100- to 1000-fold above normal and hyperbilirubinemia [4]. Positive serology often points at the diagnosis with polymerase chain reaction (PCR) confirming the diagnosis. In the era of widespread availability of PCR testing, a liver biopsy is now less commonly needed to secure the diagnosis. Common findings on liver biopsy include massive liver necrosis with almost complete absence of portal tracts and central veins. Presence of typical intranuclear viral inclusions is the hallmark finding on a liver biopsy, confirmed with immunohistochemical staining.

Given the time-sensitive nature of the disease, initiation of empiric therapy with acyclovir is indicated while awaiting diagnostic confirmation in a patient with acute liver failure.

Varicella Zoster

Varicella zoster (VZV) causes chicken pox which is a very common, albeit usually benign, contagious disease. It spreads easily from infected people via direct contact and droplets from coughing and sneezing. Individuals at highest risk include those who have never had chicken pox or are unimmunized [6].

Chicken pox occurs in epidemics among preschool and school-aged children and is characterized by generalized vesicular rash which is extremely pruritic. In addition to widespread systemic involvement, varicella may also cause a rare congenital varicella syndrome.

Similar to herpes virus, hepatitis secondary to varicella zoster can be life threatening [7, 8]. The disease severity and pattern of liver injury are similar to those seen in HSV hepatitis, and it usually occurs in the adult population that has not been previously exposed to varicella. Diagnosis is made based on serology, PCR, and liver biopsy, which show diagnostic inclusions on immunohistochemistry. Treatment is with parenteral acyclovir.

Epstein-Barr Virus

EBV is one of the most common viruses worldwide. It is usually asymptomatic, though it may cause infectious mononucleosis (IM). Its transmission is via saliva and is most common among teens and adults [6].

The pattern of liver injury is again hepatocellular, though it may rarely be cholestatic with marked hyperbilirubinemia. Majority of the patients who develop hepatitis do not have concomitant signs and symptoms of IM, though it is accompanied by lymphocytosis and/or splenomegaly. EBV hepatitis affects an older demographic compared to IM, with nearly half of patients over 60 years old. It is usually a self-limiting hepatitis which improves with supportive management [9].

Cytomegalovirus

CMV is usually spread by infected saliva, urine, and other body fluids. Most healthy individuals infected with CMV are asymptomatic, though occasionally it may cause systemic disease with primarily upper respiratory symptoms. When acquired vertically from pregnant woman to fetus it causes serious congenital disease [6].

Mild elevations in transaminases are almost always present, though the elevations are rarely higher than five times of the normal value. Patients are usually anicteric, and improve with supportive management.

Adenovirus

Adenovirus is a common virus capable of infecting multiple organ systems. It is transmitted via direct conjunctival inoculation, fecal-oral route, aerosolized droplets, or exposure to infected tissue or blood. It causes various diseases and syndromes, including acute viral gastroenteritis, acute respiratory disease, keratoconjunctivitis, and acute hemorrhagic cystitis amongst others.

It can also cause adenoviral hepatitis, which can lead to severe fulminant failure and be life threatening, typically in the immunocompromised transplant-recipient host. The injury to liver is hepatocellular, with transaminases five to ten times upper limit of normal. Serum levels of AST are often markedly more elevated than the ALT values, and may run into several thousands. Total bilirubin and GGT on the other hand are only moderately elevated [10]. Diagnosis is with secured with PCR. There is no specific treatment, though several antivirals including ribavirin, ganciclovir, cidofovir, and vidarabine have been tried in small populations with modest success [11].

Parvovirus B19

Parvovirus B19 (PV-B19) most commonly infects children and pregnant women. It spreads primarily via respiratory droplets, though infection may also occur via blood products.

It is most commonly associated with erythema infectiosum, otherwise known as the fifth disease of childhood. Its hallmark is fever and a rash classically known as "slapped-cheek appearance." Mild upper respiratory tract symptoms begin approximately 1 week after exposure to PV-B19 and last for 2–3 days. The virus then spreads to the bone marrow and enters the erythroid progenitor. It subsequently causes lysis of blood cells which leads to fever with IgM-mediated lacy exanthema. In adults it is more commonly associated with marked arthropathy, and during pregnancy may cause aplastic anemia. Post-transplant patients are another at-risk population which can manifest refractory anemia [12].

While diagnosis of erythema infectiosum is clinical, blood tests are indicated for confirmation in patients with atypical symptoms or in adults. This is typically with an enzyme-linked immunosorbent assay (ELISA) for IgM antibodies and/or PCR assay. Viral DNA is typically present in serum up to 6 months after onset of symptoms [13].

Presentation as acute hepatitis or fulminant liver failure has been mostly reported in children. While it may also occur in adults, PV-B19-associated hepatitis course is less severe than in children. The pattern of injury is typically hepatocellular, with ALT and AST often three to five times the normal value, with a preferential elevation in alanine transferase. Fulminant hepatic failure secondary to PV-B19 remains a rare clinical entity. There is no specific antiviral therapy or vaccine available for prevention.

Influenza

Influenza spreads via respiratory droplets, with humans and birds as the primary reservoir. While most flu activity occurs from October to May in the USA, it can occur year-round [6].

Influenza is often associated with mild elevations in liver enzymes, which typically resolve after clearance of the virus. This is somewhat intriguing as the virus typically infects the respiratory endothelial lining and the hepatocytes are not exposed to the viral antigen. It has been proposed that the process of CD8$^+$ T-cell infiltration of the liver in influenza infection can lead to clinically significant hepatitis [1]. The pattern of injury is typically hepatocellular with alanine aminotransferase (ALT) and aspartate aminotransferase (AST) usually two to three times above the normal limit. Alkaline phosphatase (ALKP) and gamma-glutamyl transpeptidase

(GGT) are often normal. Another observation was significantly higher serum levels of AST, ALT, and GGT in patients with pandemic influenza in 2009 caused by the H1N1 strain compared to seasonal influenza [14]. Diagnosis is confirmed with immunoassays and PCR.

Hepatitis secondary to influenza rarely progresses to acute liver failure, and when it does occur the process is more due to multiorgan failure from sepsis and ischemia than direct viral injury.

Treatment is with oseltamivir. The incidence has reduced and outbreaks have diminished in severity due to active recruitment of care providers at grassroots levels to encourage annual immunization in all with no contraindications. However, occasional viral mutations lead to resistant strains against which the efficacy of vaccine is diminished.

Severe Acute Respiratory Syndrome Coronavirus (SARS-CoV) and Middle East Respiratory Syndrome Coronavirus (MERS-CoV)

SARS-CoV is a relatively recently recognized virus, being first recognized in 2003 as the perpetrator of a massive outbreak of respiratory illness with high mortality in China. It has been virtually eradicated with no further cases reported since 2004, though CDC declared it a select agent in 2012 [6]. Another viral outbreak identified as MERS-CoV in 2012 in Saudi Arabia has bee reported recently. There is a current outbreak of the MERS-COV in South Korea since May 2015.

Both SARS- and MERS CoV-associated liver injury is reported in up to 60 % of the patients and is associated with clinically significant hepatitis. It is usually associated with focal lobular lymphocytic infiltrates and has been reported in patients with SARS. In these cases, although SARS-associated coronavirus was detected in the liver tissues by reverse transcriptase-PCR, no viral particles were seen at electron microscopy [1].

There is no specific therapy for either of the viruses. Various antivirals have been tried with little success, apart from interferon which showed modest improvement in symptoms.

Ebola Hemorrhagic Fever (EHF)

Ebola is an extremely contagious virus transmitted from direct contact with infected body fluid. Humans and primates are the primary reservoir. The most recent outbreak started in March 2014 in West Africa and is currently ongoing, and has so far resulted in over 10,000 deaths.

The disease is associated with severe fulminant liver failure, resulting in massive internal hemorrhage. Diagnosis is confirmed by IgM ELISA, PCR, and virus isolation [6].

The elevations in liver enzymes are hepatocellular in pattern, with AST being much higher than ALT. Bilirubin, ALKP, and GGT are only modestly elevated.

Treatment is supportive, with no FDA-approved specific antiviral therapy available. Experimental vaccines and treatments for Ebola are under development, but they have not yet been fully tested for safety or effectiveness [6]. Mortality remains very high.

3. *What is the management of patients who develop acute liver failure due to non-hepatotropic virus infection?*

   Acute liver failure is defined by elevation in liver enzymes, an INR >1.5, and development of encephalopathy in someone without known underlying liver disease. It is associated with rapid progression and very high mortality. The first step towards appropriate management is prompt transfer of the patient to the nearest transplant center. These patients are preferably admitted to the critical care unit, and should have close frequent monitoring of sensorium and the basic chemistry panel. Their management is very similar to management of other patients with non-acetaminophen-associated liver failure and the use of *N*-acetylcysteine may also have a role [15].

   Management of advanced encephalopathy is arguably the most challenging in acute liver failure. Management is aimed at reducing intracranial pressure. When sedation is indicated, propofol is the preferred agent as it reduces brain edema [16].

   Early transplant consideration and evaluation offer the best chance at survival in patients with acute liver failure. Even with appropriate management, mortality remains high. Prior to transplantation, most series suggested less than 15 % survival. Currently, overall short-term survival (1 year) including those undergoing transplantation is greater than 65 % [17].

4. *Do the non-hepatotropic viruses cause chronic disease or result in an elevated risk of liver cancer?*

None of the non-hepatotropic viruses, with the possible exception of PV-B19, has been shown to cause chronic liver disease. PV-B19 has been postulated as a rare and unusual etiology of chronic hepatitis. This observation is based on identification of viral DNA from the hepatocytes years after the original infection. However, the extent to which it results in actual fibrosis and chronic damage is unclear. Furthermore, interest has focused on a possible effect of co-infection with PV-B19 on the natural history of chronic hepatitis B and C [18]. Similarly, none of the above viruses have been associated with liver cancer.

References

1. Adams DH, Hubscher SG. Systemic viral infections and collateral damage in the liver. Am J Pathol. 2006;168(4):1057–9.
2. Arvin A, Campadelli-Fiume G, Mocarski E, et al., editors. Human herpesviruses: biology, therapy, and immunoprophylaxis. Chapter 36. Cambridge: Cambridge University Press; 2007.
3. Xu F, Schillinger JA, Sternberg MR, et al. Seroprevalence and coinfection with herpes simplex virus type 1 and type 2 in the United States, 1988–1994. J Infect Dis. 2002;185:1019–24.

4. Norvell JP, Blei AT, Jovanovic BD, et al. Herpes simplex virus hepatitis: an analysis of the published literature and institutional cases. Liver Transpl. 2007;13(10):1428–34.
5. Miyazaki Y, Akizuki S, Sakaoka H, Yamamoto S, Terao H. Disseminated infection of herpes simplex virus with fulminant hepatitis in a healthy adult: a case report. APMIS. 1991;99:1001–7.
6. Centers for Disease Control and Prevention (CDC). www.cdc.gov/.
7. Anderson DR, Schwartz J, Hunter NJ, et al. Varicella hepatitis: a fatal case in a previously healthy, immuno competent adult report of a case, autopsy, and review of the literature. Arch Intern Med. 1994;154(18):2101–6.
8. Roque-Afonso AM, Bralet MP, Ichai P, et al. Chickenpox-associated fulminant hepatitis that led to liver transplantation in a 63-year-old woman. Liver Transpl. 2008;14(9):1309–12.
9. Vine LJ, Shepherd K, Hunter JG, et al. Characteristics of Epstein-Barr virus hepatitis among patients with jaundice or acute hepatitis. Aliment Pharmacol Ther. 2012;36(1):16–21.
10. Cames B, Rahier J, Burtomboy G, et al. Acute adenovirus hepatitis in liver transplant recipients. J Pediatr. 1992;120(1):33–7.
11. Carter BA, Karpen SJ, Quiros-Tejeira RE, et al. Intravenous Cidofovir therapy for disseminated adenovirus in a pediatric liver transplant recipient. Transplantation. 2002;74(7):1050–2.
12. Eid AJ, Brown RA, Patel R, Razonable RR. Parvovirus B19 infection after transplantation: a review of 98 cases. Clin Infect Dis. 2006;43(1):40–8.
13. Musiani M, Zerbini M, Gentilomi G, et al. Parvovirus B19 clearance from peripheral blood after acute infection. J Infect Dis. 1995;172:1360–3.
14. Papic N, Pangercic A, Vargovic M, et al. Liver involvement during influenza infection: perspective on the 2009 influenza pandemic. Influenza Resp Viruses. 2012;6(3):e2–5.
15. Lee WM, Acute Liver Failure Study Group. Intravenous N-acetylcysteine improves transplant-free survival in early stage non-acetaminophen acute liver failure. Gastroenterology. 2009;137(3):856–64. 864.e1.
16. Wijkicks EFM, Nyberg SL. Propofol to control intracranial pressure in fulminant hepatic failure. Transplant Proc. 2002;34:1220–2.
17. AASLD Position Paper. The management of acute liver failure: update. 2011.
18. Mogensen TH, Jensen JMB, Hamilton-Dutoit S. Chronic hepatitis caused by persistent parvovirus B19 infection. BMC Infect Dis. 2010;10:246.

Chapter 13
Alcoholic Liver Disease

Ashutosh Barve, Luis S. Marsano, Dipendra Parajuli,
Matthew Cave, and Craig J. McClain

Q1: What are the typical presenting features of ALD and are there any tests that should be performed to distinguish ALD from other liver diseases.

The term alcoholic liver disease (ALD) encompasses a spectrum of disorders including simple fatty infiltration of the liver (steatosis), alcoholic hepatitis (steatohepatitis) with or without significant fibrosis, compensated cirrhosis, and decompensated cirrhosis. Steatosis can be asymptomatic or present with nonspecific symptoms such as fatigue or abdominal fullness. Alcoholic hepatitis patients also frequently complain of abdominal fullness along with other com-

A. Barve, M.D. • L.S. Marsano, M.D. • D. Parajuli, M.D.
Division of Gastroenterology, Hepatology & Nutrition, Department of Medicine,
University of Louisville School of Medicine, Louisville, KY, USA

Robley Rex Louisville VAMC, Louisville, KY, USA

M. Cave, M.D.
Division of Gastroenterology, Hepatology & Nutrition, Department of Medicine,
University of Louisville School of Medicine, Louisville, KY, USA

Robley Rex Louisville VAMC, Louisville, KY, USA

Department of Pharmacology and Toxicology, University of Louisville School of Medicine,
Center for Translational Research Building, 505 South Hancock Street, Suite 503,
Louisville, KY 40292, USA

Department of Biochemistry and Molecular Biology, University of Louisville School
of Medicine, Louisville, KY, USA

C.J. McClain, M.D. (✉)
Division of Gastroenterology, Hepatology & Nutrition, Department of Medicine,
University of Louisville School of Medicine, Louisville, KY, USA

Robley Rex Louisville VAMC, Louisville, KY, USA

Department of Pharmacology and Toxicology, University of Louisville School of Medicine,
Center for Translational Research Building, 505 South Hancock Street, Suite 503,
Louisville, KY 40292, USA
e-mail: craig.mcclain@louisville.edu; cjmccl01@louisville.edu

© Springer International Publishing Switzerland 2017
K. Saeian, R. Shaker (eds.), *Liver Disorders*,
DOI 10.1007/978-3-319-30103-7_13

plaints such as jaundice, fever, abdominal distension, gastrointestinal bleeding, changes in consciousness, and abdominal pain. Compensated cirrhotics may be asymptomatic or have anorexia, nausea, weight loss, fatigue, weakness, abnormal menstruation, loss of libido, muscle cramps, and or difficulty concentrating on mental tasks. While no specific diagnostic blood tests are available for ALD, the AST level is usually only modestly elevated (usually <300 IU/ml) and the AST/ALT ratio is usually >1.5, and most have a ratio >2. Liver biopsy is usually performed only in those patients in whom the diagnosis is in question. Diagnosis is made by clinical history, physical exam, and laboratory abnormalities in patients with evidence of liver injury and a history of significant alcohol consumption, after all the other causes of chronic liver disease have been ruled out. Other liver diseases that we routinely exclude by blood tests are shown subsequently in the text along with the corresponding initial serum assays.

Q2: What are the prognostic markers for Alcoholic Hepatitis and Alcoholic Cirrhosis.

The prognosis of patients with ALD depends on multiple factors. Chief amongst those is the seriousness of liver pathology. Patients with only fatty liver have the best outcomes, while patients with alcoholic hepatitis (AH) or cirrhosis have intermediate outcomes. Patients with AH combined with alcoholic cirrhosis have the worst outcomes. Several prognostic models have been developed to predict short-term prognosis in alcoholic hepatitis. The most commonly used one is a modified version of the *"discriminant function"* (mDF) originally described by Maddrey and Boitnott. mDF values >32 have a poor prognosis with 1 month mortality rates of 35–50 %. The prognosis of patients with mDF >32 can be further stratified based on whether or not they have hepatic encephalopathy or acute kidney injury. Two other prognostic models that successfully predict survival in alcoholic hepatitis patients are the MELD and the Glasgow Alcoholic Hepatitis scores (GAHS). A newer scoring system based on the patient's age, bilirubin, INR, and creatinine (ABIC score) separates patients into three groups with predicted 3 month survival rates of 100, 70, and 25 %. The most commonly used tool to determine the prognosis of alcoholic cirrhosis patients is the Child-Turcotte-Pugh (CTP) score. The MELD score also is a very popular prognostic model for alcoholic cirrhosis, especially in the setting of liver transplantation. These grading systems are all available online and are important for predicting factors such as need for hospitalization, risk of surgery, need/response to medical therapy, and mortality.

Q3: What are the treatment options for the different stages of ALD.

The most important treatment for ALD is abstinence from continued excess drinking. Reducing alcohol consumption even without completely stopping alcohol has been shown to improve survival. Patients who abuse alcohol or are dependent will need a referral to a qualified alcohol and substance abuse counselor for assessment and specialty treatment. The goal is sustained abstinence. Significant clinical improvement can be seen within 3 months in two-thirds of the patients, and many patients achieve complete clinical and biochemical recovery, regain muscle mass, and safely discontinue liver-related medications within 2 years. Malnutrition is common among patients with ALD. Adequate nutrition is critical in the treatment of severe ALD. It is common for patients with severe alcoholic hepatitis to have inadequate nutritional intake in the hospital. These patients often have poor appetites and are actually deprived of adequate nutrition by their caregivers due to dietary restriction of salt, water, and protein as well as intermittent interruptions to their nutrition due to various procedures. We do not hesitate to insert a nasogastric feeding tube if a calorie count proves that the patient is not consuming at least 2500 cal daily. Medications can be useful in the treatment of severe acute AH. Glucocorticoids and Pentoxifylline are two medicines presently used. Glucocorticoid therapy may improve survival in carefully selected patients, but a number of patients have obvious contraindications, a significant number of patients fail to respond, and corticosteroids often do not seem to prevent the development of acute kidney injury. Therefore, in patients with contraindications to corticosteroids or with evidence of renal injury, pentoxifylline is an alternative therapy. Combination therapy has been tested in clinical trials but with disappointing results. The most recent large trial in acute AH (STOPAH) unfortunately showed no statistically significant benefit of either steroids or pentoxifylline. Novel therapies being tested in ongoing clinical trials for severe AH include IL-1 inhibitors and a caspase inhibitor. For moderate alcoholic hepatitis, probiotics and an oral agent that inhibits absorption of endotoxin are being tested. For decompensated alcoholic cirrhosis which does not improve with abstinence, liver transplantation is a treatment option with favorable outcomes.

Introduction

Alcoholic liver disease (ALD) is a major cause of morbidity and mortality worldwide [1]. The clinical spectrum of ALD includes fatty liver, steatohepatitis with or without fibrosis, and cirrhosis. Severe Alcoholic Hepatitis (AH) is an especially important cause of morbidity, mortality, and health care costs in the United States (U.S.) and worldwide. In 2007, 56,809 patients (0.71 % of the total) were hospitalized in the U.S. with the ICD-9 diagnosis of AH [2]. Average length of stay was 6.5 days, and average hospital costs were \$37,769, which is more than twice the cost of myocardial infarction and approximately four times the cost of acute pancreatitis. A nationwide study on AH in Denmark from 1999 to 2008 [3], found that over that time period, the 28-day mortality rose from 12 to 15 %, and the 84-day mortality from 14 to 24 %. The overall 5-year mortality was 56 %; 47 % in those without cirrhosis, and 69 % in those with cirrhosis. These data from Denmark are quite similar to VA Cooperative Studies data on 4-year mortality: 42 % mortality with AH alone, and 65 % with AH plus cirrhosis [4]. Thus, despite increases in knowledge of mechanisms for AH, mortality is not improving for this important clinical problem.

The diagnosis of ALD is made in patients with evidence of liver injury based on clinical history, physical findings, and laboratory abnormalities, when there is evidence of significant alcohol consumption and after other causes of chronic liver disease have been excluded. Problems diagnosing the disease arise when the patient exhibits no symptoms or clinical findings to suggest the diagnosis, or when the patient conceals alcohol abuse. The situation is even more difficult when the patient has risk factors for other causes of liver disease, such as obesity or diabetes mellitus, or has superimposed viral hepatitis. The goal of this chapter is to review: (1) selected mechanisms of liver toxicity, (2) the clinical features that support the diagnosis of ALD, (3) the natural history and prognostic factors, and (4) potential therapy.

Mechanisms of Liver Disease

There are multiple mechanisms for alcohol-induced liver injury that are highly complex, multifactorial, and often interactive. Almost everyone who drinks heavily develops fatty liver, and subsequent (often multiple) insults then convert some patients from fatty liver to steatohepatitis and/or cirrhosis (Fig. 13.1). We address in detail the three best-established and long-standing mechanisms of ALD: (1) oxidative stress, (2) nutritional abnormalities, and (3) gut-barrier dysfunction and dysregulated cytokine signaling. These three mechanisms have provided the greatest number of targets for therapeutic interventions. We also discuss briefly selected other mechanisms, such as endoplasmic reticulum (ER) stress, genetics, and extracellular matrix.

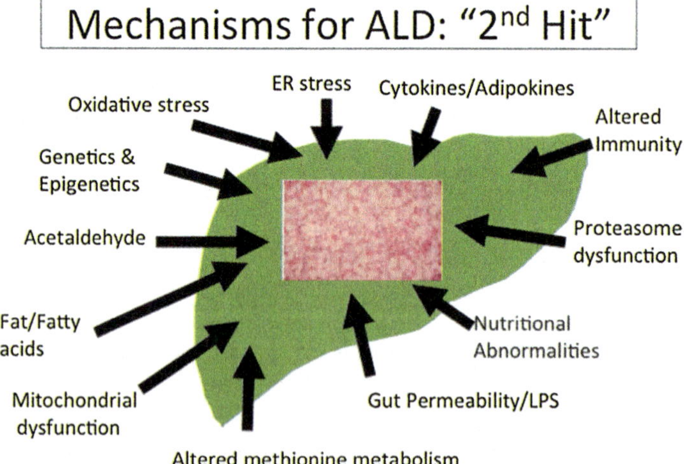

Fig. 13.1 Mechanisms for ALD: "2nd Hit"

Oxidative Stress and Lipid Peroxidation

Oxidative stress is an imbalance between pro-oxidants and antioxidants (Reviewed-[5]). Reactive oxygen species (ROS) and reactive nitrogen species (RNS) are products of normal metabolism and can be beneficial to the host (e.g., by contributing to bacterial killing) [5]. Overproduction of ROS and/or RNS or inadequate antioxidant defenses (e.g., low levels of vitamins, selenium, mitochondrial glutathione), or both, can lead to liver injury. The stimulus for oxidative stress in the liver comes from multiple sources. In hepatocytes, CYP2E1 activity increases after alcohol consumption—in part because of stabilization of messenger RNA (mRNA). Similarly, CYP2E1 activity is increased in NAFLD. The CYP2E1 system leaks electrons to initiate oxidative stress [5]. CYP2E1 is localized in the hepatic lobule in areas of alcohol-induced liver injury. Moreover, overexpression of CYP2E1 in mice and in HepG2 cells (a human hepatoma cell line) in vitro leads to enhanced alcohol hepatotoxicity. Nonparenchymal cells and infiltrating inflammatory cells (e.g., polymorphonuclear neutrophils) are another major source of pro-oxidants that are used for normal cellular processes, such as killing invading organisms. Infiltrating neutrophils use enzyme systems such as myeloperoxidase to generate hypochlorous acid (HClO–, a halide species that causes oxidative stress) and RNS.

Nutritional Abnormalities

Moderate/severe alcoholic hepatitis (AH) is regularly associated with malnutrition. In large VA Cooperative Studies, virtually every patient with AH had some degree of malnutrition [6]. Almost 50 % of severe AH patients' energy intake came from alcohol. Although calorie intake was frequently adequate, intake of protein and critical micronutrients was often deficient. In these VA cooperative studies, the severity of liver disease correlated with malnutrition. Patients were given a balanced 2500-kcal hospital diet. Voluntary oral food intake correlated in a stepwise fashion with 6-month mortality data. Thus, patients who voluntarily consumed more than 3000 kcal/day had virtually no mortality, whereas those consuming less than 1000 kcal/day had greater than 80 % 6-month mortality.

A classic example of micronutrient deficiency in ALD is zinc deficiency [7, 8]. Alcoholics regularly have decreased dietary intake of zinc, as well as poor absorption and increased excretion. Moreover, oxidative stress causes zinc to be released from critical zinc-finger proteins. These cumulative effects negatively impact critical zinc-finger functions. This can lead to liver injury, altered fat metabolism, impaired liver regeneration, etc., as well as produce classic clinical manifestations of zinc deficiency in humans such as night blindness or skin lesions.

The type of dietary fat consumed also appears to play an important role in the pathogenesis of ALD. Several studies have shown that dietary saturated fat protects against alcohol-induced liver disease in rodents, whereas dietary unsaturated fat, enriched in linoleic acid (LA), promotes alcohol-induced liver damage [9]. The mechanism(s) by which the combination of LA and alcohol promotes liver injury are not fully understood. LA is the most abundant polyunsaturated fatty acid in human diets and in human plasma and membrane lipids. Dietary intake of LA has more than tripled over the past century. LA can be enzymatically converted to bioactive oxidation products, OXLAMs, primarily via the actions of 12/15-lipoxygenase (12/15-LO), or non-enzymatically via free radical-mediated oxidation response to oxidative stress. OXLAMs (either alone or in conjunction with ethanol) can induce increased gut permeability and hepatic mitochondrial dysfunction in experimental ALD. Obesity can also accelerate ALD. As noted above, high fat diets rich in linoleic acid worsen ALD. We also have preliminary research showing that high fructose (sugared pop) diets worsen experimental ALD.

Intestinal Barrier Dysfunction/Microbiota

Alcohol, and specifically its metabolite acetaldehyde, disrupts tight junction proteins and increases gut permeability both in vitro and in vivo; and increased endotoxin levels are regularly observed in rodent models and in humans with ALD. Endotoxin stimulates the production of TNF and other proinflammatory cytokines through Toll-like receptor (TLR4) signaling, which plays a critical role in the development and progression of ALD (Fig. 13.2). Other bacteria-derived toxins, such as peptidoglycan and flagellin, may also impact TLR signaling and proinflammatory cytokine production [10]. Indeed,

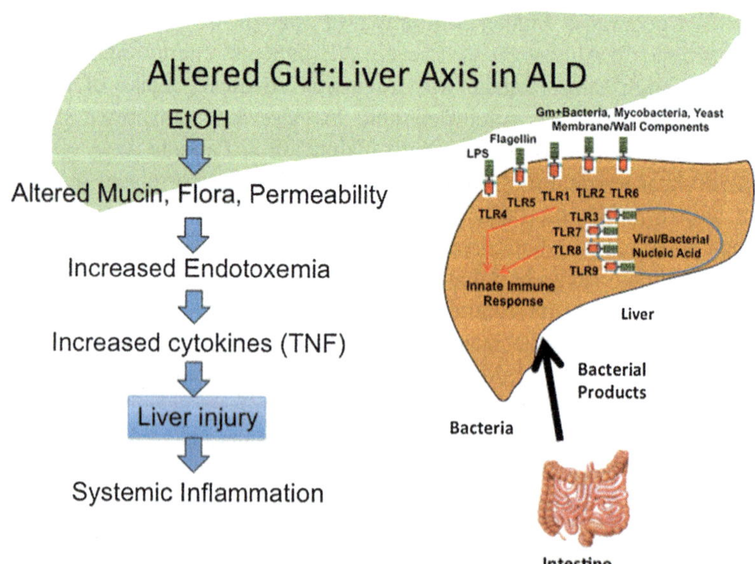

Fig. 13.2 Altered gut: liver axis in ALD

injected peptidoglycan increases liver injury/inflammation in alcohol-fed compared to control-fed mice, and ethanol feeding increases peptidoglycan levels [10, 11]. Moreover, chronic alcohol feeding increases hepatic TLRs and thus sensitizes hepatocytes to inflammation/injury induced by translocation of gut derived bacteria/toxins. Endotoxin not only plays a role in the fatty liver and liver injury of experimental ALD, but it also appears to play a role in hepatic fibrosis. In vitro assays as well as in vivo mixed chimerism studies show that endotoxin primes stellate cells for Transforming Growth Factor-β (TGF)-stimulated collagen production (reviewed-[12]). Thus, LPS also plays a role in fibrosis induction and progression.

Alterations in the gut microbiome likely play a major role in the development/ progression of gut barrier dysfunction, endotoxemia, and liver injury/fibrosis in ALD [13]. We showed that ethanol consumption caused a time-dependent decline in the abundance of both *Bacteriodetes* and *Firmicutes*, which was accompanied by a proportional increase in *Actinobacteria* and *Proteobacteria* [14]. The stability of the normal intestinal microbiome is influenced by several factors in the luminal environment including gastric acidity, gut motility, bile salts, immunological defense factors, colonic pH and competition between microorganisms for nutrients and intestinal binding sites. An altered luminal environment may lead to modifications in the microbial composition by supporting the growth of specific genera. Thus, a major increase of *Alcaligenes* (an alkaline tolerant genus) correlated with an increase in fecal pH and a decrease in fecal short-chain fatty acids (SCFA). Further, some SCFAs (e.g., butyrate) have important signaling functions and epigenetic consequences, and are a critical energy source for the intestine [15]. These alterations in gut bacteria and their metabolites represent not only major mechanisms for ALD but also therapeutic targets for intervention with agents such as probiotics and prebiotics.

Other Mechanisms

There are multiple other mechanisms that are likely important in ALD. ER stress, or the unfolded protein response (UPR) pathway, is activated by conditions of protein overload or increased unfolded proteins. Once triggered, this signaling pathway results in adaptation and recovery of homeostasis; however, severe or prolonged ER stress can ultimately result in cell death. Alcohol-induced ER stress is seen in experimental alcohol-feeding models in mice, micropigs, rats, and zebrafish [16–19]. ER stress has been also been reported in human patients with ALD [20, 21].

Fibrin/Extracellular Matrix plays a critical role in the progression of ALD. Fibrosis results from an imbalance between production and resorption of extracellular matrix (ECM) caused by a complex interplay between activation/transdifferentiation of hepatic stellate cells (HSCs), profibrogenic growth factors and cytokines, and alterations in the fibrin coagulation system. Hepatic injury in experimental models of liver disease often involves dysregulation of the fibrin cascade, resulting in the formation of fibrin clots that can cause hepatocellular death and induce inflammatory signaling in the liver. Inhibition of fibrinolysis by plasminogen activator inhibitor-1 (PAI-1) can cause fibrin-ECM to accumulate, even in the absence of enhanced fibrin deposition by the thrombin cascade. An imbalance in coagulation factors as well as elevated PAI-1 levels and hypofibrinolysis are common in patients with ALD [22].

Both genetic and epigenetic factors are important for disease pathogenesis and progression in ALD. The genetic variations are often associated with conformational changes in protein structures and functions due to single nucleotide polymorphisms (SNPs), whereas epigenetic changes are phenotypic changes due to altered gene expression without affecting the underlying DNA sequence. In ALD, polymorphisms of alcohol metabolizing enzymes such as ADH and CYP2E1, as well as antioxidant enzymes and cytokine coding genes, have shown strong correlation with the progression of ALD [23]. Important epigenetic modifications in ALD include microRNAs, DNA methylation, and histone modifications.

Clinical Features of Alcoholic Liver Disease

History

Most patients with alcoholic steatosis are asymptomatic, although some may have nonspecific symptoms such as abdominal fullness or fatigue. Patients with alcoholic hepatitis frequently have abdominal fullness (up to 80–90 % of cases), jaundice (37–60 %), fever (23–56 %), abdominal distention (35–57 %), gastrointestinal bleeding (10–23 %), changes in consciousness (18–45 %), and abdominal pain [24, 25].

Patients with compensated cirrhosis are frequently asymptomatic, but they may have anorexia, nausea, weight loss, fatigue, weakness, abnormal menstruation, loss of libido, muscular cramps, and/or difficulty concentrating on mental tasks. Patients with decompensated cirrhosis are often jaundiced, have evidence of muscle wasting, feel weak, and develop fluid retention with edema and abdominal distention. In addition, many complain of itching and others present with hematemesis or melena. Easy bruising, altered sleep pattern, and confusion are also frequent complaints.

When obtaining the history, it is important to assess the duration and amount of alcohol consumption. The most commonly employed validation tool to detect hazardous alcohol consumption is the Alcohol Use Disorders Identification Test (AUDIT). A score of 8 or more (7 or more for adults over age 65) indicates alcohol use disorder or alcohol dependence (sensitivity >90 % and specificity >80 %). A shorter screening can be done with the 3-question AUDIT-C tool that gives 0–4 points for the answer to each question and is considered positive for males with a score of ≥4 points and for females with a score of ≥3 points [26], with moderate risk being 3–5 points, high risk 6–7 points and severe risk 8–12 points.

The National Institute on Alcohol Abuse and Alcoholism has a single-question test: "How many times in the past year have you had 5 or more drinks for males, or 4 or more drinks for females, in a day?" An answer of one or more times constitutes a positive test. This question has a sensitivity of 82 % and specificity of 79 % for unhealthy alcohol use [27]. A less powerful tool is the CAGE questionnaire (the name is an acronym of its four questions) in which two or more positive answers indicate hazardous alcohol use [28].

Depending on individual susceptibility, alcohol-induced organ injury requires alcohol consumption of $\geq$20 g/day for females or $\geq$40 g/day for males; however, larger amounts than this threshold are usually needed. More than 60 % of individuals who drink more than 60 g of alcohol a day will develop fatty liver [29, 30]. A "standard" alcohol drink has 14 g of alcohol and is equivalent to 12 oz. of beer, 5 oz. of wine, 8–9 oz. of malt liquor, or 1.5 oz. of distilled spirits (whiskey, bourbon, etc.). The value of the alcohol intake history depends on the recall ability and the truthfulness of the patient. The NIAAA has highly valuable alcohol abuse information on its website entitled, "Rethinking Drinking" [http://rethinkingdrinking.niaaa.nih.gov/].

Physical Exam

On physical exam, signs of fatty liver can range from mild hepatomegaly, with blunting of the normally sharp liver edge, to massive hepatomegaly. In patients with alcoholic hepatitis, hepatomegaly (80–90 % of cases), jaundice (40–60 %), and fever (23–56 %) are very common. If the injury is severe, the patients will have ascites, hepatic encephalopathy, splenomegaly, evidence of muscle wasting, and sometimes gastrointestinal hemorrhage with portal hypertensive gastropathy or gastro-esophageal varices [24, 25].

Patients with compensated cirrhosis often have hepatomegaly with hard liver consistency and a nodular surface. They may also have splenomegaly and, less often, right upper quadrant pain. Less common findings include gynecomastia and testicular atrophy [31], amenorrhea, parotid enlargement [32], cutaneous spider angioma [33], Dupuytren's contractures [34], digital clubbing [35] (found especially in patients with hypoxemia related to hepatopulmonary syndrome), palmar erythema, and nail changes.

Patients with decompensated cirrhosis may also have mental changes of hepatic encephalopathy with variable degrees of confusion with or without asterixis, jaundice, ascites, and peripheral edema. Some patients will have evidence of gastrointestinal bleeding or other organ damage, including alcoholic gastritis or pancreatitis, alcoholic neuropathy or, less commonly, alcoholic cardiomyopathy. Signs of alcohol withdrawal are common in patients with alcoholic hepatitis who have recently discontinued alcohol.

Laboratory

Patients with ALD should have a complete blood count, international normalization ratio (INR), comprehensive metabolic panel, and GGT. Because there is the risk of overlapping viral hepatitis, serologies for current infection or past exposure to

Table 13.1 Liver Disease Differential and Appropriate Blood Tests

Disease	Blood test
Hemochromatosis	Iron/TIBC/ferritin
A1 antitrypsin deficiency	A1 genotype and levels
Wilson's disease	Ceruloplasmin
Autoimmune Hepatitis	ANA
Primary biliary cirrhosis	AMA
Hepatitis A	Hepatitis A antibody
Hepatitis B	Hepatitis B surface antigen and core antibody
Hepatitis C	Hepatitis C antibody

hepatitis A, B, and C are advised. Patients who are not immune should be vaccinated against hepatitis A and B. If the ALT is elevated, a full workup for other causes of liver disease and cirrhosis is also advisable because other immune or metabolic causes may be uncovered (Table 13.1).

Consumption of alcohol in excess of 50 g/day causes elevation of AST (sensitivity 50 %, specificity 82 %) and ALT (sensitivity 35 %, specificity 86 %) [36]. The elevation of AST is typically higher than that of ALT, and 79 % of patients with alcoholic hepatitis have an AST:ALT ratio > 2. Patients with alcoholic hepatitis with ALT > AST frequently have overlapping causes for liver disease, including superimposed viral hepatitis or drug injury (most often acetaminophen). Elevated γ-glutamyl transpeptidase (GGT) is more sensitive for alcohol abuse (56–73 %), but less specific (53–70 %) than carbohydrate deficient transferrin (CDT) or MCV [37]. Using a combination of these tests may be warranted. Elevated bilirubin, in the absence of biliary obstruction, is a marker of the severity of the alcoholic liver injury and is very important as a component of the Maddrey Discriminant Function, MELD score, Glasgow Alcoholic Hepatitis Score, the Lille model and the Child-Turcotte-Pugh Calculator index (discussed subsequently).

Liver Biopsy

In the presence of a history of alcohol abuse associated with typical liver enzyme elevations, diagnosis is very reliable with sensitivity of 91 % and specificity of 97 % [38], and liver biopsy is often not performed. Patients with atypical presentation or those who have markers of other types of liver disease (autoimmune hepatitis, hemochromatosis, viral hepatitis, etc.) are good candidates for liver biopsy. Liver biopsy helps to clarify the diagnosis and will give the stage of disease, which is useful in deciding if surveillance for hepatocellular carcinoma is needed. Patients with cirrhosis require imaging every 6 months.

Natural History and Prognosis

Chronic alcohol consumption can lead to a spectrum of liver injuries which can occur sequentially, separately, or simultaneously in the same patient [39]. Alcoholic steatosis is the initial and most common manifestation of alcoholic liver disease. It is characterized histologically by both microvesicular and macrovesicular fat accumulation within the hepatocytes, with minimal inflammatory response or hepatic fibrosis [40]. Patients with steatosis are usually asymptomatic. They typically have normal to very mild elevations of their liver enzymes, such as GGT, ALT, and AST. Serum bilirubin and markers of hepatic function (international normalized ratio (INR), albumin levels) also tend to be normal. Alcoholic steatosis is reversible with abstinence [41].

Early studies by Dr. Charles Lieber using volunteers demonstrated the relative ease with which alcohol consumption causes fatty liver [42, 43]. Indeed, volunteers who drank heavily (46% of calories as alcohol) for 1–2 weeks exhibited fatty liver on biopsy.

A subset of people who continue to drink heavily will develop AH. Why only a subset of people develop more advanced and ominous disease is unclear, but probably relates at least in part to risk factors. These risk factors can be modifiable or nonmodifiable (Table 13.2). The most important modifiable risk factor is continued drinking. Nonmodifiable risk factors include sex (females are at higher risk) and genetics (certain polymorphisms, as discussed previously in the Mechanisms section). Alcoholic Hepatitis is a necro-inflammatory process characterized by predominant neutrophilic infiltration, ballooning degeneration of hepatocytes, and hepatocyte necrosis [44]. Acutely, the development of alcoholic hepatitis is associated with a significant increase in mortality and the potential to develop portal hypertension and its complications, even without developing major fibrosis [45]. In the long term, for those who survive, this disease process is associated with an accelerated course of fibrosis progressing to cirrhosis in 40% of cases [46]. These distinctions in the natural progression of alcoholic liver disease also have therapeutic implications, explaining why a subset of alcoholics with inflammatory features are candidates for treatment with anti-inflammatory agents (i.e., corticosteroids and pentoxifyline) in an attempt to reduce proximal mortality,

Table 13.2 Risk factors

- Continued drinking
- Age, sex
- Race
- Diet/nutrition
- Genetics/epigenetics/family history
- Smoking
- Obesity
- Occupational/Environmental exposure
- Medications/drugs of abuse
- Other liver diseases

whereas patients without major inflammatory features may be better candidates for treatment geared toward reducing long-term hepatic injury/cell death, hepatic dysfunction, or possibly enhancing liver regeneration.

Due to the important acute prognostic implications of alcoholic hepatitis and possible subsequent cirrhosis, multiple scoring systems have been developed to assess the severity of liver disease in terms of patient survival in order to assign patients to proven treatment modalities. The Child-Turcotte-Pugh (CTP), the oldest scoring system, incorporates the serum bilirubin level, albumin level, PT, and the severity of ascites and hepatic encephalopathy in assigning a numerical score that is used to categorize patients (class A=scores 1–6, class B=scores 7–9, class C=scores 10–15), with a higher score denoting more severe disease [47]. It is the most widely used scoring system to evaluate severity of cirrhosis. Since 2002, the United Network for Organ Sharing (UNOS) has utilized the MELD score to grade the severity of liver disease in patients awaiting liver transplant. This represents a more objective analysis, utilizing only the serum bilirubin, creatinine, and INR [48]. This scoring system has been validated in multiple studies to accurately predict the 3 month mortality of patients with liver disease, especially those patients awaiting liver transplantation [49].

The CTP and MELD score are proven modalities to assess the gravity of liver disease due to a variety of causes. However, due to the particularly inflammatory nature and high degree of early mortality associated with acute alcoholic hepatitis, varying scoring systems have been, and continue to be, specifically developed and used in the assessment of this form of liver disease. Since its development in the in the late 1970s, the Discriminant Function (DF) of Maddrey, which incorporates the serum bilirubin and PT, has been widely used to predict short-term mortality in patients with alcoholic hepatitis and to select in an evidence-based manner, those who are likely to benefit from treatment with corticosteroids [50]. Patients are classified into those who have nonsevere alcoholic hepatitis (DF<32) and those who have severe alcoholic hepatitis (DF>32). As the proximal early mortality is 10% versus 30–60% in the groups with and without treatment, respectively [51], the latter group is usually treated with corticosteroid therapy unless contraindicated [52]. A useful link to calculate 90-day mortality in acute alcoholic hepatitis, based in the MELD score, can be found at http://www.mayoclinic.org/medical-professionals/model-end-stage-liver-disease/meld-score-90-day-mortality-rate-alcoholic-hepatitis. Other specific scoring systems include the Glasgow alcoholic hepatitis score (GAHS) which is a composite of scores related to patient age, leukocyte count, serum urea levels, serum bilirubin level, and PT ratio [53], with a score ≥9 signifying poor prognosis. In this study, patients with both, a DF>32 and a GAHS>9, had 28 day survival, if corticosteroid-treated versus corticosteroid-untreated, of 78% vs. 52%, and an 84-day survival of 59% versus 38%, respectively. If the GAHS was less than 9, there was no difference in outcome between the corticosteroid treated or untreated groups. A more recent scoring system, the ABIC score [(age×0.1)+(serum bilirubin×0.08)+(serum creatinine×0.3)+(INR×0.8)], has shown promising results in the prediction of 3 month mortality in patients with alcoholic hepatitis [54]. This model stratifies the severity of alcoholic hepatitis as low (score<6.71), intermediate (score: 6.71–8.99), and high (score≥9.0). Theses scores correspond to a 90 day survival of 100 %, 70 %, and 25 % respectively, and 1-year survival of 97 %, 64 % and 33 % respectively.

The Lille score is unique in that it is not only clinically useful in assessing the severity of patients presenting with alcoholic hepatitis, but it is also used to assess the response of patients with more severe forms of alcoholic hepatitis being treated with systemic corticosteroids. The score includes six variables: age, albumin level, bilirubin level at day 0, bilirubin level at day 7, PT, and the presence of renal insufficiency [55]. A score of <0.45 predicts a 6 month survival of $85 \pm 2.5\%$ while a score >0.45 predicts a 6 month survival of only $25 \pm 3.8\%$ (sensitivity and specificity at 81 % and 76 %, respectively) [56]. Patients with a score of ≥ 0.45 on day 7 while on therapy with corticosteroids (null responders), which represent close to 40 % of the corticosteroid treated patients, are recommended to be switched over to alternative forms of treatment because they will not benefit from the continuation of corticosteroid therapy.

Therapy

Interventions for ALD patients reside on a continuum (Fig. 13.3). All patients should control the modifiable risk factors of alcohol use, obesity, and smoking. Most with advanced disease will benefit from treating malnutrition. Some may need pharmacotherapy. Only a few will be transplant candidates, and they are patients with severely decompensated ALD who have stopped drinking.

Lifestyle Modification

When managing a patient with ALD, steps should be taken to achieve alcohol cessation. Many studies have shown that patients who quit drinking have improved survival; moreover, even cutting back on alcohol consumption can lead to some improvement in liver disease [57]. Brief-interventions, during which a patient has regular conversations with a nurse or physician focusing on feedback, responsibility, advice, empathy, and optimism, have been shown to reduce drinking [58]. Patients should be encouraged to consider behavioral programs such as Alcoholics Anonymous. For patients who continue to crave alcohol despite brief-interventions and attending behavioral programs such as Alcoholics Anonymous, pharmacologic

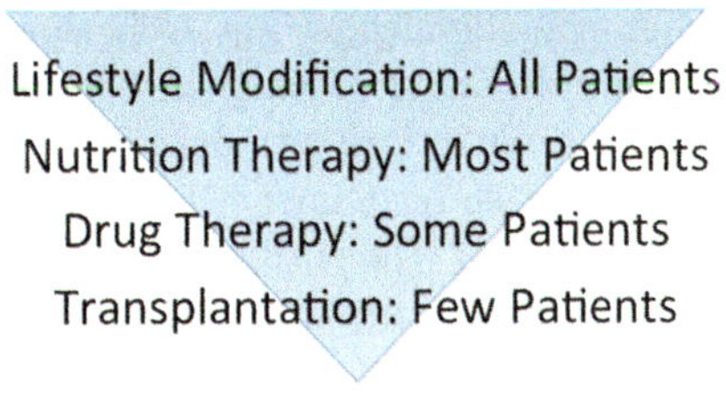

Fig. 13.3 ALD interventions

adjuncts can be offered. Baclofen is the only drug for alcohol dependence currently under investigation that has good safety data in patients with cirrhosis, making it a reasonable first-line choice in this patient population [59]. However, data are limited in ALD and more research is required.

Cigarette smoking [60] and obesity [61] are both independent risk factors for fibrosis in ALD and must also be addressed. While a patient may fit the definition of obesity (BMI > 30), he/she may still have concurrent nutritional deficiencies in macronutrients (e.g., protein) or in micronutrients (e.g., zinc), and nutrition must be evaluated.

Nutrition Therapy

Many patients with advanced ALD are malnourished, and liver disease severity correlates with the degree of malnutrition. While visceral proteins (albumin, prealbumin, and retinol binding protein) are the most common laboratory tests used to assess a patient's nutritional status, these results can be confounded by the underlying liver disease or superimposed infections. Evaluating clinical findings such as muscle wasting, edema, loss of subcutaneous fat, and glossitis/cheilosis are helpful in subjectively identifying protein energy malnutrition (PEM). Nutritional assessments of alcoholic patients can reveal adequate calorie intake. Indeed, in some studies, almost 50 % of patients' energy intake was from alcohol alone, leading to deficient protein and micronutrient intake [62]. ACG and AASLD guidelines recommend 1.2–1.5 g/kg of protein and 35–45 kcal/kg of body weight in patients with ALD [63]. For a 175 lb patient, that translates to about 96–120 g of protein a day and 2800–3600 cal a day. Adherence to sodium restriction is vital in patients starting to retain fluid (peripheral edema, ascites), which is usually seen in more advanced disease.

Patients with stable cirrhosis have nutritional deficiencies almost as severe as those found in patients with alcoholic hepatitis [64]. The frequency of malnutrition increases with the severity of disease. For example, the risk of profound malnutrition increases from 45 % in patients with Child's class A to 95 % in those with Child's C cirrhosis [64, 65]. Patients with cirrhosis who require hospitalization have a substantially higher prevalence of malnutrition compared with general medical inpatients and have significantly longer hospital stays and a twofold higher risk of in-hospital mortality [66]. Even in patients with stable, compensated cirrhosis, malnutrition is associated with higher mortality and complication rates within a year [65, 67].

Hepatic glycogen stores are depleted in patients with cirrhosis. As a result, these patients go into an early starvation mode after only 12 h of fasting compared to 48 h in normal individuals. Thus, even short periods of inadequate nutrition can result in peripheral muscle proteolysis, which contributes to protein malnutrition. Patients with decompensated cirrhosis may also be hypermetabolic. Not surprisingly, the protein intake recommended for patients with cirrhosis is higher than for healthy adults [67, 68]. The positive impact of judicious nutritional supplements in patients with cirrhosis is illustrated by a recent randomized trial showing that a nighttime

Table 13.3 Nutritional recommendations for ALD patients

• Evaluate for clinical signs of malnutrition in all ALD patients
• Daily Caloric Intake: 35–40 kcal/kg
• Daily Protein Intake: 1.2–1.5 g/kg
• Evening Snack of 700 cal and 26 g of protein for advanced disease
• Avoid n-6 unsaturated fats (linoleic acid)
• Multivitamin in most patients
– Zinc sulfate 220 mg
– Magnesium oxide 400 mg

snack of 700 kcal each evening resulted in an accrual of 2 kg of lean tissue over 12 months [69]. We stress the importance of taking a snack at about 9 pm to all our advanced cirrhotics (Table 13.3).

The increased nutritional requirements and the vulnerability to early starvation in cirrhotic patients underscore the importance of avoiding protein restriction in patients with encephalopathy. Prolonged protein restriction has no beneficial effect on encephalopathy and can be nutritionally catastrophic [64, 67, 70]. If, despite appropriate medical therapy, standard enteral formulas lead to encephalopathy, a branched chain amino acid-enriched formula can be given as a supplement to meet nitrogen needs [64, 68].

Patients with alcoholic liver disease also may have a plethora of vitamin and mineral deficiencies [64, 65]. In addition to the commonly recognized deficiencies in folate and B vitamins, deficiencies in fat soluble vitamins (A, D, and E) and minerals (magnesium, selenium, and zinc) are common causes of symptoms and physical findings in these patients [65]. Zinc deficiency, for example, may be an important component of the skin lesions, night blindness, mental irritability, confusion and hepatic encephalopathy, anorexia, altered taste and smell, hypogonadism, and altered wound healing so commonly seen in patients with alcoholic liver disease [8]. Assessment and judicious corrections of each of these deficiencies is an important aspect of the care of these patients. We advise that most patients take a multivitamin and we frequently supplement with zinc sulfate 220 mg daily, as well as magnesium oxide 400 mg daily.

Drug Therapy for Severe Alcoholic Hepatitis

A host of drugs have been tried in clinical trials to treat AH or, in some cases, alcoholic cirrhosis, and most have been ineffective (Reviewed-[1, 71–77]). Antioxidants of a variety of types including vitamin E and antioxidant cocktails have not proven to be effective in AH [73, 75, 77]. Lecithin was used in a large VA Cooperative Study to combat alcoholic fibrosis without statistically significant benefit [72]. Most recently, specific anti-TNF drugs have been ineffective in AH. Other drugs used in large trials are listed in Table 13.4 [71].

Table 13.4 Drug therapy

• PTU X
• Colchicine X
• Lecithin X
• Anabolic steroids X
• Antioxidants X
• Anti-TNFs X
• Corticosteroids
• Pentoxifylline

Corticosteroids and Pentoxifylline Therapy for Severe AH

Glucocorticoid (prednisone/prednisolone) therapy for AH has been recommended in AASLD and ACG guidelines, but some patients do not respond to steroids and have been termed "steroid resistant." Research suggests that steroid nonresponding AH patients have a 6-month mortality of approximately 60 %. Pentoxifylline (weak nonspecific PDE inhibitor) has been used in AH with some promising results, but further studies on its efficacy/mechanisms of action are needed, as well as studies on more specific PDE inhibitors [78–80]. We review data supporting the use of steroids and pentoxifylline in AH, as well as limitations of both of these drugs.

Corticosteroids have been successfully used to treat a wide variety of chronic inflammatory diseases and are the current standard of care in the treatment of severe AH. However, glucocorticoid resistance poses a challenging clinical problem. Glucocorticoids (GC) act by binding to glucocorticoid receptors (GR) in the cytoplasm, which are subsequently activated and translocate to the nucleus. There, the GR can bind to the glucocorticoid response elements (GREs) in the promoter region of the glucocorticoid responsive genes to switch on the expression of anti-inflammatory genes. Repression of inflammatory genes by GR requires recruitment of co-repressor molecules, particularly histone deacetylases (HDAC-6,-2) [81, 82]. Resistance to the anti-inflammatory effects of GC can be induced by several mechanisms which may differ between patients [83–92].

One simple and clinically utilized definition of glucocorticoid resistance in AH patients is the lack of an early change in bilirubin levels (ECBL) at 7 days [93]. The subsequently developed Lille Model also allows patients to receive a 7-day course of corticosteroids and then assesses the responsiveness previously noted [56]. These "stopping rules" have provided some greater comfort in using steroids in AH—we have criteria for drug discontinuation if it is not providing benefit.

It is important to only treat those with severe AH with steroids. Maddrey et al. first described factors associated with severe AH and devised the original Maddrey Discriminant Function (DF) [50]. Later revised and validated, several trials and meta analyses have consistently shown that patients with a Maddrey's DF score ≥ 32 or spontaneous hepatic encephalopathy who are treated with steroids have a statistically significant reduction in mortality compared to placebo [94, 95].

Pro- and anti-inflammatory cytokines (particularly TNF-α and IL-10) play an important role in the pathogenesis of AH [96]. Pentoxifylline (PTX) is a nonselective phosphodiesterase (PDE) inhibitor that has been shown to have survival benefit in initial AH studies [78, 79]. PTX treatment increases intracellular concentrations of cAMP and cGMP, and increased cAMP has been shown to positively modulate the cytokine inflammatory response. Agents that enhance cAMP (such as dbcAMP, adenylcyclase (AC) agonists, and PDE4 inhibitors) have been used in in vivo studies to protect against LPS- and alcohol-induced hepatitis [97, 98]. We have shown that chronic ethanol exposure increases LPS-inducible expression of PDE4B in monocytes/macrophages of both human and murine origin, and this is associated with enhanced NFκB activation and transcriptional activity and subsequent priming of monocytes/macrophages leading to enhanced LPS-inducible TNF-α production [99]. Initial clinical trials of patients with AH taking pentoxifylline have shown an improvement in short-term survival and a decrease in complications. In 2000, Akrividis et al. randomized 101 severe AH patients to receive either pentoxifylline (400 mg orally three times daily) or placebo for 28 days [78]. Twelve of the 49 pentoxifylline patients (24 %) died during the study period compared to 24 of 52 control patients (46.1 %, $p=0.037$). PTX was particularly effective at preventing hepatorenal syndrome.

It is important to note that combining corticosteroids and pentoxifylline does not appear to confer beneficial effects nor does switching from corticosteroids to pentoxifylline in "steroid nonresponders" [100–102]. Corticosteroids generally provide no benefit in patients with renal impairment and can increase risk of infection (especially fungal infections) [103]. The risk:benefit ratio has been improved by various models such as the early drop in bilirubin and the Lille model. However, length of steroid therapy in AH is still quite empiric.

Pentoxifylline has many theoretic advantages, including long-term safety in humans. It has hepatic anti-fibrotic effects as well as beneficial effects in some models of renal dysfunction and gut-barrier dysfunction in experimental animals [104–111]. Unfortunately, the most recent and largest study (Stop AH) comparing corticosteroids to pentoxifylline showed no benefit over placebo with either drug [112]. In contrast, a recent meta-analysis including the Stop AH data did suggest positive short-term benefits with corticosteroids and less strong benefit with pentoxifylline [113].

Our current approach for hospitalized patients with severe AH is nutritional support including feeding tube placement if necessary, and corticosteroid therapy in patients without contraindications. Patients are then reassessed at the end of 1 week for response. In patients with early renal dysfunction or steroid contraindications, pentoxifylline is used. For patients with less severe liver disease, AH (MELD under 19–20), or stable cirrhosis, we tend to use probiotic therapy (*Lactobacillus* GG) alone or in combination with pentoxifylline or zinc.

For all patients, maintaining abstinence (or at least reduced alcohol intake) is important. Patients should undergo regular surveillance (6 month imaging) for hepatocellular carcinoma and screening for esophageal varices as appropriate. Weight control, appropriate vaccinations, and elimination of smoking are also very important.

Liver Transplantation

Liver transplantation is covered in detail in the chapter on that topic. Alcoholic cirrhosis is the second most common indication for liver transplantation in the U.S. behind Hepatitis C [114]. The outcome following liver transplantation is generally quite favorable [115–117]. Important factors that reduce survival after the transplant include concurrent HCV infection, smoking, and a return to major drinking (not observed in most patients) [115, 118–120]. Many programs have a 6 month rule of abstinence before considering transplantation.

In the U.S., patients with severe AH have not been considered to be appropriate candidates for liver transplantation because of recent drinking and the risk of return to drinking [121–123]. Interesting research from France reported that carefully screened patients with severe alcoholic hepatitis who failed to respond to corticosteroid therapy had dramatic improvement in survival with early liver transplantation compared to matched controls [124]. These patients were highly selected, and this study is unlikely to translate to the U.S., especially with the severe shortage of organs.

Potential New Options

Because there is no FDA-approved therapy for any form of alcoholic liver disease, there is a pressing need for effective drug therapy. The NIH has funded a consortium to develop new molecular targets and new therapies for AH. Some of those being investigated include interleukin-1 and inflammasome inhibitors, a caspase inhibitor to block apoptosis, another interleukin-1 inhibitor in combination with pentoxifylline and zinc, and prednisone plus an anti-endotoxin. For milder disease (<20 MELD), a probiotic (*Lactobacillus* GG) is being given. Some other clinical trials include use of an extracorporeal liver assist device (ELAD) for patients who have failed steroid therapy and Granulocyte-macrophage colony-stimulating factor (GM-CSF) therapy to stimulate liver regeneration. There are also a number of anti-fibrotic agents in the pipeline. It is likely that combinations of agents will be used in the future, with varying periods of treatment. It also is likely that different drugs will be used to target different disease severity. In summary, there are several agents in clinical trials and many more in preclinical testing that make the future of ALD therapy very promising.

References

1. Carithers RL, McClain CJ. Alcoholic liver disease. In: Feldman M, Friedman LS, Brandt LJ, editors. Sleisenger and Fordtran's gastrointestinal and liver disease, vol. 2. Philadelphia, PA: Elsevier Saunders; 2016. p. 1409–27.

2. Liangpunsakul S. Clinical characteristics and mortality of hospitalized alcoholic hepatitis patients in the United States. J Clin Gastroenterol. 2011;45(8):714–9. PubMed PMID: 21085006, PubMed Central PMCID: 3135756.

3. Sandahl TD, Jepsen P, Thomsen KL, Vilstrup H. Incidence and mortality of alcoholic hepatitis in Denmark 1999-2008: a nationwide population based cohort study. J Hepatol. 2011;54(4):760–4.

4. Chedid A, Mendenhall CL, Gartside P, French SW, Chen T, Rabin L. Prognostic factors in alcoholic liver disease. VA Cooperative Study Group. Am J Gastroenterol. 1991;86(2):210–6.

5. Beier JI, McClain CJ. Mechanisms and cell signaling in alcoholic liver disease. Biol Chem. 2010;391(11):1249–64. PubMed PMID: 20868231, PubMed Central PMCID: 3755482.

6. Mendenhall C, Roselle GA, Gartside P, Moritz T. Relationship of protein calorie malnutrition to alcoholic liver disease: a reexamination of data from two Veterans Administration Cooperative Studies. Alcohol Clin Exp Res. 1995;19(3):635–41.

7. Zhong W, Zhao Y, Sun X, Song Z, McClain CJ, Zhou Z. Dietary zinc deficiency exaggerates ethanol-induced liver injury in mice: involvement of intrahepatic and extrahepatic factors. PLoS One. 2013;8(10):e76522. PubMed PMID: 24155903, PubMed Central PMCID: 3796541.

8. Mohammad MK, Zhou Z, Cave M, Barve A, McClain CJ. Zinc and liver disease. Nutr Clin Pract. 2012;27(1):8–20.

9. Kirpich IA, Feng W, Wang Y, Liu Y, Barker DF, Barve SS, et al. The type of dietary fat modulates intestinal tight junction integrity, gut permeability, and hepatic toll-like receptor expression in a mouse model of alcoholic liver disease. Alcohol Clin Exp Res. 2012;36(5):835–46. PubMed PMID: 22150547, PubMed Central PMCID: 3319492.

10. Purohit V, Bode JC, Bode C, Brenner DA, Choudhry MA, Hamilton F, et al. Alcohol, intestinal bacterial growth, intestinal permeability to endotoxin, and medical consequences: summary of a symposium. Alcohol. 2008;42(5):349–61.

11. Gustot T, Lemmers A, Moreno C, Nagy N, Quertinmont E, Nicaise C, et al. Differential liver sensitization to toll-like receptor pathways in mice with alcoholic fatty liver. Hepatology. 2006;43(5):989–1000.

12. Gao B, Seki E, Brenner DA, Friedman S, Cohen JI, Nagy L, et al. Innate immunity in alcoholic liver disease. Am J Physiol Gastrointest Liver Physiol. 2011;300(4):G516–25. PubMed PMID: 21252049, PubMed Central PMCID: 3774265.

13. Schnabl B, Brenner DA. Interactions between the intestinal microbiome and liver diseases. Gastroenterology. 2014;146(6):1513–24. PubMed PMID: 24440671, PubMed Central PMCID: 3996054.

14. Bull-Otterson L, Feng W, Kirpich I, Wang Y, Qin X, Liu Y, et al. Metagenomic analyses of alcohol induced pathogenic alterations in the intestinal microbiome and the effect of Lactobacillus rhamnosus GG treatment. PLoS One. 2013;8(1):e53028. PubMed PMID: 23326376, PubMed Central PMCID: 3541399.

15. Shi X, Wei X, Yin X, Wang Y, Zhang M, Zhao C, et al. Hepatic and fecal metabolomic analysis of the effects of lactobacillus rhamnosus GG on alcoholic fatty liver disease in mice. J Proteome Res. 2015;14(2):1174–82.

16. Esfandiari F, Villanueva JA, Wong DH, French SW, Halsted CH. Chronic ethanol feeding and folate deficiency activate hepatic endoplasmic reticulum stress pathway in micropigs. Am J Physiol Gastrointest Liver Physiol. 2005;289(1):G54–63.

17. Galligan JJ, Smathers RL, Shearn CT, Fritz KS, Backos DS, Jiang H, et al. Oxidative Stress and the ER stress response in a murine model for early-stage alcoholic liver disease. J Toxicol. 2012;2012:207594. PubMed PMID: 22829816, PubMed Central PMCID: 3399426.

18. Tsedensodnom O, Vacaru AM, Howarth DL, Yin C, Sadler KC. Ethanol metabolism and oxidative stress are required for unfolded protein response activation and steatosis in zebrafish with alcoholic liver disease. Dis Model Mech. 2013;6(5):1213–26. PubMed PMID: 23798569, PubMed Central PMCID: 3759341.

19. Tsuchiya M, Ji C, Kosyk O, Shymonyak S, Melnyk S, Kono H, et al. Interstrain differences in liver injury and one-carbon metabolism in alcohol-fed mice. Hepatology. 2012;56(1):130–9. PubMed PMID: 22307928, PubMed Central PMCID: 3350836.

20. Ramirez T, Tong M, Chen WC, Nguyen QG, Wands JR, de la Monte SM. Chronic alcohol-induced hepatic insulin resistance and endoplasmic reticulum stress ameliorated by peroxisome-proliferator activated receptor-delta agonist treatment. J Gastroenterol Hepatol. 2013;28(1):179–87. PubMed PMID: 22988930, PubMed Central PMCID: 4406771.
21. Tong M, Longato L, Ramirez T, Zabala V, Wands JR, de la Monte SM. Therapeutic reversal of chronic alcohol-related steatohepatitis with the ceramide inhibitor myriocin. Int J Exp Pathol. 2014;95(1):49–63. PubMed PMID: 24456332, PubMed Central PMCID: 3919649.
22. Dimova EY, Kietzmann T. Metabolic, hormonal and environmental regulation of plasminogen activator inhibitor-1 (PAI-1) expression: lessons from the liver. Thromb Haemost. 2008;100(6):992–1006.
23. Stickel F, Osterreicher CH. The role of genetic polymorphisms in alcoholic liver disease. Alcohol Alcohol. 2006;41(3):209–24.
24. Mendenhall CL. Alcoholic hepatitis. Clin Gastroenterol. 1981;10(2):417–41.
25. Lischner MW, Alexander JF, Galambos JT. Natural history of alcoholic hepatitis. I. The acute disease. Am J Dig Dis. 1971;16(6):481–94.
26. Bradley KA, DeBenedetti AF, Volk RJ, Williams EC, Frank D, Kivlahan DR. AUDIT-C as a brief screen for alcohol misuse in primary care. Alcohol Clin Exp Res. 2007;31(7):1208–17.
27. Smith PC, Schmidt SM, Allensworth-Davies D, Saitz R. Primary care validation of a single-question alcohol screening test. J Gen Intern Med. 2009;24(7):783–8. PubMed PMID: 19247718, PubMed Central PMCID: 2695521.
28. Ewing JA. Detecting alcoholism. The CAGE questionnaire. JAMA. 1984;252(14):1905–7.
29. Becker U, Deis A, Sorensen TI, Gronbaek M, Borch-Johnsen K, Muller CF, et al. Prediction of risk of liver disease by alcohol intake, sex, and age: a prospective population study. Hepatology. 1996;23(5):1025–9.
30. Crabb DW. Pathogenesis of alcoholic liver disease: newer mechanisms of injury. Keio J Med. 1999;48(4):184–8.
31. Van Thiel DH, Gavaler JS, Schade RR. Liver disease and the hypothalamic pituitary gonadal axis. Semin Liver Dis. 1985;5(1):35–45.
32. Dutta SK, Dukehart M, Narang A, Latham PS. Functional and structural changes in parotid glands of alcoholic cirrhotic patients. Gastroenterology. 1989;96(2 Pt 1):510–8.
33. Pirovino M, Linder R, Boss C, Kochli HP, Mahler F. Cutaneous spider nevi in liver cirrhosis: capillary microscopical and hormonal investigations. Klin Wochenschr. 1988;66(7):298–302.
34. Attali P, Ink O, Pelletier G, Vernier C, Jean F, Moulton L, et al. Dupuytren's contracture, alcohol consumption, and chronic liver disease. Arch Intern Med. 1987;147(6):1065–7.
35. Epstein O, Dick R, Sherlock S. Prospective study of periostitis and finger clubbing in primary biliary cirrhosis and other forms of chronic liver disease. Gut. 1981;22(3):203–6. PubMed PMID: 7227854, PubMed Central PMCID: 1419499.
36. Bell H, Tallaksen CM, Try K, Haug E. Carbohydrate-deficient transferrin and other markers of high alcohol consumption: a study of 502 patients admitted consecutively to a medical department. Alcohol Clin Exp Res. 1994;18(5):1103–8.
37. Yersin B, Nicolet JF, Dercrey H, Burnier M, van Melle G, Pecoud A. Screening for excessive alcohol drinking. Comparative value of carbohydrate-deficient transferrin, gamma-glutamyltransferase, and mean corpuscular volume. Arch Intern Med. 1995;155(17):1907–11.
38. Van Ness MM, Diehl AM. Is liver biopsy useful in the evaluation of patients with chronically elevated liver enzymes? Ann Intern Med. 1989;111(6):473–8.
39. Louvet A, Mathurin P. Alcoholic liver disease: mechanisms of injury and targeted treatment. Nat Rev Gastroenterol Hepatol. 2015;12(4):231–42.
40. Pateria P, de Boer B, MacQuillan G. Liver abnormalities in drug and substance abusers. Best Pract Res Clin Gastroenterol. 2013;27(4):577–96.
41. Mathurin P, Beuzin F, Louvet A, Carrie-Ganne N, Balian A, Trinchet JC, et al. Fibrosis progression occurs in a subgroup of heavy drinkers with typical histological features. Aliment Pharmacol Ther. 2007;25(9):1047–54.
42. Rubin E, Lieber CS. Alcohol-induced hepatic injury in nonalcoholic volunteers. N Engl J Med. 1968;278(16):869–76.

43. Lieber CS, Rubin E. Alcoholic fatty liver in man on a high protein and low fat diet. Am J Med. 1968;44(2):200–6.
44. MacSween RN, Burt AD. Histologic spectrum of alcoholic liver disease. Semin Liver Dis. 1986;6(3):221–32.
45. Ma C, Brunt EM. Histopathologic evaluation of liver biopsy for cirrhosis. Adv Anat Pathol. 2012;19(4):220–30.
46. Gao B, Bataller R. Alcoholic liver disease: pathogenesis and new therapeutic targets. Gastroenterology. 2011;141(5):1572–85. PubMed PMID: 21920463, PubMed Central PMCID: 3214974.
47. Said A, Holden JP, Williams JB, Musat A, Botero RC, Lucey MR. Model for end stage liver disease (MELD) scores predict mortality across a broad spectrum of liver disease in a us tertiary care-setting. Gastroenterology. 2003;124(4):A690–1.
48. Kamath PS, Wiesner RH, Malinchoc M, Kremers W, Therneau TM, Kosberg CL, et al. A model to predict survival in patients with end-stage liver disease. Hepatology. 2001;33(2):464–70.
49. Freeman Jr RB, Wiesner RH, Harper A, McDiarmid SV, Lake J, Edwards E, et al. The new liver allocation system: moving toward evidence-based transplantation policy. Liver Transpl. 2002;8(9):851–8.
50. Maddrey WC, Boitnott JK, Bedine MS, Weber Jr FL, Mezey E, White Jr RI. Corticosteroid therapy of alcoholic hepatitis. Gastroenterology. 1978;75(2):193–9.
51. Theodossi A, Eddleston AL, Williams R. Controlled trial of methylprednisolone therapy in severe acute alcoholic hepatitis. Gut. 1982;23(1):75–9. PubMed PMID: 7035299, PubMed Central PMCID: 1419581.
52. Carithers Jr RL, Herlong HF, Diehl AM, Shaw EW, Combes B, Fallon HJ, et al. Methylprednisolone therapy in patients with severe alcoholic hepatitis. A randomized multi-center trial. Ann Intern Med. 1989;110(9):685–90.
53. Forrest EH, Evans CD, Stewart S, Phillips M, Oo YH, McAvoy NC, et al. Analysis of factors predictive of mortality in alcoholic hepatitis and derivation and validation of the Glasgow alcoholic hepatitis score. Gut. 2005;54(8):1174–9. PubMed PMID: 16009691, PubMed Central PMCID: 1774903.
54. Dominguez M, Rincon D, Abraldes JG, Miquel R, Colmenero J, Bellot P, et al. A new scoring system for prognostic stratification of patients with alcoholic hepatitis. Am J Gastroenterol. 2008;103(11):2747–56.
55. Lille Model http://www.lillemodel.com/score.asp2015 (cited 2015 April 7, 2015).
56. Louvet A, Naveau S, Abdelnour M, Ramond MJ, Diaz E, Fartoux L, et al. The Lille model: a new tool for therapeutic strategy in patients with severe alcoholic hepatitis treated with steroids. Hepatology. 2007;45(6):1348–54.
57. Lucey MR. Management of alcoholic liver disease. Clin Liver Dis. 2009;13(2):267–75.
58. Lieber CS, Weiss DG, Groszmann R, Paronetto F, Schenker S. I. Veterans Affairs Cooperative Study of polyenylphosphatidylcholine in alcoholic liver disease: effects on drinking behavior by nurse/physician teams. Alcohol Clin Exp Res. 2003;27(11):1757–64.
59. Muzyk AJ, Rivelli SK, Gagliardi JP. Defining the role of baclofen for the treatment of alcohol dependence: a systematic review of the evidence. CNS Drugs. 2012;26(1):69–78.
60. Klatsky AL, Armstrong MA. Alcohol, smoking, coffee, and cirrhosis. Am J Epidemiol. 1992;136(10):1248–57.
61. Raynard B, Balian A, Fallik D, Capron F, Bedossa P, Chaput JC, et al. Risk factors of fibrosis in alcohol-induced liver disease. Hepatology. 2002;35(3):635–8.
62. Mendenhall CL, Moritz TE, Roselle GA, Morgan TR, Nemchausky BA, Tamburro CH, et al. A study of oral nutritional support with oxandrolone in malnourished patients with alcoholic hepatitis: results of a Department of Veterans Affairs cooperative study. Hepatology. 1993;17(4):564–76.
63. McCullough AJ, O'Connor JF. Alcoholic liver disease: proposed recommendations for the American College of Gastroenterology. Am J Gastroenterol. 1998;93(11):2022–36.

64. McClain CJ, Barve SS, Barve A, Marsano L. Alcoholic liver disease and malnutrition. Alcohol Clin Exp Res. 2011;35(5):815–20.
65. Singal AK, Charlton MR. Nutrition in alcoholic liver disease. Clin Liver Dis. 2012;16(4):805–26.
66. Sam J, Nguyen GC. Protein-calorie malnutrition as a prognostic indicator of mortality among patients hospitalized with cirrhosis and portal hypertension. Liver Int. 2009;29(9):1396–402.
67. Cheung K, Lee SS, Raman M. Prevalence and mechanisms of malnutrition in patients with advanced liver disease, and nutrition management strategies. Clin Gastroenterol Hepatol. 2012;10(2):117–25.
68. Plauth M, Cabre E, Riggio O, Assis-Camilo M, Pirlich M, Kondrup J, et al. ESPEN guidelines on enteral nutrition: liver disease. Clin Nutr. 2006;25(2):285–94.
69. Plank LD, Gane EJ, Peng S, Muthu C, Mathur S, Gillanders L, et al. Nocturnal nutritional supplementation improves total body protein status of patients with liver cirrhosis: a randomized 12-month trial. Hepatology. 2008;48(2):557–66.
70. Schulz GJ, Campos AC, Coelho JC. The role of nutrition in hepatic encephalopathy. Curr Opin Clin Nutr Metab Care. 2008;11(3):275–80.
71. Boetticher NC, Peine CJ, Kwo P, Abrams GA, Patel T, Aqel B, et al. A randomized, double-blinded, placebo-controlled multicenter trial of etanercept in the treatment of alcoholic hepatitis. Gastroenterology. 2008;135(6):1953–60. PubMed PMID: 18848937, PubMed Central PMCID: PMC2639749.
72. Lieber CS, Weiss DG, Groszmann R, Paronetto F, Schenker S. Veterans Affairs Cooperative Study G. II. Veterans Affairs Cooperative Study of polyenylphosphatidylcholine in alcoholic liver disease. Alcohol Clin Exp Res. 2003;27(11):1765–72.
73. Mezey E, Potter JJ, Rennie-Tankersley L, Caballeria J, Pares A. A randomized placebo controlled trial of vitamin E for alcoholic hepatitis. J Hepatol. 2004;40(1):40–6.
74. Morgan TR, Weiss DG, Nemchausky B, Schiff ER, Anand B, Simon F, et al. Colchicine treatment of alcoholic cirrhosis: a randomized, placebo-controlled clinical trial of patient survival. Gastroenterology. 2005;128(4):882–90.
75. Phillips M, Curtis H, Portmann B, Donaldson N, Bomford A, O'Grady J. Antioxidants versus corticosteroids in the treatment of severe alcoholic hepatitis--a randomised clinical trial. J Hepatol. 2006;44(4):784–90.
76. Rambaldi A, Gluud C. Meta-analysis of propylthiouracil for alcoholic liver disease--a Cochrane Hepato-Biliary Group Review. Liver. 2001;21(6):398–404.
77. Stewart S, Prince M, Bassendine M, Hudson M, James O, Jones D, et al. A randomized trial of antioxidant therapy alone or with corticosteroids in acute alcoholic hepatitis. J Hepatol. 2007;47(2):277–83.
78. Akriviadis E, Botla R, Briggs W, Han S, Reynolds T, Shakil O. Pentoxifylline improves short-term survival in severe acute alcoholic hepatitis: a double-blind, placebo-controlled trial. Gastroenterology. 2000;119(6):1637–48.
79. De BK, Gangopadhyay S, Dutta D, Baksi SD, Pani A, Ghosh P. Pentoxifylline versus prednisolone for severe alcoholic hepatitis: a randomized controlled trial. World J Gastroenterol. 2009;15(13):1613–9. PubMed PMID: 19340904, PubMed Central PMCID: 2669113.
80. Gobejishvili L, Crittenden N, Mcclain C. Controversies in hepatology: the experts analyze both sides. Thorofare, NJ: Slack, Inc.; 2011. p. 3–10.
81. De Bosscher K, Haegeman G. Minireview: latest perspectives on antiinflammatory actions of glucocorticoids. Mol Endocrinol. 2009;23(3):281–91.
82. Barnes PJ, Adcock IM. Glucocorticoid resistance in inflammatory diseases. Lancet. 2009;373(9678):1905–17.
83. Ito K, Chung KF, Adcock IM. Update on glucocorticoid action and resistance. J Allergy Clin Immunol. 2006;117(3):522–43.
84. Ito K, Yamamura S, Essilfie-Quaye S, Cosio B, Ito M, Barnes PJ, et al. Histone deacetylase 2-mediated deacetylation of the glucocorticoid receptor enables NF-kappaB suppression. J Exp Med. 2006;203(1):7–13. PubMed PMID: 16380507, PubMed Central PMCID: 2118081.

85. Ito K, Ito M, Elliott WM, Cosio B, Caramori G, Kon OM, et al. Decreased histone deacetylase activity in chronic obstructive pulmonary disease. N Engl J Med. 2005;352(19): 1967–76.
86. Wang FF, Zhu LA, Zou YQ, Zheng H, Wilson A, Yang CD, et al. New insights into the role and mechanism of macrophage migration inhibitory factor in steroid-resistant patients with systemic lupus erythematosus. Arthritis Res Ther. 2012;14(3):R103. PubMed PMID: 22551315, PubMed Central PMCID: 3446480.
87. di Mambro AJ, Parker R, McCune A, Gordon F, Dayan CM, Collins P. In vitro steroid resistance correlates with outcome in severe alcoholic hepatitis. Hepatology. 2011;53(4):1316–22.
88. Barnes PJ. Mechanisms and resistance in glucocorticoid control of inflammation. J Steroid Biochem Mol Biol. 2010;120(2-3):76–85.
89. Rajendrasozhan S, Yang SR, Edirisinghe I, Yao H, Adenuga D, Rahman I. Deacetylases and NF-kappaB in redox regulation of cigarette smoke-induced lung inflammation: epigenetics in pathogenesis of COPD. Antioxid Redox Signal. 2008;10(4):799–811. PubMed PMID: 18220485, PubMed Central PMCID: 2758554.
90. Rogatsky I, Ivashkiv LB. Glucocorticoid modulation of cytokine signaling. Tissue Antigens. 2006;68(1):1–12.
91. Hearing SD, Norman M, Probert CS, Haslam N, Dayan CM. Predicting therapeutic outcome in severe ulcerative colitis by measuring in vitro steroid sensitivity of proliferating peripheral blood lymphocytes. Gut. 1999;45(3):382–8. PubMed PMID: 10446106, PubMed Central PMCID: 1727659.
92. Kendrick SF, Henderson E, Palmer J, Jones DE, Day CP. Theophylline improves steroid sensitivity in acute alcoholic hepatitis. Hepatology. 2010;52(1):126–31.
93. Mathurin P, Abdelnour M, Ramond MJ, Carbonell N, Fartoux L, Serfaty L, et al. Early change in bilirubin levels is an important prognostic factor in severe alcoholic hepatitis treated with prednisolone. Hepatology. 2003;38(6):1363–9.
94. Mathurin P, O'Grady J, Carithers RL, Phillips M, Louvet A, Mendenhall CL, et al. Corticosteroids improve short-term survival in patients with severe alcoholic hepatitis: meta-analysis of individual patient data. Gut. 2011;60(2):255–60.
95. Rambaldi A, Saconato HH, Christensen E, Thorlund K, Wetterslev J, Gluud C. Systematic review: glucocorticosteroids for alcoholic hepatitis--a Cochrane Hepato-Biliary Group systematic review with meta-analyses and trial sequential analyses of randomized clinical trials. Aliment Pharmacol Ther. 2008;27(12):1167–78.
96. McClain CJ, Cohen DA. Increased tumor necrosis factor production by monocytes in alcoholic hepatitis. Hepatology. 1989;9(3):349–51.
97. Taguchi I, Oka K, Kitamura K, Sugiura M, Oku A, Matsumoto M. Protection by a cyclic AMP-specific phosphodiesterase inhibitor, rolipram, and dibutyryl cyclic AMP against Propionibacterium acnes and lipopolysaccharide-induced mouse hepatitis. Inflamm Res. 1999;48(7):380–5.
98. Gouillon ZQ, Miyamoto K, Donohue TM, Wan YJ, French BA, Nagao Y, et al. Role of CYP2E1 in the pathogenesis of alcoholic liver disease: modifications by cAMP and ubiquitin-proteasome pathway. Front Biosci. 1999;4:A16–25.
99. Gobejishvili L, Barve S, Joshi-Barve S, McClain C. Enhanced PDE4B expression augments LPS-inducible TNF expression in ethanol-primed monocytes: relevance to alcoholic liver disease. Am J Physiol Gastrointest Liver Physiol. 2008;295(4):G718–24. PubMed PMID: 18687753, PubMed Central PMCID: 2575909.
100. Mathurin P, Louvet A, Duhamel A, Nahon P, Carbonell N, Boursier J, et al. Prednisolone with vs without pentoxifylline and survival of patients with severe alcoholic hepatitis: a randomized clinical trial. JAMA. 2013;310(10):1033–41.
101. Sidhu SS, Goyal O, Singla P, Gupta D, Sood A, Chhina RS, et al. Corticosteroid plus pentoxifylline is not better than corticosteroid alone for improving survival in severe alcoholic hepatitis (COPE trial). Dig Dis Sci. 2012;57(6):1664–71.

102. Louvet A, Diaz E, Dharancy S, Coevoet H, Texier F, Thevenot T, et al. Early switch to pentoxifylline in patients with severe alcoholic hepatitis is inefficient in non-responders to corticosteroids. J Hepatol. 2008;48(3):465–70.
103. Singh S, Murad MH, Chandar AK, Bongiorno CM, Singal AK, Atkinson SR, et al. Comparative effectiveness of pharmacological interventions for severe alcoholic hepatitis: a systematic review and network meta-analysis. Gastroenterology. 2015;149(4):958–70.e12.
104. Asvadi I, Hajipour B, Asvadi A, Asl NA, Roshangar L, Khodadadi A. Protective effect of pentoxyfilline in renal toxicity after methotrexate administration. Eur Rev Med Pharmacol Sci. 2011;15(9):1003–9.
105. Bansal S, Wang W, Falk S, Schrier R. Combination therapy with albumin and pentoxifylline protects against acute kidney injury during endotoxemic shock in mice. Ren Fail. 2009;31(9):848–54.
106. Costantini TW, Loomis WH, Putnam JG, Drusinsky D, Deree J, Choi S, et al. Burn-induced gut barrier injury is attenuated by phosphodiesterase inhibition: effects on tight junction structural proteins. Shock. 2009;31(4):416–22. PubMed PMID: 18791495, PubMed Central PMCID: PMC3445035.
107. Costantini TW, Loomis WH, Putnam JG, Kroll L, Eliceiri BP, Baird A, et al. Pentoxifylline modulates intestinal tight junction signaling after burn injury: effects on myosin light chain kinase. J Trauma. 2009;66(1):17–24. discussion -5, PubMed PMID: 19131801, PubMed Central PMCID: PMC4251583.
108. Nasiri-Toosi Z, Dashti-Khavidaki S, Khalili H, Lessan-Pezeshki M. A review of the potential protective effects of pentoxifylline against drug-induced nephrotoxicity. Eur J Clin Pharmacol. 2013;69(5):1057–73.
109. Wattanasirichaigoon S, Menconi MJ, Fink MP. Lisofylline ameliorates intestinal and hepatic injury induced by hemorrhage and resuscitation in rats. Crit Care Med. 2000;28(5):1540–9.
110. Wystrychowski W, Wystrychowski G, Zukowska-Szczechowska E, Obuchowicz E, Grzeszczak W, Wiecek A, et al. Nephroprotective effect of pentoxifylline in renal ischemia-reperfusion in rat depends on the timing of its administration. Transplant Proc. 2014;46(8):2555–7.
111. Gobejishvili L, Barve S, Breitkopf-Heinlein K, Li Y, Zhang J, Avila DV, et al. Rolipram attenuates bile duct ligation-induced liver injury in rats: a potential pathogenic role of PDE4. J Pharmacol Exp Ther. 2013;347(1):80–90. PubMed PMID: 23887098, PubMed Central PMCID: PMC3781411.
112. Thursz MR, Richardson P, Allison M, Austin A, Bowers M, Day CP, et al. Prednisolone or pentoxifylline for alcoholic hepatitis. N Engl J Med. 2015;372(17):1619–28.
113. Hmoud BS, Patel K, Bataller R, Singal AK. Corticosteroids and occurrence of and mortality from infections in severe alcoholic hepatitis: a meta-analysis of randomized trials. Liver Int. 2016;36(5):721–8. doi: 10.1111/liv.12939. Epub 2015 Sep 14.
114. Lucey MR. Liver transplantation in patients with alcoholic liver disease. Liver Transpl. 2011;17(7):751–9.
115. Burra P, Senzolo M, Adam R, Delvart V, Karam V, Germani G, et al. Liver transplantation for alcoholic liver disease in Europe: a study from the ELTR (European Liver Transplant Registry). Am J Transplant. 2010;10(1):138–48.
116. Berlakovich GA. Challenges in transplantation for alcoholic liver disease. World J Gastroenterol. 2014;20(25):8033–9. PubMed PMID: 25009374, PubMed Central PMCID: PMC4081673.
117. Singal AK, Chaha KS, Rasheed K, Anand BS. Liver transplantation in alcoholic liver disease current status and controversies. World J Gastroenterol. 2013;19(36):5953–63. PubMed PMID: 24106395, PubMed Central PMCID: PMC3785616.
118. Pfitzmann R, Schwenzer J, Rayes N, et al. Long-term survival and predictors of relapse after orthotopic liver transplantation for alcoholic liver disease. Liver Transpl. 2007;13:197–205.
119. Cuadrado A, Fabrega E, Casafont F, Pons-Romero F. Alcohol recidivism impairs long-term patient survival after orthotopic liver transplantation for alcoholic liver disease. Liver Transpl. 2005;11(4):420–6.

120. Altamirano J, Bataller R. Cigarette smoking and chronic liver diseases. Gut. 2010;59(9):1159–62.
121. Lucey MR, Mathurin P, Morgan TR. Alcoholic hepatitis. N Engl J Med. 2009;360(26):2758–69.
122. O'Shea RS, Dasarathy S, McCullough AJ. Practice Guideline Committee of the American Association for the Study of Liver D, Practice Parameters Committee of the American College of G. Alcoholic liver disease. Hepatology. 2010;51(1):307–28.
123. Frazier TH, Stocker AM, Kershner NA, Marsano LS, McClain CJ. Treatment of alcoholic liver disease. Therap Adv Gastroenterol. 2011;4(1):63–81. PubMed PMID: 21317995, PubMed Central PMCID: 3036962.
124. Mathurin P, Moreno C, Samuel D, Dumortier J, Salleron J, Durand F, et al. Early liver transplantation for severe alcoholic hepatitis. N Engl J Med. 2011;365(19):1790–800.

Chapter 14
Nonalcoholic Fatty Liver Disease

Samer Gawrieh

Abbreviations

NAFLD   Nonalcoholic fatty liver disease
NASH   Nonalcoholic steatohepatitis
TZD   Thiazoloidinediones
CVD   Cardiovascular disease
HCC   Hepatocellular carcinoma
ALT   Alanine aminotransaminase

What Is Nonalcoholic Fatty Liver Disease (NAFLD)?

Patient-Level Answer

Nonalcoholic fatty liver disease (NAFLD) is an umbrella term used to indicate varying severities of liver disease as a consequence to increasing hepatic fat content that occur in the setting of nonsignificant alcohol intake. In the simplest and more benign form, nonalcoholic fatty liver (NAFL) also referred to as simple steatosis, there is only increase in liver fat. On the other hand, nonalcoholic steatohepatitis (NASH) is the more severe form of NAFLD, where in addition to increased hepatic fat; there is variable mixture and severity of inflammation, liver cell injury, and fibrosis.

S. Gawrieh, M.D. (✉)
Division of Gastroenterology and Hepatology, Indiana University School of Medicine,
702 Rotary Circle, Suite 225, Indianapolis, IN 46202, USA
e-mail: sgawrieh@iu.edu

© Springer International Publishing Switzerland 2017
K. Sacian, R. Shaker (eds.), *Liver Disorders*,
DOI 10.1007/978-3-319-30103-7_14

Summary of the Pertinent Literature

NAFLD is a spectrum of hepatic injury that starts with NAFL where there is an increase in intrahepatic triglycerides resulting in macrosteatosis but without hepatic necroinflammation or fibrosis. NASH is the more severe phenotype of NAFLD and is defined by histological features on liver biopsy of macrosteatosis plus findings of lobular inflammation, hepatocyte ballooning with or without fibrosis [1, 2]. These findings resemble those seen in patients with alcoholic hepatitis; however, as Dr. Ludwig originally observed, are also seen in patients who with no or nonsignificant alcohol intake [3]. The most widely used criteria for defining significant alcohol use set the thresholds at >30 g/day for men and >20 g/day for women [2, 4, 5]. Beyond these thresholds, steatosis and steatohepatitis may be related to excessive alcohol consumption.

Is NAFLD a Common Problem?

Patient-Level Answer

NAFLD is the most common liver disease worldwide. About one in three Americans has fatty liver. Many factors influence how common fatty liver is. Increasing body weight and obesity come with higher risk of NAFLD. Up to nine out of ten of the severely obese may have fatty liver. Different racial groups have different prevalence of NAFLD: Hispanics have higher chance of having fatty liver and about one in two has fatty liver, whereas African Americans have lower chance of having fatty liver and about one in four has fatty liver. Patients who have type 2 diabetes also run a higher risk and seven out of ten patients with diabetes may have fatty liver. These factors also increase the risk of having NASH with higher proportion of patients with severe obesity, diabetes, and of Hispanic ethnicity having NASH.

Summary of the Pertinent Literature

NAFLD is the most common liver disease not only in the US but also in other parts of the world. In the US, one-third of an urban population had NAFLD as defined by increased hepatic triglycerides content over 5 % by magnetic resonance spectroscopy [6]. This prevalence falls well within the range of NAFLD prevalence in the remainder of the world (6–35 %, median prevalence 20 %) [7]. The prevalence of NAFLD and NASH increases with increasing body mass index (BMI) [8]. In the morbidly obese undergoing bariatric surgery, up to 97 % have NAFLD and up to 72 % have NASH in different studies [7–9]. Patients with diabetes have a high prevalence of NAFLD with nearly 76 % of patients seen in diabetes clinics having steatosis on imaging and up to 56% of those undergoing liver biopsies having NASH despite normal aminotransferases [10–12]. Diabetes is also an independent risk factor for more severe NASH with advanced fibrosis [13–17]. The prevalence of NAFLD and NASH is impacted by race as Hispanics have higher prevalence of both compared to Whites, who in turn have higher prevalence of both than African Americans [6, 18]. The prevalence of cryptogenic cirrhosis, most commonly due to NASH, follows similar prevalence among different racial groups [19].

How Did I Get NAFLD?

Patient-Level Answer

The increase in body fat with overweight and obesity reduces insulin function in many organs. This results in the delivery of more fat in the form of free fatty acids to the liver. The liver stores the delivered fat into triglycerides to offset its toxicity. This buffer mechanism may fail in some genetically predisposed patients, who as a consequence, experience toxicity from these fatty acids leading to development of NASH with liver inflammation and fibrosis.

A small minority of patients can get fatty liver without being overweight. This can happen with a variety of conditions, such as the use of certain medications, rapid weight loss, use of intravenous nutrition, or starvation.

Summary of the Pertinent Literature

There is a linear relationship between increasing body weight and NAFLD [8]. Increasing body fat is associated with insulin resistance in adipose, muscle, and liver tissues [20, 21]. Insulin resistance is present in nearly all patients with NAFLD and is associated with increased adipose tissue lipolysis, release and delivery of free fatty acids to the liver, and increased triglycerides synthesis [22, 23]. Free fatty acids are directly hepatotoxic and promote macrophage release of inflammatory cytokines, hepatic inflammation, and apoptosis [24, 25]. The increase in fatty acid oxidation is associated with oxidative stress with increased lipid, protein, and DNA peroxidation and dysfunction in mitochondria, lysosomes, and endoplasmic reticulum, leading to hepatic inflammation, apoptosis, and fibrosis [24, 26–31].

Genome-wide association studies revealed several gene variants that alter the susceptibility to NAFLD [32–35]. The adiponutrin (patatin-like phospholipase domain-containing protein 3, PNPLA3) gene in particular has been widely tested and validated in different cohorts [36–38]. The PNPLA3 (rs738409) variant has been shown to influence hepatic triglyceride content and NAFLD severity [32–34]. The risk allele (G) for this variant has the highest frequency in Hispanics (49 %), and the lowest frequency in African Americans (17 %) while its frequency in Whites was in

Table 14.1 Causes of steatosis and steatohepatitis

Insulin resistance
Alcohol
Medications (corticosteroids, amiodarone, tamoxifen, methotrexate, anti-retrovirals, valproic acid)
Starvation
Total parenteral nutrition
Wilson Disease
Hepatitis C virus infection (genotype 3)
Lipodystrophy
Organic solvents
Abetalipoproteinemia
Acute fatty liver of pregnancy

the middle (23 %), suggesting that variants in this gene may explain at least part of the differences in susceptibility to and severity of NAFLD across racial groups [32].

Secondary causes for NAFLD should be considered when evaluating patients with hepatic steatosis or steatohepatitis who are lean and do not have the typical associated metabolic conditions (Table 14.1).

How Is the Diagnosis Made?

Patient-Level Answer

Diagnosis of NAFLD relies on abdominal imaging tests such as ultrasound or CT scan showing signs of fatty liver and excluding other conditions that can cause fatty liver or elevated liver tests. However, definitive diagnosis and determining whether a patient has NAFL or NASH currently requires doing a liver biopsy.

Summary of the Pertinent Literature

NAFLD is usually suspected based on findings of unexplained elevated amino-transferases or incidental finding of hepatic steatosis on abdominal imaging. Routine imaging studies such as ultrasound, CT scan, and MRI can only detect significant steatosis (>30 % steatosis), but cannot distinguish NAFL from NASH [39, 40]. Exclusion of concomitant chronic liver disease is done by testing for viral, autoimmune, and metabolic liver diseases. Other noninvasive methods are designed primarily to detect the fibrotic, but not the inflammatory component of NASH. These include different panels of serum markers or measurement of liver stiffness via a specially designed ultrasound or MRI (elastography) [13, 14, 41–44]. However concerns about their performance in detecting NASH and particularly NASH with advanced fibrosis are triggered by less than optimal accuracy when some of these noninvasive markers are tested in different cohort [44–46]. Liver biopsy remains the "gold standard" for the diagnosis of NAFLD and the identification of patients with NASH, despite its clinical risks and limitations [47].

My Liver Tests Are Normal; Does This Mean I Do Not Have NASH?

Patient-Level Answer

Many patients with NAFLD have normal liver tests including those at risk for NASH with advanced liver fibrosis. Routine liver tests have poor sensitivity to detect liver damage in the setting of NAFLD and NASH.

Summary of the Pertinent Literature

Normal liver tests are common in patients with NAFLD [14]. When compared to those with elevated transaminases, patients with NAFLD and normal aminotransferases had the entire spectrum of NAFLD including NASH with advanced fibrosis [16]. In a recent report for a cohort with type 2 diabetes and normal aminotransferases, NAFLD diagnosed with magnetic resonance spectroscopy was diagnosed in 76 % of the patients, and NASH was diagnosed in 56 % of the subgroup of patients that agreed to liver biopsy, highlighting the poor sensitivity of ALT as a predictor of NAFLD or NASH [12].

Do I Need to Have a Liver Biopsy to Know If I Have NASH or Severe Damage to My Liver?

Patient-Level Answer

Not every patient with NAFLD will need a liver biopsy but in some patients with NAFLD and risk factors for having NASH and significant liver fibrosis, a liver biopsy may be necessary. Such risk factors for severe NAFLD need to be carefully evaluated for by managing physician. Risk and benefits of the liver biopsy and potential change in management should also be discussed in details before proceeding with the biopsy.

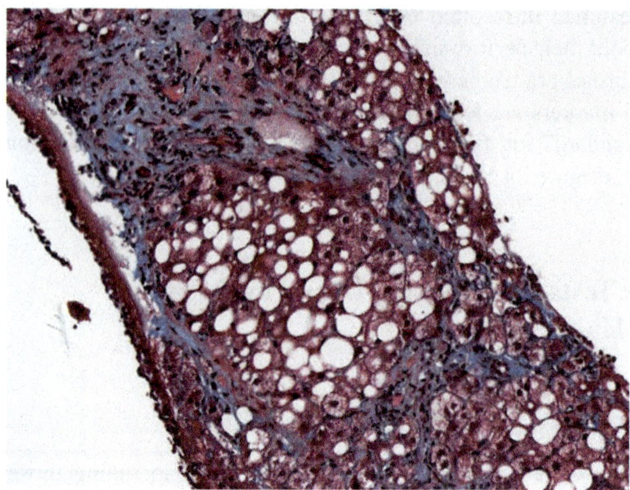

Fig. 14.1 NASH with cirrhosis. Macrosteatosis, hepatocyte ballooning, lobular inflammation, and severe fibrosis with regenerative nodule are seen in this liver biopsy

Summary of the Pertinent Literature

The definitive diagnosis of NAFLD and its subphenotypes NAFL versus NASH is based on histological analysis of a liver biopsy sample. The presence of steatosis, hepatocellular ballooning, and lobular inflammation, with or without fibrosis, are necessary criteria for diagnosis of NASH (Fig. 14.1) [1, 2]. Although liver biopsy is generally a safe procedure, its invasive nature and associated small risk of complications limits its wide scale routine use to diagnose NASH [48, 49]. Therefore, selection of patients with NAFLD for liver biopsy should be based on their estimated risk for having NASH with advanced fibrosis and after discussing the risks of liver biopsy and impact of information obtained on prognosis and management. Validated risk factors for NASH include diabetes or glucose intolerance, advanced age, high body mass index, high ALT, sleep apnea, high triglycerides, and low platelets [13, 14, 50, 51]. The current multisociety guidelines recommends using the NAFLD fibrosis score (http://nafldscore.com) as an easily accessible tool that includes many of the validated risk factors for NASH and advanced fibrosis, to choose NAFLD patients at risk for NASH with advanced fibrosis for liver biopsy [13, 47].

What Is the Outlook for My Liver If I Have NAFLD?

Patient-Level Answer

Serious liver-related complications such as cirrhosis, liver failure, and cancer may develop in some patients. Current evidence suggests that these complications are most likely to happen in patients with NASH and particularly those who have significant fibrosis. The majority of patients with NAFL will not develop these complications.

Summary of the Pertinent Literature

While patients with NAFL do not usually develop liver complications, those with NASH are at increased risk for progressive hepatic fibrosis (in 32–41 %), development of cirrhosis (in 5–25 %), liver failure (in 45–52 % of NASH cirrhosis), and hepatocellular carcinoma (HCC) (in 2.5–7 %) [52–59]. Therefore, the liver-related outcomes largely depend on the baseline NAFLD phenotype [7, 40, 47]. In patients with NASH, the single histological lesion that is most predictive of liver-related events is fibrosis and particularly advanced fibrosis [40, 59, 60]. There are emerging reports of HCC in patients with NAFLD without cirrhosis or even significant fibrosis [61–63]. While this phenomenon is interesting, it is unknown if it reflects co-occurrence of a common disease, NAFLD, with HCC which is known to occur without cirrhosis in some patients (estimated at 5 % in the US and Europe and 40 % in Asia) [64] or if it is related to sampling error of surrounding hepatic tissue resulting in underestimation of fibrosis.

Will NAFLD Affect My Overall Health?

Patient-Level Answer

NAFLD increases the risk for cardiovascular disease (CVD) and type 2 diabetes. The top three causes of death in patients with NAFLD are CVD, nonhepatic malignancies, and liver-related death, with the later tending to occur mainly in patients with NASH.

Summary of the Pertinent Literature

NAFLD, regardless of the underlying phenotype, is also an independent risk factor for CVD and type 2 diabetes [11, 40, 65–67]. CVD is the leading cause of death in patients with NAFLD followed by nonhepatic malignancies and cirrhosis-related events [52, 65, 68, 69]. Patients with NASH are at much higher risk for cirrhosis-related death than those with NAFL [40, 52, 59].

What Treatment Options Do I Have?

Patient-Level Answer

Weight loss is recommended for all patients with NAFLD. Mild to moderate weight loss of 3–7 % of baseline body weight may result in significant improvement in NAFL and NASH. Bariatric surgery in the morbidly obese patients with NAFL or NASH may result in improvement or resolution of NAFLD. For patients with biopsy proven NASH without cirrhosis or diabetes, vitamin E or pioglitazone can be considered as a treatment that may improve liver injury with long-term use.

Summary of the Pertinent Literature

The most tested effective options are weight loss, vitamin E, and pioglitazone. Mild weight loss of 3–5 % of starting body weight is sufficient to improve insulin sensitivity, aminotransferases, hepatic steatosis by various imaging modalities, and liver histology [70–88].

Improvement in NASH histological lesions such as steatosis, ballooning, and lobular inflammation usually requires more weight loss of ≥7 % of baseline weight [72, 77, 86, 87, 89, 90]. Regardless of the degree of associated weight loss, resistance or aerobic exercise can improve insulin sensitivity and hepatic steatosis [77, 80, 88, 91]. Furthermore, physical fitness predicts the risk of NAFLD and increased fitness correlates with resolution of fatty liver by magnetic resonance spectroscopy [91].

Bariatric surgery results in sustainable and considerable loss of excess weight (>30 %) in the morbidly obese, which is associated with remarkable improvement or resolution of liver injury in patients with NAFL and NASH, in addition to significant improvement in the associated metabolic comorbidities [92–102]. Certain types of bariatric surgery such as jejunoileal and biliointestinal bypasses are associated with worsening hepatic fibrosis in patients with NAFLD [95, 99, 103]. There is paucity of data about the safety of bariatric surgery in patients with NASH cirrhosis with or without portal hypertension.

Of the many antioxidants, vitamin E has been the best studied in patients with NAFLD [4, 104–108]. In the largest randomized study to date in NASH, the PIVENS, vitamin E 800 IU daily was compared to pioglitazone 30 mg daily or placebo for 96 weeks in NASH patients without underlying cirrhosis or diabetes [4]. Vitamin E and Pioglitazone resulted in improvement in hepatic steatosis, lobular inflammation, hepatocellular ballooning but without significant improvement in fibrosis. NASH resolution was observed in 43 % of subjects on vitamin E, 34 % of subjects on pioglitazone and 19 % of subjects on placebo. Unlike pioglitazone, there was no increase in weight seen in subjects taking vitamin E. The associations of vitamin E with increased mortality and prostate cancer have been subject to debate [109–114]. The safety and efficacy of vitamin E in patients with diabetes and cirrhosis is unknown. Vitamin E is considered a first line option for NASH patients without cirrhosis or diabetes according to the recent multisociety guidelines [47].

Several other studies showed similar beneficial effects of pioglitazone, a peroxisome proliferator-activated receptor gamma agonist, on NASH histology [115–117]. Concerns about long term safety of thiazoloidinediones (TZDs) in diabetic patients have been raised with reports of increased risk of congestive heart failure, bladder cancer, and bone fractures [118, 119]. The current multisociety guidelines recommend that pioglitazone may be used with caution to treat nondiabetic patients with biopsy-proven NASH [47].

A recent large randomized trial testing the effects of 72 weeks of obeticholic acid, a farnesoid X receptor portent agonist, in patients with NASH showed significant improvement in all NASH histological lesions compared to placebo [5]. While these results are encouraging, additional clinical trials are needed to confirm the efficacy and define the safety profile of obeticholic acid.

Available data from clinical trials do not convincingly show efficacy for other agents for NASH such as metformin, ursodeoxycholic acid, or long-chain polyunsaturated fatty acids and therefore these cannot be recommended for patients with NASH at the present time [107, 120–124].

Can I Take "Statins" to Lower My Cholesterol If I Have NAFLD?

Patient-Level Answer

Statins can be safely used in patients with NAFLD with or without elevated liver tests. Having NAFLD does not increase the risk for liver toxicity from statins. The benefit of cardiovascular disease risk reduction with statins far outweighs the remote risk of severe liver toxicity in patients with NAFLD.

Summary of the Pertinent Literature

The safety of statins in patients with NAFLD has been demonstrated in several studies [125–127]. The incidence of severe elevations in transaminases in patients with presumed NAFLD and underlying increased transaminases was not significantly different than that in patients with dyslipidemia and normal transaminases receiving statins or patients with liver disease and elevated transaminases who did not receive a statin [126]. Another study evaluated the course of baseline increased liver enzymes in patients with coronary artery disease who either received or did not receive statin [125]. A decline in increased liver tests with statin use was observed compared to continued increase in patients not receiving statin. The number of cardiovascular events was significantly higher in patients who did not get statin (30 % versus 10 %; relative risk reduction 68 %, $p < 0.0001$). The improvement in liver tests and potential improvement in liver histology with statins use in patients with NAFLD has been reported in other smaller studies [128–134]. Acute liver failure due to statin use necessitating liver transplantation is very rare [135]. Based on this data, the strong relationship between NAFLD and increased risk of CVD and the fact CVD is the leading cause of death in patients with NAFLD [7, 40, 65, 66, 136], there is no justification to withhold statins from NAFLD patients who have appropriate indications for their use. Statins should only be stopped in the rare situation of severe liver injury manifesting as severe elevation in the liver enzymes, jaundice, or liver failure [137].

What About My Kids?

Patient-Level Answer

NAFLD is the most common liver disease in children. A diagnosis of NAFLD in a family member, adult or child, increases the risk of NAFLD in other family members.

Summary of the Pertinent Literature

NAFLD is the most common liver disease in children in the US [138]. In an Autopsy series, 13% of children had NAFLD, of whom 18% had NASH [139]. The prevalence of NAFLD increases with age and follows the same ethnic distribution observed in adults [139]. A combination of shared environmental factors such as dietary habits and activity patterns in families, with genetic factors may increase the risk of first degree family members with NAFLD to have the disease. Family studies suggest increased frequency of NASH or cryptogenic cirrhosis in addition to obesity and diabetes in relatives of patients with NASH [140]. Another study reported one out of five patients with NASH had a first degree relative with NASH [141]. On the other hand, NAFLD in children is associated with a high risk of NAFLD in their families with a study showing 78% of parents and 59% of siblings having NAFLD [142].

Will I Need a Liver Transplant?

Patient-Level Answer

In patients with NASH cirrhosis who develop liver failure or HCC, liver transplantation should be considered as an option to improve patient survival and quality of life. Careful systematic evaluation of patients is necessary to determine candidacy. In particular, meticulous evaluation and optimization of CVD is necessary for excellent outcomes. With proper selection of candidates, and optimal control of associated obesity, cardiac and metabolic conditions, the outcomes of liver transplantation for patients with NASH are excellent.

Summary of the Pertinent Literature

Patients with NASH cirrhosis who develop liver failure or early stage HCC should be evaluated for liver transplantation. Liver transplantation for NASH is increasingly common and is currently the third most common indication for liver transplantation in the US [143–145]. Patients with NASH cirrhosis who are listed for liver transplantation are usually older, and have higher body mass index and lower incidence of HCC than those listed for other indications [143, 146]. And because they have high prevalence of CVD, a thorough cardiac evaluation prior to listing is critical to ensure optimization of the cardiac status and outcomes post-transplantation [147]. The patient survival at 1- and 3-year following transplantation for NASH cirrhosis is excellent [143–145, 148]. Patient or graft survival is not affected by NAFLD recurrence post-transplantation, which has been reported in up to 40 % of patients [145, 149–151]. Excellent control of associated metabolic comorbidities and obesity is essential for successful outcome after liver transplantation [152].

References

1. Brunt EM. Pathology of nonalcoholic fatty liver disease. Nat Rev Gastroenterol Hepatol. 2010;7(4):195–203.
2. Neuschwander-Tetri BA, Caldwell SH. Nonalcoholic steatohepatitis: summary of an AASLD Single Topic Conference. Hepatology. 2003;37(5):1202–19.
3. Ludwig J, Viggiano TR, McGill DB, Oh BJ. Nonalcoholic steatohepatitis: Mayo Clinic experiences with a hitherto unnamed disease. Mayo Clin Proc. 1980;55(7):434–8.
4. Sanyal AJ, Chalasani N, Kowdley KV, McCullough A, Diehl AM, Bass NM, et al. Pioglitazone, vitamin E, or placebo for nonalcoholic steatohepatitis. N Engl J Med. 2010;362(18):1675–85.
5. Neuschwander-Tetri BA, Loomba R, Sanyal AJ, Lavine JE, Van Natta ML, Abdelmalek MF, et al. Farnesoid X nuclear receptor ligand obeticholic acid for non-cirrhotic, non-alcoholic steatohepatitis (FLINT): a multicentre, randomised, placebo-controlled trial. Lancet. 2015;385:956.
6. Browning JD, Szczepaniak LS, Dobbins R, Nuremberg P, Horton JD, Cohen JC, et al. Prevalence of hepatic steatosis in an urban population in the United States: impact of ethnicity. Hepatology. 2004;40(6):1387–95.
7. Vernon G, Baranova A, Younossi ZM. Systematic review: the epidemiology and natural history of non-alcoholic fatty liver disease and non-alcoholic steatohepatitis in adults. Aliment Pharmacol Ther. 2011;34(3):274–85.
8. Lazo M, Clark JM. The epidemiology of nonalcoholic fatty liver disease: a global perspective. Semin Liver Dis. 2008;28(4):339–50.
9. Ong JP, Elariny H, Collantes R, Younoszai A, Chandhoke V, Reines HD, et al. Predictors of nonalcoholic steatohepatitis and advanced fibrosis in morbidly obese patients. Obes Surg. 2005;15(3):310–5.
10. Kelley DE, McKolanis TM, Hegazi RA, Kuller LH, Kalhan SC. Fatty liver in type 2 diabetes mellitus: relation to regional adiposity, fatty acids, and insulin resistance. Am J Physiol Endocrinol Metab. 2003;285(4):E906–16.
11. Targher G, Bertolini L, Padovani R, Rodella S, Tessari R, Zenari L, et al. Prevalence of non-alcoholic fatty liver disease and its association with cardiovascular disease among type 2 diabetic patients. Diabetes Care. 2007;30(5):1212–8.
12. Portillo Sanchez P, Bril F, Maximos M, Lomonaco R, Biernacki D, Orsak B, et al. High prevalence of nonalcoholic fatty liver disease in patients with type 2 diabetes mellitus and normal plasma aminotransferase levels. J Clin Endocrinol Metab. 2015;100:2231.
13. Angulo P, Hui JM, Marchesini G, Bugianesi E, George J, Farrell GC, et al. The NAFLD fibrosis score: a noninvasive system that identifies liver fibrosis in patients with NAFLD. Hepatology. 2007;45(4):846–54.

14. Ulitsky A, Ananthakrishnan AN, Komorowski R, Wallace J, Surapaneni SN, Franco J, et al. A noninvasive clinical scoring model predicts risk of nonalcoholic steatohepatitis in morbidly obese patients. Obes Surg. 2010;20(6):685–91.

15. Neuschwander-Tetri BA, Clark JM, Bass NM, Van Natta ML, Unalp-Arida A, Tonascia J, et al. Clinical, laboratory and histological associations in adults with nonalcoholic fatty liver disease. Hepatology. 2010;52(3):913–24.

16. Mofrad P, Contos MJ, Haque M, Sargeant C, Fisher RA, Luketic VA, et al. Clinical and histologic spectrum of nonalcoholic fatty liver disease associated with normal ALT values. Hepatology. 2003;37(6):1286–92.

17. Loomba R, Abraham M, Unalp A, Wilson L, Lavine J, Doo E, et al. Association between diabetes, family history of diabetes, and risk of nonalcoholic steatohepatitis and fibrosis. Hepatology. 2012;56(3):943–51.

18. Williams CD, Stengel J, Asike MI, Torres DM, Shaw J, Contreras M, et al. Prevalence of nonalcoholic fatty liver disease and nonalcoholic steatohepatitis among a largely middle-aged population utilizing ultrasound and liver biopsy: a prospective study. Gastroenterology. 2011;140(1):124–31.

19. Browning JD, Kumar KS, Saboorian MH, Thiele DL. Ethnic differences in the prevalence of cryptogenic cirrhosis. Am J Gastroenterol. 2004;99(2):292–8.

20. Schindler TH, Cardenas J, Prior JO, Facta AD, Kreissl MC, Zhang XL, et al. Relationship between increasing body weight, insulin resistance, inflammation, adipocytokine leptin, and coronary circulatory function. J Am Coll Cardiol. 2006;47(6):1188–95.

21. Shulman GI. Ectopic fat in insulin resistance, dyslipidemia, and cardiometabolic disease. N Engl J Med. 2014;371(12):1131–41.

22. Marchesini G, Brizi M, Bianchi G, Tomassetti S, Bugianesi E, Lenzi M, et al. Nonalcoholic fatty liver disease: a feature of the metabolic syndrome. Diabetes. 2001;50(8):1844–50.

23. Marchesini G, Brizi M, Morselli-Labate AM, Bianchi G, Bugianesi E, McCullough AJ, et al. Association of nonalcoholic fatty liver disease with insulin resistance. Am J Med. 1999;107(5):450–5.

24. Malhi H, Gores GJ. Molecular mechanisms of lipotoxicity in nonalcoholic fatty liver disease. Semin Liver Dis. 2008;28(4):360–9.

25. Cusi K. Role of obesity and lipotoxicity in the development of nonalcoholic steatohepatitis: pathophysiology and clinical implications. Gastroenterology. 2012;142(4):711–25.e6.

26. Malhi H, Bronk SF, Werneburg NW, Gores GJ. Free fatty acids induce JNK-dependent hepatocyte lipoapoptosis. J Biol Chem. 2006;281(17):12093–101.

27. Feldstein AE, Werneburg NW, Canbay A, Guicciardi ME, Bronk SF, Rydzewski R, et al. Free fatty acids promote hepatic lipotoxicity by stimulating TNF-alpha expression via a lysosomal pathway. Hepatology. 2004;40(1):185–94.

28. Puri P, Mirshahi F, Cheung O, Natarajan R, Maher JW, Kellum JM, et al. Activation and dysregulation of the unfolded protein response in nonalcoholic fatty liver disease. Gastroenterology. 2008;134(2):568–76.

29. Seki S, Kitada T, Yamada T, Sakaguchi H, Nakatani K, Wakasa K. In situ detection of lipid peroxidation and oxidative DNA damage in non-alcoholic fatty liver diseases. J Hepatol. 2002;37(1):56–62.

30. Li Z, Oben JA, Yang S, Lin H, Stafford EA, Soloski MJ, et al. Norepinephrine regulates hepatic innate immune system in leptin-deficient mice with nonalcoholic steatohepatitis. Hepatology. 2004;40(2):434–41.

31. Gawrieh S, Opara EC, Koch TR. Oxidative stress in nonalcoholic fatty liver disease: pathogenesis and antioxidant therapies. J Invest Med. 2004;52(8):506–14.

32. Romeo S, Kozlitina J, Xing C, Pertsemlidis A, Cox D, Pennacchio LA, et al. Genetic variation in PNPLA3 confers susceptibility to nonalcoholic fatty liver disease. Nat Genet. 2008;40(12):1461–5.

33. Speliotes EK, Yerges-Armstrong LM, Wu J, Hernaez R, Kim LJ, Palmer CD, et al. Genome-wide association analysis identifies variants associated with nonalcoholic fatty liver disease that have distinct effects on metabolic traits. PLoS Genet. 2011;7(3):e1001324.

34. Chalasani N, Guo X, Loomba R, Goodarzi MO, Haritunians T, Kwon S, et al. Genome-wide association study identifies variants associated with histologic features of nonalcoholic Fatty liver disease. Gastroenterology. 2010;139(5):1567–76. 76.e1–6.
35. Adams LA, White SW, Marsh JA, Lye SJ, Connor KL, Maganga R, et al. Association between liver-specific gene polymorphisms and their expression levels with nonalcoholic fatty liver disease. Hepatology. 2013;57(2):590–600.
36. Valenti L, Al-Serri A, Daly AK, Galmozzi E, Rametta R, Dongiovanni P, et al. Homozygosity for the patatin-like phospholipase-3/adiponutrin I148M polymorphism influences liver fibrosis in patients with nonalcoholic fatty liver disease. Hepatology. 2010;51(4):1209–17.
37. Guichelaar MM, Gawrieh S, Olivier M, Viker K, Krishnan A, Sanderson S, et al. Interactions of allelic variance of PNPLA3 with nongenetic factors in predicting nonalcoholic steatohepatitis and nonhepatic complications of severe obesity. Obesity. 2013;21(9):1935–41.
38. Sookoian S, Castano GO, Burgueno AL, Gianotti TF, Rosselli MS, Pirola CJ. A nonsynonymous gene variant in the adiponutrin gene is associated with nonalcoholic fatty liver disease severity. J Lipid Res. 2009;50(10):2111–6.
39. Saadeh S, Younossi ZM, Remer EM, Gramlich T, Ong JP, Hurley M, et al. The utility of radiological imaging in nonalcoholic fatty liver disease. Gastroenterology. 2002;123(3):745–50.
40. Musso G, Gambino R, Cassader M, Pagano G. Meta-analysis: natural history of non-alcoholic fatty liver disease (NAFLD) and diagnostic accuracy of non-invasive tests for liver disease severity. Ann Med. 2011;43(8):617–49.
41. Ratziu V, Massard J, Charlotte F, Messous D, Imbert-Bismut F, Bonyhay L, et al. Diagnostic value of biochemical markers (FibroTest-FibroSURE) for the prediction of liver fibrosis in patients with non-alcoholic fatty liver disease. BMC Gastroenterol. 2006;6:6.
42. Rosenberg WM, Voelker M, Thiel R, Becka M, Burt A, Schuppan D, et al. Serum markers detect the presence of liver fibrosis: a cohort study. Gastroenterology. 2004;127(6):1704–13.
43. Feldstein AE, Alkhouri N, De Vito R, Alisi A, Lopez R, Nobili V. Serum cytokeratin-18 fragment levels are useful biomarkers for nonalcoholic steatohepatitis in children. Am J Gastroenterol. 2013;108(9):1526–31.
44. Machado MV, Cortez-Pinto H. Non-invasive diagnosis of non-alcoholic fatty liver disease. A critical appraisal. J Hepatol. 2013;58(5):1007–19.
45. Shah AG, Lydecker A, Murray K, Tetri BN, Contos MJ, Sanyal AJ, et al. Comparison of noninvasive markers of fibrosis in patients with nonalcoholic fatty liver disease. Clin Gastroenterol Hepatol. 2009;7(10):1104–12.
46. Vuppalanchi R, Jain AK, Deppe R, Yates K, Comerford M, Masuoka HC, et al. Relationship between changes in serum levels of keratin 18 and changes in liver histology in children and adults with nonalcoholic fatty liver disease. Clin Gastroenterol Hepatol. 2014;12:2121.
47. Chalasani N, Younossi Z, Lavine JE, Diehl AM, Brunt EM, Cusi K, et al. The diagnosis and management of non-alcoholic fatty liver disease: practice guideline by the American Association for the Study of Liver Diseases, American College of Gastroenterology, and the American Gastroenterological Association. Am J Gastroenterol. 2012;107(6):811–26.
48. Bravo AA, Sheth SG, Chopra S. Liver biopsy. N Engl J Med. 2001;344(7):495–500.
49. Rockey DC, Caldwell SH, Goodman ZD, Nelson RC, Smith AD, American Association for the Study of Liver Diseases. Liver biopsy. Hepatology. 2009;49(3):1017–44.
50. Campos GM, Bambha K, Vittinghoff E, Rabl C, Posselt AM, Ciovica R, et al. A clinical scoring system for predicting nonalcoholic steatohepatitis in morbidly obese patients. Hepatology. 2008;47(6):1916–23.
51. Dixon JB, Bhathal PS, O'Brien PE. Nonalcoholic fatty liver disease: predictors of nonalcoholic steatohepatitis and liver fibrosis in the severely obese. Gastroenterology. 2001;121(1):91–100.
52. Matteoni CA, Younossi ZM, Gramlich T, Boparai N, Liu YC, McCullough AJ. Nonalcoholic fatty liver disease: a spectrum of clinical and pathological severity. Gastroenterology. 1999;116(6):1413–9.
53. Harrison SA, Torgerson S, Hayashi PH. The natural history of nonalcoholic fatty liver disease: a clinical histopathological study. Am J Gastroenterol. 2003;98(9):2042–7.

54. Fassio E, Alvarez E, Dominguez N, Landeira G, Longo C. Natural history of nonalcoholic steatohepatitis: a longitudinal study of repeat liver biopsies. Hepatology. 2004;40(4):820–6.
55. Adams LA, Sanderson S, Lindor KD, Angulo P. The histological course of nonalcoholic fatty liver disease: a longitudinal study of 103 patients with sequential liver biopsies. J Hepatol. 2005;42(1):132–8.
56. Ekstedt M, Franzen LE, Mathiesen UL, Thorelius L, Holmqvist M, Bodemar G, et al. Long-term follow-up of patients with NAFLD and elevated liver enzymes. Hepatology. 2006;44(4):865–73.
57. Hui JM, Kench JG, Chitturi S, Sud A, Farrell GC, Byth K, et al. Long-term outcomes of cirrhosis in nonalcoholic steatohepatitis compared with hepatitis C. Hepatology. 2003;38(2):420–7.
58. Sanyal AJ, Banas C, Sargeant C, Luketic VA, Sterling RK, Stravitz RT, et al. Similarities and differences in outcomes of cirrhosis due to nonalcoholic steatohepatitis and hepatitis C. Hepatology. 2006;43(4):682–9.
59. Younossi ZM, Stepanova M, Rafiq N, Makhlouf H, Younoszai Z, Agrawal R, et al. Pathologic criteria for nonalcoholic steatohepatitis: interprotocol agreement and ability to predict liver-related mortality. Hepatology. 2011;53(6):1874–82.
60. Angulo P, Bugianesi E, Bjornsson ES, Charatcharoenwitthaya P, Mills PR, Barrera F, et al. Simple non-invasive systems predict long-term outcomes of patients with nonalcoholic fatty liver disease. Gastroenterology. 2013;145:782.
61. Yasui K, Hashimoto E, Komorizono Y, Koike K, Arii S, Imai Y, et al. Characteristics of patients with nonalcoholic steatohepatitis who develop hepatocellular carcinoma. Clin Gastroenterol Hepatol. 2011;9(5):428–33. quiz e50.
62. Baffy G, Brunt EM, Caldwell SH. Hepatocellular carcinoma in non-alcoholic fatty liver disease: an emerging menace. J Hepatol. 2012;56(6):1384–91.
63. Bullock RE, Zaitoun AM, Aithal GP, Ryder SD, Beckingham IJ, Lobo DN. Association of non-alcoholic steatohepatitis without significant fibrosis with hepatocellular carcinoma. J Hepatol. 2004;41(4):685–6.
64. Forner A, Llovet JM, Bruix J. Hepatocellular carcinoma. Lancet. 2012;379(9822):1245–55.
65. Targher G, Day CP, Bonora E. Risk of cardiovascular disease in patients with nonalcoholic fatty liver disease. N Engl J Med. 2010;363(14):1341–50.
66. Targher G, Bertolini L, Rodella S, Tessari R, Zenari L, Lippi G, et al. Nonalcoholic fatty liver disease is independently associated with an increased incidence of cardiovascular events in type 2 diabetic patients. Diabetes Care. 2007;30(8):2119–21.
67. Sung KC, Kim SH. Interrelationship between fatty liver and insulin resistance in the development of type 2 diabetes. J Clin Endocrinol Metab. 2011;96(4):1093–7.
68. Ong JP, Pitts A, Younossi ZM. Increased overall mortality and liver-related mortality in non-alcoholic fatty liver disease. J Hepatol. 2008;49(4):608–12.
69. Rafiq N, Bai C, Fang Y, Srishord M, McCullough A, Gramlich T, et al. Long-term follow-up of patients with nonalcoholic fatty liver. Clin Gastroenterol Hepatol. 2009;7(2):234–8.
70. Kugelmas M, Hill DB, Vivian B, Marsano L, McClain CJ. Cytokines and NASH: a pilot study of the effects of lifestyle modification and vitamin E. Hepatology. 2003;38(2):413–9.
71. Ryan MC, Abbasi F, Lamendola C, Carter S, McLaughlin TL. Serum alanine aminotransferase levels decrease further with carbohydrate than fat restriction in insulin-resistant adults. Diabetes Care. 2007;30(5):1075–80.
72. Nobili V, Manco M, Devito R, Di Ciommo V, Comparcola D, Sartorelli MR, et al. Lifestyle intervention and antioxidant therapy in children with nonalcoholic fatty liver disease: a randomized, controlled trial. Hepatology. 2008;48(1):119–28.
73. Catalano D, Trovato GM, Martines GF, Randazzo M, Tonzuso A. Bright liver, body composition and insulin resistance changes with nutritional intervention: a follow-up study. Liver Int. 2008;28(9):1280–7.
74. Larson-Meyer DE, Newcomer BR, Heilbronn LK, Volaufova J, Smith SR, Alfonso AJ, et al. Effect of 6-month calorie restriction and exercise on serum and liver lipids and markers of liver function. Obesity (Silver Spring). 2008;16(6):1355–62.

75. Zhang X, Yeung DC, Karpisek M, Stejskal D, Zhou ZG, Liu F, et al. Serum FGF21 levels are increased in obesity and are independently associated with the metabolic syndrome in humans. Diabetes. 2008;57(5):1246–53.
76. Lazo M, Solga SF, Horska A, Bonekamp S, Diehl AM, Brancati FL, et al. Effect of a 12-month intensive lifestyle intervention on hepatic steatosis in adults with type 2 diabetes. Diabetes Care. 2010;33(10):2156–63.
77. Promrat K, Kleiner DE, Niemeier HM, Jackvony E, Kearns M, Wands JR, et al. Randomized controlled trial testing the effects of weight loss on nonalcoholic steatohepatitis. Hepatology. 2010;51(1):121–9.
78. Elias MC, Parise ER, de Carvalho L, Szejnfeld D, Netto JP. Effect of 6-month nutritional intervention on non-alcoholic fatty liver disease. Nutrition. 2010;26(11-12):1094–9.
79. Browning JD, Baker JA, Rogers T, Davis J, Satapati S, Burgess SC. Short-term weight loss and hepatic triglyceride reduction: evidence of a metabolic advantage with dietary carbohydrate restriction. Am J Clin Nutr. 2011;93(5):1048–52.
80. Hallsworth K, Fattakhova G, Hollingsworth KG, Thoma C, Moore S, Taylor R, et al. Resistance exercise reduces liver fat and its mediators in non-alcoholic fatty liver disease independent of weight loss. Gut. 2011;60(9):1278–83.
81. Sevastianova K, Santos A, Kotronen A, Hakkarainen A, Makkonen J, Silander K, et al. Effect of short-term carbohydrate overfeeding and long-term weight loss on liver fat in overweight humans. Am J Clin Nutr. 2012;96(4):727–34.
82. de Piano A, de Mello MT, Sanches Pde L, da Silva PL, Campos RM, Carnier J, et al. Long-term effects of aerobic plus resistance training on the adipokines and neuropeptides in nonalcoholic fatty liver disease obese adolescents. Eur J Gastroenterol Hepatol. 2012;24(11):1313–24.
83. Sullivan S, Kirk EP, Mittendorfer B, Patterson BW, Klein S. Randomized trial of exercise effect on intrahepatic triglyceride content and lipid kinetics in nonalcoholic fatty liver disease. Hepatology. 2012;55(6):1738–45.
84. Wong VW, Chan RS, Wong GL, Cheung BH, Chu WC, Yeung DK, et al. Community-based lifestyle modification programme for non-alcoholic fatty liver disease: a randomized controlled trial. J Hepatol. 2013;59(3):536–42.
85. Scaglioni F, Marino M, Ciccia S, Procaccini A, Busacchi M, Loria P, et al. Short-term multidisciplinary non-pharmacological intervention is effective in reducing liver fat content assessed non-invasively in patients with nonalcoholic fatty liver disease (NAFLD). Clin Res Hepatol Gastroenterol. 2013;37(4):353–8.
86. Ueno T, Sugawara H, Sujaku K, Hashimoto O, Tsuji R, Tamaki S, et al. Therapeutic effects of restricted diet and exercise in obese patients with fatty liver. J Hepatol. 1997;27(1):103–7.
87. Vilar Gomez E, Rodriguez De Miranda A, Gra Oramas B, Arus Soler E, Llanio Navarro R, Calzadilla Bertot L, et al. Clinical trial: a nutritional supplement Viusid, in combination with diet and exercise, in patients with nonalcoholic fatty liver disease. Aliment Pharmacol Ther. 2009;30(10):999–1009.
88. Thoma C, Day CP, Trenell MI. Lifestyle interventions for the treatment of non-alcoholic fatty liver disease in adults: a systematic review. J Hepatol. 2012;56(1):255–66.
89. Harrison SA, Fecht W, Brunt EM, Neuschwander-Tetri BA. Orlistat for overweight subjects with nonalcoholic steatohepatitis: a randomized, prospective trial. Hepatology. 2009;49(1):80–6.
90. Zelber-Sagi S, Kessler A, Brazowsky E, Webb M, Lurie Y, Santo M, et al. A double-blind randomized placebo-controlled trial of orlistat for the treatment of nonalcoholic fatty liver disease. Clin Gastroenterol Hepatol. 2006;4(5):639–44.
91. Kantartzis K, Thamer C, Peter A, Machann J, Schick F, Schraml C, et al. High cardiorespiratory fitness is an independent predictor of the reduction in liver fat during a lifestyle intervention in non-alcoholic fatty liver disease. Gut. 2009;58(9):1281–8.
92. Silverman EM, Sapala JA, Appelman HD. Regression of hepatic steatosis in morbidly obese persons after gastric bypass. Am J Clin Pathol. 1995;104(1):23–31.
93. Clark JM, Alkhuraishi AR, Solga SF, Alli P, Diehl AM, Magnuson TH. Roux-en-Y gastric bypass improves liver histology in patients with non-alcoholic fatty liver disease. Obes Res. 2005;13(7):1180–6.

94. Mattar SG, Velcu LM, Rabinovitz M, Demetris AJ, Krasinskas AM, Barinas-Mitchell E, et al. Surgically-induced weight loss significantly improves nonalcoholic fatty liver disease and the metabolic syndrome. Ann Surg. 2005;242(4):610–7. discussion 8–20.
95. Mathurin P, Gonzalez F, Kerdraon O, Leteurtre E, Arnalsteen L, Hollebecque A, et al. The evolution of severe steatosis after bariatric surgery is related to insulin resistance. Gastroenterology. 2006;130(6):1617–24.
96. Liu X, Lazenby AJ, Clements RH, Jhala N, Abrams GA. Resolution of nonalcoholic steatohepatits after gastric bypass surgery. Obes Surg. 2007;17(4):486–92.
97. Caiazzo R, Lassailly G, Leteurtre E, Baud G, Verkindt H, Raverdy V, et al. Roux-en-Y gastric bypass versus adjustable gastric banding to reduce nonalcoholic fatty liver disease: a 5-year controlled longitudinal study. Ann Surg. 2014;260(5):893–9.
98. Dixon JB, Bhathal PS, Hughes NR, O'Brien PE. Nonalcoholic fatty liver disease: improvement in liver histological analysis with weight loss. Hepatology. 2004;39(6):1647–54.
99. Mathurin P, Hollebecque A, Arnalsteen L, Buob D, Leteurtre E, Caiazzo R, et al. Prospective study of the long-term effects of bariatric surgery on liver injury in patients without advanced disease. Gastroenterology. 2009;137(2):532–40.
100. Mummadi RR, Kasturi KS, Chennareddygari S, Sood GK. Effect of bariatric surgery on nonalcoholic fatty liver disease: systematic review and meta-analysis. Clin Gastroenterol Hepatol. 2008;6(12):1396–402.
101. Chavez-Tapia NC, Tellez-Avila FI, Barrientos-Gutierrez T, Mendez-Sanchez N, Lizardi-Cervera J, Uribe M. Bariatric surgery for non-alcoholic steatohepatitis in obese patients. Cochrane Database Syst Rev 2010; (1):CD007340.
102. Puzziferri N, Roshek 3rd TB, Mayo HG, Gallagher R, Belle SH, Livingston EH. Long-term follow-up after bariatric surgery: a systematic review. JAMA. 2014;312(9):934–42.
103. Hocking MP, Duerson MC, O'Leary JP, Woodward ER. Jejunoileal bypass for morbid obesity. Late follow-up in 100 cases. N Engl J Med. 1983;308(17):995–9.
104. Bugianesi E, Gentilcore E, Manini R, Natale S, Vanni E, Villanova N, et al. A randomized controlled trial of metformin versus vitamin E or prescriptive diet in nonalcoholic fatty liver disease. Am J Gastroenterol. 2005;100(5):1082–90.
105. Dufour JF, Oneta CM, Gonvers JJ, Bihl F, Cerny A, Cereda JM, et al. Randomized placebo-controlled trial of ursodeoxycholic Acid with vitamin e in nonalcoholic steatohepatitis. Clin Gastroenterol Hepatol. 2006;4(12):1537–43.
106. Harrison SA, Torgerson S, Hayashi P, Ward J, Schenker S. Vitamin E and vitamin C treatment improves fibrosis in patients with nonalcoholic steatohepatitis. Am J Gastroenterol. 2003;98(11):2485–90.
107. Lavine JE, Schwimmer JB, Van Natta ML, Molleston JP, Murray KF, Rosenthal P, et al. Effect of vitamin E or metformin for treatment of nonalcoholic fatty liver disease in children and adolescents: the TONIC randomized controlled trial. JAMA. 2011;305(16):1659–68.
108. Pacana T, Sanyal AJ. Vitamin E and nonalcoholic fatty liver disease. Curr Opin Clin Nutr Metab Care. 2012;15(6):641–8.
109. Miller 3rd ER, Pastor-Barriuso R, Dalal D, Riemersma RA, Appel LJ, Guallar E. Meta-analysis: high-dosage vitamin E supplementation may increase all-cause mortality. Ann Intern Med. 2005;142(1):37–46.
110. Bjelakovic G, Nikolova D, Gluud LL, Simonetti RG, Gluud C. Mortality in randomized trials of antioxidant supplements for primary and secondary prevention: systematic review and meta-analysis. JAMA. 2007;297(8):842–57.
111. Gerss J, Kopcke W. The questionable association of vitamin E supplementation and mortality--inconsistent results of different meta-analytic approaches. Cell Mol Biol. 2009;55(Suppl):OL1111–20.
112. Berry D, Wathen JK, Newell M. Bayesian model averaging in meta-analysis: vitamin E supplementation and mortality. Clin Trials. 2009;6(1):28–41.
113. Dietrich M, Jacques PF, Pencina MJ, Lanier K, Keyes MJ, Kaur G, et al. Vitamin E supplement use and the incidence of cardiovascular disease and all-cause mortality in the Framingham Heart Study: does the underlying health status play a role? Atherosclerosis. 2009;205(2):549–53.

114. Klein EA, Thompson Jr IM, Tangen CM, Crowley JJ, Lucia MS, Goodman PJ, et al. Vitamin E and the risk of prostate cancer: the Selenium and Vitamin E Cancer Prevention Trial (SELECT). JAMA. 2011;306(14):1549–56.
115. Aithal GP, Thomas JA, Kaye PV, Lawson A, Ryder SD, Spendlove I, et al. Randomized, placebo-controlled trial of pioglitazone in nondiabetic subjects with nonalcoholic steatohepatitis. Gastroenterology. 2008;135(4):1176–84.
116. Belfort R, Harrison SA, Brown K, Darland C, Finch J, Hardies J, et al. A placebo-controlled trial of pioglitazone in subjects with nonalcoholic steatohepatitis. N Engl J Med. 2006;355(22):2297–307.
117. Promrat K, Lutchman G, Uwaifo GI, Freedman RJ, Soza A, Heller T, et al. A pilot study of pioglitazone treatment for nonalcoholic steatohepatitis. Hepatology. 2004;39(1):188–96.
118. Azoulay L, Yin H, Filion KB, Assayag J, Majdan A, Pollak MN, et al. The use of pioglitazone and the risk of bladder cancer in people with type 2 diabetes: nested case-control study. BMJ. 2012;344:e3645.
119. Bennett WL, Maruthur NM, Singh S, Segal JB, Wilson LM, Chatterjee R, et al. Comparative effectiveness and safety of medications for type 2 diabetes: an update including new drugs and 2-drug combinations. Ann Intern Med. 2011;154(9):602–13.
120. Rakoski MO, Singal AG, Rogers MA, Conjeevaram H. Meta-analysis: insulin sensitizers for the treatment of non-alcoholic steatohepatitis. Aliment Pharmacol Ther. 2010;32(10):1211–21.
121. Leuschner UF, Lindenthal B, Herrmann G, Arnold JC, Rossle M, Cordes HJ, et al. High-dose ursodeoxycholic acid therapy for nonalcoholic steatohepatitis: a double-blind, randomized, placebo-controlled trial. Hepatology. 2010;52(2):472–9.
122. Lindor KD, Kowdley KV, Heathcote EJ, Harrison ME, Jorgensen R, Angulo P, et al. Ursodeoxycholic acid for treatment of nonalcoholic steatohepatitis: results of a randomized trial. Hepatology. 2004;39(3):770–8.
123. Scorletti E, Bhatia L, McCormick KG, Clough GF, Nash K, Hodson L, et al. Effects of purified eicosapentaenoic and docosahexaenoic acids in non-alcoholic fatty liver disease: results from the *WELCOME study. Hepatology. 2014;60:1211.
124. Sanyal AJ, Abdelmalek MF, Suzuki A, Cummings OW, Chojkier M. No significant effects of ethyl-eicosapentanoic acid on histologic features of nonalcoholic steatohepatitis in a phase 2 trial. Gastroenterology. 2014;147(2):377–84.e1.
125. Athyros VG, Tziomalos K, Gossios TD, Griva T, Anagnostis P, Kargiotis K, et al. Safety and efficacy of long-term statin treatment for cardiovascular events in patients with coronary heart disease and abnormal liver tests in the Greek Atorvastatin and Coronary Heart Disease Evaluation (GREACE) Study: a post-hoc analysis. Lancet. 2010;376(9756):1916–22.
126. Chalasani N, Aljadhey H, Kesterson J, Murray MD, Hall SD. Patients with elevated liver enzymes are not at higher risk for statin hepatotoxicity. Gastroenterology. 2004;126(5):1287–92.
127. Lewis JH, Mortensen ME, Zweig S, Fusco MJ, Medoff JR, Belder R. Efficacy and safety of high-dose pravastatin in hypercholesterolemic patients with well-compensated chronic liver disease: results of a prospective, randomized, double-blind, placebo-controlled, multicenter trial. Hepatology. 2007;46(5):1453–63.
128. Athyros VG, Mikhailidis DP, Didangelos TP, Giouleme OI, Liberopoulos EN, Karagiannis A, et al. Effect of multifactorial treatment on non-alcoholic fatty liver disease in metabolic syndrome: a randomised study. Curr Med Res Opin. 2006;22(5):873–83.
129. Han KH, Rha SW, Kang HJ, Bae JW, Choi BJ, Choi SY, et al. Evaluation of short-term safety and efficacy of HMG-CoA reductase inhibitors in hypercholesterolemic patients with elevated serum alanine transaminase concentrations: PITCH study (PITavastatin versus atorvastatin to evaluate the effect on patients with hypercholesterolemia and mild to moderate hepatic damage). J Clin Lipidol. 2012;6(4):340–51.
130. Hatzitolios A, Savopoulos C, Lazaraki G, Sidiropoulos I, Haritanti P, Lefkopoulos A, et al. Efficacy of omega-3 fatty acids, atorvastatin and orlistat in non-alcoholic fatty liver disease with dyslipidemia. Indian J Gastroenterol. 2004;23(4):131–4.
131. Kiyici M, Gulten M, Gurel S, Nak SG, Dolar E, Savci G, et al. Ursodeoxycholic acid and atorvastatin in the treatment of nonalcoholic steatohepatitis. Can J Gastroenterol. 2003;17(12):713–8.

132. Ekstedt M, Franzen LE, Mathiesen UL, Holmqvist M, Bodemar G, Kechagias S. Statins in non-alcoholic fatty liver disease and chronically elevated liver enzymes: a histopathological follow-up study. J Hepatol. 2007;47(1):135–41.
133. Hyogo H, Tazuma S, Arihiro K, Iwamoto K, Nabeshima Y, Inoue M, et al. Efficacy of atorvastatin for the treatment of nonalcoholic steatohepatitis with dyslipidemia. Metabolism. 2008;57(12):1711–8.
134. Nelson A, Torres DM, Morgan AE, Fincke C, Harrison SA. A pilot study using simvastatin in the treatment of nonalcoholic steatohepatitis: a randomized placebo-controlled trial. J Clin Gastroenterol. 2009;43(10):990–4.
135. Chalasani N. Statins and hepatotoxicity: focus on patients with fatty liver. Hepatology. 2005;41(4):690–5.
136. Bacchi E, Negri C, Targher G, Faccioli N, Lanza M, Zoppini G, et al. Both resistance training and aerobic training reduce hepatic fat content in type 2 diabetic subjects with nonalcoholic fatty liver disease (the RAED2 Randomized Trial). Hepatology. 2013;58(4):1287–95.
137. Chalasani NP, Hayashi PH, Bonkovsky HL, Navarro VJ, Lee WM, Fontana RJ. ACG Clinical Guideline: the diagnosis and management of idiosyncratic drug-induced liver injury. Am J Gastroenterol. 2014;109(7):950–66. quiz 67.
138. Patton HM, Sirlin C, Behling C, Middleton M, Schwimmer JB, Lavine JE. Pediatric nonalcoholic fatty liver disease: a critical appraisal of current data and implications for future research. J Pediatr Gastroenterol Nutr. 2006;43(4):413–27.
139. Schwimmer JB, Deutsch R, Kahen T, Lavine JE, Stanley C, Behling C. Prevalence of fatty liver in children and adolescents. Pediatrics. 2006;118(4):1388–93.
140. Struben VM, Hespenheide EE, Caldwell SH. Nonalcoholic steatohepatitis and cryptogenic cirrhosis within kindreds. Am J Med. 2000;108(1):9–13.
141. Willner IR, Waters B, Patil SR, Reuben A, Morelli J, Riely CA. Ninety patients with nonalcoholic steatohepatitis: insulin resistance, familial tendency, and severity of disease. Am J Gastroenterol. 2001;96(10):2957–61.
142. Schwimmer JB, Celedon MA, Lavine JE, Salem R, Campbell N, Schork NJ, et al. Heritability of nonalcoholic fatty liver disease. Gastroenterology. 2009;136(5):1585–92.
143. Charlton MR, Burns JM, Pedersen RA, Watt KD, Heimbach JK, Dierkhising RA. Frequency and outcomes of liver transplantation for nonalcoholic steatohepatitis in the United States. Gastroenterology. 2011;141(4):1249–53.
144. Singal AK, Guturu P, Hmoud B, Kuo YF, Salameh H, Wiesner RH. Evolving frequency and outcomes of liver transplantation based on etiology of liver disease. Transplantation. 2013;95(5):755–60.
145. Agopian VG, Kaldas FM, Hong JC, Whittaker M, Holt C, Rana A, et al. Liver transplantation for nonalcoholic steatohepatitis: the new epidemic. Ann Surg. 2012;256(4):624–33.
146. O'Leary JG, Landaverde C, Jennings L, Goldstein RM, Davis GL. Patients with NASH and cryptogenic cirrhosis are less likely than those with hepatitis C to receive liver transplants. Clin Gastroenterol Hepatol. 2011;9(8):700–4.e1.
147. Newsome PN, Allison ME, Andrews PA, Auzinger G, Day CP, Ferguson JW, et al. Guidelines for liver transplantation for patients with non-alcoholic steatohepatitis. Gut. 2012;61(4):484–500.
148. Afzali A, Berry K, Ioannou GN. Excellent posttransplant survival for patients with nonalcoholic steatohepatitis in the United States. Liver Transpl. 2012;18(1):29–37.
149. Tanaka T, Sugawara Y, Tamura S, Kaneko J, Takazawa Y, Aoki T, et al. Living donor liver transplantation for non-alcoholic steatohepatitis: a single center experience. Hepatol Res. 2014;44(10):E3–e10.
150. El Atrache MM, Abouljoud MS, Divine G, Yoshida A, Kim DY, Kazimi MM, et al. Recurrence of non-alcoholic steatohepatitis and cryptogenic cirrhosis following orthotopic liver transplantation in the context of the metabolic syndrome. Clin Transplant. 2012;26(5):E505–12.
151. Dureja P, Mellinger J, Agni R, Chang F, Avey G, Lucey M, et al. NAFLD recurrence in liver transplant recipients. Transplantation. 2011;91(6):684–9.
152. Said A. Non-alcoholic fatty liver disease and liver transplantation: outcomes and advances. World J Gastroenterol. 2013;19(48):9146–55.

Chapter 15
Autoimmune Liver Diseases: Autoimmune Hepatitis

Albert J. Czaja

Patient Questions

1. What is autoimmune hepatitis?
2. How is autoimmune hepatitis treated?
3. How will I do?

Answers

1. What is autoimmune hepatitis?

   Autoimmune hepatitis is a chronic inflammation of the liver of uncertain cause that is characterized by features of immunological activity. Autoantibodies, increased serum levels of immunoglobulin, especially immunoglobulin G (IgG), and histological findings that disclose localized infiltrations of lymphocytes, frequently in conjunction with plasma cells, and a damage pattern called interface hepatitis are typical findings. Autoimmune hepatitis is frequently associated with other concurrent immune-mediated diseases, especially autoimmune thyroid disorders (autoimmune thyroiditis, Graves' disease), and its occurrence has been ascribed to a loss of immune tolerance for self-antigens and the development of an auto-reactive state. Autoimmune hepatitis usually does not resolve without treatment, and the principal concern is that it can progress to cirrhosis and liver failure. The disease does not have an identifiable cause, and genetic factors may influence susceptibility to the disease. Autoimmune hepatitis is not transmitted by a

A.J. Czaja, M.D. (✉)
Division of Gastroenterology and Hepatology, Mayo Clinic College of Medicine,
200 First Street S.W., Rochester, MN 55905, USA
e-mail: czaja.albert@mayo.edu

© Springer International Publishing Switzerland 2017
K. Sacian, R. Shaker (eds.), *Liver Disorders*,
DOI 10.1007/978-3-319-30103-7_15

single gene, but the propensity for auto-reactivity may be present in family members. Other chronic liver diseases can have clinical features that resemble those of autoimmune hepatitis, and the diagnosis requires exclusion of viral, drug-related, metabolic (nonalcoholic fatty liver disease), hereditary (Wilson disease, hemochromatosis, alpha-1 antitrypsin disease), and cholestatic liver diseases (primary biliary cholangitis, primary sclerosing cholangitis).

2. How is autoimmune hepatitis treated?

Prednisone or prednisolone in conjunction with azathioprine is the mainstay treatment for autoimmune hepatitis. Initial doses of the corticosteroid are gradually reduced during a 4-week induction period to a dose that is then maintained until clinical, laboratory, and histological resolution. Prednisone or prednisolone can be administered alone in higher dose for patients with azathioprine intolerance, absence of thiopurine methyltransferase activity, or concerns about drug effects on pregnancy, and budesonide in combination with azathioprine can be considered for non-cirrhotic patients with mild uncomplicated disease or findings that might be worsened by therapy with prednisone or prednisolone (obesity, diabetes, osteopenia, or hypertension). Drug intolerance, progressive disease despite compliance with therapy (treatment failure), and improvement but not resolution of symptoms and laboratory tests after protracted therapy (incomplete response) are justifications for treatment modifications. Mycophenolate mofetil and the calcineurin inhibitors (cyclosporine and tacrolimus) have been used as salvage agents for drug intolerance and steroid-refractory disease, and liver transplantation should be considered in patients with features of liver failure (ascites, encephalopathy). The standard and nonstandard drugs for autoimmune hepatitis are unlicensed in the United States, and they have been used for off-label indications.

3. How will I do?

Symptoms and laboratory tests improve within 2 weeks, and the laboratory findings can be normal or near-normal within 3 months. The average duration of treatment until normal or near-normal laboratory tests and liver tissue is 22 months. Treatment can be withdrawn in >60 % of patients, and the frequency of achieving a treatment-free state of at least 3 years duration is 19–40 %. Relapse after drug withdrawal occurs in 28–87 %, usually within 3 months, and its occurrence is lowest in individuals who have normal laboratory tests and liver tissue prior to drug withdrawal. Corticosteroid-induced complications that warrant drug withdrawal or dose adjustment occur in 12–29 %, and cytopenia attributable to therapy with azathioprine develops in 6 %. Fourteen percent of patients improve but not to normal or near-normal laboratory tests (incomplete response), and 7 % worsen during treatment (treatment failure). Cirrhosis develops in 12 % after 10 years and 34 % after 20 years, and its occurrence relates to the rapidity and completeness of the treatment response. Hepatic fibrosis can improve, stabilize, or disappear if inflammatory activity is rapidly and completely suppressed, and the 10-year survival is 80–89 %.

Table 15.1 Codified international criteria for the diagnosis of autoimmune hepatitis

Features	Definite autoimmune hepatitis	Probable autoimmune hepatitis
Abnormal serum AST, ALT and AP levels	Abnormal serum AST and ALT levels of any degree with less pronounced serum AP abnormality	Abnormal serum AST and ALT levels of any degree with less pronounced serum AP abnormality
Serum α_1-antitrypsin, copper, and ceruloplasmin levels	Normal serum levels	Any abnormal serum level provided Wilson disease excluded
Abnormal serum globulin, γ-globulin or IgG level	Serum globulin or γ-globulin or IgG level greater than 1.5-fold ULN	Serum globulin or γ-globulin or IgG level greater than ULN
ANA, SMA, or anti-LKM1 positive	Serum titers >1:80 by IIF or levels strongly positive by ELISA	Serum titers or levels weakly positive or negative and supplemented by positivity for other nonstandard antibodies
AMA titer or level	AMA negative	AMA negative
IgM anti-HAV, HBsAg, HBV DNA, anti-HCV and HCV RNA negative	All markers negative for active viral infection	All markers negative for active viral infection
Interface hepatitis on histological examination	Moderate-to-severe interface hepatitis without destructive biliary changes, granulomas or other prominent features that suggest alternative diagnosis	Moderate-to-severe interface hepatitis without destructive biliary changes, granulomas or other prominent features that suggest alternative diagnosis
No other etiological factors	Alcohol <25 g/day	Alcohol <50 g/day
	No recent exposure to hepatotoxic drugs	Some drug or alcohol exposure
	No celiac disease	Celiac disease concurrent but unlikely primary cause of liver injury

ALT alanine aminotransferase, *AMA* antimitochondrial antibodies, *ANA* antinuclear antibodies, *AP* alkaline phosphatase, *AST* aspartate aminotransferase, *DNA* deoxyribonucleic acid, *ELISA* enzyme-linked immunosorbent assay, *HAV* hepatitis A virus, *HBsAg* hepatitis B surface antigen, *HBV* hepatitis B virus, *HCV* hepatitis C virus, *IgG* immunoglobulin G, *IgM* immunoglobulin M, *IIF* indirect immunofluorescence, *RNA* ribonucleic acid, *ULN* upper limit of normal range
Adapted from the Journal of Hepatology 1999;31:929–938 with permission of Elsevier BV and the European Association for the Study of the Liver

Diagnostic Criteria

The diagnosis requires the presence of clinical, laboratory, and histological features that typify the disease and the exclusion of other liver diseases that resemble it [1, 2]. Diagnostic criteria have been codified by an international panel, and they ensure uniformity of the diagnosis [3] (Table 15.1). Chronic viral hepatitis, drug-induced chronic liver disease (commonly associated with minocycline or nitrofurantoin), nonalcoholic fatty liver disease (NAFLD), hereditary liver disease (especially

Table 15.2 Comprehensive diagnostic scoring system of the international autoimmune hepatitis group

Clinical features	Points	Clinical features	Points
Female	+2	Average alcohol intake	
		<25 g/day	+2
		>60 g/day	−2
AP:AST (or ALT) ratio		Histologic findings	
<1.5	+2	Interface hepatitis	+3
1.5–3.0	0	Lymphoplasmacytic infiltrate	+1
>3.0	−2	Rosette formation	+1
		Biliary changes	−3
		Other atypical changes	−3
		None of above	−5
Serum globulin or IgG level above ULN		Concurrent immune disease,	
>2.0	+3	including celiac disease	+2
1.5–2.0	+2	Other autoantibodies	+2
1.0–1.5	+1	HLA DRB1*03 or DRB1*04	+1
<1.0	0		
ANA, SMA, or anti-LKM1		Response to corticosteroids	
>1:80	+3	Complete	+2
1:80	+2	Relapse after drug withdrawal	+3
1:40	+1		
<1:40	0		
AMA positive	−4		
Hepatitis markers		Aggregate score pre-treatment	
Positive	−3	Definite autoimmune hepatitis	>15
Negative	+3	Probable autoimmune hepatitis	10–15
Hepatotoxic drug exposure		Aggregate score post-treatment	
Positive	−4	Definite autoimmune hepatitis	>17
Negative	+1	Probable autoimmune hepatitis	12–17

ALT alanine aminotransferase, *AMA* antimitochondrial antibodies, *ANA* antinuclear antibodies, *AP* alkaline phosphatase, *AST* aspartate aminotransferase, *HLA* human leukocyte antigen, *IgG* immunoglobulin G, *LKM1* liver/kidney microsome type 1, *SMA* smooth muscle antibodies, *ULN* upper limit of the normal range

Adapted from the Journal of Hepatology 31:929–938, 1999 with permission of Elsevier BV and the European Association for the Study of the Liver

Wilson disease), and the immune-mediated cholangiopathies (primary biliary cholangitis [PBC] and primary sclerosing cholangitis [PSC]) must be excluded [1, 2, 4].

Diagnostic scoring systems can support the clinical judgment. A comprehensive scoring system, originally designed to ensure the homogeneity of study populations, provides a diagnostic template that indicates the key clinical, laboratory, and histological features of autoimmune hepatitis [3] (Table 15.2). Each feature is graded, and the strength of the diagnosis is determined before and after corticosteroid

Table 15.3 Simplified diagnostic scoring system of the international autoimmune hepatitis group

Category	Scoring elements	Results	Points
Autoantibodies	ANA or SMA	1:40 by IIF	+1
	ANA or SMA	≥1:80 by IIF	+2
	Anti-LKM1 (alternative to ANA and SMA)	≥1:40 by IIF	+2
	Anti-SLA (alternative to ANA, SMA and LKM1)	Positive	+2
Immunoglobulins	Immunoglobulin G level	>ULN	+1
		>1.1 times ULN	+2
Histological findings	Interface hepatitis	Compatible features	+1
		Typical features	+2
Viral markers	IgM anti-HAV, HBsAg, HBV DNA, HCV RNA	No viral markers	+2
		Probable diagnosis	≥6
		Definite diagnosis	≥7

ANA antinuclear antibodies, *DNA* deoxyribonucleic acid, *HAV* hepatitis A virus, *HBsAg* hepatitis B surface antigen, *HBV* hepatitis B virus, *HCV* hepatitis C virus, *IIF* indirect immunofluorescence, *IgM* immunoglobulin M, *LKM1* liver microsome type 1, *RNA* ribonucleic acid, *SLA* soluble liver antigen, *SMA* smooth muscle antibodies, *ULN* upper limit of the normal range
Adapted from Hepatology 48:169–176, 2008 with permission of John Wiley & Sons, Inc. and the American Association for the Study of Liver Disease

therapy. A simplified scoring system facilitates clinical application of the diagnostic tool, and it does not score treatment response [5] (Table 15.3).

The comprehensive scoring system has greater sensitivity for the diagnosis of autoimmune hepatitis than the simplified scoring system (100 % versus 95 %), and the simplified scoring system has greater specificity (90 % versus 73 %) and accuracy (92 % versus 82 %) [6]. The scoring systems have not been validated by prospective studies, and each system depends on antibody assessments by indirect immunofluorescence (IIF). Clinical judgment is the gold standard against which the scoring systems have been measured, and scoring results can never supersede clinical judgment.

Typical Features

Autoimmune hepatitis occurs in all age groups [7–9], genders (female-to-male ratio, 3.7:1) [10, 11], and ethnic populations [12], and it must be considered in all patients with an acute or chronic inflammatory liver disease of uncertain cause [13–16], including patients with graft dysfunction after liver transplantation [17–19].

Clinical Presentations

Autoimmune hepatitis may present as a chronic indolent liver disease characterized by fatigue, myalgia, and jaundice [1, 2], an acute hepatitis [20, 21], an acute severe (fulminant) liver failure [22–24], or an asymptomatic chronic liver disorder [25–27]. Patients with chronic symptomatic liver disease frequently have cirrhosis at presentation (29 %) [28], and they may present because of a spontaneous exacerbation of inflammatory activity [29]. Patients with acute severe (fulminant) liver failure may have histological findings of centrilobular necrosis, absent or low titers of autoantibodies, and normal or mildly abnormal serum levels of immunoglobulin G [24, 30]. Asymptomatic patients frequently have histological features of moderate-to-severe interface hepatitis (91 %) and fibrosis (41 %) that are not reflected in their clinical phenotype [25].

Autoantibodies

Antinuclear antibodies (ANA), smooth muscle antibodies (SMA), and antibodies to liver kidney microsome type 1 (anti-LKM1) are the standard serological markers of autoimmune hepatitis [1, 4], and they can be assessed by IIF or enzyme-linked immunosorbent assays (ELISAs) [31]. ANA are the sole markers of autoimmune hepatitis in 32 % of patients, and SMA characterize the disease in 16 % [32, 33] (Table 15.4). ANA and SMA occur together in 43 % of patients with autoimmune hepatitis, and these concurrent findings have superior diagnostic value than the presence of ANA or SMA alone. The specificity of concurrent ANA and SMA for autoimmune hepatitis is 99 %; the positive predictability is 97 %; the negative predictability is 69 %; and the diagnostic accuracy is 74 % [32]. ANA are directed against nuclear antigens, including centromere, ribonucleoproteins, and ribonucleoprotein complexes [34], and they may appear and disappear during the course of the disease with no prognostic connotation [33].

SMA are directed against actin and non-actin components of the cytoskeleton, and they lack disease- and organ-specificity [35–37]. They support the diagnosis of autoimmune hepatitis, especially when present with ANA [32]. Their sensitivity for autoimmune hepatitis when present as the sole marker in patients with chronic liver disease is 16 %. The specificity of an isolated finding is 96 %; the positive predictability is 76 %; the negative predictability is 60 %; and diagnostic accuracy is 61 % [32]. Both ANA and SMA can support the diagnosis of autoimmune hepatitis, but their detection alone or together is insufficient to establish the diagnosis. Like ANA, SMA can appear or disappear during the course of the disease without prognostic implications [33]. In autoimmune hepatitis, SMA are directed, mainly but not exclusively, against actin (75 % versus 25 %) [38].

Anti-LKM1 occur in only 1–4 % of North American adults with autoimmune hepatitis [32, 39], but when present they have a diagnostic specificity of 99 % [32]

Table 15.4 Autoantibodies associated with autoimmune hepatitis

Autoantibodies	Antigenic target	Clinical relevance
ANA	Diverse nuclear antigens (centromere, ribonucleoproteins, ribonucleoprotein complexes) [34]	Isolated finding in AIH, 32% [32]
		Concurrent with SMA in AIH, 43% [32]
		Diagnostic specificity with SMA, 99% [32]
		Diagnostic accuracy with SMA, 74% [32]
		Characterizes type 1 AIH [44]
SMA	Actin and non-actin antigens (tubulin, desmin, vimentin, skeletin) [35–37]	Isolated finding in AIH, 16% [32]
		Concurrent with ANA in AIH, 43% [32]
		Diagnostic specificity with ANA, 99% [32]
		Characterizes type 1 AIH [44]
Anti-LKM1	Cytochrome mono-oxygenase (CYP2D6) [42]	Rare in North American adults, 1–4% [39]
		Mainly in European children, 14–38% [7, 40]
		Concurrence with ANA or SMA, 1–3% [39]
		High diagnostic specificity, 99% [32]
		Low diagnostic sensitivity, 1% [32]
		Characterizes type 2 AIH [40, 44]
Anti-SLA	Transfer ribonucleoprotein complex (Sep [O-phosphoserine] tRNA:sec [selenocysteine] tRNA synthase) [48, 49]	High diagnostic specificity, 99% [50, 51]
		Low diagnostic sensitivity, 7–19% [51]
		Associated with relapse and severity [53, 55]
		Concurrent with HLA DRB1*0301, 83% [53]
		Frequent in cryptogenic hepatitis, 26% [51]
		Associated with anti-Ro/SSA, 77–96% [56]

(continued)

Table 15.4 (continued)

Autoantibodies	Antigenic target	Clinical relevance
Anti-actin	Filamentous (F) actin [57]	Diagnostic indices may exceed SMA [58, 62]
		Absent in 14% of AIH with SMA [38]
		Anti-α-actinin associated with severity [59]
Atypical pANCA	Neutrophilic nuclear membrane (beta-tubulin isotype 5) [63, 68]	Frequent in type 1 AIH, 49–92% [65, 66]
		Absent in type 2 AIH [67]
		Present in CUC and PSC [68]
		May suggest AIH or overlap syndrome [66]

AIH autoimmune hepatitis, *ANA* antinuclear antibodies, *IgA* immunoglobulin A, *CUC* chronic ulcerative colitis, *LKM1* antibodies to liver kidney microsome type 1, *pANCA* perinuclear anti-neutrophil cytoplasmic antibodies, *PSC* primary sclerosing cholangitis, *Ro/SSA* ribonucleoprotein/ Sjogren's syndrome A antigen, *SLA* antibodies to soluble liver antigen, *SMA* smooth muscle antibodies

Numbers in brackets are references

(Table 15.4). The low sensitivity of anti-LKM1 for autoimmune hepatitis in North American adults (1–4%) contributes to the low diagnostic accuracy of these antibodies in this population (57%) [32]. Anti-LKM1 occur mainly in European children (14–38%) [7, 40, 41], and they coexist with ANA or SMA in only 1–3% of adults with autoimmune hepatitis [32, 39]. Anti-LKM1 are directed against the cytochrome mono-oxygenase, CYP2D6, and this antigen has been implicated as a key target in autoimmune hepatitis [42, 43].

The exclusivity of the serological findings has justified the designations of type 1 autoimmune hepatitis, characterized by ANA and SMA, and type 2 autoimmune hepatitis, characterized by anti-LKM1 [40, 44]. These designations are clinical descriptors rather than valid pathological entities, and they have not been endorsed by the International Autoimmune Hepatitis Group (IAIHG) [3]. The two types of autoimmune hepatitis do not have distinctive clinical and histological findings, treatments, and outcomes. The designations are useful to describe serological phenotypes and to define homogeneous patient populations in research projects.

Nonstandard Autoantibodies

The nonstandard autoantibodies used in the diagnosis of autoimmune hepatitis are antibodies to soluble liver antigen (anti-SLA), antibodies to actin (anti-actin), and atypical perinuclear anti-neutrophil cytoplasmic antibodies (pANCA) [45–47] (Table 15.4). Testing for these serological markers has not been incorporated into a codified diagnostic algorithm, and these antibodies are sought mainly in patients who lack the conventional serological markers or who have an uncertain diagnosis [1].

Antibodies to soluble liver antigen are directed against a transfer ribonucleoprotein complex (tRNP$^{(Ser)Sec}$) that has been designated SEPSECS (Sep[O-phosphoserine] tRNA:sec [selenocysteine] tRNA synthase) [48, 49] (Table 15.4). Antibodies to SLA have exquisite diagnostic specificity for autoimmune hepatitis [50–52], but they occur in only 7–19 % of patients depending on ethnic background [51]. The antibodies have been associated with a propensity to relapse after corticosteroid withdrawal (frequency of relapse, 74–100 %) [51, 53, 54], and they characterize patients with severe disease [55] and HLA DRB1*0301 [53]. Antibodies to SLA have been detected in 26 % of patients who lack the conventional autoantibodies, and they may allow re-classification of patients with chronic cryptogenic hepatitis as autoimmune hepatitis [51]. Antibodies to SLA commonly coexist with antibodies to ribonucleoprotein/Sjogren's syndrome A (Ro/SSA) (frequency of concurrence, 77–96 %) [52, 56].

Antibodies to actin (anti-actin) are directed against filamentous actin, and this reactivity is closely associated with autoimmune hepatitis [38, 57] (Table 15.4). Smooth muscle antibodies react against actin and non-actin components [35], and antibodies to actin detected by ELISA have greater specificity for autoimmune hepatitis than SMA detected by IIF (90 % versus 75 %) [58]. Antibodies to actin detected by ELISA have a similar diagnostic sensitivity for autoimmune hepatitis as SMA detected by IIF (74 % versus 71 %), but anti-actin have a greater positive predictability (58 % versus 37 %) [58]. Virtually all patients with anti-actin (99 %) have SMA, but up to 14 % with SMA lack anti-actin [38]. Antibodies against both actin and α-actinin, which is the predominant epitope of the actin molecule, identify patients with severe disease, and double reactivity by this investigational assay may have prognostic implications [54, 59, 60]. The preferred assay for anti-actin has not been standardized, and the discrepancies between studies assessing performance parameters may be assay-dependent [57, 58, 61, 62].

Atypical perinuclear anti-neutrophil cytoplasmic antibodies (pANCA) are directed against proteins within the nuclear membrane of neutrophils [63, 64], and they are present in 49–92 % of patients with autoimmune hepatitis, often in extremely high titer [65–67] (Table 15.4). Beta-tubulin isotype 5 is the primary target antigen, and it cross-reacts with an evolutionary bacterial protein (FtsZ), suggesting that intestinal micro-organisms trigger the immune response. Atypical pANCA are useful in supporting the diagnosis of autoimmune hepatitis in patients who lack the conventional autoantibodies. Atypical pANCA also occur in PSC and chronic ulcerative colitis, and their presence in autoimmune hepatitis warrants the exclusion of these diseases [68]. Atypical pANCA are absent in patients with type 2 (anti-LKM1-positive) autoimmune hepatitis [67]. Other nonstandard autoantibodies, including antibodies to asialoglycoprotein receptor (anti-ASGPR) [69, 70], liver cytosol type 1 (anti-LC1) [71], and antibodies to liver kidney type 3 (anti-LKM3) [72], are mainly investigational, not generally available, or in some populations, rarely present [46] (Table 15.4).

Histological Findings

A liver tissue examination is required to establish the diagnosis [1, 5, 73–76]. Studies suggesting otherwise have not assessed the number of patients with compatible clinical features but other diagnoses that would have been excluded by liver tissue examination [77].

The histological hallmark of autoimmune hepatitis is interface hepatitis [1–3]. Lymphocytes, frequently in association with plasma cells, infiltrate the portal tract, and the limiting plate of the portal tract is disrupted with spillage of the dense lymphocytic infiltrate into the hepatic lobule. Plasma cells are abundantly present in 66 % of liver tissue specimens, but they are not requisites for the diagnosis [78] (Fig. 15.1). Other features that can distinguish autoimmune hepatitis, especially from drug-induced liver injury, are hepatocyte rosette formation and emperiopolesis (penetration of one cell into and through a larger cell) [75].

Lymphoid and pleomorphic cholangitis are present in 7–9 % of patients [79, 80], and isolated bile duct lesions, including destructive cholangitis, are consistent with the diagnosis in the absence of a cholestatic syndrome [80, 81]. Centrilobular (zone 3) necrosis occurs in 29 % of patients with autoimmune hepatitis, including those with cirrhosis [82]. In 78 % of patients with centrilobular necrosis, interface hepatitis is also present [83]. Centrilobular necrosis has been associated with an acute onset [23, 83], but it is also a reflection of disease severity [82].

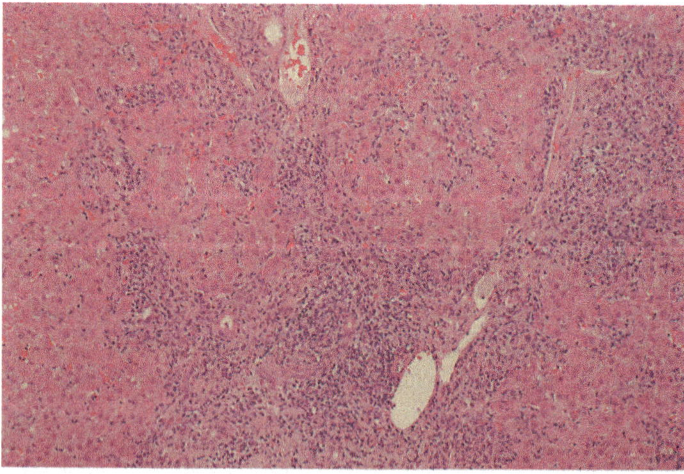

Fig. 15.1 Interface hepatitis. Lymphoplasmacytic infiltrate of the portal tract, disruption of the limiting plate (interface hepatitis), and spillage of mononuclear cells into the hepatic lobule with periportal inflammation and early bridging between portal tracts and central veins constitute the classical histological pattern of autoimmune hepatitis. The damage pattern is not disease-specific and chronic viral, drug-related, and hereditary (Wilson disease) liver diseases must be excluded. Hematoxylin-eosin, original magnification, ×200. Re-published from *MacSween's Pathology of the Liver*, Fifth Edition, 2007, Chapter 10, Autoimmune hepatitis, Figure 10.2, by Albert J. Czaja, MD and Herschel A. Carpenter, MD, with permission from Churchill Livingstone Elsevier, Inc.

Concurrent Immune Diseases

One or more immune-mediated diseases coexist with autoimmune hepatitis in 14–44 % of patients [9, 84–86]. The frequency and nature of the concurrent diseases are influenced by age and genetic predisposition [9, 85]. Autoimmune thyroid diseases (30 % versus 13 %) and rheumatic diseases (13 % versus 0 %), including rheumatoid arthritis, Sjogren's syndrome, and systemic lupus erythematosus, are more common in patients aged ≥60 years than in young adults aged ≤30 years. In contrast, adult patients aged ≤30 years have concurrent ulcerative colitis more frequently (10 % versus 0 %) [9, 84]. HLA DRB1*04 has been associated with the propensity for concurrent disease in white North American patients [87, 88], and this HLA phenotype is more common in the elderly [9]. In other populations, autoimmune hepatitis is mainly a disease of the young [89], and the frequency of concurrent disease is low (14–18 %) [85]. The concurrent immune diseases must be managed independently, and only ulcerative colitis and celiac disease can directly influence the nature, behavior, and treatment of the liver disease.

Ulcerative colitis occurs in 16 % of adults with autoimmune hepatitis, and these patients should undergo cholangiography to exclude primary sclerosing cholangitis (PSC) [90]. Cholangiograms can suggest the diagnosis of PSC in 10–42 % of adults with otherwise typical autoimmune hepatitis [90, 91], and these patients respond variably to conventional corticosteroid therapy [90]. Similar changes ("autoimmune cholangitis") are evident in 50 % of children with autoimmune hepatitis [41]. Corticosteroid treatment ameliorates the disease in children, but the biliary disease frequently progresses, liver transplantation may be required, and recurrent disease after transplantation is common [92]. Hepatic fibrosis commonly distorts the bile ducts, and these distortions can be confused with PSC by endoscopic and magnetic resonance cholangiography [93]. Focal bile duct strictures and dilations are the radiographic hallmarks of PSC.

Celiac disease occurs in 1–4 % of patients with autoimmune hepatitis [94–96], frequently in the absence of overt gastrointestinal symptoms, and acute, severe, and chronic hepatitis can occur in patients with celiac disease that is responsive to gluten restriction [97–101]. Serological assessment for celiac disease by assays for immunoglobulin A (IgA) antibodies to tissue transglutaminase or endomysium can identify a treatable coexistent immune-mediated disease or another basis for the liver dysfunction that might improve during gluten restriction [102].

Treatment Regimens

All patients with autoimmune hepatitis are candidates for therapy regardless of symptom status or disease severity [1, 2]. Symptoms emerge in 26–70 % of asymptomatic patients, and an asymptomatic state does not preclude progressive liver disease or the need for treatment [25–27]. Untreated patients with mild autoimmune hepatitis can improve spontaneously, but they do so less commonly (12 % versus 63 %) than treated patients during 77 ± 31 months of observation [27]. Asymptomatic disease can progress to cirrhosis and liver failure, and the 10-year survival of untreated patients with mild disease is lower than that of treated patients with severe disease (67 % versus 98 %).

Prednisone or prednisolone in combination with azathioprine is the standard treatment of autoimmune hepatitis [1, 2, 103]. The corticosteroids are administered in high initial dose during a 4-week induction phase in conjunction with a fixed dose of azathioprine [104, 105] (Table 15.5). The dose of corticosteroids is reduced during this period from 30 mg daily to 10 mg daily while the dose of azathioprine remains fixed at 50 mg daily. A maintenance phase follows during which the doses of prednisone or prednisolone, 10 mg daily, and azathioprine, 50 mg daily, are continued. Prednisolone is preferred over prednisone in Europe, and the doses of prednisolone (as high as 1 mg/kg daily) and azathioprine (1–2 mg/kg daily) are weight-based [2, 106, 107]. The prednisolone dose is reduced gradually over 2–3 months to 10 mg daily. This regimen is designed to produce rapid reductions in the serum aminotransferase levels, especially in non-cirrhotic patients, but it may be associated with more corticosteroid-induced side effects [2].

Prednisone or prednisolone can be administered without azathioprine in patients with known azathioprine intolerance, severe cytopenia (leukocyte count, $<2.5 \times 10^9/l$; platelet count, $<50 \times 10^9/l$), absent thiopurine methyltransferase activity, or concerns about the effects of azathioprine on active malignancy or pregnancy [1].

Table 15.5 Frontline treatment regimens for autoimmune hepatitis

Preferred regimen	Monotherapy for azathioprine intolerance	Alternative regimen in highly selected patients
Prednisone or prednisolone [1]	Prednisone or prednisolone [1]	Budesonide [109]
30 mg daily × 1 week	60 mg daily × 1 week	6–9 mg daily until end point
20 mg daily × 1 week	40 mg daily × 1 week	
15 mg daily × 2 weeks	30 mg daily × 2 weeks	
10 mg daily until end point	20 mg daily until end point	
Azathioprine [1]	Azathioprine [1]	Azathioprine [109]
50 mg daily from outset until end point	None	1–2 mg/kg body weight from outset

European preference: Prednisolone, up to 1 mg/kg daily, in combination with azathioprine, 1–2 mg/kg daily. The prednisolone dose is reduced gradually over 2–3 months to 10 mg daily [2, 106, 107]

Treatment end points: Normalization of laboratory tests and liver tissue; improvement but not to normalization of liver tests after 36 months of therapy; worsening of laboratory tests despite compliance with treatment regimen; drug intolerance (severe cosmetic or metabolic changes, vertebral compression, severe cytopenia) [1]

Emerging selection criteria for alternative budesonide and azathioprine regimen: Treatment-naïve, non-cirrhotic, uncomplicated patients with mild inflammatory activity or pre-morbid conditions at risk during conventional corticosteroid therapy [111–113]

Numbers in brackets are references

Monotherapy is as effective as combination therapy [108]. A higher dose of prednisone or prednisolone is required, and corticosteroid-induced side effects (mainly, cosmetic) occur more commonly than with combination therapy (44 % versus 10 %) [108]. The corticosteroid dose during the 4-week induction phase is reduced from 60 mg daily to 20 mg daily, and the dose is continued at 20 mg daily during the maintenance phase [104, 105] (Table 15.5).

Budesonide (6–9 mg daily) in combination with azathioprine (1–2 mg/kg body weight daily) can be considered as an alternative frontline therapy in highly selected patients (Table 15.5). Serum aspartate (AST) and alanine (ALT) aminotransferase levels normalized more frequently (47 % versus 18 %) and side effects occurred less often (28 % versus 53 %) in patients randomized to the budesonide regimen compared to patients randomized to prednisone (40 mg daily tapered to 10 mg daily) in combination with azathioprine (1–2 mg/kg body weight daily) [109]. The treatment duration was 6 months; the frequency of histological resolution was not assessed; and the durability of the response was not established. Furthermore, the poor results in the patients receiving conventional therapy were unexplained [109], and improved outcomes (except for less weight gain) were not evident in the budesonide-treated children [110]. The performance characteristics of budesonide are incompletely understood in autoimmune hepatitis, and the use of budesonide should be highly selective and cautious.

Budesonide therapy has not been effective as a salvage regimen for corticosteroid-dependent or refractory patients [111], and it has been associated with typical steroid-related side effects in patients with cirrhosis [112, 113]. The target population for budesonide therapy is undefined, but treatment-naïve, uncomplicated, non-cirrhotic patients with mild disease or with osteopenia, diabetes, hypertension, or obesity are prime candidates for this therapy.

Outcomes

Treatment is continued until resolution of clinical, laboratory and histological findings, or until there is clinical evidence that the treatment is inadequate or harmful [1]. Patients may progress to cirrhosis or liver failure [114], develop hepatocellular carcinoma or other malignancies [115], or relapse after drug withdrawal [116]. Five-year survival exceeds 90 % in most studies [28, 117, 118], and 10- and 20-year survivals from liver-related disease have been at least 80 % and 70 %, respectively [28, 117, 119, 120].

Resolution

Normalization of liver tests and liver tissue is the ideal treatment response [1, 121], and it justifies an attempt to withdraw treatment in the hope of establishing a treatment-free state [1, 122] (Table 15.6). The frequency of achieving a treatment-free state is 19–40 % in studies of at least 3 years duration [121, 123, 124], and it has been possible for at

Table 15.6 Outcomes of treatment in autoimmune hepatitis

Outcomes	Features	Consequences
Resolution	Frequency, 22 % [121]	Treatment-free ≥3 years, 19–40 % [121, 123]
Incomplete response	Frequency, 14 % [121, 131]	Treatment-dependence [201]
	Activity ≥36 months of therapy [131]	
Treatment failure	Frequency, 7 % [132]	Disease progression and liver failure [132]
Drug toxicity	Corticosteroid-related, 12–29 % [27]	Azathioprine-related cytopenia, ≤10 % [138]
	Azathioprine-related, 5–10 % [136, 138]	Bone marrow failure rare [139, 140]
	Budesonide-related, 28 % [109]	TPMT testing before azathioprine [2, 146]
	Azathioprine, category D drug [149]	Azathioprine unnecessary during pregnancy in AIH [1, 146]
	Azathioprine safe in pregnant IBD [152, 153]	
	Pre-term delivery and low birth weight with early azathioprine exposure [151]	
Cirrhosis	Frequency, 16 % (1–27 years) [117]	Corticosteroid-treatment effective [28, 155]
	Occurrence, 12–34 % after 10–20 years [117]	10-year survival, 80–89 % [28, 117]
Hepatocellular carcinoma	Frequency, 1–9 % [158–160]	Outcome reflects stage and condition [162]
	SIR, 23.3 (95 % CI, 7.3–54.3) [161]	Surveillance with hepatic ultrasonography every 6 months, especially if predictive factors present [115, 146]
	Annual incidence, 1.1–1.9 % [158–160]	
	Cirrhosis required (1–16 years) [158]	
	Predictive factors: portal hypertension, therapy ≥3 years, cirrhosis ≥10 years [157]	
Extrahepatic cancer	Frequency, 5 % [147]	Prognosis generally good [147]
	Diverse cell types, SIR 2.7 [148]	Outcome depends on nature and stage [147]
	Non-melanoma skin cancers most common, SIR 5–28.5 [163]	Routine health exams indefinitely [115]
	Associated with azathioprine [164, 166]	

(continued)

Table 15.6 (continued)

Outcomes	Features	Consequences
Relapse	Frequency, 28–87 % [116, 121, 169]	Progression to cirrhosis, 10 % [175]
	Associated mainly with incomplete histological resolution [121, 172, 173]	Liver failure, 3 % [175]
		Poor outcomes with repeat events [175]

AIH autoimmune hepatitis, *IBD* inflammatory bowel disease, *SIR* standardized incidence ratio, *TPMT* thiopurine methyltransferase

Numbers in brackets are references

least 5 years in 36 % of patients treated to normal or near-normal liver tissue prior to drug withdrawal [125]. The major difficulty in establishing a treatment-free state is to normalize the liver tissue. Reversion to normal liver tissue is achievable in only 22 % of patients who are treated with conventional corticosteroid regimens, and multiple liver tissue examinations may be necessary to document the occurrence [121, 122, 126].

Laboratory tests typically improve within 2 weeks of therapy [127], and they may return to normal or near-normal levels after a mean treatment duration of 3 ± 3 months [118]. Histological improvement lags behind laboratory resolution by 3–8 months [128–130], and only 11 % of patients achieve normal or near-normal liver tissue within 6 months [131]. The average duration of treatment until normal or near-normal laboratory tests and liver tissue is 22 months in the United States [131] and 24 months in Europe [2].

Incomplete Response

Fourteen percent of patients improve, but they do not achieve normal or near-normal laboratory and histological examinations [121, 131] (Table 15.6). These patients are on long-term corticosteroid therapy and at increasing risk for drug-induced complications. The inability to achieve laboratory and histological resolution after 36 months of continuous treatment constitutes an incomplete response, and it justifies a change in management objectives [131]. The goals must be to suppress and stabilize the inflammatory activity while avoiding drug-induced complications. Normal liver tests and liver tissue can still be achieved [124], but they are not aggressively pursued with full-dose treatment regimens [1, 2].

Treatment Failure

Seven percent of patients worsen despite compliance with the treatment regimen, and they are at risk for disease progression and liver failure [132] (Table 15.6). The accuracy of the original diagnosis must be reconfirmed, and alternative or superimposed diseases (steatosis, drug-induced liver injury, and overlap syndrome) excluded. The original treatment regimen must be altered to treat the refractory disease. High dose regimens of prednisone or prednisolone with or without high dose azathioprine are first-line options, and other salvage therapies (calineurin inhibitors and mycophenolate mofetil) can also be considered [133, 134]. Liver transplantation is the preferred therapy for liver failure [135].

Drug Toxicity

Corticosteroid-induced side effects relate in part to the dose of the drug and the duration of the treatment. Eighty percent of patients taking prednisone or prednisolone, ≥ 10 mg daily, for ≥ 24 months experience some cosmetic changes (weight gain, acne, hirsutism, or striae), and the development of side effects (intolerable cosmetic changes, obesity, mental instability, hypertension, diabetes, or vertebral compression) compels dose reduction or drug withdrawal in 12–29 % [27, 121, 136] (Table 15.6). Therapy with budesonide has produced similar changes in 28 % over 6 months in a randomized clinical trial [109], and budesonide-treated patients with cirrhosis may be at increased risk for budesonide-related complications [112, 113]. Cirrhosis may increase the propensity for corticosteroid-induced side effects because of reduced binding sites for free prednisolone [137] or decreased hepatic clearance of budesonide [112].

Azathioprine intolerance compels dose reduction or discontinuation of the drug in 5–10 % of patients, and the principal side effects are cytopenia, nausea, vomiting, rash, and pancreatitis [136, 138] (Table 15.6). Cholestatic liver injury is uncommon, but it must be considered in patients who worsen during treatment. Bone marrow failure is a rare complication, but a justification for assessing thiopurine methyltransferase (TPMT) activity prior to treatment [139, 140]. Routine screening for TPMT has not been promulgated in autoimmune hepatitis [1, 2], because TPMT activity has not been predictive of drug toxicity [141–144]. The value of screening for TPMT activity is mainly to detect the 0.3 % of the population who have absent enzyme activity and are at risk for drug-induced bone marrow failure [145]. This reassurance before treatment can strengthen confidence in the treatment regimen, especially in patients with cirrhosis and pretreatment cytopenia, and it supports the pretreatment assessment of TPMT activity [146]. Complete blood counts should be performed at 3–6 month intervals in all patients receiving azathioprine to monitor for myelosuppression [1].

The incidence of extra-hepatic malignancy in treated patients with autoimmune hepatitis is 1 per 194 patient years of surveillance [147]; the 10-year probability of occurrence is 3 % [147]; and the standardized incidence ratio (SIR) for extra-hepatic malignancy is 2.7 (95 % confidence interval, 1.8–3.9) [148]. Chronic immunosuppressive therapy in general is associated with an increased risk of malignancy, and a rigorous tumor surveillance strategy must be maintained [115].

Azathioprine is listed as a category D drug for pregnancy. Multiple congenital malformations have been described in animals [149]; 6-thioguanine metabolites pass the human placenta [150]; and infants exposed in early pregnancy may be more prone to have preterm delivery, low birth weight, small size for gestational age, and ventricular or atrial septal defects [151]. Congenital abnormalities have not been attributed to azathioprine therapy in pregnant women treated for inflammatory bowel disease, and the risk of azathioprine toxicity during pregnancy may be minimal or nonexistent in this population [152, 153]. Furthermore, the severity of the maternal illness rather than the drug may be the basis for growth restriction and preterm delivery [151]. Azathioprine is a nonessential drug in the management of autoimmune hepatitis, and it is reasonable to avoid its use in pregnancy by adjusting the corticosteroid dose [146, 154].

Progressive Fibrosis and Cirrhosis

Progressive hepatic fibrosis and the development of cirrhosis are common consequences of autoimmune hepatitis [28, 114, 117, 155, 156]. The fibrotic process is driven in part by persistent hepatic inflammation, and the frequency of cirrhosis is 54 % if therapy has failed to fully suppress inflammatory activity within 36 months [131] (Table 15.6). The frequency of cirrhosis is 16 % during 1–27 years of observation (median, 5.7 years), and cirrhosis develops in 12 % after 10 years and 34 % after 20 years [117]. The 10-year survival of patients with histological cirrhosis is 80–89 % [28, 117, 118, 155], and the longevity of patients with cirrhosis may contribute to the late occurrence of hepatocellular malignancy [123, 157, 158].

Hepatocellular Carcinoma

Hepatocellular carcinoma develops in 1–9 % of patients with autoimmune hepatitis and cirrhosis, and the annual incidence is 1.1–1.9 % [158–160] (Table 15.6). The standardized incidence ratio (SIR) for hepatocellular carcinoma in Swedish patients with autoimmune hepatitis is 23.3 (95 % confidence interval, 7.5–54.3) [161]. Cirrhosis is a prerequisite for hepatocellular carcinoma, and the duration of cirrhosis before the occurrence of hepatocellular carcinoma ranges from 1 to 16 years (mean interval, 8.5 years) [158]. Surveillance has not been formally recommended because the annual incidence of hepatocellular carcinoma in autoimmune hepatitis does not exceed the threshold of 1.5 % for cost-effectiveness [162]. Men with autoimmune hepatitis and cirrhosis and those patients with features of portal hypertension, immunosuppressive treatment for $\geq$3 years, treatment failure, and cirrhosis of $\geq$10 years duration have risk factors that distinguish them from other patients, and these features have been proposed as indications for annual screening with hepatic ultrasonography [115, 146, 157, 158].

Extrahepatic Malignancies

Extrahepatic malignancies develop in 5 % of patients with autoimmune hepatitis; the incidence is 1 case per 194 patient-years; and the risk is 1.4-fold greater than in an age- and gender-matched healthy population [147] (Table 15.6). Tumors are of diverse cell types (bladder, blood, breast, cervix, lymphatic tissue, skin, soft tissue, and stomach), and non-melanoma skin cancers are probably the most common [115, 163]. The SIR for extrahepatic malignancy in treated patients with autoimmune hepatitis is 2.7 (95 % confidence interval, 1.8–3.9) [148]; the SIR for squamous cell carcinoma of the skin is 28.5 (95 % confidence interval, 9.9–43.1) [163]; and the SIR for basal cell carcinoma is 5.0 (95 % confidence interval, 1–8.9) [163]. Outcomes are related to the nature and stage of the tumor at diagnosis [115, 147]. The predisposition for the malignancies is unclear, but it may relate to the immunosuppressive treatment or the autoimmune liver disease [115]. Non-melanoma skin cancers have been associated with the type and duration of immunosuppressive therapy (especially mercaptopurine and azathioprine) in inflammatory bowel disease and after organ transplantation [164–166]. Autoimmune diseases may also predispose to the development of malignancy without implicating a predisposing treatment [167, 168]. Routine health screening measures should be maintained in all patients with autoimmune hepatitis.

Relapse After Drug Withdrawal

Relapse occurs in 28–87 % of patients, usually within 3 months after drug withdrawal, and it warrants re-institution of treatment [116, 121, 169–171] (Table 15.6). A serum aspartate aminotransferase level (AST) ≥3-fold the upper limit of the normal range (ULN) is invariably associated with recurrent interface hepatitis on histological examination, and the laboratory finding alone is sufficient to restart therapy [129]. The propensity for relapse has been associated with incomplete histological resolution, especially residual plasma cell infiltration [121, 172, 173], progression to cirrhosis during therapy [172], genetic predisposition [53], and rapid corticosteroid withdrawal [174]. The occurrence is not predictable or preventable, but its frequency can be reduced to 28 % in patients who achieve normal laboratory tests and liver tissue before drug withdrawal [121].

Retreatment with corticosteroids induces laboratory resolution in 94 % after 4 ± 1 months and histological improvement to normal or near normal in 59 % after 8 ± 2 months [170]. Relapse may result in cirrhosis (10 %) or liver failure (3 %), but these infrequent consequences may be reduced by early laboratory detection of relapse and prompt re-treatment [175]. Discontinuation of medication after an initial relapse is typically followed by another relapse, and multiple relapses and retreatments are associated with increased frequencies of cirrhosis (38 %) and death from hepatic failure or requirement for liver transplantation (20 %) [175].

The pursuit of a treatment-free state must be balanced against the risks associated with relapse and those associated with indefinite immunosuppressive therapy [122]. Since relapse can be recognized quickly by standard laboratory tests and re-treated effectively, the withdrawal of treatment in those patients who achieve normal tests and liver tissue has been advocated [1]. The occurrence of relapse under these ideal withdrawal conditions justifies re-treatment that is maintained indefinitely [176, 177].

Treatment Strategies for Suboptimal Responses

Suboptimal responses to conventional corticosteroid therapy warrant a revised treatment strategy that may include higher doses of standard treatment, calcineurin inhibitors, mycophenolate mofetil, long-term maintenance therapy, or liver transplantation [178].

Treatment Failure

High doses of prednisone or prednisolone alone or in combination with high dose azathioprine is the preferred management strategy for treatment failure [1, 104, 134] (Table 15.7). The dose of prednisone or prednisolone is 30 mg daily in conjunction with azathioprine, 150 mg daily. Treatment is maintained at fixed doses for at least 1 month. The regimen is then modified after each month of laboratory improvement by reducing the dose of prednisone or prednisolone by 10 mg and the dose of azathioprine by 50 mg until conventional maintenance doses are achieved (prednisone or prednisolone, 10 mg daily, and azathioprine, 50 mg daily) [104]. Prednisone or prednisolone, 60 mg daily, can be substituted for the combination regimen in azathioprine-intolerant patients and those with severe cytopenia [134]. The corticosteroid dose is reduced by 10 mg after each month of laboratory improvement until a conventional maintenance dose of 20 mg daily is achieved (Table 15.7). Laboratory tests improve to normal or near-normal in >70 % of patients within 2 years, but histological improvement to normal or near-normal liver tissue is achieved in only 14–20 %. Cirrhosis develops in 82 %, drug-induced side effects are common, treatment is indefinite, and 5-year survival is 41 % [132, 133, 179].

The calcineurin inhibitors have been used as salvage therapies for decades, but the regimens have not been enthusiastically endorsed in part because they may paradoxically increase immune reactivity [180] (Table 15.7). They have also been variably effective in treating autoimmune hepatitis after liver transplantation [181]; they have been associated with serious side effects, especially neurotoxicity [182, 183]; head-to-head comparison studies with conventional corticosteroid based salvage regimens have not been performed [184]; and the optimal dosing schedule and drug monitoring strategy have been unclear [184]. Nevertheless, the composite

Table 15.7 Salvage therapies in autoimmune hepatitis

Salvage therapy	Regimen	Results
High dose combination	Indication: worsening disease [1]	Normal or near-normal laboratory tests, >70 % [179]
	Prednisone or prednisolone, 30 mg daily, and azathioprine, 150 mg daily × 1 month [104, 134, 178]	Normal or near-normal liver tissue, 14–20 % [179]
	Steroid dose reduction × 10 mg and azathioprine reduction × 50 mg each month of improvement until standard maintenance dose [104, 134, 178]	Cirrhosis, 82 % [132, 133]
		Side effects, common [132, 133]
		5-year survival, 41 % [132, 133]
High dose monotherapy	Indication: worsening disease [1]	Same as with high dose combination [132, 133, 179]
	Prednisone or prednisolone, 60 mg daily × 1 month [104, 134, 178]	Preferred if severe cytopenia, absent TPMT activity, or known azathioprine intolerance [1, 134]
	Steroid dose reduction × 10 mg each month of improvement until standard maintenance dose [104, 134, 178]	
Cyclosporine	Indication: worsening disease [134]	Composite experiences (10 reports): [184]
	Neoral, 2–5 mg/kg daily [178, 188]	Laboratory improvement, 94 % [184, 185]
	Trough levels, 100–300 ng/ml [188]	Ineffective or poorly tolerated, 6 % [184, 185]
Tacrolimus	Indication: worsening disease [134]	Composite experiences (3 reports): [184]
	Initial dose, 0.5–1 mg daily [190, 191]	Laboratory improvement, 98 % [184, 185]
	Maintenance, ≤3 mg twice daily [184]	Ineffective or poorly tolerated, 2 % [184, 185]
	Serum, 3 ng/ml (1.7–10.7 ng/ml) [184]	
Mycophenolate mofetil	Indications: worsening disease and azathioprine intolerance [134, 194]	Composite experiences (11 reports): [184–186]
	Initial dose, 1 g daily [184]	Laboratory improvement, 47 % [184]
	Maintenance, 1.5–2 g daily [184]	Ineffective or poorly tolerated, 53 % [184]
	Avoid in pregnancy [184]	Azathioprine intolerance, 58 % [194, 196]
		Refractory disease, 12 % [194, 196]
		Steroid dose reduction or withdrawal, 40 % [184]

(continued)

Table 15.7 (continued)

Salvage therapy	Regimen	Results
Liver transplantation	Indications: MELD ≥ 16, fulminant presentation, intractable symptoms, drug intolerance, or liver cancer [203]	5-year survival (adults), 75–79 % [135, 204, 205]
		Recurrence, 8–12 % at 1 year, 36–68 % at 5 years [207]
		Re-transplantation, 13–23 % [17, 210, 211]
		5-year survival after recurrence, 89–100 % [212]

MELD model of end-stage liver disease

Numbers in brackets are references

results from small, single-center, clinical experiences with cyclosporine and tacrolimus have supported their efficacy, and they are a consideration for steroid-refractory patients [184–186].

Cyclosporine therapy has improved laboratory tests in 94 % of 32 patients treated for corticosteroid-intolerance or refractory liver disease in a composite of results reported in ten studies since 1985 [184–187]. The treatment was ineffective or poorly tolerated in 6 % [184] (Table 15.7). Cyclosporine was administered mainly as Neoral®, 2–5 mg/kg daily, with dose adjustments to achieve trough levels of 100–300 ng/ml [178, 184, 188].

Tacrolimus has been similarly effective as a salvage therapy, inducing a positive response of any degree in 98 % and a negative response, defined as no response or treatment-ending drug intolerance, in 2 % of 41 patients reported in three studies since 1995 [184, 189–191]. Tacrolimus has been administered mainly at an initial dose of 0.5–1 mg daily with dose adjustments to a maintenance level of 1 mg daily to 3 mg twice daily and a serum level of 3 ng/ml (range, 1.7–10.7 ng/ml) [178, 184].

Mycophenolate mofetil, a next generation purine antagonist, is another drug that has been used in small clinical trials as a salvage therapy for corticosteroid-refractory and azathioprine-intolerant patients [184–186] (Table 15.7). A compilation of recent experiences indicates that the drug induces laboratory improvement in 47 % and no response or drug intolerance in 53 % when used in combination with prednisone or prednisolone and in lieu of azathioprine [184]. Patients treated for azathioprine intolerance have improved more commonly than patients treated for refractory liver disease (58 % versus 12 %), and these findings suggest that the effectiveness of mycophenolate mofetil as a salvage agent could be improved by better patient selection [184, 192–197]. Complete corticosteroid withdrawal was possible in 40 % of patients reported in 11 studies, and the overall frequency of treatment ending side effects was 15 % [184].

The dose of mycophenolate mofetil in autoimmune hepatitis has ranged from 500 mg daily to 3 g daily [184–186] (Table 15.7). The drug is usually started in a dose of 1 g daily and increased as tolerated to a maintenance dose of 1.5–2 g daily. The most common side effects have been nausea and leukopenia [198, 199], and the drug must be avoided in pregnancy [184]. Mycophenolate mofetil has been associated with miscarriages and congenital defects of the face and heart that reflect abnormalities in the migration of the fetal cranial neural crest [200].

Incomplete Response

Patients who improve but fail to normalize their laboratory tests and liver tissue after 36 months are unlikely to achieve an optimal end point by continuing standard therapy [131] (Table 15.7). The management strategy must be modified to prevent disease progression and treatment-related side effects by suppressing liver inflammation on the lowest dose of medication possible. The dose of prednisone or prednisolone can be reduced in a gradual fashion by decrements as low as 2.5 mg daily as the dose of azathioprine is increased to 2 mg/kg daily [124, 176]. Complete withdrawal from corticosteroids and long-term maintenance on azathioprine alone may be possible. Low dose corticosteroid therapy has been maintained for 7–43 years (mean, 16 years) in 42 patients [201], and it has generally been well tolerated except for isolated cases of cryptococcal meningitis and aseptic necrosis of the hip. Progression to cirrhosis has occurred in 54 %, and the need for liver transplantation has been rare (2 %) [201].

Drug Toxicity

The incriminated medication is reduced in dose or discontinued depending on the severity of the toxicity [1]. The tolerated medication is then adjusted in dose to compensate for the altered regimen. Side effects, including mild cytopenia, can commonly be corrected by dose reduction. Determination of TPMT activity is warranted before continuing azathioprine in cytopenic patients [1]. Mycophenolate mofetil has been effective in patients with azathioprine intolerance [194, 196], but one of its important side effects is myelosuppression [198, 199, 202]. The mechanisms of bone marrow toxicity are probably different in patients taking azathioprine [140] and those taking mycophenolate mofetil [198, 199], but some caution is warranted when considering the use of mycophenolate mofetil in any form of drug-induced bone marrow toxicity.

Relapse After Corticosteroid Withdrawal

Relapse is managed by restarting the original treatment regimen that had induced disease resolution (Table 15.7). Treatment is continued until normalization of laboratory tests reflective of liver inflammation (serum aminotransferase, γ-globulin, and immunoglobulin G levels). The dose of prednisone or prednisolone is then gradually decreased as the dose of azathioprine is increased to 2 mg/kg daily. Corticosteroids are finally withdrawn, and treatment with azathioprine is maintained indefinitely. Eight-five percent of patients have remained inactive on azathioprine therapy during a 10-year observation period [177].

Patients not taking azathioprine or azathioprine intolerant can be managed on low dose prednisone or prednisolone [176]. The corticosteroid dose is reduced gradually by 2.5 mg to the lowest dose necessary to prevent laboratory instability (typical dose, ≤10 mg daily; median dose, 7.5 mg daily) [176]. Corticosteroid-related complications acquired during conventional therapy improve in 85 % of patients treated with low dose regimens; the frequency of death from hepatic failure or requirement for liver transplantation is similar to that of patients treated with conventional regimens after relapse (9 % versus 10 %); and 36 % of patients improve to normal or near-normal liver tests and liver tissue with protracted treatment [176].

Liver Transplantation

Liver transplantation is the preferred salvage therapy for patients with features of liver failure [134], and it should be considered if the model of end-stage liver disease (MELD) score exceeds 16 points, the presentation is fulminant, features of hepatic decompensation emerge, symptoms are intractable, treatment is poorly tolerated, or liver cancer is suspected [203] (Table 15.7). Ten percent of patients with corticosteroid-refractory disease require this intervention [135]. The 5-year patient survival is 75–79 % in adults [135, 204, 205] and 86 % in children [206]. Autoimmune hepatitis recurs in the allograft in 8–12 % after 1 year and 36–68 % after 5 years [207–209], and graft failure may warrant re-transplantation in 13–23 % [17, 210, 211]. The actuarial 5-year survival of adults with recurrent autoimmune hepatitis is 89–100 % [211, 212], and the possibility of recurrence should not defeat the prospect of liver transplantation for a suitable candidate.

Overview

Autoimmune hepatitis is an immune-mediated inflammatory liver disease of unknown cause that may progress to cirrhosis or liver failure. Diagnostic criteria have been codified, and the diagnosis requires the confident exclusion of other liver diseases that may resemble it. Liver biopsy examination is an essential component of the evaluation. Treatment with prednisone or prednisolone in combination with azathioprine is the mainstay therapy, and it improves laboratory tests and liver tissue to normal or near-normal in most patients after 22–24 months. Budesonide in combination with prednisone or prednisolone can be considered in non-cirrhotic patients with mild, uncomplicated liver disease or pre-morbid conditions that would be aggravated by conventional corticosteroid regimens.

Corticosteroid-induced side effects are mainly cosmetic, but the possibility of osteopenia and vertebral compression, especially in post-menopausal women, justifies a bone maintenance strategy that emphasizes regular exercise, calcium and vitamin D supplementation, periodic bone densitometry, and bisphosphonates as necessary. Pretreatment assessment of TPMT activity should be considered in all patients who will be treated with azathioprine, especially those with cytopenia, and leukocyte and platelet counts must be monitored at 3–6 month intervals in all azathioprine treated patients.

Treatment can be withdrawn in patients who have normalized liver tests and liver tissue, but relapse is always possible (frequency, $\geq 28\%$) and serum AST and γ-globulin levels must be monitored closely to detect this occurrence. Re-treatment after relapse induces resolution of the liver dysfunction, and indefinite therapy with azathioprine (2 mg/kg daily) is warranted. A treatment-free state is possible in 19–40 % of patients. Other outcomes include treatment failure (7 %), incomplete response (14 %), drug toxicity (12–29 %), cirrhosis (54 %), hepatocellular carcinoma (1–9 %), and extrahepatic malignancies (5 %). Treatments with high doses of corticosteroids alone or with azathioprine, calcineurin inhibitors, and mycophenolate mofetil are salvage therapies that must be used for off-label indications in a highly individualized and well-monitored fashion. Autoimmune hepatitis is a treatable chronic liver disease, and the survival expectation is high.

Acknowledgement This review did not receive financial support from a funding agency or institution, and Albert J. Czaja, MD has no conflict of interests to declare.

References

1. Manns MP, Czaja AJ, Gorham JD, Krawitt EL, Mieli-Vergani G, Vergani D, et al. Diagnosis and management of autoimmune hepatitis. Hepatology. 2010;51:2193–213.
2. Gleeson D, Heneghan MA. British Society of Gastroenterology (BSG) guidelines for management of autoimmune hepatitis. Gut. 2011;60:1611–29.
3. Alvarez F, Berg PA, Bianchi FB, Bianchi L, Burroughs AK, Cancado EL, et al. International Autoimmune Hepatitis Group Report: review of criteria for diagnosis of autoimmune hepatitis. J Hepatol. 1999;31:929–38.
4. Czaja AJ. Autoimmune hepatitis. Part B: diagnosis. Expert Rev Gastroenterol Hepatol. 2007;1:129–43.
5. Hennes EM, Zeniya M, Czaja AJ, Pares A, Dalekos GN, Krawitt EL, et al. Simplified criteria for the diagnosis of autoimmune hepatitis. Hepatology. 2008;48:169–76.
6. Czaja AJ. Performance parameters of the diagnostic scoring systems for autoimmune hepatitis. Hepatology. 2008;48:1540–8.
7. Gregorio GV, Portmann B, Reid F, Donaldson PT, Doherty DG, McCartney M, et al. Autoimmune hepatitis in childhood: a 20-year experience. Hepatology. 1997;25:541–7.
8. Al-Chalabi T, Boccato S, Portmann BC, McFarlane IG, Heneghan MA. Autoimmune hepatitis (AIH) in the elderly: a systematic retrospective analysis of a large group of consecutive patients with definite AIH followed at a tertiary referral centre. J Hepatol. 2006;45:575–83.
9. Czaja AJ, Carpenter HA. Distinctive clinical phenotype and treatment outcome of type 1 autoimmune hepatitis in the elderly. Hepatology. 2006;43:532–8.

10. Czaja AJ, Donaldson PT. Gender effects and synergisms with histocompatibility leukocyte antigens in type 1 autoimmune hepatitis. Am J Gastroenterol. 2002;97:2051–7.
11. Al-Chalabi T, Underhill JA, Portmann BC, McFarlane IG, Heneghan MA. Impact of gender on the long-term outcome and survival of patients with autoimmune hepatitis. J Hepatol. 2008;48:140–7.
12. Czaja AJ. Autoimmune hepatitis in diverse ethnic populations and geographical regions. Expert Rev Gastroenterol Hepatol. 2013;7:365–85.
13. Czaja AJ, Carpenter HA, Santrach PJ, Moore SB, Homburger HA. The nature and prognosis of severe cryptogenic chronic active hepatitis. Gastroenterology. 1993;104:1755–61.
14. Heringlake S, Schutte A, Flemming P, Schmiegel W, Manns MP, Tillmann HL. Presumed cryptogenic liver disease in Germany: high prevalence of autoantibody-negative autoimmune hepatitis, low prevalence of NASH, no evidence for occult viral etiology. Z Gastroenterol. 2009;47:417–23.
15. Czaja AJ. Cryptogenic chronic hepatitis and its changing guise in adults. Dig Dis Sci. 2011;56:3421–38.
16. Czaja AJ. Autoantibody-negative autoimmune hepatitis. Dig Dis Sci. 2012;57:610–24.
17. Czaja AJ. Diagnosis, pathogenesis, and treatment of autoimmune hepatitis after liver transplantation. Dig Dis Sci. 2012;57:2248–66.
18. Liberal R, Longhi MS, Grant CR, Mieli-Vergani G, Vergani D. Autoimmune hepatitis after liver transplantation. Clin Gastroenterol Hepatol. 2012;10:346–53.
19. Liberal R, Zen Y, Mieli-Vergani G, Vergani D. Liver transplantation and autoimmune liver diseases. Liver Transpl. 2013;19:1065–77.
20. Nikias GA, Batts KP, Czaja AJ. The nature and prognostic implications of autoimmune hepatitis with an acute presentation. J Hepatol. 1994;21:866–71.
21. Crapper RM, Bhathal PS, Mackay IR, Frazer IH. 'Acute' autoimmune hepatitis. Digestion. 1986;34:216–25.
22. Kessler WR, Cummings OW, Eckert G, Chalasani N, Lumeng L, Kwo PY. Fulminant hepatic failure as the initial presentation of acute autoimmune hepatitis. Clin Gastroenterol Hepatol. 2004;2:625–31.
23. Stravitz RT, Lefkowitch JH, Fontana RJ, Gershwin ME, Leung PS, Sterling RK, et al. Autoimmune acute liver failure: proposed clinical and histological criteria. Hepatology. 2011;53:517–26.
24. Czaja AJ. Acute and acute severe (fulminant) autoimmune hepatitis. Dig Dis Sci. 2013;58:897–914.
25. Kogan J, Safadi R, Ashur Y, Shouval D, Ilan Y. Prognosis of symptomatic versus asymptomatic autoimmune hepatitis: a study of 68 patients. J Clin Gastroenterol. 2002;35:75–81.
26. Feld JJ, Dinh H, Arenovich T, Marcus VA, Wanless IR, Heathcote EJ. Autoimmune hepatitis: effect of symptoms and cirrhosis on natural history and outcome. Hepatology. 2005;42:53–62.
27. Czaja AJ. Features and consequences of untreated type 1 autoimmune hepatitis. Liver Int. 2009;29:816–23.
28. Roberts SK, Therneau TM, Czaja AJ. Prognosis of histological cirrhosis in type 1 autoimmune hepatitis. Gastroenterology. 1996;110:848–57.
29. Burgart LJ, Batts KP, Ludwig J, Nikias GA, Czaja AJ. Recent-onset autoimmune hepatitis. Biopsy findings and clinical correlations. Am J Surg Pathol. 1995;19:699–708.
30. Yasui S, Fujiwara K, Yonemitsu Y, Oda S, Nakano M, Yokosuka O. Clinicopathological features of severe and fulminant forms of autoimmune hepatitis. J Gastroenterol. 2011;46:378–90.
31. Vergani D, Alvarez F, Bianchi FB, Cancado EL, Mackay IR, Manns MP, et al. Liver autoimmune serology: a consensus statement from the committee for autoimmune serology of the International Autoimmune Hepatitis Group. J Hepatol. 2004;41:677–83.
32. Czaja AJ. Performance parameters of the conventional serological markers for autoimmune hepatitis. Dig Dis Sci. 2011;56:545–54.

33. Czaja AJ. Behavior and significance of autoantibodies in type 1 autoimmune hepatitis. J Hepatol. 1999;30:394–401.
34. Czaja AJ, Nishioka M, Morshed SA, Hachiya T. Patterns of nuclear immunofluorescence and reactivities to recombinant nuclear antigens in autoimmune hepatitis. Gastroenterology. 1994;107:200–7.
35. Toh BH. Smooth muscle autoantibodies and autoantigens. Clin Exp Immunol. 1979;38:621–8.
36. Kurki P, Miettinen A, Linder E, Pikkarainen P, Vuoristo M, Salaspuro MP. Different types of smooth muscle antibodies in chronic active hepatitis and primary biliary cirrhosis: their diagnostic and prognostic significance. Gut. 1980;21:878–84.
37. Kurki P, Miettinen A, Salaspuro M, Virtanen I, Stenman S. Cytoskeleton antibodies in chronic active hepatitis, primary biliary cirrhosis, and alcoholic liver disease. Hepatology. 1983;3:297–302.
38. Czaja AJ, Cassani F, Cataleta M, Valentini P, Bianchi FB. Frequency and significance of antibodies to actin in type 1 autoimmune hepatitis. Hepatology. 1996;24:1068–73.
39. Czaja AJ, Manns MP, Homburger HA. Frequency and significance of antibodies to liver/kidney microsome type 1 in adults with chronic active hepatitis. Gastroenterology. 1992;103:1290–5.
40. Homberg JC, Abuaf N, Bernard O, Islam S, Alvarez F, Khalil SH, et al. Chronic active hepatitis associated with antiliver/kidney microsome antibody type 1: a second type of "autoimmune" hepatitis. Hepatology. 1987;7:1333–9.
41. Gregorio GV, Portmann B, Karani J, Harrison P, Donaldson PT, Vergani D, et al. Autoimmune hepatitis/sclerosing cholangitis overlap syndrome in childhood: a 16-year prospective study. Hepatology. 2001;33:544–53.
42. Manns MP, Griffin KJ, Sullivan KF, Johnson EF. LKM-1 autoantibodies recognize a short linear sequence in P450IID6, a cytochrome P-450 monooxygenase. J Clin Invest. 1991;88:1370–8.
43. Ma Y, Thomas MG, Okamoto M, Bogdanos DP, Nagl S, Kerkar N, et al. Key residues of a major cytochrome P4502D6 epitope are located on the surface of the molecule. J Immunol. 2002;169:277–85.
44. Czaja AJ, Manns MP. The validity and importance of subtypes in autoimmune hepatitis: a point of view. Am J Gastroenterol. 1995;90:1206–11.
45. Czaja AJ, Norman GL. Autoantibodies in the diagnosis and management of liver disease. J Clin Gastroenterol. 2003;37:315–29.
46. Czaja AJ, Shums Z, Norman GL. Nonstandard antibodies as prognostic markers in autoimmune hepatitis. Autoimmunity. 2004;37:195–201.
47. Czaja AJ. Autoantibodies in autoimmune liver disease. Adv Clin Chem. 2005;40:127–64.
48. Costa M, Rodriguez-Sanchez JL, Czaja AJ, Gelpi C. Isolation and characterization of cDNA encoding the antigenic protein of the human tRNP(Ser)Sec complex recognized by autoantibodies from patients withtype-1 autoimmune hepatitis. Clin Exp Immunol. 2000;121:364–74.
49. Volkmann M, Luithle D, Zentgraf H, Schnolzer M, Fiedler S, Heid H, et al. SLA/LP/tRNP((Ser)Sec) antigen in autoimmune hepatitis: identification of the native protein in human hepatic cell extract. J Autoimmun. 2010;34:59–65.
50. Wies I, Brunner S, Henninger J, Herkel J, Kanzler S, Meyer zum Buschenfelde KH, et al. Identification of target antigen for SLA/LP autoantibodies in autoimmune hepatitis. Lancet. 2000;355:1510–5.
51. Baeres M, Herkel J, Czaja AJ, Wies I, Kanzler S, Cancado EL, et al. Establishment of standardised SLA/LP immunoassays: specificity for autoimmune hepatitis, worldwide occurrence, and clinical characteristics. Gut. 2002;51:259–64.
52. Eyraud V, Chazouilleres O, Ballot E, Corpechot C, Poupon R, Johanet C. Significance of antibodies to soluble liver antigen/liver pancreas: a large French study. Liver Int. 2009;29:857–64.

53. Czaja AJ, Donaldson PT, Lohse AW. Antibodies to soluble liver antigen/liver pancreas and HLA risk factors for type 1 autoimmune hepatitis. Am J Gastroenterol. 2002;97:413–9.
54. Czaja AJ. Autoantibodies as prognostic markers in autoimmune liver disease. Dig Dis Sci. 2010;55:2144–61.
55. Ma Y, Okamoto M, Thomas MG, Bogdanos DP, Lopes AR, Portmann B, et al. Antibodies to conformational epitopes of soluble liver antigen define a severe form of autoimmune liver disease. Hepatology. 2002;35:658–64.
56. Montano-Loza AJ, Shums Z, Norman GL, Czaja AJ. Prognostic implications of antibodies to Ro/SSA and soluble liver antigen in type 1 autoimmune hepatitis. Liver Int. 2012;32:85–92.
57. Granito A, Muratori L, Muratori P, Pappas G, Guidi M, Cassani F, et al. Antibodies to filamentous actin (F-actin) in type 1 autoimmune hepatitis. J Clin Pathol. 2006;59:280–4.
58. Aubert V, Pisler IG, Spertini F. Improved diagnoses of autoimmune hepatitis using an anti-actin ELISA. J Clin Lab Anal. 2008;22:340–5.
59. Gueguen P, Dalekos G, Nousbaum JB, Zachou K, Putterman C, Youinou P, et al. Double reactivity against actin and alpha-actinin defines a severe form of autoimmune hepatitis type 1. J Clin Immunol. 2006;26:495–505.
60. Renaudineau Y, Dalekos GN, Gueguen P, Zachou K, Youinou P. Anti-alpha-actinin antibodies cross-react with anti-ssDNA antibodies in active autoimmune hepatitis. Clin Rev Allergy Immunol. 2008;34:321–5.
61. Czaja AJ, Manns MP. Advances in the diagnosis, pathogenesis and management of autoimmune hepatitis. Gastroenterology. 2010;139:58–72.
62. Frenzel C, Herkel J, Luth S, Galle PR, Schramm C, Lohse AW. Evaluation of F-actin ELISA for the diagnosis of autoimmune hepatitis. Am J Gastroenterol. 2006;101:2731–6.
63. Terjung B, Herzog V, Worman HJ, Gestmann I, Bauer C, Sauerbruch T, et al. Atypical anti-neutrophil cytoplasmic antibodies with perinuclear fluorescence in chronic inflammatory bowel diseases and hepatobiliary disorders colocalize with nuclear lamina proteins. Hepatology. 1998;28:332–40.
64. Terjung B, Worman HJ, Herzog V, Sauerbruch T, Spengler U. Differentiation of antineutrophil nuclear antibodies in inflammatory bowel and autoimmune liver diseases from antineutrophil cytoplasmic antibodies (p-ANCA) using immunofluorescence microscopy. Clin Exp Immunol. 2001;126:37–46.
65. Targan SR, Landers C, Vidrich A, Czaja AJ. High-titer antineutrophil cytoplasmic antibodies in type-1 autoimmune hepatitis. Gastroenterology. 1995;108:1159–66.
66. Bansi D, Chapman R, Fleming K. Antineutrophil cytoplasmic antibodies in chronic liver diseases: prevalence, titre, specificity and IgG subclass. J Hepatol. 1996;24:581–6.
67. Zauli D, Ghetti S, Grassi A, Descovich C, Cassani F, Ballardini G, et al. Anti-neutrophil cytoplasmic antibodies in type 1 and 2 autoimmune hepatitis. Hepatology. 1997;25:1105–7.
68. Terjung B, Spengler U, Sauerbruch T, Worman HJ. "Atypical p-ANCA" in IBD and hepatobiliary disorders react with a 50-kilodalton nuclear envelope protein of neutrophils and myeloid cell lines. Gastroenterology. 2000;119:310–22.
69. Czaja AJ, Pfeifer KD, Decker RH, Vallari AS. Frequency and significance of antibodies to asialoglycoprotein receptor in type 1 autoimmune hepatitis. Dig Dis Sci. 1996;41:1733–40.
70. Hausdorf G, Roggenbuck D, Feist E, Buttner T, Jungblut PR, Conrad K, et al. Autoantibodies to asialoglycoprotein receptor (ASGPR) measured by a novel ELISA--revival of a disease-activity marker in autoimmune hepatitis. Clin Chim Acta. 2009;408:19–24.
71. Bridoux-Henno L, Maggiore G, Johanet C, Fabre M, Vajro P, Dommergues JP, et al. Features and outcome of autoimmune hepatitis type 2 presenting with isolated positivity for anti-liver cytosol antibody. Clin Gastroenterol Hepatol. 2004;2:825–30.
72. Fabien N, Desbos A, Bienvenu J, Magdalou J. Autoantibodies directed against the UDP-glucuronosyltransferases in human autoimmune hepatitis. Autoimmun Rev. 2004;3:1–9.
73. Adams LA, Lindor KD, Angulo P. The prevalence of autoantibodies and autoimmune hepatitis in patients with nonalcoholic fatty liver disease. Am J Gastroenterol. 2004;99:1316–20.

74. Fujiwara K, Fukuda Y, Yokosuka O. Precise histological evaluation of liver biopsy specimen is indispensable for diagnosis and treatment of acute-onset autoimmune hepatitis. J Gastroenterol. 2008;43:951–8.
75. Suzuki A, Brunt EM, Kleiner DE, Miquel R, Smyrk TC, Andrade RJ, et al. The use of liver biopsy evaluation in discrimination of idiopathic autoimmune hepatitis versus drug-induced liver injury. Hepatology. 2011;54:931–9.
76. Efe C, Ozaslan E, Purnak T, Ozseker B, Kav T, Bayraktar Y. Liver biopsy is a superior diagnostic method in some patients showing the typical laboratory features of autoimmune hepatitis. Clin Res Hepatol Gastroenterol. 2012;36:185–8.
77. Bjornsson E, Talwalkar J, Treeprasertsuk S, Neuhauser M, Lindor K. Patients with typical laboratory features of autoimmune hepatitis rarely need a liver biopsy for diagnosis. Clin Gastroenterol Hepatol. 2011;9:57–63.
78. Czaja AJ, Carpenter HA. Sensitivity, specificity, and predictability of biopsy interpretations in chronic hepatitis. Gastroenterology. 1993;105:1824–32.
79. Ludwig J, Czaja AJ, Dickson ER, LaRusso NF, Wiesner RH. Manifestations of nonsuppurative cholangitis in chronic hepatobiliary diseases: morphologic spectrum, clinical correlations and terminology. Liver. 1984;4:105–16.
80. Czaja AJ, Carpenter HA. Autoimmune hepatitis with incidental histologic features of bile duct injury. Hepatology. 2001;34:659–65.
81. Czaja AJ, Muratori P, Muratori L, Carpenter HA, Bianchi FB. Diagnostic and therapeutic implications of bile duct injury in autoimmune hepatitis. Liver Int. 2004;24:322–9.
82. Miyake Y, Iwasaki Y, Terada R, Onishi T, Okamoto R, Takaguchi K, et al. Clinical features of Japanese type 1 autoimmune hepatitis patients with zone III necrosis. Hepatol Res. 2007;37:801–5.
83. Okano N, Yamamoto K, Sakaguchi K, Miyake Y, Shimada N, Hakoda T, et al. Clinicopathological features of acute-onset autoimmune hepatitis. Hepatol Res. 2003;25:263–70.
84. Czaja AJ. Clinical features, differential diagnosis and treatment of autoimmune hepatitis in the elderly. Drugs Aging. 2008;25:219–39.
85. Bittencourt PL, Farias AQ, Porta G, Cancado EL, Miura I, Pugliese R, et al. Frequency of concurrent autoimmune disorders in patients with autoimmune hepatitis: effect of age, gender, and genetic background. J Clin Gastroenterol. 2008;42:300–5.
86. Efe C, Wahlin S, Ozaslan E, Berlot AH, Purnak T, Muratori L, et al. Autoimmune hepatitis/primary biliary cirrhosis overlap syndrome and associated extrahepatic autoimmune diseases. Eur J Gastroenterol Hepatol. 2012;24:531–4.
87. Czaja AJ, Carpenter HA, Santrach PJ, Moore SB. Significance of HLA DR4 in type 1 autoimmune hepatitis. Gastroenterology. 1993;105:1502–7.
88. Czaja AJ, Strettell MD, Thomson LJ, Santrach PJ, Moore SB, Donaldson PT, et al. Associations between alleles of the major histocompatibility complex and type 1 autoimmune hepatitis. Hepatology. 1997;25:317–23.
89. Czaja AJ, Souto EO, Bittencourt PL, Cancado EL, Porta G, Goldberg AC, et al. Clinical distinctions and pathogenic implications of type 1 autoimmune hepatitis in Brazil and the United States. J Hepatol. 2002;37:302–8.
90. Perdigoto R, Carpenter HA, Czaja AJ. Frequency and significance of chronic ulcerative colitis in severe corticosteroid-treated autoimmune hepatitis. J Hepatol. 1992;14:325–31.
91. Abdalian R, Dhar P, Jhaveri K, Haider M, Guindi M, Heathcote EJ. Prevalence of sclerosing cholangitis in adults with autoimmune hepatitis: evaluating the role of routine magnetic resonance imaging. Hepatology. 2008;47:949–57.
92. Mieli-Vergani G, Vergani D. Autoimmune liver diseases in children - what is different from adulthood? Best Pract Res Clin Gastroenterol. 2011;25:783–95.
93. Lewin M, Vilgrain V, Ozenne V, Lemoine M, Wendum D, Paradis V, et al. Prevalence of sclerosing cholangitis in adults with autoimmune hepatitis: a prospective magnetic resonance imaging and histological study. Hepatology. 2009;50:528–37.

94. Mirzaagha F, Azali SH, Islami F, Zamani F, Khalilipour E, Khatibian M, et al. Coeliac disease in autoimmune liver disease: a cross-sectional study and a systematic review. Dig Liver Dis. 2010;42:620–3.
95. van Gerven NM, Bakker SF, de Boer YS, Witte BI, Bontkes H, van Nieuwkerk CM, et al. Seroprevalence of celiac disease in patients with autoimmune hepatitis. Eur J Gastroenterol Hepatol. 2014;26:1104. doi:10.1097/MEG.0000000000000172.
96. Volta U, De Franceschi L, Molinaro N, Cassani F, Muratori L, Lenzi M, et al. Frequency and significance of anti-gliadin and anti-endomysial antibodies in autoimmune hepatitis. Dig Dis Sci. 1998;43:2190–5.
97. Abdo A, Meddings J, Swain M. Liver abnormalities in celiac disease. Clin Gastroenterol Hepatol. 2004;2:107–12.
98. Kaukinen K, Halme L, Collin P, Farkkila M, Maki M, Vehmanen P, et al. Celiac disease in patients with severe liver disease: gluten-free diet may reverse hepatic failure. Gastroenterology. 2002;122:881–8.
99. Mugica F, Castiella A, Otazua P, Munagorri A, Recasens M, Barrio J, et al. Prevalence of coeliac disease in unexplained chronic hypertransaminasemia. Rev Esp Enferm Dig. 2001;93:707–14.
100. Rubio-Tapia A, Murray JA. Liver involvement in celiac disease. Minerva Med. 2008;99:595–604.
101. Volta U, Granito A, De Franceschi L, Petrolini N, Bianchi FB. Anti tissue transglutaminase antibodies as predictors of silent coeliac disease in patients with hypertransaminasaemia of unknown origin. Dig Liver Dis. 2001;33:420–5.
102. Volta U. Pathogenesis and clinical significance of liver injury in celiac disease. Clin Rev Allergy Immunol. 2009;36:62–70.
103. Czaja AJ. Drug choices in autoimmune hepatitis: Part A - steroids. Expert Rev Gastroenterol Hepatol. 2012;6:603–15.
104. Czaja AJ. Current and prospective pharmacotherapy for autoimmune hepatitis. Expert Opin Pharmacother. 2014;15:1715–36.
105. Czaja AJ. Diagnosis and management of autoimmune hepatitis. Clin Liver Dis. 2015;19:57.
106. Schramm C, Weiler-Normann C, Wiegard C, Hellweg S, Muller S, Lohse AW. Treatment response in patients with autoimmune hepatitis. Hepatology. 2010;52:2247–8.
107. Lohse AW, Mieli-Vergani G. Autoimmune hepatitis. J Hepatol. 2011;55:171–82.
108. Summerskill WH, Korman MG, Ammon HV, Baggenstoss AH. Prednisone for chronic active liver disease: dose titration, standard dose, and combination with azathioprine compared. Gut. 1975;16:876–83.
109. Manns MP, Woynarowski M, Kreisel W, Lurie Y, Rust C, Zuckerman E, et al. Budesonide induces remission more effectively than prednisone in a controlled trial of patients with auto-immune hepatitis. Gastroenterology. 2010;139:1198–206.
110. Woynarowski M, Nemeth A, Baruch Y, Koletzko S, Melter M, Rodeck B, et al. Budesonide versus prednisone with azathioprine for the treatment of autoimmune hepatitis in children and adolescents. J Pediatr. 2013;163:1347–53.e1.
111. Czaja AJ, Lindor KD. Failure of budesonide in a pilot study of treatment-dependent autoimmune hepatitis. Gastroenterology. 2000;119:1312–6.
112. Geier A, Gartung C, Dietrich CG, Wasmuth HE, Reinartz P, Matern S. Side effects of budesonide in liver cirrhosis due to chronic autoimmune hepatitis: influence of hepatic metabolism versus portosystemic shunts on a patient complicated with HCC. World J Gastroenterol. 2003;9:2681–5.
113. Efe C, Ozaslan E, Kav T, Purnak T, Shorbagi A, Ozkayar O, et al. Liver fibrosis may reduce the efficacy of budesonide in the treatment of autoimmune hepatitis and overlap syndrome. Autoimmun Rev. 2012;11:330–4.
114. Czaja AJ, Carpenter HA. Progressive fibrosis during corticosteroid therapy of autoimmune hepatitis. Hepatology. 2004;39:1631–8.
115. Czaja AJ. Hepatocellular cancer and other malignancies in autoimmune hepatitis. Dig Dis Sci. 2013;58:1459–76.

116. van Gerven NM, Verwer BJ, Witte BI, van Hoek B, Coenraad MJ, van Erpecum KJ, et al. Relapse is almost universal after withdrawal of immunosuppressive medication in patients with autoimmune hepatitis in remission. J Hepatol. 2013;58:141–7.
117. Hoeroldt B, McFarlane E, Dube A, Basumani P, Karajeh M, Campbell MJ, et al. Long-term outcomes of patients with autoimmune hepatitis managed at a nontransplant center. Gastroenterology. 2011;140:1980–9.
118. Kanzler S, Lohr H, Gerken G, Galle PR, Lohse AW. Long-term management and prognosis of autoimmune hepatitis (AIH): a single center experience. Z Gastroenterol. 2001;39:339–41. 44-8.
119. Floreani A, Niro G, Rosa Rizzotto E, Antoniazzi S, Ferrara F, Carderi I, et al. Type I autoimmune hepatitis: clinical course and outcome in an Italian multicentre study. Aliment Pharmacol Ther. 2006;24:1051–7.
120. Delgado JS, Vodonos A, Malnick S, Kriger O, Wilkof-Segev R, Delgado B, et al. Autoimmune hepatitis in southern Israel: a 15-year multicenter study. J Dig Dis. 2013;14:611–8.
121. Czaja AJ, Davis GL, Ludwig J, Taswell HF. Complete resolution of inflammatory activity following corticosteroid treatment of HBsAg-negative chronic active hepatitis. Hepatology. 1984;4:622–7.
122. Czaja AJ. Review article: permanent drug withdrawal is desirable and achievable for autoimmune hepatitis. Aliment Pharmacol Ther. 2014;39:1043–58.
123. Seo S, Toutounjian R, Conrad A, Blatt L, Tong MJ. Favorable outcomes of autoimmune hepatitis in a community clinic setting. J Gastroenterol Hepatol. 2008;23:1410–4.
124. Czaja AJ, Menon KV, Carpenter HA. Sustained remission after corticosteroid therapy for type 1 autoimmune hepatitis: a retrospective analysis. Hepatology. 2002;35:890–7.
125. Czaja AJ, Beaver SJ, Shiels MT. Sustained remission after corticosteroid therapy of severe hepatitis B surface antigen-negative chronic active hepatitis. Gastroenterology. 1987;92:215–9.
126. Czaja AJ. Advances in the current treatment of autoimmune hepatitis. Dig Dis Sci. 2012;57:1996–2010.
127. Czaja AJ, Rakela J, Ludwig J. Features reflective of early prognosis in corticosteroid-treated severe autoimmune chronic active hepatitis. Gastroenterology. 1988;95:448–53.
128. Soloway RD, Summerskill WH, Baggenstoss AH, Geall MG, Gitnick GL, Elveback IR, et al. Clinical, biochemical, and histological remission of severe chronic active liver disease: a controlled study of treatments and early prognosis. Gastroenterology. 1972;63:820–33.
129. Czaja AJ, Wolf AM, Baggenstoss AH. Laboratory assessment of severe chronic active liver disease during and after corticosteroid therapy: correlation of serum transaminase and gamma globulin levels with histologic features. Gastroenterology. 1981;80:687–92.
130. Luth S, Herkel J, Kanzler S, Frenzel C, Galle PR, Dienes HP, et al. Serologic markers compared with liver biopsy for monitoring disease activity in autoimmune hepatitis. J Clin Gastroenterol. 2008;42:926–30.
131. Czaja AJ. Rapidity of treatment response and outcome in type 1 autoimmune hepatitis. J Hepatol. 2009;51:161–7.
132. Montano-Loza AJ, Carpenter HA, Czaja AJ. Features associated with treatment failure in type 1 autoimmune hepatitis and predictive value of the model of end-stage liver disease. Hepatology. 2007;46:1138–45.
133. Czaja AJ, Carpenter HA. Empiric therapy of autoimmune hepatitis with mycophenolate mofetil: comparison with conventional treatment for refractory disease. J Clin Gastroenterol. 2005;39:819–25.
134. Czaja AJ. Management of recalcitrant autoimmune hepatitis. Curr Hepat Rep. 2013;12:66–77.
135. Vogel A, Heinrich E, Bahr MJ, Rifai K, Flemming P, Melter M, et al. Long-term outcome of liver transplantation for autoimmune hepatitis. Clin Transplant. 2004;18:62–9.
136. Czaja AJ. Safety issues in the management of autoimmune hepatitis. Expert Opin Drug Saf. 2008;7:319–33.

137. Uribe M, Go VL, Kluge D. Prednisone for chronic active hepatitis: pharmacokinetics and serum binding in patients with chronic active hepatitis and steroid major side effects. J Clin Gastroenterol. 1984;6:331–5.
138. Bajaj JS, Saeian K, Varma RR, Franco J, Knox JF, Podoll J, et al. Increased rates of early adverse reaction to azathioprine in patients with Crohn's disease compared to autoimmune hepatitis: a tertiary referral center experience. Am J Gastroenterol. 2005;100:1121–5.
139. Bacon BR, Treuhaft WH, Goodman AM. Azathioprine-induced pancytopenia. Occurrence in two patients with connective-tissue diseases. Arch Intern Med. 1981;141:223–6.
140. Ben Ari Z, Mehta A, Lennard L, Burroughs AK. Azathioprine-induced myelosuppression due to thiopurine methyltransferase deficiency in a patient with autoimmune hepatitis. J Hepatol. 1995;23:351–4.
141. Langley PG, Underhill J, Tredger JM, Norris S, McFarlane IG. Thiopurine methyltransferase phenotype and genotype in relation to azathioprine therapy in autoimmune hepatitis. J Hepatol. 2002;37:441–7.
142. Czaja AJ, Carpenter HA. Thiopurine methyltransferase deficiency and azathioprine intolerance in autoimmune hepatitis. Dig Dis Sci. 2006;51:968–75.
143. Heneghan MA, Allan ML, Bornstein JD, Muir AJ, Tendler DA. Utility of thiopurine methyltransferase genotyping and phenotyping, and measurement of azathioprine metabolites in the management of patients with autoimmune hepatitis. J Hepatol. 2006;45:584–91.
144. Ferucci ED, Hurlburt KJ, Mayo MJ, Livingston S, Deubner H, Gove J, et al. Azathioprine metabolite measurements are not useful in following treatment of autoimmune hepatitis in Alaska Native and other non-Caucasian people. Can J Gastroenterol. 2011;25:21–7.
145. Szumlanski CL, Honchel R, Scott MC, Weinshilboum RM. Human liver thiopurine methyltransferase pharmacogenetics: biochemical properties, liver-erythrocyte correlation and presence of isozymes. Pharmacogenetics. 1992;2:148–59.
146. Czaja AJ. Review article: the management of autoimmune hepatitis beyond consensus guidelines. Aliment Pharmacol Ther. 2013;38:343–64.
147. Wang KK, Czaja AJ, Beaver SJ, Go VL. Extrahepatic malignancy following long-term immunosuppressive therapy of severe hepatitis B surface antigen-negative chronic active hepatitis. Hepatology. 1989;10:39–43.
148. Ngu JH, Gearry RB, Frampton CM, Stedman CA. Mortality and the risk of malignancy in autoimmune liver diseases: a population-based study in Canterbury, New Zealand. Hepatology. 2012;55:522–9.
149. Rosenkrantz JG, Githens JH, Cox SM, Kellum DL. Azathioprine (Imuran) and pregnancy. Am J Obstet Gynecol. 1967;97:387–94.
150. de Boer NK, Jarbandhan SV, de Graaf P, Mulder CJ, van Elburg RM, van Bodegraven AA. Azathioprine use during pregnancy: unexpected intrauterine exposure to metabolites. Am J Gastroenterol. 2006;101:1390–2.
151. Cleary BJ, Kallen B. Early pregnancy azathioprine use and pregnancy outcomes. Birth Defects Res A Clin Mol Teratol. 2009;85:647–54.
152. Casanova MJ, Chaparro M, Domenech E, Barreiro-de Acosta M, Bermejo F, Iglesias E, et al. Safety of thiopurines and anti-TNF-alpha drugs during pregnancy in patients with inflammatory bowel disease. Am J Gastroenterol. 2013;108:433–40.
153. Akbari M, Shah S, Velayos FS, Mahadevan U, Cheifetz AS. Systematic review and meta-analysis on the effects of thiopurines on birth outcomes from female and male patients with inflammatory bowel disease. Inflamm Bowel Dis. 2013;19:15–22.
154. Aggarwal N, Chopra S, Suri V, Sikka P, Dhiman RK, Chawla Y. Pregnancy outcome in women with autoimmune hepatitis. Arch Gynecol Obstet. 2011;284:19–23.
155. Davis GL, Czaja AJ, Ludwig J. Development and prognosis of histologic cirrhosis in corticosteroid-treated hepatitis B surface antigen-negative chronic active hepatitis. Gastroenterology. 1984;87:1222–7.
156. Czaja AJ. Hepatic inflammation and progressive liver fibrosis in chronic liver disease. World J Gastroenterol. 2014;20:2515–32.

157. Montano-Loza AJ, Carpenter HA, Czaja AJ. Predictive factors for hepatocellular carcinoma in type 1 autoimmune hepatitis. Am J Gastroenterol. 2008;103:1944–51.
158. Yeoman AD, Al-Chalabi T, Karani JB, Quaglia A, Devlin J, Mieli-Vergani G, et al. Evaluation of risk factors in the development of hepatocellular carcinoma in autoimmune hepatitis: implications for follow-up and screening. Hepatology. 2008;48:863–70.
159. Wang KK, Czaja AJ. Hepatocellular carcinoma in corticosteroid-treated severe autoimmune chronic active hepatitis. Hepatology. 1988;8:1679–83.
160. Park SZ, Nagorney DM, Czaja AJ. Hepatocellular carcinoma in autoimmune hepatitis. Dig Dis Sci. 2000;45:1944–8.
161. Werner M, Almer S, Prytz H, Lindgren S, Wallerstedt S, Bjornsson E, et al. Hepatic and extrahepatic malignancies in autoimmune hepatitis. A long-term follow-up in 473 Swedish patients. J Hepatol. 2009;50:388–93.
162. Bruix J, Sherman M. Management of hepatocellular carcinoma: an update. Hepatology. 2011;53:1020–2.
163. Leung J, Dowling L, Obadan I, Davis J, Bonis PA, Kaplan MM, et al. Risk of non-melanoma skin cancer in autoimmune hepatitis. Dig Dis Sci. 2010;55:3218–23.
164. Jensen P, Hansen S, Moller B, Leivestad T, Pfeffer P, Geiran O, et al. Skin cancer in kidney and heart transplant recipients and different long-term immunosuppressive therapy regimens. J Am Acad Dermatol. 1999;40:177–86.
165. Long MD, Herfarth HH, Pipkin CA, Porter CQ, Sandler RS, Kappelman MD. Increased risk for non-melanoma skin cancer in patients with inflammatory bowel disease. Clin Gastroenterol Hepatol. 2010;8:268–74.
166. Long MD, Martin CF, Pipkin CA, Herfarth HH, Sandler RS, Kappelman MD. Risk of melanoma and nonmelanoma skin cancer among patients with inflammatory bowel disease. Gastroenterology. 2012;143:390–9.
167. Varoczy L, Gergely L, Zeher M, Szegedi G, Illes A. Malignant lymphoma-associated autoimmune diseases--a descriptive epidemiological study. Rheumatol Int. 2002;22:233–7.
168. Brown LM, Gridley G, Check D, Landgren O. Risk of multiple myeloma and monoclonal gammopathy of undetermined significance among white and black male United States veterans with prior autoimmune, infectious, inflammatory, and allergic disorders. Blood. 2008;111:3388–94.
169. Hegarty JE, Nouri Aria KT, Portmann B, Eddleston AL, Williams R. Relapse following treatment withdrawal in patients with autoimmune chronic active hepatitis. Hepatology. 1983;3:685–9.
170. Czaja AJ, Ammon HV, Summerskill WH. Clinical features and prognosis of severe chronic active liver disease (CALD) after corticosteroid-induced remission. Gastroenterology. 1980;78:518–23.
171. Czaja AJ. Late relapse of type 1 autoimmune hepatitis after corticosteroid withdrawal. Dig Dis Sci. 2010;55:1761–9.
172. Verma S, Gunuwan B, Mendler M, Govindrajan S, Redeker A. Factors predicting relapse and poor outcome in type I autoimmune hepatitis: role of cirrhosis development, patterns of transaminases during remission and plasma cell activity in the liver biopsy. Am J Gastroenterol. 2004;99:1510–6.
173. Czaja AJ, Carpenter HA. Histological features associated with relapse after corticosteroid withdrawal in type 1 autoimmune hepatitis. Liver Int. 2003;23:116–23.
174. Takahashi A, Ohira H, Abe K, Miyake Y, Abe M, Yamamoto K, et al. Rapid corticosteroid tapering: important risk factor for type 1 autoimmune hepatitis relapse in Japan. Hepatol Res. 2015;45:638. doi:10.1111/hepr.12397.
175. Montano-Loza AJ, Carpenter HA, Czaja AJ. Consequences of treatment withdrawal in type 1 autoimmune hepatitis. Liver Int. 2007;27:507–15.
176. Czaja AJ. Low-dose corticosteroid therapy after multiple relapses of severe HBsAg-negative chronic active hepatitis. Hepatology. 1990;11:1044–9.

177. Johnson PJ, McFarlane IG, Williams R. Azathioprine for long-term maintenance of remission in autoimmune hepatitis. N Engl J Med. 1995;333:958–63.
178. Selvarajah V, Montano-Loza AJ, Czaja AJ. Systematic review: managing suboptimal treatment responses in autoimmune hepatitis with conventional and nonstandard drugs. Aliment Pharmacol Ther. 2012;36:691–707.
179. Schalm SW, Ammon HV, Summerskill WH. Failure of customary treatment in chronic active liver disease: causes and management. Ann Clin Res. 1976;8:221–7.
180. Hess AD, Fischer AC, Horwitz LR, Laulis MK. Cyclosporine-induced autoimmunity: critical role of autoregulation in the prevention of major histocompatibility class II-dependent auto-aggression. Transplant Proc. 1993;25:2811–3.
181. Lohse AW, Weiler-Norman C, Burdelski M. De novo autoimmune hepatitis after liver transplantation. Hepatol Res. 2007;37 Suppl 3:S462.
182. Serkova NJ, Christians U, Benet LZ. Biochemical mechanisms of cyclosporine neurotoxicity. Mol Interv. 2004;4:97–107.
183. Toledo Perdomo K, Navarro Cabello MD, Perez Saez MJ, Ramos Perez MJ, Aguera Morales ML, Aljama GP. Reversible acute encephalopathy with mutism, induced by calcineurin inhibitors after renal transplantation. J Nephrol. 2012;25:839. doi:10.5301/jn.5000080.
184. Czaja AJ. Drug choices in autoimmune hepatitis: Part B - nonsteroids. Expert Rev Gastroenterol Hepatol. 2012;6:617–35.
185. Czaja AJ. Nonstandard drugs and feasible new interventions for autoimmune hepatitis. Part-I. Inflamm Allergy Drug Targets. 2012;11:337–50.
186. Czaja AJ. Autoimmune hepatitis: focusing on treatments other than steroids. Can J Gastroenterol. 2012;26:615–20.
187. Mistilis SP, Vickers CR, Darroch MH, McCarthy SW. Cyclosporin, a new treatment for autoimmune chronic active hepatitis. Med J Aust. 1985;143:463–5.
188. Malekzadeh R, Nasseri-Moghaddam S, Kaviani MJ, Taheri H, Kamalian N, Sotoudeh M. Cyclosporin A is a promising alternative to corticosteroids in autoimmune hepatitis. Dig Dis Sci. 2001;46:1321–7.
189. Van Thiel DH, Wright H, Carroll P, Abu-Elmagd K, Rodriguez-Rilo H, McMichael J, et al. Tacrolimus: a potential new treatment for autoimmune chronic active hepatitis: results of an open-label preliminary trial. Am J Gastroenterol. 1995;90:771–6.
190. Aqel BA, Machicao V, Rosser B, Satyanarayana R, Harnois DM, Dickson RC. Efficacy of tacrolimus in the treatment of steroid refractory autoimmune hepatitis. J Clin Gastroenterol. 2004;38:805–9.
191. Larsen FS, Vainer B, Eefsen M, Bjerring PN, Adel Hansen B. Low-dose tacrolimus ameliorates liver inflammation and fibrosis in steroid refractory autoimmune hepatitis. World J Gastroenterol. 2007;13:3232–6.
192. Devlin SM, Swain MG, Urbanski SJ, Burak KW. Mycophenolate mofetil for the treatment of autoimmune hepatitis in patients refractory to standard therapy. Can J Gastroenterol. 2004;18:321–6.
193. Inductivo-Yu I, Adams A, Gish RG, Wakil A, Bzowej NH, Frederick RT, et al. Mycophenolate mofetil in autoimmune hepatitis patients not responsive or intolerant to standard immunosuppressive therapy. Clin Gastroenterol Hepatol. 2007;5:799–802.
194. Hennes EM, Oo YH, Schramm C, Denzer U, Buggisch P, Wiegard C, et al. Mycophenolate mofetil as second line therapy in autoimmune hepatitis? Am J Gastroenterol. 2008;103:3063–70.
195. Hlivko JT, Shiffman ML, Stravitz RT, Luketic VA, Sanyal AJ, Fuchs M, et al. A single center review of the use of mycophenolate mofetil in the treatment of autoimmune hepatitis. Clin Gastroenterol Hepatol. 2008;6:1036–40.
196. Sharzehi K, Huang MA, Schreibman IR, Brown KA. Mycophenolate mofetil for the treatment of autoimmune hepatitis in patients refractory or intolerant to conventional therapy. Can J Gastroenterol. 2010;24:588–92.

197. Baven-Pronk AM, Coenraad MJ, van Buuren HR, de Man RA, van Erpecum KJ, Lamers MM, et al. The role of mycophenolate mofetil in the management of autoimmune hepatitis and overlap syndromes. Aliment Pharmacol Ther. 2011;34:335–43.
198. Matsui K, Shibagaki Y, Sasaki H, Chikaraishi T, Yasuda T, Kimura K. Mycophenolate mofetil-induced agranulocytosis in a renal transplant recipient. Clin Exp Nephrol. 2010;14:637–40.
199. von Vietinghoff S, Ouyang H, Ley K. Mycophenolic acid suppresses granulopoiesis by inhibition of interleukin-17 production. Kidney Int. 2010;78:79–88.
200. Lin AE, Singh KE, Strauss A, Nguyen S, Rawson K, Kimonis VE. An additional patient with mycophenolate mofetil embryopathy: cardiac and facial analyses. Am J Med Genet A. 2011;155A:748–56.
201. Seela S, Sheela H, Boyer JL. Autoimmune hepatitis type 1: safety and efficacy of prolonged medical therapy. Liver Int. 2005;25:734–9.
202. Shin BC, Chung JH, Kim HL. Sirolimus: a switch option for mycophenolate mofetil-induced leukopenia in renal transplant recipients. Transplant Proc. 2013;45:2968–9.
203. Tripathi D, Neuberger J. Autoimmune hepatitis and liver transplantation: indications, results, and management of recurrent disease. Semin Liver Dis. 2009;29:286–96.
204. Neuberger J. Transplantation for autoimmune hepatitis. Semin Liver Dis. 2002;22:379–86.
205. Nunez-Martinez O, De la Cruz G, Salcedo M, Molina J, De Diego A, Ripoll C, et al. Liver transplantation for autoimmune hepatitis: fulminant versus chronic hepatitis presentation. Transplant Proc. 2003;35:1857–8.
206. Martin SR, Alvarez F, Anand R, Song C, Yin W. Outcomes in children who underwent transplantation for autoimmune hepatitis. Liver Transpl. 2011;17:393–401.
207. Campsen J, Zimmerman MA, Trotter JF, Wachs M, Bak T, Steinberg T, et al. Liver transplantation for autoimmune hepatitis and the success of aggressive corticosteroid withdrawal. Liver Transpl. 2008;14:1281–6.
208. Prados E, Cuervas-Mons V, de la Mata M, Fraga E, Rimola A, Prieto M, et al. Outcome of autoimmune hepatitis after liver transplantation. Transplantation. 1998;66:1645–50.
209. Montano-Loza AJ, Mason AL, Ma M, Bastiampillai RJ, Bain VG, Tandon P. Risk factors for recurrence of autoimmune hepatitis after liver transplantation. Liver Transpl. 2009;15:1254–61.
210. Birnbaum AH, Benkov KJ, Pittman NS, McFarlane-Ferreira Y, Rosh JR, LeLeiko NS. Recurrence of autoimmune hepatitis in children after liver transplantation. J Pediatr Gastroenterol Nutr. 1997;25:20–5.
211. Ratziu V, Samuel D, Sebagh M, Farges O, Saliba F, Ichai P, et al. Long-term follow-up after liver transplantation for autoimmune hepatitis: evidence of recurrence of primary disease. J Hepatol. 1999;30:131–41.
212. Yusoff IF, House AC, De Boer WB, Ferguson J, Garas G, Heath D, et al. Disease recurrence after liver transplantation in Western Australia. J Gastroenterol Hepatol. 2002;17:203–7.

Chapter 16
Autoimmune Liver Diseases: Primary Biliary Cholangitis

Ahmad H. Ali, Elizabeth J. Carey, and Keith D. Lindor

Patient Questions and Answers

1. What does Primary Biliary Cholangitis do to me?

   Primary biliary Cholangitis (or PBC for short) is a chronic, or long-lasting, disease that causes the small bile ducts in the liver to become inflamed and damaged and ultimately disappear. This damage to the liver tissue can lead to cirrhosis, a condition in which the liver slowly deteriorates and is unable to function normally. In cirrhosis, scar tissue replaces healthy liver tissue, partially blocking the flow of blood through the liver. PBC can cause fatigue (feeling tired), itching of the skin, and dry eyes and mouth. Some patients with PBC have jaundice, a condition that causes yellowish discoloration of the skin and the whites of the eye. Some patients with PBC also have hypothyroidism (a condition in which the thyroid gland releases low amounts of the thyroid hormone), hyperthyroidism (a condition in which the thyroid gland releases excessive amounts of the thyroid hormone), osteopenia (weak bones, people with this condition are more likely to develop bone fractures), hyperlipidemia (high blood cholesterol), Raynaud's disease (a painful condition in which the fingers turn blue in color), and vitamin deficiency (vitamins A, D, E, and K).

2. Is it treatable?

   Treatment for PBC depends on how early a health care provider diagnoses the disease and whether complications are present. In the early stages of PBC,

A.H. Ali, M.B.B.S. • E.J. Carey, M.D.
Division of Gastroenterology and Hepatology, Mayo Clinic, Phoenix, AZ, USA

K.D. Lindor, M.D. (✉)
Division of Gastroenterology and Hepatology, Mayo Clinic, Phoenix, AZ, USA

College of Health Solutions, Arizona State University,
550 North 3rd Street, Phoenix, AZ 85004, USA
e-mail: keith.lindor@asu.edu

© Springer International Publishing Switzerland 2017
K. Saeian, R. Shaker (eds.), *Liver Disorders*,
DOI 10.1007/978-3-319-30103-7_16

treatment can slow the progression of liver damage to cirrhosis. In the early stages of cirrhosis, the goals of treatment are to slow the progression of tissue scarring in the liver and prevent complications. As cirrhosis progresses, a person may need additional treatments and hospitalization to manage complications.

Ursodeoxycholic acid (Ursodiol) is the only therapy approved by the FDA for PBC. It is taken orally and the dose is calculated based on the person's weight. Ursodiol is a nontoxic bile acid. It replaces the bile acids that are toxic to the liver. Ursodiol provides the most benefit in patients with early stages of PBC, as it reduces the likelihood of needing a liver transplant and improves the survival. However, treatment with ursodiol in the late stages of PBC can still slow the progression of the disease. Although ursodiol decreases the likelihood of needing a liver transplant, it does not cure the disease.

3. Are there other problems I can expect?

Yes, there are complications that you should expect if you have PBC. Most complications of PBC occur in the final stages of the disease, when PBC progresses to cirrhosis of the liver.

(a) Portal hypertension

Portal hypertension develops when the scar tissue in the liver blocks the normal blood flow to the liver. When this happens, you may develop one or more of the following symptoms: edema (lower limb swelling due to fluid accumulation in the lower limbs), ascites (fluid accumulation inside the abdominal cavity), and splenomegaly (enlargement of the spleen). Spontaneous bacterial peritonitis is a rare but serious complication that requires immediate attention.

(b) Varices

Portal hypertension may cause enlargement of the blood vessels in the esophagus, stomach, or both. These vessels can burst, resulting in hemorrhage, requiring immediate medical attention.

(c) Hepatic encephalopathy

Cirrhosis of the liver can lead to symptoms of brain dysfunction such memory and concentration problems, personality problems, sleep disturbance, and in extreme cases, coma.

(d) Metabolic bone disease

PBC can lead to weakening of the bones, a condition called osteopenia. When the bones become weaker, the condition is referred to as osteoporosis. Patients with this condition are more likely to develop bone fractures.

(e) Hepatocellular carcinoma

Hepatocellular carcinoma is a type of liver cancer that occurs mainly in cirrhotic patients. It has a high mortality and treatment options are very limited. For these reasons, it is recommended for patients with cirrhosis to be screened for hepatocellular carcinoma every 6–12 months. Detecting this cancer in an early stage increases the chances of survival.

Summary

Primary biliary cholangitis (PBC) is a chronic cholestatic liver disease characterized by destruction of small intra-hepatic bile ducts, leading to fibrosis and eventually liver cirrhosis and its consequent complications. The serological hallmark of PBC is the antimitochondrial antibody (AMA), a highly disease-specific antibody found in ~95 % of cases of PBC. Since the introduction of ursodeoxycholic acid (UDCA), the natural history of PBC has changed significantly. Several randomized placebo-controlled studies have shown that UDCA improves the transplant-free survival in PBC patients. Patients with early stages of PBC seem to benefit the most from UDCA therapy, as they live just as long as the health population. UDCA therapy should be continued indefinitely. In this chapter, we review the natural history of PBC before and after the introduction of UDCA, diagnosis, clinical manifestations, etiology, epidemiology, and complications of PBC. We also review the management of PBC and its related symptoms associated conditions, and special cases related to PBC, focusing on AMA-negative PBC and diagnosis and management of the PBC-Autoimmune hepatitis overlap syndrome.

Introduction

Primary Biliary Cholangitis (PBC) is a chronic progressive disease of the liver characterized by destruction of the small intra-hepatic bile ducts and periportal inflammation and fibrosis, leading ultimately to cirrhosis and its consequent complications such as liver failure and portal hypertension [1]. It was first described in 1851 by Addison, but it was not until 1949 that Ahren introduced the term "primary biliary cirrhosis" [2] and the name was only recently changed to primary biliary cholangitis to better reflect the disease in which cirrhosis is not universally present. The serological hallmark of PBC is the antimitochondrial antibody (AMA) [3, 4]; an autoimmune antibody that targets a family of mitochondrial enzymes named the 2-oxo-acid dehydrogenase complexes [5–7]. AMA is present in ~95 % of PBC patients [8, 9], and is rarely detected in healthy individuals [10]. The diagnosis of PBC is established in the setting of a cholestatic liver profile picture, exclusion of all other causes of cholestasis, and presence of AMA [11]. In some, particularly in patients who are AMA-negative, liver biopsy might be needed to establish a diagnosis of PBC. PBC affects mainly middle-aged women, with a female-to-male ratio of 10:1 [1]. Ursodeoxycholic acid (UDCA) is the only medical therapy approved by the Food and Drug Administration (FDA) for treatment of PBC. About 40 % of PBC patients do not respond adequately to UDCA [12]. Newer therapies which have shown promising preliminary results are being investigated in PBC patients with an inadequate response to UDCA. In this chapter we review the natural history, clinical presentation, diagnosis, etiology, and clinical outcomes of PBC. We also review current clinical trials of new therapies in PBC.

Natural History

Patterns of Clinical Disease and Natural History in the Pre-UDCA Era

The presentation of PBC varies from asymptomatic disease with only biochemical evidence of PBC, to symptomatic PBC or decompensated cirrhosis. PBC is usually asymptomatic at the time of diagnosis due to the widespread use of screening liver chemistries and AMA. The prevalence of asymptomatic PBC has increased from as low as 20 % in early series [13–15] to as high as 61 % in the recently published literature [16]. Mahl et al. [17] reported the clinical outcomes of 247 PBC patients, of whom 85.8 % were symptomatic at presentation. The median duration of follow-up from diagnosis was 6.4 years for the group with symptoms (range: 0.04–24.2 years) and 12.2 years for the group without symptoms at diagnosis (range: 1.1–19.2 years). The median survival of PBC patients in this study from the time of diagnosis was twice as long for patients who presented without symptoms compared to symptomatic patients (16 years versus 7.5 years) [17]. In addition, the 10-year survival was significantly worse in the symptomatic group compared to the patients who had no symptoms at the time of diagnosis (78 % versus 38 %) [17]. Furthermore, of the 36 patients who were asymptomatic at presentation, 64 % developed symptoms over a median time interval of 5.3 years [17]. Patients who remained asymptomatic had a considerably longer life span when compared to patients who developed symptoms (median survival 16.7 years versus 12.6 years). The overall survival of asymptomatic patients was diminished compared to a matched control population [17]. Moreover, the 10-year survival of PBC patients who developed symptoms during the follow-up period was significantly worse than that of the patients who remained symptomatic (90 % versus 70 %) [17]. In another study, Springer et al. [18] examined the natural history of 91 patients referred to the Toronto Hospital between 1983 and 1994 with abnormal liver biochemistries and liver biopsy-compatible, AMA-positive PBC. Median follow-up was 61.2 months. During this period, 36.2 % developed PBC symptoms (pruritus in 24.1 %, and jaundice in 7.7 %) [18]. Of the 91 patients, 9.9 % reached an end-point; 7.7 % underwent liver transplantation, and 2.2 % died from liver failure [18]. The median time interval to develop symptoms from presentation was 50.6 months (range: 3.5–156.8 months) [18]. The 10-year survival (Fig. 16.1) was significantly lower in the entire PBC group (80 %) when compared to a matched population (92 %) [18]. PBC patients who remained asymptomatic had a survival equal to that of the general population (Fig. 16.2) [18]. Moreover, PBC patients who became symptomatic had a 10-year survival significantly shorter than the general population (73 % versus 94 %, Fig. 16.2) [18]. These studies indicate that PBC is a progressive disease in the majority of patients, PBC patients (regardless of symptoms) have a shorter life span than the general population, a significant proportion of asymptomatic PBC patients will develop symptoms, and PBC patients who have symptoms at diagnosis have a poorer prognosis than patients who are asymptomatic at presentation. In addition, these studies also indicate that PBC patients who remain symptom-free have an excellent prognosis.

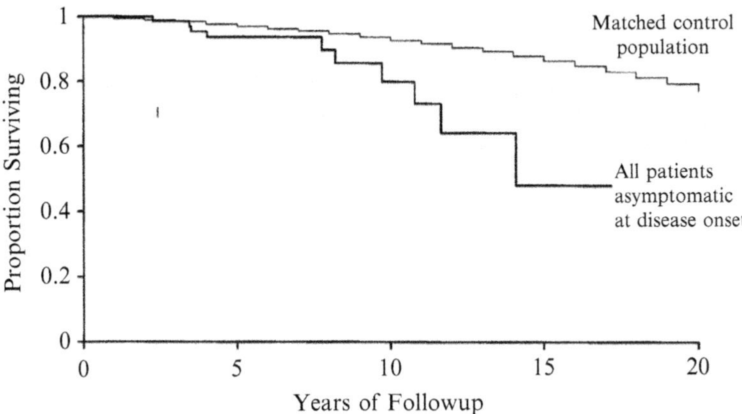

Fig. 16.1 Asymptomatic primary biliary cirrhosis: a study of its natural history and prognosis. Spring J, Cauch-Dudek K, O'Rourke K, et al. Am J Gastro. 1999; 94(1): 47–53

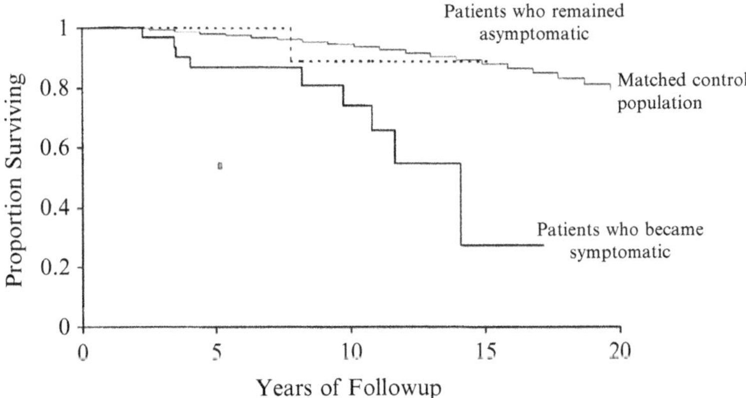

Fig. 16.2 Asymptomatic primary biliary cirrhosis: a study of its natural history and prognosis. Spring J, Cauch-Dudek K, O'Rourke K, et al. Am J Gastro. 1999; 94(1): 47–53

Patients with symptomatic PBC show a more rapid progression to end-stage liver disease and have a worse prognosis than that observed in the asymptomatic patients [16, 18–20]. In the late phase of the disease, serum bilirubin levels increase [21] and clinical features of liver failure such as portal hypertension and hepatic encephalopathy develop [20]. The mean survival times in symptomatic patients vary between 6 and 10 years [22, 23]. In a 28-year follow-up study of a large cohort that included 770 PBC patients [19], the percentage of patients who developed liver failure was 15.4 % and 26.4 % after 5 years and 10 years of diagnosis, respectively [19]. Of all the variables, serum bilirubin is the best predictor of survival in PBC patients [21, 24–28]. Advanced age, male gender, advanced histological stage, elevated serum ALP, low serum albumin, development of esophageal varices, and prolonged prothrombin time have also been associated with poor prognosis in patients with PBC [20].

In some patients, presence of AMA may be the only evidence of PBC. In an early report [29], patients incidentally discovered to have positive AMA (titers ≥ 1:40) but no symptoms of liver disease and normal hepatic biochemistries were followed for over 18 years. Liver biopsies were compatible with or diagnostic of PBC in 83 % of patients at baseline [29]. During the follow-up period, 76 % of patients developed PBC symptoms, and 83 % had persistently elevated serum alkaline phosphatase (ALP) levels [30]. Repeat liver biopsies in 10 patients showed that two patients progressed histologically by one stage, and two other patients progressed by two stages [30]. None of the patients during the follow-up period died from liver disease [30]. This study suggests that patients who test positive for AMA but have no liver-related symptoms and normal hepatic biochemistries might eventually develop symptomatic but slowly progressive PBC. These findings, however, need to be confirmed in a larger cohort of patients.

Natural History in the UDCA Era

The natural history of PBC has significantly changed since the introduction of UDCA. Responders to UDCA demonstrate survival comparable to age- and sex-matched healthy subjects [31]. Studies have shown that UDCA delays histological progression [32], delays development of esophageal varices [33], and improves the transplant-free survival of PBC patients [34–42]. Data compiled from three clinical trials in which PBC patients were randomly assigned to receive either UDCA or placebo for up to 4 years have shown that the survival free of liver transplantation was significantly improved in the UDCA-treated arm compared to the controls (Fig. 16.3) [43]. The effect of UDCA on the development of esophageal varices has been evaluated in a prospective clinical trial of 180 patients who received either UDCA or placebo for 4 years [33]. At baseline, 22.8 % had varices. After 4 years of treatment, the risk of developing varices in the UDCA- versus placebo-treated patients was 16 % versus 58 %, respectively [33].

Survival

A Markov model, using death, liver transplantation, and histological stage progression as the main clinical end points, was used to assess the survival of 262 PBC patients (Fig. 16.4) [44]. In this prospective follow-up study, patients received UDCA at a dose of 13–15 mg/kg daily for a mean of 8 years (range: 1–22 years). The overall 10- and 20-year survival rate was substantially better than that predicted by the model [44]. The predicted survival rate was 92 % at 10 years and 82 % at 20 years [44]. The predicted survival rate without liver

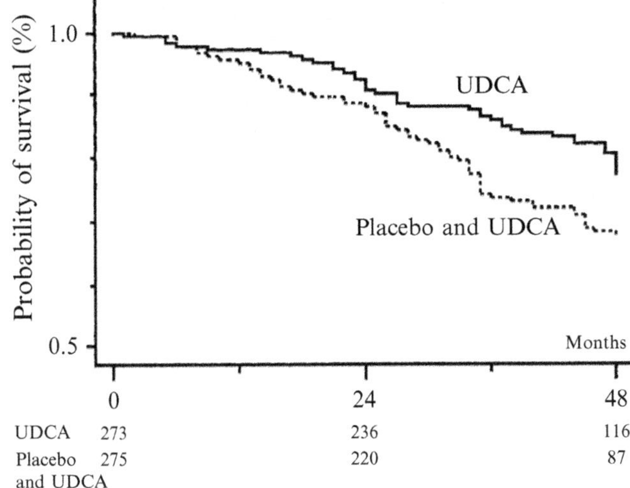

Fig. 16.3 Combined analysis of randomized controlled trials of ursodeoxycholic acid in primary biliary cirrhosis. Poupon RE, Lindor KD, Cauch-Dudek C, et al. Gastroenterology. 1997; 113: 884–890

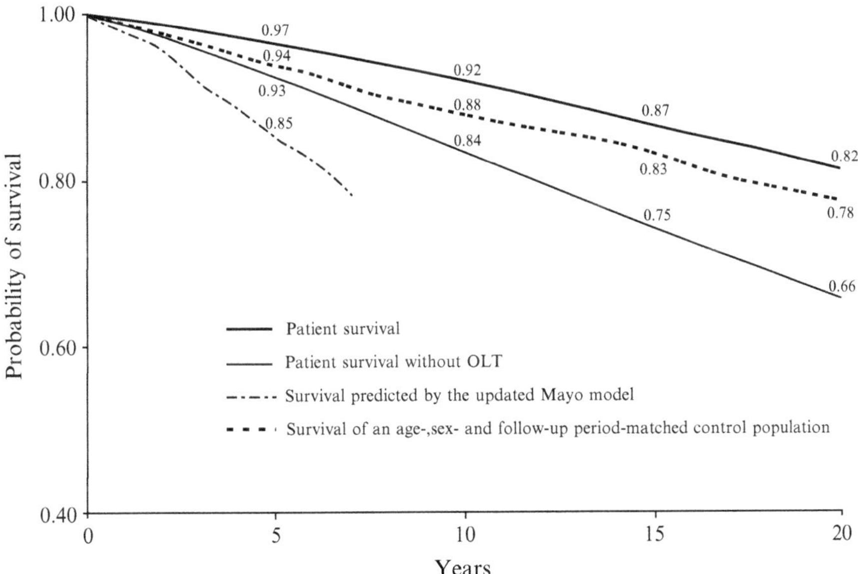

Fig. 16.4 The effect of urosdeoxycholic acid therapy on the natural course of primary biliary cirrhosis. Corpechot C, Carrat F, Bahr A, et al. Gastroenterology. 2005; 128(2): 297–303

transplantation was 84 % at 10 years and 66 % at 20 years [44]. The survival predicted by the updated Mayo model was far poorer than the survival predicted on UDCA therapy [44]. In patients with early histological-stage PBC, the predicted survival rate was 97 % at 10 years and 88 % at 20 years. In the same group, the predicted survival without liver transplantation was 93 % at 10 years and 77 % at 20 years, which was similar to that of a matched control population [44]. However, patients with late histological stage PBC had worse 10- and 20-year survival rate without liver transplantation compared to that of a matched control group (68 % and 48 % versus 82 % and 71 %, respectively) [44].

Models using time-fixed Cox proportional hazards have been developed to assess the survival in PBC patients. The Mayo PBC risk score [26] is the most widely used model to assess the survival in PBC patients. This model helps determine treatment success in clinical trials of PBC and also guides timing for liver transplantation. Recently, serum ALP and bilirubin have been shown to be excellent predictors of long-term outcomes (death or liver transplantation) in PBC [45]. These biochemical markers are useful surrogate endpoints when designing clinical trials assessing newer therapies in PBC [45].

Diagnosis of PBC

Liver Biochemical Tests

Elevated serum ALP is the most frequent serum biochemical abnormality detected in patients with PBC [15, 16, 19, 22, 46–48]. Other biochemical abnormalities in PBC patients are mildly elevated levels of liver transaminases and elevated immunoglobulin M (IgM) levels [11]. Elevated serum bilirubin is rarely seen in early PBC; levels tend to increase as the clinical and histological stage of the disease progress [21]. In addition to the liver-related serum biochemistries, PBC patients frequently have elevated serum lipids, namely serum cholesterol levels [49].

Autoantibodies

The serological hallmark of PBC is the presence of AMA; a highly disease-specific autoantibody found in nearly 95 % of cases of PBC [8, 9]. An AMA titer of $\geq 1{:}40$ is indicative of PBC. This autoantibody targets members of a family of mitochondrial enzymes, the 2-oxo-acid dehydrogenase complexes, and include pyruvate dehydrogenase complex (PDC-E2), branched chain 2-oxo-acid dehydrogenase complex (BCOADC-E2), and 2-oxo-glutaric acid dehydrogenase complex (OADC-E2) [5–7]. More specifically, the lipoylated domains of the E2 and E3 binding protein (E3BP) components of the PDC-E2 and the E2 components of the OADC-E2 and

BCOADC-E2 are the epitopes recognized by the AMAs [5, 6]. In HEp-2 cell mono-layers, AMAs typically exhibit cytoplasmic "string of pearls" fluorescence staining with a coarse, filamentous, granular, and speckled pattern [50]. The presence of AMA in the sera of patients with PBC was first described in 1965 [4], and in 1987, the AMA antigens were cloned and identified [7, 51, 52]. Enzyme-linked immuno-sorbent assay (ELISA) is the most widely used method of detection of AMA in commercial laboratories [12]. The magnitude of antibody level correlates poorly with the stage of PBC [11], and may persist after liver transplantation [53]. AMAs are rarely found in healthy individuals. In an Italian study involving 1530 individu-als, 0.5 % tested positive for AMA [10].

In addition to AMA, antinuclear antibodies (ANAs) may also be detected in patients with PBC [54]. Some ANAs have been found to be of diagnostic and prognostic value. Anti-Sp100 antibodies (present in 17–41 % of PBC cases) [55–61], anti-Sp140 antibod-ies (present in 11–15 % of PBC cases) [62], and antinucleoporin p62 antibodies (present in 13–32 % of PBC cases) [63, 64] are thought to be specific for PBC, therefore, they can be useful when the diagnosis of PBC is uncertain. In a Japanese study that included 276 PBC patients [65], the presence of anti-gp210 antibodies was identified as an important risk factor for progression to liver failure and need for transplantation [65], whereas the presence of anti-centromere antibodies was identified as an important risk factor for development of esophageal varices and hepatocellular carcinoma [65]. Other ANAs found in the sera of PBC patients are the anti-promyelocytic leukemia proteins antibod-ies [66], anti-SUMO antibodies [67], and anti-lamin B receptor antibodies [68–70]. The clinical significance of the latter ANAs is yet to be determined.

Histology

PBC is characterized by chronic, nonsuppurative cholangitis that mainly affects the interlobular and septal bile ducts [71]. The term "florid duct lesion" is used to describe the intense inflammatory lesions around the bile ducts [72–74]. The intense inflammatory infiltrate consists of lymphocytes, plasma cells, macrophages, poly-morphonuclear cells, and in some cases, epithelioid granulomas [75–79]. Histological staging systems in PBC have been developed by Rubin, Popper, and Schaffner [80], Scheuer [81], and Ludwig [71]. Of all the staging systems available, Ludwig's stag-ing system is the most widely used, in which stage I is characterized by inflammation limited to the portal space, stage II is characterized by inflammation involving the periportal areas as well, stage III is characterized by septal fibrosis or inflammatory bridging, and stage IV represents cirrhosis. Nodular regenerative hyperplasia (NRH) is a known complication in PBC [82–86] and should be differentiated from cirrhosis. Liver biopsy is not routinely used in clinical practice to diagnose PBC, as ~95 % of cases of PBC are AMA-positive. Biopsy may be indicated when the suspicion for PBC is high in the absence of AMA [11]. Liver biopsy may also be indicated in patients in whom the suspicion for PBC-Autoimmune hepatitis (AIH) overlap syn-drome is high [11]. In these circumstances, patients may have histological features of AIH such as periportal or periseptal lymphocytic piecemeal necrosis [87].

Role of Imaging

Imaging is not necessary to establish the diagnosis of PBC, but may be performed at the time of presentation to exclude biliary obstruction. Ultrasound or magnetic resonance cholangiography (MRC) are typically performed. In a study of 117 PBC patients, all extra-hepatic ducts were normal on cholangiograms [47]. The intra-hepatic ducts, however, were abnormal in 9% of patients, revealing mild tapering, narrowing, and irregularity [47]. Transient elastography (TE), a simple and noninvasive procedure, has been shown to be useful for assessing liver fibrosis in PBC when compared with other surrogate markers of liver fibrosis [88]. Larger and longer-term studies are needed to validate these findings.

Diagnostic Approach

The diagnosis of PBC can be made when two of the three following criteria are met (the American Association for the Study of Liver Disease (AASLD) Guidelines) [11]:

(a) Biochemical evidence of cholestasis, mainly elevated serum ALP
(b) Presence of AMA
(c) Histopathological evidence of PBC, when liver biopsy is performed.

Clinical Manifestations of PBC

Symptoms

Fatigue

Fatigue is the most common symptom in PBC, affecting nearly 80% of individuals [89]. Severe fatigue can have a severe negative impact and has been associated with an increased mortality, depression, and poor quality of life [90–97]. Fatigue in PBC does not correlate with disease activity and seems not to respond to therapies, including UDCA [96]. The etiology of fatigue in PBC is poorly understood. It is, however, thought that chronic cholestasis that occurs in PBC causes degenerative changes in areas in the brain that regulate autonomic functions, ultimately resulting in impaired delivery of oxygen to the peripheral tissue which in turn leads to expression of fatigue and its associated cognitive impairment through secondary dysfunction of peripheral muscles [96, 98]. Evidence in favor of an organic central nervous system process in PBC comes from neurophysiological studies which suggest organic brain changes in PBC. Newton et al. [99] found that 53% of PBC patients had concentration and memory problems, and that they repetitively failed neuropsychiatric testing. These findings progressed over a 2-year follow-up period [99]. Patients with symptomatic PBC have worse outcomes when compared to patients with asymptomatic PBC [100]. Current therapies seem to be ineffective in the treatment of fatigue in PBC, including liver transplantation, as a significant proportion of patients with PBC continue to suffer severe fatigue even after liver transplantation [101]. This highlights the need to understand the underlying mechanism(s) of fatigue in PBC, as it will help develop therapies for this debilitating symptom.

Pruritus

Pruritus is a less frequent, but more specific, symptom than fatigue in patients with PBC [102, 103]. It affects 20–70 % of PBC patients [102–106]. The pruritus of cholestasis tends to be generalized. It leads to scratching, sometimes violent, resulting in excoriations and prurigo nodularis [107]. This type of pruritus can lead to sleep deprivation, depression, and in some patients, to suicidal ideations [107]. A survey was conducted in 239 PBC patients to understand how patients with cholestatic pruritus perceive pruritus [108]. Of these, 69 % reported itching. Seventeen percent reported that itch was "relentless" or so severe that it lead to wanting to "tear the skin off", and 3.6 % of patients reported that they itched until they bled [108]. Seventy-four percent of the 162 respondents who addressed the question reported that itch affected sleep, 65 % that the itch was worst at night, and 11 % reported that nothing provided relief [108]. The etiology of pruritus in cholestasis is unknown. Accumulation of bile acids in tissues [109, 110], excess of histamine in patients with liver disease and pruritus [111], and excess of substance P [112, 113] (an excitatory neurotransmitter) have been proposed as mechanisms by which pruritus is triggered in patients with liver disease. More recently, lysophosphatidic acid (LPA) and autotaxin, the serum enzyme converting lysophosphatidylcholine into LPA, have been found in higher concentrations in the sera of patients with cholestatic disorders, including PBC, compared to control subjects, suggesting that LPA and autotaxin play a role in the pathogenesis of cholestatic pruritus [114]. The natural history of pruritus in PBC has been inadequately studied and most data is derived from clinical trials of therapies in PBC. Talwalkar et al. [103] examined the natural course of pruritus in PBC patients enrolled in a multicenter, randomized, placebo-controlled clinical trial of UDCA in PBC. They reported that the overall prevalence of pruritus in the placebo group did not differ between study entry and follow-up at 36 months (56 % versus 49 %) [103]. In addition, 30 % of patients in the UDCA group reported symptom improvement compared to 24 % of the placebo-treated patients after 1 year of therapy [103]. Conversely, only 7.9 % of patients in the UDCA group reported development of pruritus compared to 14.5 % patients in the placebo group after 1 year of therapy [103]. Similar to fatigue, pruritus can have a negative impact on the patients' quality of lives [107].

Other Conditions and Symptoms Associated with PBC

A number of conditions are associated with PBC [115]. These include Hashimoto's thyroiditis (12.5 %), Grave's disease (1.9 %), Raynaud's disease (18 %), Sjogren's syndrome (34.3 %), systemic lupus erythematosus (2.2 %), scleroderma/CREST (6.1 %), rheumatoid arthritis (6.1 %), cutaneous autoimmune diseases (5 %), celiac disease (1.4 %), and vasculitis (2.2 %) [115]. Female patients are more likely to have PBC in association with these conditions than male patients [115]. The presence of these conditions does not reduce the survival in PBC patients [115].

Physical Examination

The physical examination in patients with PBC is usually normal. Signs of hyperlipidemia such as xanthomas and xanthelasmas can be found. Ascites, splenomegaly, hepatomegaly, and spider angiomata are frequently found when PBC is complicated by portal hypertension [11, 116]. Jaundice and hepatic encephalopathy are signs of advanced disease [20].

Portal Hypertension

Portal hypertension is a feared complication of PBC. The development and burden of esophageal varices in PBC has been prospectively examined in 265 patients with PBC (69 % had stage III and IV PBC at baseline) enrolled in a clinical trial [117]. Patients were followed for a median of 5.6 years. Esophageal varices developed in 31 % of patients, 48 % of whom experienced ≥1 episodes of variceal bleeding. After the development of varices, the 3-year survival was 59 %, and after the initial variceal bleeding episode, the 3-year survival was 46 % [117]. Unlike other liver diseases, patients with PBC can develop portal hypertension and gastroesophageal varices in the pre-cirrhotic stages of PBC [84, 86]. In a study of 325 patients with PBC enrolled in two clinical trials, 127 patients were identified as early-stage (stage I and II) PBC at baseline; 6 % of those with early-stage PBC had gastroesophageal varices at baseline [118]. A number of noninvasive tools using simple biochemical markers have been developed to assist clinicians in identifying PBC patients whom might benefit from screening upper endoscopy for gastroesophageal varices. Patanwala et al. [119] developed the Newcastle Varices in PBC (NVP) score that uses the following parameters: serum ALP, serum albumin, and platelet count. This noninvasive tool has been developed in a large well-characterized cohort of PBC and has been validated internally and externally with excellent performance (93 % sensitivity, 93 % negative predictive value, and a discriminating value "AUROC" of 0.86).

Bone Disease

Osteoporosis is a frequent complication of PBC [120]. Numerous studies have reported a strong association between low bone mass and PBC [121–126]. The finding of lower levels of osteocalcin (a marker of bone formation) and higher levels of urinary hydroxyproline (a marker of bone resorption) among PBC patients than in controls lends support to this phenomenon [127]. Studies have reported a prevalence of 20–35 % of osteoporosis among the PBC population [121, 127, 128]. Patients with PBC have a 30-fold increased risk of osteoporosis when compared to the normal population, and patients with advanced-stage PBC have a 5.4-fold increased risk of developing osteoporosis compared to their counterparts with early-stage PBC [128]. Reports evaluating the risk factors for developing osteoporosis in PBC have identified increasing age, low body mass index, previous fractures, increasing serum bilirubin, severity of cholestasis, and advanced histological stage of PBC as independent risk factors for osteoporosis in PBC [127, 128]. The rate of bone loss during the early histological course of PBC is slower than that in patients with advanced histological-stage PBC [128]. As the histological course in patients with early PBC progresses, the rate of bone loss equals that in patients with advanced histological-stage PBC [128]. Typically, PBC patients suffer from osteoporosis of the lumbar spine and hip area, and the rate of bone loss in the lumbar spine correlates with that in the hip bone [128].

Hyperlipidemia

Hyperlipidemia is commonly associated with PBC, occurring in 75 95 % of cases [129]. Typically, patients with PBC have markedly elevated total cholesterol (up to 1775 mg/dL has been reported [130]), elevated high-density lipoprotein (HDL), and elevated low-density lipoprotein (LDL) [130]. Patients with advanced PBC tend to have higher LDL levels when compared to patients with early PBC [130]. The mechanisms of hyperlipidemia in PBC are different than those in other conditions. In vitro studies suggest that biliary cholestasis, lipid reflux from the biliary ducts into the bloodstream, and an increased cholesterol synthesis lead to the hyperlipidemia seen in cholestatic disorders [131–136]. Hyperlipidemia associated with PBC does not place PBC patients at increased risk for atherosclerotic-related deaths. In one study, the reported percentage of atherosclerosis-related deaths in a cohort of 312 patients with PBC whom were followed for 7.4 years was only 2.2 % [130]. Importantly, the incidence of atherosclerosis death among the PBC patients was not different when compared with a matched U.S. control population [130].

Vitamin Deficiency

PBC patients may have decreased bile acid secretion into the intestines, leading to an increased risk for lipid malabsorption. Clinically important deficiencies of fat-soluble vitamins A, D, E, and K are uncommon in PBC patients [137–141]. Fat-soluble vitamins may be decreased in patients with advanced PBC, leading to night blindness, neuropathy, and prolonged prothrombin time [11, 141].

Etiology of PBC

The etiology of PBC is poorly understood. Findings from several studies suggest a role for genetics and environmental factors in the pathogenesis of PBC. Family studies revealed that the prevalence of PBC is ~0.72 % and 1.2 % in first-degree relatives and offspring of affected individuals respectively [142, 143]. A large study of first-degree relatives of PBC patients found that 20 % of sisters, 15 % of mothers, and 10 % of daughters of PBC patients were positive for AMA [144]. Several genome-wide association studies (GWAS) have identified loci (such as *HLA*, *IL12A*, and *IL12RB2*, *SPIB*, *IRF5-TNPO3* and 17q12-21, *STAT4*, *DENND1B*, *CD80*, *IL7R*, *CXCR5*, *TNFRSF1A*, *CLEC16A*, and *NFKB1*) strongly associated with PBC [145–149]. Specific mutations of the X chromosome, particularly X monosomy, have been linked to the development of PBC [150].

Data from several studies suggest that environmental factors may play a role in the development of PBC. Infections, particularly urinary tract infections caused by *E. coli*, and the xenobiotics have been linked to the development of PBC [143]. An early association between PBC and UTI has been reported, as in one study, 59 % of 1032 PBC patients reported a history of UTI [151]. Interestingly, PBC patients' sera react with both *E. coli* and PDC-E2, and there is cross-reactivity between antibodies in PBC patients and enzymes secreted by *E. coli* [152, 153]. The xenobiotic 2-octynoic acid, used as a food additive and in manufacturing nail polish, reacts to AMA, and when injected into mice, it results in high titers of AMA and development of PBC-like histological lesions [154, 155]. The clustering of cases of PBC around areas of superfund toxic waste sites has been recently reported [156], suggesting that toxin exposure may play a role in the development of PBC. Smoking cigarettes and use of hormone replacement therapies have also been associated with PBC [12, 143].

Epidemiology of PBC

Studies report a prevalence of PBC ranging from 19 to 365 cases per million in the United States, Canada, Australia, and Europe [157–159]. In Olmsted County, Minnesota, the reported age-adjusted incidence of PBC per million persons was 45 for women and 7 for men, with an overall incidence of 27 per million persons [158]. In a recent Canadian epidemiological study [160], the reported overall age- and sex-adjusted annual incidence of PBC in the Calgary Health Region was 30.3 cases per million (48.4 per million in women and 10.4 per million in men) [160]. European epidemiological studies have estimated PBC incidence rates of 4–58 per million persons-years [161–167]. Recent reports suggest that the incidence and prevalence of PBC might be increasing. In Sheffield, United Kingdom, the incidence of PBC has increased from 5.8 to 20.5 cases per million between the years 1980 and 1999 [46, 168]. In Finland, the incidence and prevalence of PBC increased from 12 cases to 17 cases and from 103 cases per million to 180 cases per million, respectively, in the time period between 1988 and 1999 [159]. In the Calgary Health Region, Canada, the prevalence increased from 100 cases per million in 1996 to 227 cases per million in 2002 [160]. It is still unknown whether the trends in the PBC epidemiology reflect true increase in the frequency of PBC cases or an increase in awareness of the disease by physicians and, perhaps, prolonged survival of PBC patients after UDCA has been introduced. Indeed, recent reports suggest that the absolute number of PBC patients undergoing transplantation for PBC has been decreasing [169], reflecting a change in the natural history of PBC following the introduction of UDCA.

Therapy for PBC

Food and Herbals

No clinical evidence exists to support the use or avoidance of specific foods or herbal supplements in PBC patients.

Herbal and alternative medicines have seldom been examined in patients with PBC. Silymarin has tested in combination with UDCA in PBC but offered little benefit [170]. Currently, no clinical evidence exists regarding safety or efficacy of other herbal products.

UDCA

In addition to being safe, several randomized controlled clinical studies reported that the use of UDCA in patients with PBC not only improves liver biochemistries, but also delays histological progression, delays the development of esophageal varices, improves the liver-transplantation-free survival, and in a selected group of PBC patients, it improves the survival [32–34, 36–41, 43, 44, 171]. At least four mechanisms have been proposed by which UDCA exerts its therapeutic effects: (1) UDCA inhibits the intestinal absorption of toxic bile acids [172–176], (2) UDCA stimulates biliary secretion of bile acids and organic anions, thereby preventing cholestasis induced by toxic bile acids [177–180], (3) UDCA exerts cytoprotective effects against the hepatotoxic effects of the toxic bile acids [181–185], and (4) UDCA may have anti-inflammatory and immunomodulatory properties, based on results from animal experiments [186, 187]. UDCA is the only medical therapy approved by the FDA for treatment of PBC. The recommended dose is 13–15 mg/kg/day, and it should be started in all patients with PBC regardless of the stage of the disease, as long as liver biochemistries are abnormal [11]. Lifelong treatment with UDCA is recommended. Biochemical response to UDCA at 1 year of treatment is a strong predictor of long-term prognosis [38, 188, 189]. Biochemical response has been defined by numerous criteria: the Mayo Clinic criteria (decrease in serum ALP<2 times the upper limit of normal (ULN)) [190], the Spanish criteria (decrease in ALP<40% from baseline or to normal value) [38], the French criteria (decrease in ALP<3 times ULN, decrease in aspartate aminotransferase <2 times ULN, and decrease in bilirubin <1.0 mg/dL) [188], and the Dutch criteria (normalization of bilirubin and/or albumin after treatment if one or both were abnormal at baseline) [189] have been commonly used. Approximately 40% of PBC patients have incomplete response to UDCA. This group of patients is at high risk for serious outcomes [191].

UDCA is generally safe; no serious adverse events have been reported. Weight gain, loose stools, and hair thinning have been infrequently reported and have not raised issues of patients' noncompliance to therapy [11, 192].

Management of Symptoms of PBC

Fatigue

A supportive positive approach to the management of symptoms in PBC, in particular fatigue, is vital and in itself can lead to improvements in quality of life. The two most important features associated with fatigue in PBC are excessive daytime sleepiness and autonomic dysfunction [96]. Therefore, it is crucial to rule out other causes of excessive daytime sleepiness and autonomic dysfunction such as obstructive sleep apnea, anemia, malabsorption, cardiac failure, hypothyroidism, adrenal insufficiency, diabetes mellitus, and use of sleep aid medicines, sedatives, narcotics, and antihypertensive medicines.

UDCA, Ondansetron (a serotonin receptor 3 antagonist) and Fluoxetine (a selective serotonin reuptake inhibitor) have not improved PBC-associated fatigue [193, 194]. Modafinil, a stimulant, has been investigated as a treatment option in PBC patients suffering fatigue [195]. In an open label study using modafinil [196], 14 PBC patients achieved objective short-term benefits in terms of daytime excessive sleepiness and fatigue. At 14 months follow-up, 66% of patients failed to tolerate modafinil long-term [196]. Larger and longer-term placebo-controlled studies are needed to investigate the role of modafinil in PBC-associated fatigue. A small placebo controlled clinical trial did not show benefit [197].

Liver transplantation is reserved for PBC patients with fatigue who failed conservative therapies. Although it has been reported that liver transplantation improves fatigue in patients with PBC [101], a considerable proportion of patients with PBC continue to suffer from severe fatigue after liver transplantation [101].

Pruritus

UDCA does not relieve pruritus in patients with PBC. The effects of several anti-pruritic agents have been investigated in patients with PBC. Liver transplantation is reserved for patients with intractable pruritus after they fail all existing therapies.

Procedures That Remove the Pruritogens from the Body

The most commonly used drug in this class is Cholestyramine [198]. It is a resin that is not absorbed from the intestines and binds anions in the small intestines increasing their fecal excretion, including bile acids and cholesterol [199]. The use of cholestyramine has been associated with improvement of pruritus in patients with PBC [198, 200]. The recommended dose in PBC-related pruritus is 4 g per dose and not exceed 16 g/day, given 2–4 h before or after UDCA [11]. The side effects of this resin tend to be minor (mainly bloating and diarrhea) [199]. It is recommended to take cholestyramine immediately before and after breakfast, as the rationale for its use is to bind the pruritogens that accumulate in the gallbladder during the overnight fast and that are secreted into the small intestine after breaking the fast. Coleavalam, also a resin, was tested in a placebo-controlled clinical trial. The effect of this resin was not better than that of placebo [201].

Rifampicin

The use of Rifampicin, an antibiotic, has been associated with relief of pruritus in PBC patients [202–205]. The mechanism of action of this antibiotic as an antipruritic agent is poorly understood. The recommended dose ranges between 300 mg daily and 600 mg (in 2 divided doses) daily [11]. It was concluded in a meta-analysis study of several clinical trials that rifampicin is safe [206]; however, there is a risk of hepatotoxicity [207], severe hemolytic anemia and nephrotoxicity [204] with the use of rifampicin, but these are rare events. Serial liver chemistries and renal function tests are recommended in patients using this drug.

Opiate Antagonists

Naloxone and Naltrexone are opioid antagonists used for the treatment of the pruritus of cholestasis [208–217]. They act by decreasing the opioidergic tone [112]. To decrease the probability of an opiate withdrawal-like reaction (characterized by tachycardia, abdominal pain, high blood pressure, goose bumps, nightmares, and depersonalization) that some patients experience, it is recommended by some experts to initiate treatment in a controlled environment (surgery suite, specialty clinic, etc.) using intravenous infusions before instituting the oral forms [199]. The dose should be increased gradually to avoid opiate withdrawal-like reactions, until relief of pruritus is achieved.

The metabolism of naltrexone is slow in patients with cirrhosis [218], therefore caution should be exercised when using this drug in this population. A rare but serious adverse event associated with using naltrexone is hepatic failure [219], therefore, routine liver chemistries are recommended in patients using this medication.

Other Agents

Serotonin Antagonists

The serotonin system participates in the neurotransmission of nociceptive stimuli. Odansetron, a serotonin receptor 3 antagonist, has been examined in PBC patients with pruritus but provided only minimal relief of pruritus [220–223].

Antidepressants

Selective serotonin reuptake inhibitors have been shown to have antipruritic effects. Sertraline (75–100 mg daily) has been associated with relief of pruritus in PBC patients [224].

Phenobarbital

Phenobarbital has been shown to have antipruritic effects [225, 226]. The sedative effect of phenobarbital may also be associated with its ameliorating effects on pruritus.

Antihistamines

Antihistamines have been associated with relief of pruritus in PBC patients [227]. The sedative effect of antihistamines may also help patients sleep, as deprivation of sleep is a significant problem in PBC patients suffering pruritus.

Other Options

A transient relief of pruritus has been reported in association with anion adsorption and plasma separation, and the extracorporeal liver support systems [228–230]. This option should be reserved only for patients with intractable pruritus who failed other therapies.

Plasmapheresis seems to be effective in relieving pruritus in PBC patients who have intractable pruritus and failed medical therapy. Old reports have shown that plasmapheresis results in prompt relief of pruritus, decrease in serum bilirubin, and a decrease in the bile acid pool [231, 232]. The duration of clinical response may vary; up to 5 months of pruritus relief following plasmapheresis has been reported by a few patients [232]. Unfortunately, patients reported return of symptom to the pre-plasmapheresis degree 2–3 weeks after the last session of plasmapharesis. The mechanism by which plasmapheresis results in pruritus relief is removal of pruritgens, immune complexes, and bile salts, but this is not clear yet [231]. Most patients with PBC tolerated plasmapheresis quite well, and no adverse events related to plasmapheresis in PBC patients have been reported [233].

Management of Sicca Syndrome

Patients with Sicca syndrome generally suffer from dry eyes and dry mouths, with their consequent complications. Therefore, measures should be taken to prevent complications of these symptoms. The use of artificial tears and humidification of the house environment are recommended [11]. Cyclosporine ophthalmic solution can be used under the supervision of an ophthalmologist when conservative measures fail [234]. Measures to improve oral health include regular visits to the dentist, use of fluoride-containing toothpastes, daily flossing, and avoidance of sugar-containing snacks between meals [235, 236]. Chewing sugar-free gum can improve saliva production as well as the use of cholinergic agents such as pilocarpine and cevimeline [11]. Oral candidiasis can occur as a complication of dry mouth and requires specific intervention [11]. In mild cases, nystatin solution might help reduce the symptoms and duration of infections. Oral and systemic antifungals such as fluconazole are indicated in severe cases of oral candidiasis.

Management of Sjogren's Syndrome and CREST Syndrome

The management of CREST (C-calcinosis, R-Raynaud's, E-esophageal dysfunction, S-sclerdactyly, T-telangiectasia) requires a specialized team effort and these patients should be referred to rheumatologists and other appropriate subspecialties.

Complications Related to Cirrhosis

Hepatocellular Carcinoma

Hepatocellular carcinoma (HCC) is a recognizable complication of PBC. The exact frequency of HCC in the PBC population is unknown but is estimated to be between 0.7 and 5.9 % [237–242]. HCC development significantly affects the survival of patients with PBC. The reported 5- and 10-year survival times for patients with PBC who did not develop HCC versus those who did develop HCC was 95 % vs. 75 % and 85 % vs. 45 %, respectively [242]. Older age, male sex, previous blood transfusion, presence of portal hypertension, and advanced histological stage of PBC have been identified as independent risk factors for development of HCC in patients with PBC [240–242]. Recently, it has been reported that patients with PBC who developed HCC and underwent liver transplantation had better survival than those who did not undergo liver transplantation [238]. Regular screening for HCC with cross-sectional imaging with or without alpha fetoprotein at 6- to 12-month intervals is recommended for all patients with liver cirrhosis [243].

Portal Hypertension

Portal hypertension is a frequent complication in cirrhotic patients. There is still a debate on timing of screening PBC patients for esophageal varices. A number of noninvasive tools have been proposed to be used as indicators for the presence of esophageal varices in PBC patients: (a) a platelet count of <200,000/mm^3, an albumin level <4.0 g/dL, and a bilirubin level >1.2 mg/dL [244], (b) a Mayo risk score of ≥4.0 [190], (c) a platelet count <140,000/mm^3 and/or a Mayo risk score of ≥4.5 [245], (d) the MABPT model (M-male sex, A-albumin <3.5 g/dL, B-bilirubin ≥1.2 mg/dL, PT-prothrombin time ≥12.9 s) [118], (e) the Newcastle Varices PBC score (uses platelet count, albumin, and ALP level) [119]. Only two scores have been cross-validated in independent sets of PBC patients [119, 245].

Management of Portal Hypertension

The management of esophageal varices in patients with PBC follows the guidelines published by the AASLD [246]. Screening upper endoscopy is indicated all PBC patients when the diagnosis of cirrhosis is made. Nonselective beta blocker therapy (propranolol or nadolol) or endoscopic variceal ligation is recommended in patients who have medium to large varices that have not bled and have a high risk of hemorrhage (Child score B/C or variceal red wale markings on endoscopy) [246].

Unlike other liver diseases, varices can develop in the early histological stages of PBC [118, 247]. In patients with pre-cirrhotic PBC and varices who fail traditional therapies (i.e. nonselective beta blockers, ligation, or both), a distal splenorenal shunt (DSRS) might be an alternative to prevent recurrent bleeding [248]. This approach does not deprive the liver of its blood supply and helps preserve the hepatic function in patients with PBC [248]. DSRS is rarely performed nowadays for this indication.

Complications Related to Chronic Cholestasis

Osteopenia and Osteoporosis

Patients with PBC are at significantly higher risk for osteopenia and osteoporosis and their consequent complications when compared to a matched population [120, 127, 128, 249]. Dual-energy X-ray absorptiometry (DXA) is used to measure the bone mineral density (BMD) and is the gold standard for diagnosis of osteopenia and osteoporosis. A baseline screening DXA is recommended in all patients when a diagnosis of PBC is confirmed, with follow-up DXA every 2–3 years [11]. Calcium (1500 mg daily) and vitamin D (1000 IU daily) supplements may be used if there is no history of renal stones [11]. Weight-bearing and muscle-strengthening exercise, smoking cessation, and avoidance of excessive alcohol intake are generally recommended [250]. Bisphosphonate therapy (namely alendronate 70 mg orally weekly) is recommended in PBC patients with osteoporosis. In a randomized controlled clinical trial, alendronate significantly improved bone mineral density when compared to etidronate and placebo [251–253]. Alendronate should not be used in patients with acid reflux or known varices [11].

Hyperlipidemia

PBC is frequently complicated by hypercholesterolemia, which poses no additional risk for atherosclerotic-related death [49, 130]. When classic risk factors for cardiovascular and cerebrovascular diseases are present, such as family history of myocardial infarction, diabetes mellitus, and hypertension, the use of statins is appropriate provided no contraindications to their use exists. The use of statins in PBC is safe [129], even in the presence of abnormal liver biochemistries. UDCA might be helpful in reducing serum cholesterol levels in PBC patients. In a randomized placebo-controlled clinical trial of 177 PBC patients with hypercholesterolemia, UDCA significantly reduced serum total cholesterol levels compared to placebo [254].

Liver Transplantation

In the 1980s, PBC was the leading indication for liver transplantation across North America and Europe [11]. Following the introduction of UDCA, the natural history of PBC has changed significantly [31]. With the use of UDCA in PBC patients, the transplant-free survival rates have considerably improved, even among patients with advanced stages of PBC when they demonstrate biochemical response to UDCA, as defined by various international groups. Patients with early-stage PBC on UDCA live

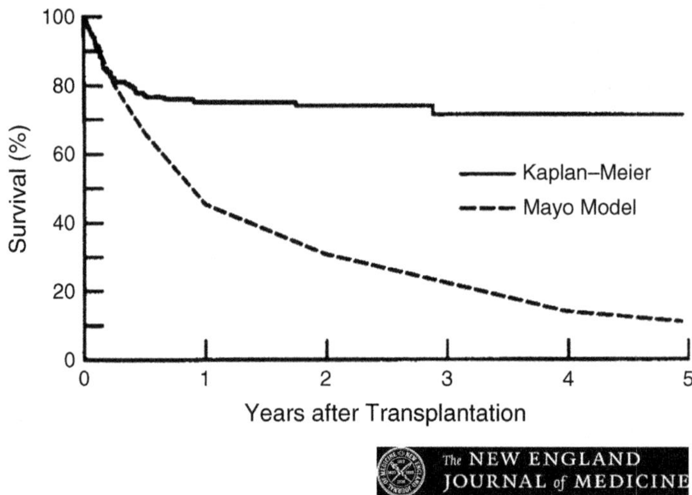

Fig. 16.5 Actual (Kaplan–Meier) survival after transplantation in 161 patients with primary biliary cirrhosis and estimated survival without transplantation as predicted by the Mayo Model (simulated control). Markus BH et al. N Engl J Med 1989; 320: 1709–1713

just as long as the healthy population [31, 44]. In the United States the burden of PBC on liver transplantation has reduced over a 12-year period. Lee et al. [169] reported that the absolute number of liver transplants for PBC has decreased an average of 5.4 transplants per year and the absolute number of cases of PBC added to the liver transplant waiting list has also significantly decreased between the years 1995 and 2006 [169]. Despite these facts, 40 % of PBC patients have inadequate response to UDCA and are at high risk for adverse outcomes and many progress to end-stage liver disease [191].

Liver transplantation remains the only curative option for PBC patients with end-stage liver disease and is the sixth leading indication for liver transplantation (Fig. 16.5) [11, 255]. The reported 5-year survival in PBC patients who underwent liver transplantation in North America and Europe in the late 1990s ranged between 78 and 87 % [255–257]. Acute rejection of the transplanted graft occurs in 46–56 % of PBC patients but is rarely of clinical significance, as it responds very well to increasing the immunosuppression [258–260]. Chronic rejection of the transplanted graft is a more serious but rare problem, occurring in 2–9.3 % [261].

About 20–25 % of PBC patients who undergo liver transplantation develop recurrent PBC [11]. Liver biopsy remains the gold standard for diagnosis of recurrent PBC in the transplanted graft, as AMAs may persist in the sera of PBC patients even after liver transplantation [53]. Tacrolimus-based immunosuppression posttransplantation, male sex and advanced recipient's age have been identified as risk factors for recurrent PBC in the transplanted graft [258, 260]. It has been reported that liver transplantation improves fatigue and pruritus in PBC patients [101]. However, a significant proportion of PBC patients continue to suffer from severe debilitating fatigue after liver transplantation [101].

General Advice

Pregnancy, Hormone Replacement, and PBC

Because up to 25 % of cases of PBC present younger than the age of 50, some women with PBC will be of childbearing age at the time of diagnosis [262]. Pregnancy in women with PBC is frequently symptomatic, with up to 53 % of pregnant women with PBC developing de novo pruritus, and up to 71 % requiring symptom-specific therapy [263]. Liver biochemistries remain stable through the pregnancy in 70 % of cases, however, 72 % of PBC cases develop biochemical flare up in the post-partum period [263]. Pregnancy in PBC women is mostly uneventful, with 91 % of women reporting at least one successful live birth [263]. Moreover, UDCA appears to be safe during pregnancy and lactation. In one study, 6 women with PBC took UDCA at various time points during pregnancy without adverse fetal consequences [263].

As with all other women with cirrhosis who become pregnant, it is advisable to screen for varices in the second trimester [11]. Nonselective beta blockers are safe during pregnancy [11].

Estrogens promote cholestasis, so oral contraceptives and pregnancy can induce or worsen pruritus in patients with PBC [11].

Screening Family Members

First-degree family members of PBC patients are at increased risk for developing PBC [144]. Screening for PBC is done by measuring serum ALP and AMA. The clinical value of screening family members of patients with PBC is unclear.

Long-Term Follow-Up

UDCA should be continued indefinitely [11]. Liver biochemistries should be assessed at 3- to 6-month intervals. Thyroid function tests should be performed annually or when suspicion for hypothyroidism or hyperthyroidism is high [11]. Patients with a new diagnosis of cirrhosis should undergo screening endoscopy for esophageal varices [246]. No consensus exists on screening pre-cirrhotic PBC patients for esophageal varices; using any of the noninvasive markers as a guiding tool for screening for esophageal varices is reasonable. DXA at baseline and every 2–3 years is recommended in all patients with PBC to screen for osteopenia and osteoporosis and to monitor bisphosphonate therapy [11]. Cross-sectional imaging with or without measuring alpha fetoprotein level every 6–12 months in PBC patients with cirrhosis is recommended [243].

Special Cases of PBC

AMA-Negative PBC

AMAs are present in 95 % of PBC patients. Five percent of PBC cases are AMA-negative [264]. In these circumstances, a liver biopsy is indicated to establish the diagnosis. PBC-specific ANAs might also be helpful in this setting. The percentage of AMA-negative patients might decrease in the future with the development of newer, more sensitive ELISA screening techniques [265]. The natural course of patients with AMA-negative PBC is similar to that observed in patients with classic AMA-positive PBC [266]. All patients with AMA-negative PBC should receive UDCA, and treatment should continue indefinitely [11]. The same screening procedures and long-term care in patients with classic PBC apply to patients with AMA-negative PBC.

PBC/AIH Overlap Syndrome

The diagnosis of PBC/AIH overlap is suspected when patients demonstrate features of both diseases. The true prevalence of this condition is unknown; however, the reported estimated prevalence ranges between 2 and 20 % [87]. Hispanics may be more likely to have PBC/AIH overlap syndrome than non-Hispanics [267].

Diagnosis of PBC/AIH

Diagnosis of PBC/AIH is challenging, largely due to the lack of consensus on the diagnostic criteria for this syndrome. The two most widely used criteria for the diagnosis of PBC/AIH overlap syndrome are the Paris Study Group Criteria [268] and the International Autoimmune Hepatits Group (IAIHG) [269]. The diagnosis of the PBC/AIH overlap syndrome is based on the presence of at least two of the three diagnostic criteria for each disease [87]. For PBC, the diagnostic criteria are (1) ALP levels >2 times ULN, (2) positive AMA, and (3) liver biopsy showing bile duct lesions consistent with PBC. For AIH, the diagnostic criteria are (1) ALT levels >5 times ULN, (2) serum immunoglobulin G >2 times ULN, and (3) liver biopsy showing periportal and/or periseptal lymphocytic piecemeal necrosis. In addition to the mentioned diagnostic criteria, some of the serological markers have been found to be of diagnostic value. The anti-dsDNA antibodies are found more frequently in patients with PBC/AIH overlap syndrome (60 %) than in patients with PBC alone (3 %) or AIH alone (26 %) [270], and positivity for both AMA and anti-dsDNA antibodies have been found in 47 % of cases of overlap syndrome as opposed to 1 % in AIH and 3 % in PBC [270].

Clinical Course of PBC/AIH

The natural history of PBC/AIH is poorly understood. It has been reported that patients with PBC/AIH overlap syndrome had worse outcomes in terms of complications of portal hypertension and need for liver transplantation when compared to patients with PBC alone [271]. More recently, Levy et al. [267] reported that Hispanic subjects with PBC/AIH had worse outcomes in terms of development of portal hypertension, variceal hemorrhage, need for liver transplantation, or death, when compared to a non-Hispanic group of patients with PBC/AIH.

At this time, there is no consensus on the management of patients with PBC/AIH. A combination of UDCA and immunosuppression is a reasonable approach. Given the rarity of this combination, randomized clinical trials are unlikely to occur.

Consecutive PBC/AIH

Rarely, PBC may morph into AIH over time. A review of 282 cases of PBC followed long term suggest that 4.3% (12/282) develop features of AIH [272]. Of those who developed AIH following PBC, 16.6% died from hepatic failure secondary to HCC [272].

AMA-Positive AIH

There are case reports of patients with AIH who test positive for AMA, but on long-term follow-up, these patients did not develop PBC [273].

Future Therapies

Obeticholic acid (OCA, INT-747) is a farnesoid X receptor (FXR) agonist [274] that has shown promising results in early clinical trials in patients with PBC who had inadequate response to UDCA [275, 276]. Preliminary reports from the ongoing phase III randomized placebo-controlled clinical trial of OCA in PBC patients showed that 47% of patients in the 5 g—OCA arm and 46% of patients in the 5 mg—followed by 10 mg-OCA arm reached the composite primary endpoint of a reduction of ALP to <1.67 times ULN, a total bilirubin within normal limits, and at least a 15% decrease in serum ALP, compared to only 10% of patients who received placebo (data presented in the European Association for the Study of Liver 2014 meeting).

NGM282, a novel specific inhibitor of the cholesterol 7α hydroxylase enzyme (the rate-limiting enzyme in bile acid synthesis), is currently evaluated in a phase II clinical trial in PBC patients.

Expert Commentary

Primary biliary cholangitis (PBC), a progressive disease of the biliary tree characterized by cholestasis and damage of the small bile ducts, can lead to cirrhosis and liver failure. The introduction of ursodeoxycholic acid (UDCA) has favorably changed the natural course of PBC. Once a leading indication for liver transplantation, PBC is now the sixth leading indication for liver transplantation. UDCA has been shown to prolong the survival of PBC patients without liver transplantation. In patients with early stages of PBC, institution of UDCA early in the course of the disease can improve the survival. Despite the documented efficacy of UDCA, approximately 40 % of PBC patients show inadequate response to UDCA. These patients have are at high risk for serious complications. Liver transplantation, the only curative option in patients with end-stage liver disease due to PBC, is an invasive procedure and expensive procedure. PBC recurs in the transplanted graft in up to 25 % of cases. These facts underscore the need for newer, more effective therapies for PBC. Obeticholic acid (OCA), a first-in-class farnesoid X receptor (FXR) agonist, has shown promising results during the first year of an ongoing phase III clinical trial in patients with PBC. The use of the genome-wide association studies (GWAS) might help us identify loci of therapeutic importance, which would help us identify future potential therapeutic agents.

References

1. Talwalkar JA, Lindor KD. Primary biliary cirrhosis. Lancet. 2003;362:53–61.
2. Ahrens Jr EH, Payne MA, Kunkel HG, et al. Primary biliary cirrhosis. Medicine (Baltimore). 1950;29:299–364.
3. Hadziyannis S, Scheuer PJ, Feizi T, et al. Immunological and histological studies in primary biliary cirrhosis. J Clin Pathol. 1970;23:95–8.
4. Walker JG, Doniach D, Roitt IM, et al. Serological tests in diagnosis of primary biliary cirrhosis. Lancet. 1965;1:827–31.
5. Cha S, Leung PS, Gershwin ME, et al. Combinatorial autoantibodies to dihydrolipoamide acetyltransferase, the major autoantigen of primary biliary cirrhosis. Proc Natl Acad Sci U S A. 1993;90:2527–31.
6. Mutimer DJ, Fussey SP, Yeaman SJ, et al. Frequency of IgG and IgM autoantibodies to four specific M2 mitochondrial autoantigens in primary biliary cirrhosis. Hepatology. 1989;10:403–7.
7. Gershwin ME, Mackay IR, Sturgess A, et al. Identification and specificity of a cDNA encoding the 70 kd mitochondrial antigen recognized in primary biliary cirrhosis. J Immunol. 1987;138:3525–31.
8. Baum H, Palmer C. The PBC-specific antigen. Mol Aspects Med. 1985;8:201–34.
9. Frazer IH, Mackay IR, Jordan TW, et al. Reactivity of anti-mitochondrial autoantibodies in primary biliary cirrhosis: definition of two novel mitochondrial polypeptide autoantigens. J Immunol. 1985;135:1739–45.
10. Mattalia A, Quaranta S, Leung PS, et al. Characterization of antimitochondrial antibodies in health adults. Hepatology. 1998;27:656–61.
11. Lindor KD, Gershwin ME, Poupon R, et al. Primary biliary cirrhosis. Hepatology. 2009;50:291–308.

12. Bowlus CL, Gershwin ME. The diagnosis of primary biliary cirrhosis. Autoimmun Rev. 2014;13:441–4.
13. Klatskin G, Kantor FS. Mitochondrial antibody in primary biliary cirrhosis and other diseases. Ann Intern Med. 1972;77:533–41.
14. Sherlock S. Primary billiary cirrhosis (chronic intrahepatic obstructive jaundice). Gastroenterology. 1959;37:574–86.
15. Sherlock S, Scheuer PJ. The presentation and diagnosis of 100 patients with primary biliary cirrhosis. N Engl J Med. 1973;289:674–8.
16. Prince MI, Chetwynd A, Craig WL, et al. Asymptomatic primary biliary cirrhosis: clinical features, prognosis, and symptom progression in a large population based cohort. Gut. 2004;53:865–70.
17. Mahl TC, Shockcor W, Boyer JL. Primary biliary cirrhosis: survival of a large cohort of symptomatic and asymptomatic patients followed for 24 years. J Hepatol. 1994;20:707–13.
18. Springer J, Cauch-Dudek K, O'Rourke K, et al. Asymptomatic primary biliary cirrhosis: a study of its natural history and prognosis. Am J Gastroenterol. 1999;94:47–53.
19. Prince M, Chetwynd A, Newman W, et al. Survival and symptom progression in a geographically based cohort of patients with primary biliary cirrhosis: follow-up for up to 28 years. Gastroenterology. 2002;123:1044–51.
20. Pares A, Rodes J. Natural history of primary biliary cirrhosis. Clin Liver Dis. 2003;7:779–94.
21. Shapiro JM, Smith H, Schaffner F. Serum bilirubin: a prognostic factor in primary biliary cirrhosis. Gut. 1979;20:137–40.
22. Christensen E, Crowe J, Doniach D, et al. Clinical pattern and course of disease in primary biliary cirrhosis based on an analysis of 236 patients. Gastroenterology. 1980;78:236–46.
23. Locke 3rd GR, Therneau TM, Ludwig J, et al. Time course of histological progression in primary biliary cirrhosis. Hepatology. 1996;23:52–6.
24. Bonnand AM, Heathcote EJ, Lindor KD, et al. Clinical significance of serum bilirubin levels under ursodeoxycholic acid therapy in patients with primary biliary cirrhosis. Hepatology. 1999;29:39–43.
25. Christensen E, Neuberger J, Crowe J, et al. Beneficial effect of azathioprine and prediction of prognosis in primary biliary cirrhosis. Final results of an international trial. Gastroenterology. 1985;89:1084–91.
26. Dickson ER, Grambsch PM, Fleming TR, et al. Prognosis in primary biliary cirrhosis: model for decision making. Hepatology. 1989;10:1–7.
27. Keiding S, Ericzon BG, Eriksson S, et al. Survival after liver transplantation of patients with primary biliary cirrhosis in the Nordic countries. Comparison with expected survival in another series of transplantations and in an international trial of medical treatment. Scand J Gastroenterol. 1990;25:11–8.
28. Rydning A, Schrumpf E, Abdelnoor M, et al. Factors of prognostic importance in primary biliary cirrhosis. Scand J Gastroenterol. 1990;25:119–26.
29. Mitchison HC, Bassendine MF, Hendrick A, et al. Positive antimitochondrial antibody but normal alkaline phosphatase: is this primary biliary cirrhosis? Hepatology. 1986;6:1279–84.
30. Metcalf JV, Mitchison HC, Palmer JM, et al. Natural history of early primary biliary cirrhosis. Lancet. 1996;348:1399–402.
31. Imam MH, Lindor KD. The natural history of primary biliary cirrhosis. Semin Liver Dis. 2014;34:329–33.
32. Angulo P, Batts KP, Therneau TM, et al. Long-term ursodeoxycholic acid delays histological progression in primary biliary cirrhosis. Hepatology. 1999;29:644–7.
33. Lindor KD, Jorgensen RA, Therneau TM, et al. Ursodeoxycholic acid delays the onset of esophageal varices in primary biliary cirrhosis. Mayo Clin Proc. 1997;72:1137–40.
34. Combes B, Carithers Jr RL, Maddrey WC, et al. A randomized, double-blind, placebo-controlled trial of ursodeoxycholic acid in primary biliary cirrhosis. Hepatology. 1995;22:759–66.

35. Corpechot C, Carrat F, Bonnand AM, et al. The effect of ursodeoxycholic acid therapy on liver fibrosis progression in primary biliary cirrhosis. Hepatology. 2000;32:1196–9.
36. Heathcote EJ, Cauch-Dudek K, Walker V, et al. The Canadian Multicenter Double-blind Randomized Controlled Trial of ursodeoxycholic acid in primary biliary cirrhosis. Hepatology. 1994;19:1149–56.
37. Lindor KD, Therneau TM, Jorgensen RA, et al. Effects of ursodeoxycholic acid on survival in patients with primary biliary cirrhosis. Gastroenterology. 1996;110:1515–8.
38. Pares A, Caballeria L, Rodes J. Excellent long-term survival in patients with primary biliary cirrhosis and biochemical response to ursodeoxycholic Acid. Gastroenterology. 2006;130:715–20.
39. Poupon RE, Balkau B, Eschwege E, et al. A multicenter, controlled trial of ursodiol for the treatment of primary biliary cirrhosis. UDCA-PBC Study Group. N Engl J Med. 1991;324:1548–54.
40. Poupon RE, Poupon R, Balkau B. Ursodiol for the long-term treatment of primary biliary cirrhosis. The UDCA-PBC Study Group. N Engl J Med. 1994;330:1342–7.
41. Lindor KD, Dickson ER, Baldus WP, et al. Ursodeoxycholic acid in the treatment of primary biliary cirrhosis. Gastroenterology. 1994;106:1284–90.
42. Batts KP, Jorgensen RA, Dickson ER, et al. Effects of ursodeoxycholic acid on hepatic inflammation and histological stage in patients with primary biliary cirrhosis. Am J Gastroenterol. 1996;91:2314–7.
43. Poupon RE, Lindor KD, Cauch-Dudek K, et al. Combined analysis of randomized controlled trials of ursodeoxycholic acid in primary biliary cirrhosis. Gastroenterology. 1997;113:884–90.
44. Corpechot C, Carrat F, Bahr A, et al. The effect of ursodeoxycholic acid therapy on the natural course of primary biliary cirrhosis. Gastroenterology. 2005;128:297–303.
45. Lammers WJ, van Buuren HR, Hirschfield GM, et al. Levels of alkaline phosphatase and bilirubin are surrogate endpoints of outcomes of patients with primary biliary cirrhosis - an international follow-up study. Gastroenterology. 2014;147:1338.
46. Triger DR. Primary biliary cirrhosis: an epidemiological study. Br Med J. 1980;281:772–5.
47. Wiesner RH, LaRusso NF, Ludwig J, et al. Comparison of the clinicopathologic features of primary sclerosing cholangitis and primary biliary cirrhosis. Gastroenterology. 1985;88:108–14.
48. Jeffrey GP, Reed WD, Shilkin KB. Primary biliary cirrhosis: clinicopathological characteristics and outcome. J Gastroenterol Hepatol. 1990;5:639–45.
49. Sorokin A, Brown JL, Thompson PD. Primary biliary cirrhosis, hyperlipidemia, and atherosclerotic risk: a systematic review. Atherosclerosis. 2007;194:293–9.
50. Koh WH, Dunphy J, Whyte J, et al. Characterisation of anticytoplasmic antibodies and their clinical associations. Ann Rheum Dis. 1995;54:269–73.
51. Fussey SP, Guest JR, James OF, et al. Identification and analysis of the major M2 autoantigens in primary biliary cirrhosis. Proc Natl Acad Sci U S A. 1988;85:8654–8.
52. Yeaman SJ, Fussey SP, Danner DJ, et al. Primary biliary cirrhosis: identification of two major M2 mitochondrial autoantigens. Lancet. 1988;1:1067–70.
53. Dubel L, Farges O, Bismuth H, et al. Kinetics of anti-M2 antibodies after liver transplantation for primary biliary cirrhosis. J Hepatol. 1995;23:674–80.
54. Kaplan MM, Gershwin ME. Primary biliary cirrhosis. N Engl J Med. 2005;353:1261–73.
55. Muratori P, Muratori L, Cassani F, et al. Anti-multiple nuclear dots (anti-MND) and anti-SP100 antibodies in hepatic and rheumatological disorders. Clin Exp Immunol. 2002;127:172–5.
56. Muratori P, Muratori L, Ferrari R, et al. Characterization and clinical impact of antinuclear antibodies in primary biliary cirrhosis. Am J Gastroenterol. 2003;98:431–7.
57. Powell F, Schroeter AL, Dickson ER. Antinuclear antibodies in primary biliary cirrhosis. Lancet. 1984;1:288–9.
58. Remmel T, Piirsoo A, Koiveer A, et al. Clinical significance of different antinuclear antibodies patterns in the course of primary biliary cirrhosis. Hepatogastroenterology. 1996;43:1135–40.
59. Rigopoulou EI, Davies ET, Pares A, et al. Prevalence and clinical significance of isotype specific antinuclear antibodies in primary biliary cirrhosis. Gut. 2005;54:528–32.

60. Szostecki C, Krippner H, Penner E, et al. Autoimmune sera recognize a 100 kD nuclear protein antigen (sp-100). Clin Exp Immunol. 1987;68:108–16.
61. Zuchner D, Sternsdorf T, Szostecki C, et al. Prevalence, kinetics, and therapeutic modulation of autoantibodies against Sp100 and promyelocytic leukemia protein in a large cohort of patients with primary biliary cirrhosis. Hepatology. 1997;26:1123–30.
62. Granito A, Yang WH, Muratori L, et al. PML nuclear body component Sp140 is a novel autoantigen in primary biliary cirrhosis. Am J Gastroenterol. 2010;105:125–31.
63. Wesierska-Gadek J, Hohenuer H, Hitchman E, et al. Autoantibodies against nucleoporin p62 constitute a novel marker of primary biliary cirrhosis. Gastroenterology. 1996;110:840–7.
64. Wesierska-Gadek J, Penner E, Battezzati PM, et al. Correlation of initial autoantibody profile and clinical outcome in primary biliary cirrhosis. Hepatology. 2006;43:1135–44.
65. Nakamura M, Kondo H, Mori T, et al. Anti-gp210 and anti-centromere antibodies are different risk factors for the progression of primary biliary cirrhosis. Hepatology. 2007;45:118–27.
66. Sternsdorf T, Guldner HH, Szostecki C, et al. Two nuclear dot-associated proteins, PML and Sp100, are often co-autoimmunogenic in patients with primary biliary cirrhosis. Scand J Immunol. 1995;42:257–68.
67. Janka C, Selmi C, Gershwin ME, et al. Small ubiquitin-related modifiers: a novel and independent class of autoantigens in primary biliary cirrhosis. Hepatology. 2005;41:609–16.
68. Courvalin JC, Lassoued K, Worman HJ, et al. Identification and characterization of autoantibodies against the nuclear envelope lamin B receptor from patients with primary biliary cirrhosis. J Exp Med. 1990;172:961–7.
69. Worman HJ, Yuan J, Blobel G, et al. A lamin B receptor in the nuclear envelope. Proc Natl Acad Sci U S A. 1988;85:8531–4.
70. Nickowitz RE, Worman HJ. Autoantibodies from patients with primary biliary cirrhosis recognize a restricted region within the cytoplasmic tail of nuclear pore membrane glycoprotein Gp210. J Exp Med. 1993;178:2237–42.
71. Ludwig J, Dickson ER, McDonald GS. Staging of chronic nonsuppurative destructive cholangitis (syndrome of primary biliary cirrhosis). Virchows Arch A Pathol Anat Histol. 1978;379:103–12.
72. Nakanuma Y, Ohta G, Takeshita H, et al. Florid duct lesions and extensive bile duct loss of the intrahepatic biliary tree in chronic liver diseases other than primary biliary cirrhosis. Acta Pathol Jpn. 1983;33:1095–104.
73. Nakanuma Y, Ohta G, Kono N, et al. Electron microscopic observation of destruction of biliary epithelium in primary biliary cirrhosis. Liver. 1983;3:238–48.
74. Nakanuma Y, Ohta G. Quantitation of hepatic granulomas and epithelioid cells in primary biliary cirrhosis. Hepatology. 1983;3:423–7.
75. Nakanuma Y. Distribution of B lymphocytes in nonsuppurative cholangitis in primary biliary cirrhosis. Hepatology. 1993;18:570–5.
76. Nakanuma Y, Harada K. Florid duct lesion in primary biliary cirrhosis shows highly proliferative activities. J Hepatol. 1993;19:216–21.
77. Nakanuma Y. Necroinflammatory changes in hepatic lobules in primary biliary cirrhosis with less well-defined cholestatic changes. Hum Pathol. 1993;24:378–83.
78. Terasaki S, Nakanuma Y, Yamazaki M, et al. Eosinophilic infiltration of the liver in primary biliary cirrhosis: a morphological study. Hepatology. 1993;17:206–12.
79. Lee RG, Epstein O, Jauregui H, et al. Granulomas in primary biliary cirrhosis: a prognostic feature. Gastroenterology. 1981;81:983–6.
80. Rubin E, Schaffner F, Popper H. Primary Biliary Cirrhosis. Chronic Non-Suppurative Destructive Cholangitis. Am J Pathol. 1965;46:387–407.
81. Scheuer P. Primary biliary cirrhosis. Proc R Soc Med. 1967;60:1257–60.
82. Hauftova D, Jezdinska V, Fischer J, et al. Primary biliary cirrhosis, CRST syndrome, Sjogren's syndrome and nodular regenerative liver hyperplasia. Cesk Gastroenterol Vyz. 1982;36:429–36.
83. Chazouilleres O, Andreani T, Legendre C, et al. Nodular regenerative hyperplasia of the liver and primary biliary cirrhosis. A fortuitous association? Gastroenterol Clin Biol. 1986;10:764–6.

84. Nakanuma Y, Ohta G. Nodular hyperplasia of the liver in primary biliary cirrhosis of early histological stages. Am J Gastroenterol. 1987;82:8–10.
85. Castellano G, Colina F, Moreno D, et al. Nodular regenerative hepatic hyperplasia associated with primary biliary cirrhosis. Rev Clin Esp. 1992;191:433–4.
86. Colina F, Pinedo F, Solis JA, et al. Nodular regenerative hyperplasia of the liver in early histological stages of primary biliary cirrhosis. Gastroenterology. 1992;102:1319–24.
87. Floreani A, Franceschet I, Cazzagon N. Primary biliary cirrhosis: overlaps with other autoimmune disorders. Semin Liver Dis. 2014;34:352–60.
88. Floreani A, Cazzagon N, Martines D, et al. Performance and utility of transient elastography and noninvasive markers of liver fibrosis in primary biliary cirrhosis. Dig Liver Dis. 2011;43:887–92.
89. Newton JL, Bhala N, Burt J, et al. Characterisation of the associations and impact of symptoms in primary biliary cirrhosis using a disease specific quality of life measure. J Hepatol. 2006;44:776–83.
90. Jones DE, Bhala N, Burt J, et al. Four year follow up of fatigue in a geographically defined primary biliary cirrhosis patient cohort. Gut. 2006;55:536–41.
91. Jones DE, Bhala N, Newton JL. Reflections on therapeutic trials in primary biliary cirrhosis: a quality of life oriented counter-view. Hepatology. 2006;43:633. author reply 634.
92. Newton JL, Gibson GJ, Tomlinson M, et al. Fatigue in primary biliary cirrhosis is associated with excessive daytime somnolence. Hepatology. 2006;44:91–8.
93. Stanca CM, Bach N, Krause C, et al. Evaluation of fatigue in U.S. patients with primary biliary cirrhosis. Am J Gastroenterol. 2005;100:1104–9.
94. Bjornsson E, Kalaitzakis E, Neuhauser M, et al. Fatigue measurements in patients with primary biliary cirrhosis and the risk of mortality during follow-up. Liver Int. 2010;30:251–8.
95. Jones DE, Al-Rifai A, Frith J, et al. The independent effects of fatigue and UDCA therapy on mortality in primary biliary cirrhosis: results of a 9 year follow-up. J Hepatol. 2010;53:911–7.
96. Newton JL. Fatigue in primary biliary cirrhosis. Clin Liver Dis. 2008;12:367–83. ix.
97. Zein CO, McCullough AJ. Association between fatigue and decreased survival in primary biliary cirrhosis. Gut. 2007;56:1165–6. author reply 1166.
98. Hollingsworth KG, Newton JL, Taylor R, et al. Pilot study of peripheral muscle function in primary biliary cirrhosis: potential implications for fatigue pathogenesis. Clin Gastroenterol Hepatol. 2008;6:1041–8.
99. Newton JL, Hollingsworth KG, Taylor R, et al. Cognitive impairment in primary biliary cirrhosis: symptom impact and potential etiology. Hepatology. 2008;48:541–9.
100. Quarneti C, Muratori P, Lalanne C, et al. Fatigue and pruritus at onset identify a more aggressive subset of primary biliary cirrhosis. Liver Int. 2014;35:636.
101. Carbone M, Bufton S, Monaco A, et al. The effect of liver transplantation on fatigue in patients with primary biliary cirrhosis: a prospective study. J Hepatol. 2013;59:490–4.
102. Witt-Sullivan H, Heathcote J, Cauch K, et al. The demography of primary biliary cirrhosis in Ontario, Canada. Hepatology. 1990;12:98–105.
103. Talwalkar JA, Souto E, Jorgensen RA, et al. Natural history of pruritus in primary biliary cirrhosis. Clin Gastroenterol Hepatol. 2003;1:297–302.
104. Jones EA, Bergasa NV. The pruritus of cholestasis. Hepatology. 1999;29:1003–6.
105. Crowe J, Christensen E, Doniach D, et al. Early features of primary biliary cirrhosis: an analysis of 85 patients. Am J Gastroenterol. 1985;80:466–8.
106. Ng VL, Ryckman FC, Porta G, et al. Long-term outcome after partial external biliary diversion for intractable pruritus in patients with intrahepatic cholestasis. J Pediatr Gastroenterol Nutr. 2000;30:152–6.
107. Beuers U, Kremer AE, Bolier R, et al. Pruritus in cholestasis: facts and fiction. Hepatology. 2014;60:399–407.
108. Rishe E, Azarm A, Bergasa NV. Itch in primary biliary cirrhosis: a patients' perspective. Acta Derm Venereol. 2008;88:34–7.
109. Lloyd-Thomas HG, Sherlock S. Testosterone therapy for the pruritus of obstructive jaundice. Br Med J. 1952;2:1289–91.

110. Stiehl A. Bile acids and bile acid sulfates in the skin of patients with cholestasis and pruritus. Z Gastroenterol. 1974;12:121–4.
111. Gittlen SD, Schulman ES, Maddrey WC. Raised histamine concentrations in chronic cholestatic liver disease. Gut. 1990;31:96–9.
112. Jones EA, Bergasa NV. The pruritus of cholestasis: from bile acids to opiate agonists. Hepatology. 1990;11:884–7.
113. Trivedi M, Bergasa NV. Serum concentrations of substance P in cholestasis. Ann Hepatol. 2010;9:177–80.
114. Kremer AE, Martens JJ, Kulik W, et al. Lysophosphatidic acid is a potential mediator of cholestatic pruritus. Gastroenterology. 2010;139:1008–18. 1018.e1.
115. Floreani A, Franceschet I, Cazzagon N, et al. Extrahepatic autoimmune conditions associated with primary biliary cirrhosis. Clin Rev Allergy Immunol. 2015;48:192.
116. Runyon BA. Introduction to the revised American Association for the Study of Liver Diseases Practice Guideline management of adult patients with ascites due to cirrhosis 2012. Hepatology. 2013;57:1651–3.
117. Gores GJ, Wiesner RH, Dickson ER, et al. Prospective evaluation of esophageal varices in primary biliary cirrhosis: development, natural history, and influence on survival. Gastroenterology. 1989;96:1552–9.
118. Ali AH, Sinakos E, Silveira MG, et al. Varices in early histological stage primary biliary cirrhosis. J Clin Gastroenterol. 2011;45:e66–71.
119. Patanwala I, McMeekin P, Walters R, et al. A validated clinical tool for the prediction of varices in PBC: the Newcastle Varices in PBC Score. J Hepatol. 2013;59:327–35.
120. Levy C, Lindor KD. Management of osteoporosis, fat-soluble vitamin deficiencies, and hyperlipidemia in primary biliary cirrhosis. Clin Liver Dis. 2003;7:901–10.
121. Lindor KD, Janes CH, Crippin JS, et al. Bone disease in primary biliary cirrhosis: does ursodeoxycholic acid make a difference? Hepatology. 1995;21:389–92.
122. Kehayoglou AK, Holdsworth CD, Agnew JE, et al. Bone disease and calcium absorption in primary biliary cirrhosis with special reference to vitamin-D therapy. Lancet. 1968;1:715–8.
123. Matloff DS, Kaplan MM, Neer RM, et al. Osteoporosis in primary biliary cirrhosis: effects of 25-hydroxyvitamin D3 treatment. Gastroenterology. 1982;83:97–102.
124. Mitchison HC, Malcolm AJ, Bassendine MF, et al. Metabolic bone disease in primary biliary cirrhosis at presentation. Gastroenterology. 1988;94:463–70.
125. Maddrey WC. Bone disease in patients with primary biliary cirrhosis. Prog Liver Dis. 1990;9:537–54.
126. Rosen H. Primary biliary cirrhosis and bone disease. Hepatology. 1995;21:253–5.
127. Guanabens N, Pares A, Ros I, et al. Severity of cholestasis and advanced histological stage but not menopausal status are the major risk factors for osteoporosis in primary biliary cirrhosis. J Hepatol. 2005;42:573–7.
128. Menon KV, Angulo P, Weston S, et al. Bone disease in primary biliary cirrhosis: independent indicators and rate of progression. J Hepatol. 2001;35:316–23.
129. Cash WJ, O'Neill S, O'Donnell ME, et al. Randomized controlled trial assessing the effect of simvastatin in primary biliary cirrhosis. Liver Int. 2013;33:1166–74.
130. Crippin JS, Lindor KD, Jorgensen R, et al. Hypercholesterolemia and atherosclerosis in primary biliary cirrhosis: what is the risk? Hepatology. 1992;15:858–62.
131. Sabesin SM. Cholestatic lipoproteins--their pathogenesis and significance. Gastroenterology. 1982;83:704–9.
132. Jahn CE, Schaefer EJ, Taam LA, et al. Lipoprotein abnormalities in primary biliary cirrhosis. Association with hepatic lipase inhibition as well as altered cholesterol esterification. Gastroenterology. 1985;89:1266–78.
133. Quarfordt SH, Oelschlaeger H, Krigbaum WR, et al. Effect of biliary obstruction on canine plasma and biliary lipids. Lipids. 1973;8:522–30.
134. Byers SO, Friedman M. Observations concerning the production and excretion of cholesterol in mammals. V. The relation of biliary retention of cholesterol, distention of the biliary tract,

the shunting of bile to the vena cava, and the removal of the gastro-intestinal tract to the hypercholesteremia consequent on biliary obstruction. J Exp Med. 1952;95:19–24.
135. Back P, Gerok W. Bile acids in human diseases: [mit] 40 tables. II. Bile Acid Meeting, Freiburg i Br., June 30-July 1, 1972, Stuttgart. New York, NY: Schattauer; 1972.
136. Fredrickson DS, Loud AV, Hinkelman BT, et al. The effect of ligation of the common bile duct on cholesterol synthesis in the rat. J Exp Med. 1954;99:43–53.
137. Kaplan MM, Elta GH, Furie B, et al. Fat-soluble vitamin nutriture in primary biliary cirrhosis. Gastroenterology. 1988;95:787–92.
138. Lanspa SJ, Chan AT, Bell 3rd JS, et al. Pathogenesis of steatorrhea in primary biliary cirrhosis. Hepatology. 1985;5:837–42.
139. Kowdley KV, Emond MJ, Sadowski JA, et al. Plasma vitamin K1 level is decreased in primary biliary cirrhosis. Am J Gastroenterol. 1997;92:2059–61.
140. Phillips JR, Angulo P, Petterson T, et al. Fat-soluble vitamin levels in patients with primary biliary cirrhosis. Am J Gastroenterol. 2001;96:2745–50.
141. Jeffrey GP, Muller DP, Burroughs AK, et al. Vitamin E deficiency and its clinical significance in adults with primary biliary cirrhosis and other forms of chronic liver disease. J Hepatol. 1987;4:307–17.
142. Hirschfield GM, Invernizzi P. Progress in the genetics of primary biliary cirrhosis. Semin Liver Dis. 2011;31:147–56.
143. Hirschfield GM, Gershwin ME. The immunobiology and pathophysiology of primary biliary cirrhosis. Annu Rev Pathol. 2013;8:303–30.
144. Lazaridis KN, Juran BD, Boe GM, et al. Increased prevalence of antimitochondrial antibodies in first-degree relatives of patients with primary biliary cirrhosis. Hepatology. 2007;46:785–92.
145. Donaldson PT, Baragiotta A, Heneghan MA, et al. HLA class II alleles, genotypes, haplotypes, and amino acids in primary biliary cirrhosis: a large-scale study. Hepatology. 2006;44:667–74.
146. Hirschfield GM, Liu X, Han Y, et al. Variants at IRF5-TNPO3, 17q12-21 and MMEL1 are associated with primary biliary cirrhosis. Nat Genet. 2010;42:655–7.
147. Hirschfield GM, Liu X, Xu C, et al. Primary biliary cirrhosis associated with HLA, IL12A, and IL12RB2 variants. N Engl J Med. 2009;360:2544–55.
148. Liu X, Invernizzi P, Lu Y, et al. Genome-wide meta-analyses identify three loci associated with primary biliary cirrhosis. Nat Genet. 2010;42:658–60.
149. Mells GF, Floyd JA, Morley KI, et al. Genome-wide association study identifies 12 new susceptibility loci for primary biliary cirrhosis. Nat Genet. 2011;43:329–32.
150. Invernizzi P, Miozzo M, Battezzati PM, et al. Frequency of monosomy X in women with primary biliary cirrhosis. Lancet. 2004;363:533–5.
151. Gershwin ME, Selmi C, Worman HJ, et al. Risk factors and comorbidities in primary biliary cirrhosis: a controlled interview-based study of 1032 patients. Hepatology. 2005;42:1194–202.
152. Fussey SP, Ali ST, Guest JR, et al. Reactivity of primary biliary cirrhosis sera with Escherichia coli dihydrolipoamide acetyltransferase (E2p): characterization of the main immunogenic region. Proc Natl Acad Sci U S A. 1990;87:3987–91.
153. Bogdanos DP, Baum H, Grasso A, et al. Microbial mimics are major targets of crossreactivity with human pyruvate dehydrogenase in primary biliary cirrhosis. J Hepatol. 2004;40:31–9.
154. Rieger R, Leung PS, Jeddeloh MR, et al. Identification of 2-nonynoic acid, a cosmetic component, as a potential trigger of primary biliary cirrhosis. J Autoimmun. 2006;27:7–16.
155. Wakabayashi K, Lian ZX, Leung PS, et al. Loss of tolerance in C57BL/6 mice to the autoantigen E2 subunit of pyruvate dehydrogenase by a xenobiotic with ensuing biliary ductular disease. Hepatology. 2008;48:531–40.
156. Ala A, Stanca CM, Bu-Ghanim M, et al. Increased prevalence of primary biliary cirrhosis near Superfund toxic waste sites. Hepatology. 2006;43:525–31.
157. Boonstra K, Kunst AE, Stadhouders PH, et al. Rising incidence and prevalence of primary biliary cirrhosis: a large population-based study. Liver Int. 2014;34:e31–8.

158. Kim WR, Lindor KD, Locke 3rd GR, et al. Epidemiology and natural history of primary biliary cirrhosis in a US community. Gastroenterology. 2000;119:1631–6.
159. Rautiainen H, Salomaa V, Niemela S, et al. Prevalence and incidence of primary biliary cirrhosis are increasing in Finland. Scand J Gastroenterol. 2007;42:1347–53.
160. Myers RP, Shaheen AA, Fong A, et al. Epidemiology and natural history of primary biliary cirrhosis in a Canadian health region: a population-based study. Hepatology. 2009;50:1884–92.
161. Danielsson A, Boqvist L, Uddenfeldt P. Epidemiology of primary biliary cirrhosis in a defined rural population in the northern part of Sweden. Hepatology. 1990;11:458–64.
162. Eriksson S, Lindgren S. The prevalence and clinical spectrum of primary biliary cirrhosis in a defined population. Scand J Gastroenterol. 1984;19:971–6.
163. Hamlyn AN, Macklon AF, James O. Primary biliary cirrhosis: geographical clustering and symptomatic onset seasonality. Gut. 1983;24:940–5.
164. James OF, Bhopal R, Howel D, et al. Primary biliary cirrhosis once rare, now common in the United Kingdom? Hepatology. 1999;30:390–4.
165. Lofgren J, Jarnerot G, Danielsson D, et al. Incidence and prevalence of primary biliary cirrhosis in a defined population in Sweden. Scand J Gastroenterol. 1985;20:647–50.
166. Myszor M, James OF. The epidemiology of primary biliary cirrhosis in north-east England: an increasingly common disease? Q J Med. 1990;75:377–85.
167. Remmel T, Remmel H, Uibo R, et al. Primary biliary cirrhosis in Estonia. With special reference to incidence, prevalence, clinical features, and outcome. Scand J Gastroenterol. 1995;30:367–71.
168. Ray-Chadhuri DRE, MacComack K. Epidemiology of PBC in Sheffield updated: demographics and relation to water supply. London: British Association for the Study of the Liver; 2001. p. 42.
169. Lee J, Belanger A, Doucette JT, et al. Transplantation trends in primary biliary cirrhosis. Clin Gastroenterol Hepatol. 2007;5:1313–5.
170. Angulo P, Patel T, Jorgensen RA, et al. Silymarin in the treatment of patients with primary biliary cirrhosis with a suboptimal response to ursodeoxycholic acid. Hepatology. 2000;32:897–900.
171. Poupon RE, Lindor KD, Pares A, et al. Combined analysis of the effect of treatment with ursodeoxycholic acid on histologic progression in primary biliary cirrhosis. J Hepatol. 2003;39:12–6.
172. Beuers U, Spengler U, Zwiebel FM, et al. Effect of ursodeoxycholic acid on the kinetics of the major hydrophobic bile acids in health and in chronic cholestatic liver disease. Hepatology. 1992;15:603–8.
173. Chazouilleres O, Marteau P, Haniche M, et al. Ileal absorption of bile acids in patients with chronic cholestasis: SeHCAT test results and effect of ursodeoxycholic acid (UDCA). Dig Dis Sci. 1996;41:2417–22.
174. Jazrawi RP, de Caestecker JS, Goggin PM, et al. Kinetics of hepatic bile acid handling in cholestatic liver disease: effect of ursodeoxycholic acid. Gastroenterology. 1994;106:134–42.
175. Lanzini A, De Tavonatti MG, Panarotto B, et al. Intestinal absorption of the bile acid analogue 75Se-homocholic acid-taurine is increased in primary biliary cirrhosis, and reverts to normal during ursodeoxycholic acid administration. Gut. 2003;52:1371–5.
176. Stiehl A. Intestinal absorption of bile acids: effect of ursodeoxycholic acid treatment. Ital J Gastroenterol. 1995;27:193–5.
177. Ikebuchi Y, Shimizu H, Ito K, et al. Ursodeoxycholic acid stimulates the formation of the bile canalicular network. Biochem Pharmacol. 2012;84:925–35.
178. Paumgartner G, Beuers U. Mechanisms of action and therapeutic efficacy of ursodeoxycholic acid in cholestatic liver disease. Clin Liver Dis. 2004;8:67–81. vi.
179. Poupon R. Ursodeoxycholic acid and bile-acid mimetics as therapeutic agents for cholestatic liver diseases: an overview of their mechanisms of action. Clin Res Hepatol Gastroenterol. 2012;36 Suppl 1:S3–12.
180. Uriz M, Saez E, Prieto J, et al. Ursodeoxycholic acid is conjugated with taurine to promote secretin-stimulated biliary hydrocholeresis in the normal rat. PLoS One. 2011;6:e28717.

181. Bernstein C, Payne CM, Bernstein H, et al. Activation of the metallothionein IIA promoter and other key stress response elements by ursodeoxycholate in HepG2 cells: relevance to the cytoprotective function of ursodeoxycholate. Pharmacology. 2002;65:2–9.
182. Guldutuna S, Zimmer G, Imhof M, et al. Molecular aspects of membrane stabilization by ursodeoxycholate [see comment]. Gastroenterology. 1993;104:1736–44.
183. Mitsuyoshi H, Nakashima T, Sumida Y, et al. Ursodeoxycholic acid protects hepatocytes against oxidative injury via induction of antioxidants. Biochem Biophys Res Commun. 1999;263:537–42.
184. Rodrigues CM, Fan G, Ma X, et al. A novel role for ursodeoxycholic acid in inhibiting apoptosis by modulating mitochondrial membrane perturbation. J Clin Invest. 1998;101:2790–9.
185. Rodrigues CM, Fan G, Wong PY, et al. Ursodeoxycholic acid may inhibit deoxycholic acid-induced apoptosis by modulating mitochondrial transmembrane potential and reactive oxygen species production. Mol Med. 1998;4:165–78.
186. Kikuchi K, Hsu W, Hosoya N, et al. Ursodeoxycholic acid reduces CpG-induced IgM production in patients with primary biliary cirrhosis. Hepatol Res. 2009;39:448–54.
187. Yoshikawa M, Tsujii T, Matsumura K, et al. Immunomodulatory effects of ursodeoxycholic acid on immune responses. Hepatology. 1992;16:358–64.
188. Corpechot C, Abenavoli L, Rabahi N, et al. Biochemical response to ursodeoxycholic acid and long-term prognosis in primary biliary cirrhosis. Hepatology. 2008;48:871–7.
189. Kuiper EM, Hansen BE, de Vries RA, et al. Improved prognosis of patients with primary biliary cirrhosis that have a biochemical response to ursodeoxycholic acid. Gastroenterology. 2009;136:1281–7.
190. Angulo P, Lindor KD, Therneau TM, et al. Utilization of the Mayo risk score in patients with primary biliary cirrhosis receiving ursodeoxycholic acid. Liver. 1999;19:115–21.
191. Carey EJ. Cholestatic liver disease. New York, NY: Springer; 2014.
192. Siegel JL, Jorgensen R, Angulo P, et al. Treatment with ursodeoxycholic acid is associated with weight gain in patients with primary biliary cirrhosis. J Clin Gastroenterol. 2003;37:183–5.
193. Theal JJ, Toosi MN, Girlan L, et al. A randomized, controlled crossover trial of ondansetron in patients with primary biliary cirrhosis and fatigue. Hepatology. 2005;41:1305–12.
194. Talwalkar JA, Donlinger JJ, Gossard AA, et al. Fluoxetine for the treatment of fatigue in primary biliary cirrhosis: a randomized, double-blind controlled trial. Dig Dis Sci. 2006;51:1985–91.
195. Kaplan MM, Bonis PA. Modafinil for the treatment of fatigue in primary biliary cirrhosis. Ann Intern Med. 2005;143:546–7.
196. Hardy T, MacDonald C, Jones DE, et al. A follow-up study of modafinil for the treatment of daytime somnolence and fatigue in primary biliary cirrhosis. Liver Int. 2010;30:1551–2.
197. Jones DE, Newton JL. An open study of modafinil for the treatment of daytime somnolence and fatigue in primary biliary cirrhosis. Aliment Pharmacol Ther. 2007;25:471–6.
198. Datta DV, Sherlock S. Cholestyramine for long term relief of the pruritus complicating intrahepatic cholestasis. Gastroenterology. 1966;50:323–32.
199. Bergasa NV. Pruritus of cholestasis. In: Carstens E, Akiyama T, editors. Itch: mechanisms and treatment. Boca Raton, FL: CRC Press/Taylor & Francis; 2014.
200. Van Itallie TB, Hashim SA, Crampton RS, et al. The treatment of pruritus and hypercholesteremia of primary biliary cirrhosis with cholestyramine. N Engl J Med. 1961;265:469–74.
201. Kuiper EM, van Erpecum KJ, Beuers U, et al. The potent bile acid sequestrant colesevelam is not effective in cholestatic pruritus: results of a double-blind, randomized, placebo-controlled trial. Hepatology. 2010;52:1334–40.
202. Hoensch HP, Balzer K, Dylewizc P, et al. Effect of rifampicin treatment on hepatic drug metabolism and serum bile acids in patients with primary biliary cirrhosis. Eur J Clin Pharmacol. 1985;28:475–7.
203. Ghent CN, Carruthers SG. Treatment of pruritus in primary biliary cirrhosis with rifampin. Results of a double-blind, crossover, randomized trial. Gastroenterology. 1988;94:488–93.
204. Bachs L, Pares A, Elena M, et al. Comparison of rifampicin with phenobarbitone for treatment of pruritus in biliary cirrhosis. Lancet. 1989;1:574–6.

205. Podesta A, Lopez P, Terg R, et al. Treatment of pruritus of primary biliary cirrhosis with rifampin. Dig Dis Sci. 1991;36:216–20.
206. Khurana S, Singh P. Rifampin is safe for treatment of pruritus due to chronic cholestasis: a meta-analysis of prospective randomized-controlled trials. Liver Int. 2006;26:943–8.
207. Prince MI, Burt AD, Jones DE. Hepatitis and liver dysfunction with rifampicin therapy for pruritus in primary biliary cirrhosis. Gut. 2002;50:436–9.
208. Thornton JR, Losowsky MS. Opioid peptides and primary biliary cirrhosis. BMJ. 1988;297:1501–4.
209. Bergasa NV, Schmitt JM, Talbot TL, et al. Open-label trial of oral nalmefene therapy for the pruritus of cholestasis. Hepatology. 1998;27:679–84.
210. Bergasa NV, Alling DW, Talbot TL, et al. Oral nalmefene therapy reduces scratching activity due to the pruritus of cholestasis: a controlled study. J Am Acad Dermatol. 1999;41:431–4.
211. Terg R, Coronel E, Sorda J, et al. Efficacy and safety of oral naltrexone treatment for pruritus of cholestasis, a crossover, double blind, placebo-controlled study. J Hepatol. 2002;37:717–22.
212. Mansour-Ghanaei F, Taheri A, Froutan H, et al. Effect of oral naltrexone on pruritus in cholestatic patients. World J Gastroenterol. 2006;12:1125–8.
213. Jones EA, Bergasa NV. The pruritus of cholestasis and the opioid system. JAMA. 1992;268:3359–62.
214. Bergasa NV, Talbot TL, Alling DW, et al. A controlled trial of naloxone infusions for the pruritus of chronic cholestasis. Gastroenterology. 1992;102:544–9.
215. Bergasa NV, Alling DW, Talbot TL, et al. Effects of naloxone infusions in patients with the pruritus of cholestasis. A double-blind, randomized, controlled trial. Ann Intern Med. 1995;123:161–7.
216. Carson KL, Tran TT, Cotton P, et al. Pilot study of the use of naltrexone to treat the severe pruritus of cholestatic liver disease. Am J Gastroenterol. 1996;91:1022–3.
217. Wolfhagen FH, Sternieri E, Hop WC, et al. Oral naltrexone treatment for cholestatic pruritus: a double-blind, placebo-controlled study. Gastroenterology. 1997;113:1264–9.
218. Bertolotti M, Ferrari A, Vitale G, et al. Effect of liver cirrhosis on the systemic availability of naltrexone in humans. J Hepatol. 1997;27:505–11.
219. Mitchell JE. Naltrexone and hepatotoxicity. Lancet. 1986;1:1215.
220. Jones EA. Pruritus and fatigue associated with liver disease: is there a role for ondansetron? Expert Opin Pharmacother. 2008;9:645–51.
221. Raderer M, Muller C, Scheithauer W. Ondansetron for pruritus due to cholestasis. N Engl J Med. 1994;330:1540.
222. Schworer H, Ramadori G. Improvement of cholestatic pruritus by ondansetron. Lancet. 1993;341:1277.
223. Jones EA, Molenaar HA, Oosting J. Ondansetron and pruritus in chronic liver disease: a controlled study. Hepatogastroenterology. 2007;54:1196–9.
224. Mayo MJ, Handem I, Saldana S, et al. Sertraline as a first-line treatment for cholestatic pruritus. Hepatology. 2007;45:666–74.
225. Bloomer JR, Boyer JL. Phenobarbital effects in cholestatic liver diseases. Ann Intern Med. 1975;82:310–7.
226. Ghent CN, Bloomer JR, Hsia YE. Efficacy and safety of long-term phenobarbital therapy of familial cholestasis. J Pediatr. 1978;93:127–32.
227. Greaves MW. Antihistamines in dermatology. Skin Pharmacol Physiol. 2005;18:220–9.
228. Pusl T, Denk GU, Parhofer KG, et al. Plasma separation and anion adsorption transiently relieve intractable pruritus in primary biliary cirrhosis. J Hepatol. 2006;45:887–91.
229. Sturm E, Franssen CF, Gouw A, et al. Extracorporal albumin dialysis (MARS) improves cholestasis and normalizes low apo A-I levels in a patient with benign recurrent intrahepatic cholestasis (BRIC). Liver. 2002;22 Suppl 2:72–5.
230. Doria C, Mandala L, Smith J, et al. Effect of molecular adsorbent recirculating system in hepatitis C virus-related intractable pruritus. Liver Transpl. 2003;9:437–43.
231. Cohen LB, Ambinder EP, Wolke AM, et al. Role of plasmapheresis in primary biliary cirrhosis. Gut. 1985;26:291–4.

232. Lauterburg BH, Taswell HF, Pineda AA, et al. Treatment of pruritus of cholestasis by plasma perfusion through USP-charcoal-coated glass beads. Lancet. 1980;2:53–5.
233. Ambinder EP, Cohen LB, Wolke AM, et al. The clinical effectiveness and safety of chronic plasmapheresis in patients with primary biliary cirrhosis. J Clin Apher. 1985;2:219–23.
234. Tatlipinar S, Akpek EK. Topical ciclosporin in the treatment of ocular surface disorders. Br J Ophthalmol. 2005;89:1363–7.
235. Richards A, Rooney J, Prime S, et al. Primary biliary cirrhosis. Sole presentation with rampant dental caries. Oral Surg Oral Med Oral Pathol. 1994;77:16–8.
236. Mang FW, Michieletti P, O'Rourke K, et al. Primary biliary cirrhosis, sicca complex, and dysphagia. Dysphagia. 1997;12:167–70.
237. Deutsch M, Papatheodoridis GV, Tzakou A, et al. Risk of hepatocellular carcinoma and extrahepatic malignancies in primary biliary cirrhosis. Eur J Gastroenterol Hepatol. 2008;20:5–9.
238. Imam MH, Silveira MG, Sinakos E, et al. Long-term outcomes of patients with primary biliary cirrhosis and hepatocellular carcinoma. Clin Gastroenterol Hepatol. 2012;10:182–5.
239. Jones DE, Metcalf JV, Collier JD, et al. Hepatocellular carcinoma in primary biliary cirrhosis and its impact on outcomes. Hepatology. 1997;26:1138–42.
240. Silveira MG, Suzuki A, Lindor KD. Surveillance for hepatocellular carcinoma in patients with primary biliary cirrhosis. Hepatology. 2008;48:1149–56.
241. Suzuki A, Lymp J, Donlinger J, et al. Clinical predictors for hepatocellular carcinoma in patients with primary biliary cirrhosis. Clin Gastroenterol Hepatol. 2007;5:259–64.
242. Tomiyama Y, Takenaka K, Kodama T, et al. Risk factors for survival and the development of hepatocellular carcinoma in patients with primary biliary cirrhosis. Intern Med. 2013;52:1553–9.
243. Bruix J, Sherman M, American Association for the Study of Liver Diseases. Management of hepatocellular carcinoma: an update. Hepatology. 2011;53:1020–2.
244. Bressler B, Pinto R, El-Ashry D, et al. Which patients with primary biliary cirrhosis or primary sclerosing cholangitis should undergo endoscopic screening for oesophageal varices detection? Gut. 2005;54:407–10.
245. Levy C, Zein CO, Gomez J, et al. Prevalence and predictors of esophageal varices in patients with primary biliary cirrhosis. Clin Gastroenterol Hepatol. 2007;5:803–8.
246. Garcia-Tsao G, Sanyal AJ, Grace ND, et al. Prevention and management of gastroesophageal varices and variceal hemorrhage in cirrhosis. Hepatology. 2007;46:922–38.
247. Ikeda F, Okamoto R, Baba N, et al. Prevalence and associated factors with esophageal varices in early primary biliary cirrhosis. J Gastroenterol Hepatol. 2012;27:1320–8.
248. Boyer TD, Kokenes DD, Hertzler G, et al. Effect of distal splenorenal shunt on survival of patients with primary biliary cirrhosis. Hepatology. 1994;20:1482–6.
249. Springer JE, Cole DE, Rubin LA, et al. Vitamin D-receptor genotypes as independent genetic predictors of decreased bone mineral density in primary biliary cirrhosis. Gastroenterology. 2000;118:145–51.
250. Watts NB, Bilezikian JP, Camacho PM, et al. American Association of Clinical Endocrinologists Medical Guidelines for Clinical Practice for the diagnosis and treatment of postmenopausal osteoporosis: executive summary of recommendations. Endocr Pract. 2010;16:1016–9.
251. Guanabens N, Pares A, Ros I, et al. Alendronate is more effective than etidronate for increasing bone mass in osteopenic patients with primary biliary cirrhosis. Am J Gastroenterol. 2003;98:2268–74.
252. Guanabens N, Monegal A, Cerda D, et al. Randomized trial comparing monthly ibandronate and weekly alendronate for osteoporosis in patients with primary biliary cirrhosis. Hepatology. 2013;58:2070–8.
253. Zein CO, Jorgensen RA, Clarke B, et al. Alendronate improves bone mineral density in primary biliary cirrhosis: a randomized placebo-controlled trial. Hepatology. 2005;42:762–71.
254. Balan V, Dickson ER, Jorgensen RA, et al. Effect of ursodeoxycholic acid on serum lipids of patients with primary biliary cirrhosis. Mayo Clin Proc. 1994;69:923–9.
255. MacQuillan GC, Neuberger J. Liver transplantation for primary biliary cirrhosis. Clin Liver Dis. 2003;7:941–56. ix.

256. Liermann Garcia RF, Evangelista Garcia C, McMaster P, et al. Transplantation for primary biliary cirrhosis: retrospective analysis of 400 patients in a single center. Hepatology. 2001;33:22–7.
257. Neuberger J, Gunson B, Hubscher S, et al. Immunosuppression affects the rate of recurrent primary biliary cirrhosis after liver transplantation. Liver Transpl. 2004;10:488–91.
258. Charatcharoenwitthaya P, Pimentel S, Talwalkar JA, et al. Long-term survival and impact of ursodeoxycholic acid treatment for recurrent primary biliary cirrhosis after liver transplantation. Liver Transpl. 2007;13:1236–45.
259. Milkiewicz P, Gunson B, Saksena S, et al. Increased incidence of chronic rejection in adult patients transplanted for autoimmune hepatitis: assessment of risk factors. Transplantation. 2000;70:477–80.
260. Jacob DA, Neumann UP, Bahra M, et al. Long-term follow-up after recurrence of primary biliary cirrhosis after liver transplantation in 100 patients. Clin Transplant. 2006;20:211–20.
261. Milkiewicz P. Liver transplantation in primary biliary cirrhosis. Clin Liver Dis. 2008;12:461–72. xi.
262. Efe C, Kahramanoglu-Aksoy E, Yilmaz B, et al. Pregnancy in women with primary biliary cirrhosis. Autoimmun Rev. 2014;13:931–5.
263. Trivedi PJ, Kumagi T, Al-Harthy N, et al. Good maternal and fetal outcomes for pregnant women with primary biliary cirrhosis. Clin Gastroenterol Hepatol. 2014;12:1179–85.e1.
264. Lacerda MA, Ludwig J, Dickson ER, et al. Antimitochondrial antibody-negative primary biliary cirrhosis. Am J Gastroenterol. 1995;90:247–9.
265. Oertelt S, Rieger R, Selmi C, et al. A sensitive bead assay for antimitochondrial antibodies: chipping away at AMA-negative primary biliary cirrhosis. Hepatology. 2007;45:659–65.
266. Mendes F, Lindor KD. Antimitochondrial antibody-negative primary biliary cirrhosis. Gastroenterol Clin North Am. 2008;37:479–84. viii.
267. Levy C, Naik J, Giordano C, et al. Hispanics with primary biliary cirrhosis are more likely to have features of autoimmune hepatitis and reduced response to ursodeoxycholic acid than non-Hispanics. Clin Gastroenterol Hepatol. 2014;12:1398–405.
268. Chazouilleres O, Wendum D, Serfaty L, et al. Primary biliary cirrhosis-autoimmune hepatitis overlap syndrome: clinical features and response to therapy. Hepatology. 1998;28:296–301.
269. Hennes EM, Zeniya M, Czaja AJ, et al. Simplified criteria for the diagnosis of autoimmune hepatitis. Hepatology. 2008;48:169–76.
270. Muratori P, Granito A, Pappas G, et al. The serological profile of the autoimmune hepatitis/primary biliary cirrhosis overlap syndrome. Am J Gastroenterol. 2009;104:1420–5.
271. Silveira MG, Talwalkar JA, Angulo P, et al. Overlap of autoimmune hepatitis and primary biliary cirrhosis: long-term outcomes. Am J Gastroenterol. 2007;102:1244–50.
272. Poupon R, Chazouilleres O, Corpechot C, et al. Development of autoimmune hepatitis in patients with typical primary biliary cirrhosis. Hepatology. 2006;44:85–90.
273. O'Brien C, Joshi S, Feld JJ, et al. Long-term follow-up of antimitochondrial antibody-positive autoimmune hepatitis. Hepatology. 2008;48:550–6.
274. Adorini L, Pruzanski M, Shapiro D. Farnesoid X receptor targeting to treat nonalcoholic steatohepatitis. Drug Discov Today. 2012;17:988–97.
275. Kowdley KV, Luketic V, Chapman R. An international study evaluating the farnesoid x receptor agonist obeticholic acid as monotherapy in PBC. J Hepatol. 2011;54:S13.
276. Mason A, Luketic V, Lindor K, Hirschfield G, Gordon S, Mayo M, et al. Farnesoid-X receptor agonists: a new class of drugs for the treatment of PBC? An international study evaluating the addition of INT-747 to ursodeoxycholic acid. J Hepatol. 2010;52:S1–21.

Chapter 17
Autoimmune Liver Diseases: Primary Sclerosing Cholangitis

José Franco

Abbreviations

AIDS	Acquired immune deficiency syndrome
ALT	Alanine aminotransferase
AST	Aspartate aminotransferase
CT	Computerized tomography
DEXA	Dual energy X-ray absorptiometry
ERC	Endoscopic retrograde cholangiography
FISH	Fluorescent in situ hybridization
IBD	Inflammatory bowel disease
IgG4	Immunoglobulin G4
MELD	Model for end-stage liver disease
MRC	Magnetic resonance cholangiography
MRI	Magnetic resonance imaging
P-ANCA	Perinuclear antineutrophil cytoplasmic antibodies
PSC	Primary sclerosing cholangitis
PTC	Percutaneous transhepatic cholangiography
SAM-E	S-adenosylmethionine
TIPS	Transjugular intrahepatic portosystemic shunt
UDCA	Ursodeoxycholic acid
UNOS	United Network for Organ Sharing

J. Franco, M.D. (✉)
Division of Gastroenterology and Hepatology, Medical College of Wisconsin,
8700 West Wisconsin Avenue, Milwaukee, WI 53226, USA
e-mail: jfranco@mcw.edu

© Springer International Publishing Switzerland 2017
K. Saeian, R. Shaker (eds.), *Liver Disorders*,
DOI 10.1007/978-3-319-30103-7_17

Patient Questions and Answers

1. *What is Primary Sclerosing Cholangitis and how did I get it?*

    Primary sclerosing cholangitis, or PSC for short, is a chronic liver disease that leads to strictures or narrowing of the large and small bile ducts in the liver. The bile ducts are the plumbing of the liver and serve to move products produced in the liver to the small intestine, where they perform functions necessary for survival. While the exact cause of PSC remains unclear, it is frequently classified as an autoimmune disease. This means that it may be the result of an overactive or abnormal immune system. Patients with PSC frequently have other autoimmune disorders with the most common being inflammation of the colon, or colitis. Unfortunately, there is no effective therapy that prevents the progression of PSC and many patients will develop advanced liver disease and possibly cirrhosis which is severe, irreversible scarring of the liver. It is important to recognize that PSC is not associated with alcohol use, specific diets or behaviors. Primary sclerosing cholangitis is not the result of an infection or exposure to other individuals. You cannot transmit PSC to other individuals.

2. *What can I do to treat Primary Sclerosing Cholangitis?*

    It is important to remember that your PSC is not the result of anything you have done wrong. While not related to alcohol, it is important to avoid alcohol as regular alcohol use can by itself lead to liver damage. As with all chronic liver diseases, you should be checked for immunity or protection to hepatitis A and B. If tests show that you are not protected, you should undergo vaccination. Both of these vaccines are safe and effective. It is important to maintain a healthy diet as patients who are able to accomplish this are better able to tolerate chronic illnesses, including PSC. Because of the strong association with colitis (inflammation of the colon), you should undergo a colonoscopy (a test to examine your colon) unless you have already had one. Primary sclerosing cholangitis can also lead to difficulty absorbing certain vitamins such as vitamin D. When patients have low vitamin D levels it can lead to thinning of the bones, osteoporosis, and possible bone fractures. Because of this, you should undergo a test known as a bone densitometry to determine whether you are at risk for developing bone disease.

    There is no specific medicine that has been shown to be effective in slowing the progression of PSC. While it is classified as an autoimmune disorder, it does not respond to medications that are effective against other autoimmune conditions. While you may want to explore alternative or natural therapies such as herbal therapies, I would discourage you from using these substances as they are frequently not regulated by the Food and Drug Administration and in some cases have also been shown to be harmful to the liver. You should always let all of your doctors know of any medicine you are taking, as some medicines may not be as well tolerated by patients with liver disease such as PSC.

3. *Will I need a liver transplant?*

    The natural history of PSC is highly variable. Some patients present at a young age and have an aggressive course leading to the need for liver transplantation, while others will carry a diagnosis of PSC for many years and not require liver transplantation or die from this condition. Since PSC is a progressive disease and there is no known effective medical therapy, it will be important that you follow-up with a hepatologist or liver doctor on a regular basis even if you do not have any symptoms. During these visits you will be asked about symptoms as well as undergo a physical exam and blood tests that will allow your hepatologist to determine the overall status of the PSC and when a liver transplant evaluation should be considered. Your hepatologist may determine that a repeat examination of your bile ducts is necessary, particularly if there is suspicion that a cancer has developed in the bile ducts. Cancer of the bile ducts is known as cholangiocarcinoma. You should have an ultrasound of the liver and gallbladder every year as there in an increased risk of developing both liver and gallbladder cancer. You should contact your physicians immediately if you experience symptoms including jaundice or yellowing of the eyes and skin, worsening itching throughout your body which is most noticeable at night, fever, weight loss, and abdominal pain which most commonly occurs in the area over your liver.

Autoimmune Liver Diseases: Primary Sclerosing Cholangitis

Summary

Primary sclerosing cholangitis (PSC) is a chronic condition characterized by inflammation, fibrosis, and obliteration involving the intra- as well as extrahepatic bile ducts. Initially described in 1924 and once considered a rare condition, the condition can no longer be considered rare as advancements in cholangiography have led to more frequent diagnosis. While the etiology remains elusive, it is commonly classified as an autoimmune liver disease and other immune-mediated conditions, most notably inflammatory bowel disease, are frequently concurrently encountered. Genetic predisposition also appears to play a contributory role based on the finding of associated as well as protective haplotypes. Complications of PSC are both nonspecific and associated with chronic cholestatic liver disease as well as those specific to PSC. The natural history is highly variable with the potential for progression to cirrhosis, end-stage liver disease, and the need for liver transplantation. Patients with PSC are also at an increased risk for the development of cholangiocarcinoma as well as colorectal, gallbladder, and hepatocellular carcinoma. Despite the evaluations of multiple pharmacologic agents, there is currently no medical therapy that has been shown to alter the timeline to death or the need for liver transplantation. Liver transplantation is the only effective therapy for long-term survival in those who develop complications of end-stage liver disease and is associated with excellent long-term results. Variants of PSC include small-duct PSC, overlap PSC and autoimmune hepatitis, and immunoglobulin G cholangiopathy.

Epidemiology

Various epidemiological studies have placed the incidence of PSC from 0.9 to 1.31 cases per 100,000 person-years and the prevalence at 8.5 to 13.6 cases per 100,000 persons [1, 2]. There is, however, significant regional variability which supports the theory of genetic predisposition playing a role. Sixty to 70% of affected patients have underlying inflammatory bowel disease (IBD), more frequently chronic Ulcerative Colitis than Crohn Disease with colonic involvement [3, 4]. The IBD is typically diagnosed several years prior to PSC [5]. In addition, while associated with IBD, the two disorders' activity level and progression do not necessarily correlate. Approximately two-thirds of those affected with PSC are male with the median age at diagnosis of approximately 37 [2].

Etiology

While the exact etiology of PSC remains unknown, it appears that both genetic and immunologic factors play prominent roles.

Genetics

Evidence supporting a genetic cause includes strong familial patterns as well as a strong association with specific haplotypes, most notably B8DR3, B8DR13, and B8DR15. Conversely, haplotypes DRB1*040, DRB1*070, and MICA*002 are associated with a decreased risk of developing PSC [6–9].

Immune-Mediated

An immune mechanism is supported by the findings of serum autoantibodies in a large number of those with PSC, the most common being perinuclear antineutrophil cytoplasmic antibodies (p-ANCA) which are found in up to two-thirds of patients. Other autoantibodies occasionally encountered include antinuclear and anti-smooth muscle antibodies [10]. Additionally, hypergammaglobulinemia is common, as is the association with other autoimmune disorders, most notably inflammatory bowel disease.

Other potential etiologies that may play minor roles in PSC include infectious causes, toxin exposure, and vascular complications.

Infectious

The association of PSC with IBD has led to the theory that damaged colonic mucosa leads to translocation of bacteria that enter the blood stream and bile ducts. The failure to identify specific organisms, the absence of portal phlebitis, failure of antibiotics or colectomy to alter the natural history and the fact that not all patients with PSC have IBD argues against an infectious etiology.

Toxin-Mediated

Toxin exposure as a cause of PSC is based on the theory that imbalances between hydrophilic and hydrophobic bile acids, such as lithocolic acid, can lead to biliary epithelial damage and strictures. Other toxic agents that have been evaluated include iron and copper, both of which are shown to be elevated in many patients with PSC. Elevated iron and copper levels, however, are nonspecific findings and can be associated with both hepatocellular and cholestatic disorders.

Vascular Injury

Vascular injury to the hepatic artery has long been associated with biliary strictures in liver transplant recipients; however, examination of the hepatic vasculature in PSC has failed to demonstrate damage either to the hepatic artery, portal vein, or hepatic vein.

Clinical Presentation

The clinical presentation of patients affected by PSC is highly variable. At one end of the spectrum is the asymptomatic patient who is diagnosed based on cholestatic hepatic biochemistries obtained in the setting of IBD. The majority of patients with PSC will be diagnosed when presenting with symptoms that lead to further investigation. The most common presenting symptoms are pruritus, jaundice, right upper quadrant abdominal pain and acute cholangitis. Unfortunately, some patients will present with advanced liver disease manifested by weight loss, ascites, hepatic encephalopathy, portal hypertensive bleeding, or cholangiocarcinoma.

Diagnosis

Laboratories

The majority of patients with PSC will demonstrate cholestasis on hepatic biochemistries. Alkaline phosphatase values greater than 2.5-fold normal values are seen in the majority of patients. As a result, elevated alkaline phosphatase values which are confirmed to be of biliary origin should result in a thorough evaluation and consideration for PSC. Total bilirubin values are elevated in over 50 % of affected patients and 90 % demonstrate a two to threefold elevation in alanine aminotransferase (ALT) and aspartate aminotransferase (AST). Serum iron and copper values are frequently elevated, but as previously mentioned, are nonspecific and therefore not helpful for diagnostic purposes. Despite the finding of p-ANCA autoantibodies in the majority of PSC patients, their presence is nonspecific and should not be utilized to make a diagnosis of PSC. This is in contrast to other autoimmune hepatic disorders such as autoimmune hepatitis and primary biliary cirrhosis where serum autoantibodies play a pivotal role in diagnosis.

Cholangiography

The diagnosis of PSC is made based on the classic cholangiographic findings of diffuse strictures with intervening areas of normal appearing bile ducts leading to the so-called "beading." Seventy-five percent of strictures involve both the intra and extrahepatic bile ducts, with 15 % having strictures limited to the extrahepatic system. The cystic duct and gallbladder are involved in approximately 15 % of patients and a smaller number have pancreatic duct involvement [11–13]. Dominant strictures, defined as a diameter less than 1.5 mm in the common bile duct and less than 1.0 mm in the hepatic duct, are present in approximately half of PSC patients. Pseudodiverticula, particularly in the common bile duct are occasionally seen. While initially used as exclusionary criteria in PSC patients, the presence of biliary stones are now well-recognized as a common finding and frequent cause of cholangitis. There are three current modalities that can be used to image the biliary system. Endoscopic retrograde cholangiography (ERC) allows direct biliary visualization as well as also providing the opportunity to perform cytologic analysis, stricture dilation, removal of stones, and biliary stenting. Potential complications of ERC include bleeding, cholangitis, and pancreatitis [14]. Percutaneous hepatic cholangiography (PTC) also allows direct access to the biliary system but has similar complications to ERC and requires experienced radiologists as intrahepatic bile ducts are generally not dilated in PSC. The test of choice when attempting to make a diagnosis of PSC is the magnetic resonance cholangiography (MRC). The noninvasive nature of MRC limits complications and is more cost-effective than ERC or PTC. These advantages must be weighed against the fact that MRC unlike ERC and PTC does not offer the opportunity to perform biliary brushings for cytology nor intervene therapeutically. Magnetic resonance cholangiography also lacks sensitivity compared to ERC when assessing for peripheral bile duct changes. Once a diagnosis of PSC is established, there is no indication for further instrumentation of the biliary system unless there is a change in the patient's clinical status.

Histology

Liver biopsy at the present is not felt to be necessary to establish a diagnosis of PSC, nor to determine disease severity. Liver biopsy should be considered in all patients suspected of having small-duct PSC or overlap syndrome with autoimmune hepatitis. The classic finding when a liver biopsy is performed in PSC patients is the concentric fibrosis (onion-skinning) involving the periductal region. This lesion, however, is observed in only a minority of patients [12]. Additionally, biopsy sampling variation may fail to detect these lesions in patients who otherwise have classic cholangiographic findings.

Natural History

The natural history of PSC is highly variable and while it is a progressive disease, the rate of progression per year varies significantly in individual patients. Multiple studies have attempted to determine the time period from diagnosis to the need for liver transplantation or death and estimates range from 7 to 18 years from presentation [4, 15, 16]. Much of this variability is associated with the fact that some patients present early in their disease course without symptoms but have abnormal liver biochemistries, while others' initial presentation may be a complication of advanced disease with portal hypertension or cholangiocarcinoma.

Various prognostic models have been utilized in an attempt to predict future outcomes but their value is questionable in this clinical setting due the highly variable nature of PSC. The most common employed of these prognostic models is one proposed by the Mayo Clinic and utilizes the following variables; total bilirubin, age, presence or absence of variceal bleeding, serum albumin, and aspartate aminotransferase values [17].

Primary Sclerosing Cholangitis Variants

Small-Duct Primary Sclerosing Cholangitis

Small-duct PSC is characterized by cholestatic biochemistries with a normal cholangiogram. Liver biopsy is essential in this group for diagnostic purposes and may demonstrate the periductal damage and onion-skinning previously described. Small-duct PSC represents approximately 10 % of all PSC cases. Small-duct PSC patients may have symptoms but a greater percentage are asymptomatic when compared to large-duct PSC. Approximately 10–15 % of those with small-duct PSC will progress to large-duct PSC, typically over 5–10 years. Patients with small-duct PSC have a better long-term prognosis with fewer complications when compared to their large-duct counterparts [18, 19].

Overlap Syndrome with Autoimmune Hepatitis

Between 1 and 17% of patients with PSC will also have an overlap syndrome with autoimmune hepatitis [20–22]. These patients will present with a hepatocellular injury as well as cholestasis and have detectable antinuclear antibodies and anti-smooth muscle antibodies. Immunoglobulin G elevations, as in classical autoimmune hepatitis, are typically seen. Liver biopsy should therefore be performed in all patients with PSC who have aminotransferase values greater than five times the upper limit of normal or IgG values greater than two times the upper limit of normal. Liver biopsy demonstrates histologic findings of both conditions; the periductal "onion-skinning" damage seen in PSC and the interface hepatitis and prominent plasma cell infiltration which is classically described in autoimmune hepatitis. The autoimmune hepatitis component unlike the PSC component is responsive to immunosuppression, with the most common agents utilized being corticosteroids and azathioprine. Patients with overlap PSC and autoimmune hepatitis may progress more rapidly than those affected by PSC alone due to the combination of the hepatocellular and cholestatic components.

Primary Sclerosing Cholangitis in Association with Autoimmune Pancreatitis

Autoimmune pancreatitis is a manifestation of a systemic disorder affecting multiple organs and is associated with an elevated serum immunoglobulin G4 (IgG4). Histology of the pancreas shows a predominantly lymphocyte and plasma cell infiltrate. Pancreatic abnormalities include lesions that are frequently difficult to differentiate from malignancy as well as pancreatic duct strictures. A subset of these patients will have biliary strictures similar to those seen in PSC occasionally in the absence of pancreatic abnormalities, a condition occasionally referred to as IgG4 cholangiopathy. Those with IgG4 cholangiopathy tend to have a more aggressive disease course compared to those with PSC and normal IgG4 values [23, 24]. Primary sclerosing cholangitis associated with elevated IgG4 levels are frequently responsive to corticosteroid therapy and it is recommended to measure IgG4 levels in all newly diagnosed PSC patients [25].

Secondary Sclerosing Cholangitis

There are various conditions that can affect the biliary system and produce findings that mimic the strictures seen in PSC. Prior to making a diagnosis of PSC these secondary causes must be carefully looked for and eliminated as potential etiologies. Secondary causes include congenital biliary tract disorders such as biliary atresia and

Caroli's Disease, AIDS cholangiopathy, ischemic strictures, biliary malignancies such as cholangiocarcinoma not associated with PSC, previous biliary injuries as a result of surgery and chemical exposure to toxins such as fluxoridine, a pyrimidine analogue infused via the hepatic artery in patients with metastatic colon cancer to the liver [26].

Complications of Primary Sclerosing Cholangitis

Complications of PSC can be classified as those that are related to the cholestatic nature of the disorder and those that are unique to PSC.

Complications of Cholestatic Liver Disease

Cholestasis-related complications include pruritus, bone disease, fat soluble vitamin deficiency, and portal hypertension.

Pruritus

Pruritus can be one of the most disabling complications of cholestatic liver diseases with failure to respond to therapy frequently leading to frustration in both patients and clinicians. While much attention has been focused on the accumulation of biliary compounds in various tissues, the exact mechanism remains unknown [27]. There does not appear to be a strong correlation with the severity of liver disease and patients with mild to moderate biliary strictures may have the most severe symptoms. The subjective nature of pruritus makes accurate measurement difficult and while multiple tools including visual aids are available, they are not generally utilized in clinical practice. The treatment of pruritus generally involves a stepwise approach. First line therapy typically involves anion exchange resins such as cholestyramine initially at four grams twice daily (before and after breakfast if the gallbladder is present) and increasing to four times daily as necessary [28]. Patients must communicate with their pharmacist in order to ensure that cholestyramine does not interfere with the absorption of other medications or fat-soluble vitamins. Side effects include mild constipation, diarrhea, abdominal pain, flatulence, nausea, and vomiting. If the pruritus remains refractory, rifampin at doses of 150–300 mg twice daily can be added with careful monitoring of serum liver and renal biochemistries [29]. Additional first line agents include Sertraline, a selective serotonin uptake inhibitor, at 100 mg daily and nighttime antihistamines due to their sedative side-effect profile. Second line therapies include naltrexone, an opioid antagonist, at 50 mg daily and phenobarbital at doses of 60–100 mg nightly [30]. Third line therapies include plasmapheresis which is effective but cumbersome. Therapies that have been proposed but lack supporting data include dronabinol, ondansetron, ultraviolet light, and S-adenosylmethionine (SAM-E). Liver transplant has been proposed for patients with severe, refractory pruritus despite low Model for End Stage Liver Disease (MELD) scores. Exception points for patients with low MELD scores can be requested due to refractory pruritus but the subjective nature of this complication has led to few exceptions being granted.

Bone Disease

Bone disease in the setting of chronic liver diseases is frequently referred to as hepatic osteodystrophy and includes osteopenia and osteoporosis. Both are now recognized as a frequent finding in all patients with chronic liver diseases but are most pronounced in those with cholestasis [31]. The mechanism for bone disease in PSC is likely multifactorial and includes decreased formation and increased resorption. Vitamin D deficiency may play a minor role. Longer duration of IBD, older age, female gender, and low body weight are other contributing factors. All patients with newly diagnosed PSC should undergo bone mineral density assessment (DEXA) and at intervals of 2–3 years based on initial results [32, 33]. Treatment includes calcium 1200 mg daily and vitamin D 1000 IU supplementation. This supplementation should be in conjunction with a regular exercise regimen. Hormone replacement while effective is not generally employed due to the side-effect profile. Bisphosphonate therapy is beneficial in patients with osteoporosis and primary biliary cirrhosis and is also indicated for those with osteoporosis and PSC [34]. Bisphosphonates should be avoided in those patients with esophageal varices as they have been shown to increase the risk of bleeding due to esophageal ulcerations. Intravenous bisphosphonates are effective options in those with osteoporosis who have contraindications to oral therapy due to esophageal varices.

Fat-Soluble Vitamin Deficiency

Patients with cholestatic hepatic disorders including PSC are at risk for developing malabsorption and deficiency of vitamins A, D, E, and K due to decrease in the availability of bile salts [35]. While bile salt production from cholesterol and bile acids is normal, the impaired flow of bile salts due to biliary strictures results in a relative deficiency in bile salt function in the small intestine. Vitamin A deficiency is rarely of clinical consequence. Levels can be measured and effective supplementation is available. Care must be taken to avoid vitamin A toxicity from over-supplementation. Vitamin D deficiency is the most clinically significant of all the fat-soluble vitamin deficiencies. As previously mentioned, by itself it is not responsible for bone disease, but likely plays a contributing role. Vitamin D levels are also easily measured and supplemented. Vitamin E deficiency is rare and can be supplemented if serum levels are decreased. Vitamin K deficiency can lead to elevated prothrombin times and typically responds well to supplementation.

Portal Hypertension

Patients with PSC frequently progress to cirrhosis and develop portal hypertension complicated by esophageal and gastric varices, ascites, and hepatic encephalopathy. These patients should be treated similar to non-PSC cirrhotic patients. While current recommendations are for all patients with cirrhosis to undergo an upper endoscopy to evaluate for varices, those affected by PSC are also at risk for the development of pre-cirrhotic, pre-sinusoidal portal hypertension and should therefore undergo endoscopic evaluation. Nonselective beta blockade for primary prophylaxis of documented varices is effective with band ligation utilized in those intolerant of beta blockers. Sodium restricted diets in combination with diuretics, most commonly spironolactone and furosemide, are the standard of care in patients with ascites. Beta blockers should be avoided in PSC patients with refractory ascites due to concerns for the development of acute kidney injury. Avoidance of factors that precipitate hepatic encephalopathy including intravascular volume depletion, infections, gastrointestinal bleeding, and electrolyte disturbances are paramount. Minimal hepatic encephalopathy, as well as overt encephalopathy, should be treated with lactulose and if necessary the addition of rifaximin as a second agent.

Complications Specific to Primary Sclerosing Cholangitis

Disease-specific complications associated with PSC include IBD and colorectal cancer, peristomal varices, dominant strictures, biliary stones, gallbladder carcinoma, and cholangiocarcinoma.

Inflammatory Bowel Disease and Colorectal Carcinoma

The majority of patients with PSC will have concurrent IBD, more frequently ulcerative colitis than Crohn Disease with colonic involvement. Up to 7.5 % of IBD patients will be affected by PSC [3, 4]. The IBD is typically diagnosed prior to PSC in the majority of patients, but can vary with some patients' first symptoms of IBD being years after the diagnosis of PSC or even following liver transplantation. Inflammatory Bowel Disease in the setting of PSC differs from those not affected by PSC with more rectal sparing, greater right-sided disease, more backwash ileitis and more quiescent disease in those with PSC [36, 37]. While all patients with chronic colitis are at increased risk for the development of colorectal cancer, those IBD patients with PSC are at a much greater risk [38]. Current recommendations include colonoscopy every one to 2 years in those IBD patients who also carry a diagnosis of PSC. Colon biopsies should always be obtained to evaluate for dysplastic changes. The use of ursodeoxycholic acid (UDCA) has been advocated by some as decreasing the risk of colonic dysplasia and colorectal carcinoma based on two small studies [39, 40], but subsequent studies have not supported its effectiveness. Patients with PSC and IBD who undergo liver transplant have been shown as a group to have more difficult to manage IBD despite the fact that their post-transplant medical regimen includes one or more immunosuppressive agents.

Peristomal Varices

Patients with concurrent IBD and PSC have frequently undergone proctocolectomy with ileostomy formation due to refractory colitis or colorectal cancer. These patients will occasionally develop peristomal varices. While not associated with the mortality seen in patients with esophageal or gastric variceal bleeding, the morbidity and impact on quality of life can be significant. Local temporizing measures have been of limited efficacy with transjugular intrahepatic portosystemic shunt (TIPS) proving to be beneficial in refractory cases if no contraindications exist.

Dominant Biliary Strictures

Dominant strictures, defined as a diameter less than 1.5 mm in the common bile duct and less than 1 mm in the hepatic duct, are seen in up to half of all PSC patients [41, 42]. The length of these strictures varies but is typically short. Dominant strictures can result in deterioration of previously stable disease and lead to worsening jaundice, pruritus, and cholangitis. Strictures should be promptly addressed with endoscopic therapy being the preferred method. Following sphincterotomy, balloon dilation of the stricture with stent placement is frequently necessary. The need for stents, their associated exchanges and instrumentation increases the risk of cholangitis and mandates the need for pre and post-procedure antibiotics. Unfortunately, strictures in the intrahepatic region are not always accessible endoscopically and may require a percutaneous approach. Finally, it is imperative to perform brush cytology of dominant strictures whether by endoscopic or percutaneous approaches to differentiate dominant nonmalignant strictures from cholangiocarcinoma.

Biliary Stones

As previously mentioned, biliary stones, once considered exclusionary for PSC, are now recognized as a common finding. Strictures, in particular dominant strictures, and impaired bile flow play key roles in stone formation. Complications include pain, cholangitis, and clinical deterioration. Aggressive antibiotic use particularly for biliary pathogens and prompt endoscopic stone retrieval are indicated. While there may be a role for UDCA to prevent stone formation and improve bile flow, little data currently exists.

Gallbladder Disease Including Adenocarcinoma

Primary sclerosing cholangitis involves the gallbladder as well as the cystic duct in 15 % of patients. Gallstones, which are common in the general population, are seen in up to 26 % of PSC patients [13]. Patients with PSC are also at risk for the development of mass lesions. Gallbladder polyps in particular are common and can lead to dysplasia and adenocarcinoma [43]. Current recommendations include performing annual gallbladder ultrasounds to evaluate for mass lesions and if present for the patients to undergo cholecystectomy regardless of the size of the lesion unless contraindications exists [32].

Cholangiocarcinoma

One of the most feared complications of PSC is the development of cholangiocarcinoma. Approximately 50 % of patients diagnosed with cholangiocarcinoma will be diagnosed within one year of their PSC diagnosis. Afterwards the annual risk is 0.5–1.0 % with a 10-year risk of 7–10 % [44–47]. Unfortunately, a large number have advanced disease including loco-regional as well as distant disease at the time of diagnosis. It remains unclear as to what specific factors in PSC patients predispose patients to develop cholangiocarcinoma. The differentiation between benign strictures and cholangiocarcinoma, particularly in dominant strictures, remains a challenge. Biochemical testing with CA19-9 is limited by the fact that it is nonspecific and can be elevated from benign strictures and cholangitis. Patients who lack the Lewis antigen will not demonstrate detectable CA19-9 even in the presence of cholangiocarcinoma. Imaging studies with computerized tomography, ultrasound, MRC, and ERC fail to consistently differentiate benign from malignant strictures. Biliary brushing done at the time of ERC has long been recognized to have good specificity but sensitivities under 50 %. Newer approaches to aid in the diagnosis of cholangiocarcinoma include fluorescent in situ hybridization (FISH). This technique evaluates cells obtained from suspicious lesions by brush cytology and evaluates for polysomy (the duplication of two or more chromosomes) in greater than five cells [48]. At the present time, there are no formal recommendations from any society regarding cholangiocarcinoma screening and surveillance with CA19-9, MRC, cholangioscopy during ERC or other imaging modalities.

Treatment of cholangiocarcinoma has traditionally been limited. The diffuse biliary nature of PSC has made surgical resection an option for a limited few and chemotherapy has not been shown to be of significant benefit. More recently, liver transplant in a highly selected group of patients with hilar lesions less than three cm in diameter and without evidence of spread has been evaluated. These patients undergo external beam as well as brachytherapy in conjunction with chemotherapy. Percutaneous transhepatic cholangiography should be avoided in these patients for fear of seeding the peritoneum with malignant cells. Some centers are reporting 5-year survival comparable to non-cholangiocarcinoma patients [49]. Transplant centers with an active protocol in place can petition regional review boards for MELD exception points for these patients.

Hepatocellular Carcinoma

While not unique to cholestatic liver diseases or PSC, patients with established cirrhosis are at risk for developing hepatocellular carcinoma (HCC). Screening and surveillance for HCC is indicated in all cirrhotic patients regardless of age and involves ultrasound examination every 6 months with suspicious lesions warranting further evaluation with a dynamic study such as CT or MRI [50]. The role of alpha fetoprotein for screening of HCC remains controversial and no recommendations can be made at this time.

Medical Therapy in Primary Sclerosing Cholangitis

Numerous agents have been evaluated in the treatment of PSC and there is no evidence to suggest that there is effective medical therapy. Agents that have been evaluated in small trials include corticosteroids, cyclosporine, tacrolimus, azathioprine, methotrexate, penicillamine, and colchicine. Antibiotics while indicated for invasive procedures and for episodes of cholangitis, do not alter the natural history of PSC. The most studied of all agents is ursodeoxycholic acid (UDCA) which has been shown to slow disease progression and alter the natural history in patients with primary biliary cirrhosis (PBC) at doses ranging from 13 to 15 mg/kg/day [51]. Similar doses in PSC patients resulted in biochemical improvement but failed to alter the natural history [52]. Due to the large bile duct involvement in PSC relative to PBC, it was theorized that greater doses would be necessary for a benefit to be seen. Despite increasing doses, this benefit did not materialize and a multicenter trial evaluating doses of 28–30 mg/kg/day was terminated early due to an increased frequency of decompensation, need for transplant and death in the treatment group [53]. As previously mentioned, corticosteroid therapy is indicated in patients with IgG4- associated cholangitis and in combination with azathioprine in those with PSC-AIH overlap.

Liver Transplantation for Primary Sclerosing Cholangitis

Liver transplantation has been shown to be the only effective therapy that alters the natural history of PSC with approximately 250 transplants performed annually in the United States for PSC. Listing for liver transplantation is overseen and regulated by the United Network for Organ Sharing (UNOS) and utilizes the MELD score to determine listing priority. Refractory pruritus, recurrent bacterial cholangitis, and cholangiocarcinoma are PSC-specific complications that will be considered by regional review boards for MELD exception points [54]. Due to the diffuse biliary strictures associated with PSC as well as the risk of future cholangiocarcinoma in the recipient remnant bile duct, the biliary anastomosis performed at the time of transplantation is a Roux-Y-choledochojejunostomy. Overall results following liver transplant for PSC are excellent with 5-year survival of approximately 85%. Recurrent PSC in the transplant liver occurs in approximately 20% of patients and will occasionally result in the need for retransplantation [55, 56]. Biliary strictures which can be due to other factors including ischemia and hepatic artery injury are frequently difficult to differentiate from recurrent PSC strictures. Biliary access for interventional purposes following liver transplant typically involves a percutaneous approach due to the Roux-Y-choledochojejunostomy biliary anastomosis.

Future Trends

There are three major areas in PSC that will require greater attention if we are to make significant impact on morbidity and mortality.

First, there is no effective medical therapy and this requires immediate attention. Large, multicenter, randomized controlled trials are urgently needed. Without medical therapy, physicians are forced to address complications while taking a wait and see approach regarding liver transplantation.

Second, consensus recommendations regarding cholangiocarcinoma screening and surveillance need to be developed. Imaging studies and/or biomarkers that are both cost-effective and have acceptable sensitivity and specificity are currently lacking. This has resulted in multiple imaging modalities usually in combination with CA 19-9 being employed despite lack of supporting data.

Finally, once a lesion that is suspicious for cholangiocarcinoma develops, current diagnostic testing including brush cytology and FISH are suboptimal. While the negative predictive value for the combination of brush cytology and FISH is 90%, the positive predictive value is only 50% [48]. Liver transplantation is now an effective therapy in selected patients with cholangiocarcinoma. It is essential that patients with cholangiocarcinoma be identified as early as possible in order to undergo transplant evaluation at centers with established protocols.

References

1. Bambha K, Kim WR, Tawalkar J, et al. Incidence, clinical spectrum, and outcomes of primary sclerosing cholangitis in a United States community. Gastroenterology. 2003;125(5):1364–9.
2. Boberg KM, Aadland E, Jahnsen J, et al. Incidence and prevalence of primary biliary cirrhosis, primary sclerosing cholangitis, and autoimmune hepatitis in a Norwegian population. Scand J Gastroenterol. 1999;33(1):99–103.
3. Schrumpf E, Fausa O, Elgio K, et al. Hepatobiliary complications of inflammatory bowel disease. Semin Liver Dis. 1988;8:201–9.
4. Wiesner R, Grambsch P, Dickson E, et al. Primary sclerosing cholangitis: natural history, prognostic factors and survival analysis. Hepatology. 1989;10:430–6.

5. Loftus E, Harewood G, Loftus C, et al. PSC-IBD: a unique form of inflammatory bowel disease associated with primary sclerosing cholangitis. Gut. 2005;54:91–6.
6. Jorge A, Esley C, Ahamuda J. Family incidence of primary sclerosing cholangitis associated with immunologic diseases. Endoscopy. 1987;19:114–7.
7. Donaldson P, Farrant J, Wilkinson M, et al. Dual association of HLA DR2 and DR3 with primary sclerosing cholangitis. Hepatology. 1991;13:129–33.
8. Donaldson P, Doherty D, Haylar K, et al. Susceptibility to autoimmune chronic active hepatitis: human leukocyte antigens DR4 and A1-B8-DR3 are independent risk factors. Hepatology. 1991;13:701–6.
9. Norris S, Elli K, Collins R, et al. Mapping MHC-encoded susceptibility and resistance in primary sclerosing cholangitis: the role of MICA polymorphism. Gastroenterology. 2001;120(6):1475–82.
10. Hov J, Boberg K, Karlsen T. Autoantibodies in primary sclerosing cholangitis. World J Gastroenterol. 2008;14:3781–91.
11. MacCarty R, LaRusso N, Wiesner R, et al. Primary sclerosing cholangitis: findings on cholangiography and pancreatography. Radiology. 1983;149:39–44.
12. Lee Y, Kaplan M. Primary sclerosing cholangitis. N Engl J Med. 1995;332:924–33.
13. Brandt D, MacCarty R, Charboneau J, et al. Gallbladder disease in patients with primary sclerosing cholangitis. Am J Roentgenol. 1988;150:571–4.
14. Navaneethan U, Jegadeesan R, Nayak S, et al. ERCP-related adverse events in patients with primary sclerosing cholangitis. Gastrointest Endosc. 2015;81:410–9.
15. Aadland E, Schrumpf E, Fausa O, et al. Primary sclerosing cholangitis: a long-term follow-up study. Scand J Gastroenterol. 1997;22:655–64.
16. Farrant J, Hayllar K, Wilkinson M, et al. Natural history and prognostic variables in primary sclerosing cholangitis. Gastroenterology. 1991;100:1710–7.
17. http://www.mayoclinic.org/gi-rst/mayomodel3.html.
18. Wee A, Ludwig J. Pericholangitis in chronic ulcerative colitis; primary sclerosing cholangitis of the small bile ducts? Ann Intern Med. 1985;102:581–7.
19. Chapman R. Small duct primary sclerosing cholangitis. J Hepatol. 2002;36:692–4.
20. Van Buuren H, Hoogstraten H, Terkivatan T, et al. High prevalence of autoimmune hepatitis among patients with primary sclerosing cholangitis. J Hepatol. 2000;33:543–8.
21. Kaya M, Angulo P, Lindor K. Overlap of autoimmune hepatitis and primary sclerosing cholangitis: an evaluation of a modified scoring system. J Hepatol. 2000;33:537–42.
22. Floreani A, Rizzotto E, Ferrerra F, et al. Clinical course and outcome of autoimmune hepatitis/primary sclerosing cholangitis overlap syndrome. Am J Gastroenterol. 2005;100:1516–22.
23. Bjornsson E, Chari S, Smyrk T, et al. Immunoglobulin G4 associated cholangitis: description an emerging clinical entity based on review of the literature. Hepatology. 2007;45:1547–54.
24. Mendes F, Jorgensen R, Keach J, et al. Elevated serum IgG4 concentration in patients with primary sclerosing cholangitis. Am J Gastroenterol. 2006;101:2070–5.
25. Hamano H, Kawa S, Horiuchi A, et al. High serum IgG4 concentrations in patients with sclerosing pancreatitis. N Engl J Med. 2001;344:732–8.
26. Iman M, Talwalkar J, Lindor K. Secondary sclerosing cholangitis; pathogenesis, diagnosis and management. Clin Liver Dis. 2013;17:269–77.
27. Jones E, Vergasa N. The pruritus of cholestasis and the opioid system. JAMA. 1992;268:3359–62.
28. Datta D, Sherlock S. Treatment of pruritus of obstructive jaundice with cholestyramine. Br Med J. 1963;1:216–9.
29. Bachs L, Pares A, Elena M, et al. Effects of long-term rifampicin administration in primary biliary cirrhosis. Gastroenterology. 1992;102:2077–80.
30. Bloomer J, Boyer J. Phenobarbital effects in cholestatic liver diseases. Ann Intern Med. 1975;82:310–7.
31. Sokhi R, Anantharaju A, Kondaveeti R, et al. Bone mineral density among cirrhotic patients awaiting liver transplantation. Liver Transpl. 2004;10:648–53.
32. Chapman R, Fevery J, Kalloo A, et al. Diagnosis and management of primary sclerosing cholangitis. AASLD practice guidelines. Hepatology. 2010;51:660–78.

33. Crippin J, Jorgensen R, Dickson E, et al. Hepatic osteodystrophy in primary biliary cirrhosis; effects of medical treatment. Am J Gastroenterol. 1994;89:47–50.
34. Zein C, Lindor K, Angulo P. Alendronate improves bone mineral density in primary biliary cirrhosis: a randomized placebo-controlled trial. Hepatology. 2005;42:62–771.
35. Phillips J, Angulo P, Petterson T, et al. Fat-soluble vitamin levels in patients with primary biliary cirrhosis. Am J Gastroenterol. 2001;96:2745–50.
36. Broome U, Bergquist A. Primary sclerosing cholangitis, inflammatory bowel disease, and colon cancer. Semin Liver Dis. 2006;26:31–41.
37. Schrumpf E, Elgio K, Fausa O, et al. Sclerosing cholangitis in ulcerative colitis. Scand J Gastroenterol. 1980;15:689–97.
38. Broome U, Lofberg R, Beress B, et al. Primary sclerosing cholangitis and ulcerative colitis: evidence for increased neoplastic potential. Hepatology. 1995;22:1404–8.
39. Pardi D, Loftus E, Kremers W, et al. Ursodeoxycholic acid as a chemopreventive agent in patients with ulcerative colitis and primary sclerosing cholangitis. Gastroenterology. 2003;124:889–93.
40. Tung B, Edmond M, Haggitt R, et al. Ursodiol use is associated with lower prevalence of colonic neoplasia in patients with ulcerative colitis and primary sclerosing cholangitis. Ann Intern Med. 2001;134:89–95.
41. Stiehl A, Rudolph G, Kloters-Plachky P, et al. Development of dominant bile duct stenosis in patients with primary sclerosing cholangitis treated with ursodeoxycholic acid: outcome after endoscopic treatment. J Hepatol. 2002;36:151–6.
42. Bjornsson E, Lindqvist-Ottosson J, Asztely M, et al. Dominant strictures in patients with primary sclerosing cholangitis. Am J Gastroenterol. 2004;99:502–8.
43. Lewis J, Talwalkar J, Rosen C, et al. Prevalence and risk factors for gallbladder neoplasia in patients with primary sclerosing cholangitis; evidence for a metaplasia-dysplasia-carcinoma sequence. Am J Surg Pathol. 2007;31:907–13.
44. Boberg K, Lind G. Primary sclerosing cholangitis and malignancy. Best Pract Res Clin Gastroenterol. 2011;25:753–64.
45. Bergquist A, Ekborn A, Olsson R, et al. Hepatic and extrahepatic malignancies in primary sclerosing cholangitis. J Hepatol. 2002;36:321–7.
46. Burak K, Angulo P, Pasha T, et al. Incidence and risk factors for cholangiocarcinoma in primary sclerosing cholangitis. Am J Gastroenterol. 2004;99:523–6.
47. Boberg K, Bergquist A, Mitchell S. Cholangiocarcinoma in primary sclerosing cholangitis: risk factors and clinical presentation. Scand J Gastroenterol. 2003;37:1205–11.
48. Moreno L, Kipp B, Halling K, et al. Advanced cytologic techniques for the detection of malignant pancreatobiliary strictures. Gastroenterology. 2006;131:1064–72.
49. Rea D, Heimbach J, Rosen C, et al. Liver transplantation with neoadjuvant chemoradiation is more effective than resection for hilar cholangiocarcinoma. Ann Surg. 2005;242:451–8.
50. Bruix J, Sherman M. Management of hepatocellular carcinoma; an update. AASLD practice guidelines. Hepatology. 2005;42:1208–36.
51. Coperchot C, Carrat F, Bahr A, et al. The effect of ursodeoxycholic acid therapy on the natural history of primary biliary cirrhosis. Gastroenterology. 2005;128:297–303.
52. Lindor K. Ursodiol for primary sclerosing cholangitis. Mayo Primary Sclerosing Cholangitis-Ursodeoxycholic Acid Study Group. N Engl J Med. 1997;336:691–5.
53. Lindor K, Kowdley K, Velimir A, et al. High-dose ursodeoxycholic acid for the treatment of primary sclerosing cholangitis. Hepatology. 2008;50:808–14.
54. Gores G, Nagorney D, Rosen C. Cholangiocarcinoma: is transplantation an option? For whom? Hepatology. 2007;47:455–9.
55. Graziadei I, Wiesner R, Marotta P, et al. Long-term results of patients undergoing liver transplantation for primary sclerosing cholangitis. Hepatology. 1999;30:1121–7.
56. Campsen J, Zimmerman M, Trotter J, et al. Clinically recurrent primary sclerosing cholangitis following liver transplantation; a time course. Liver Transpl. 2008;14:181–5.

Chapter 18
Autoimmune Liver Diseases: Overlap Syndromes

Albert J. Czaja

Patient Questions

1. What is an overlap syndrome?
2. How are overlap syndromes treated?
3. How will I do?

Answers

1. What is an overlap syndrome?

   An overlap syndrome has mixed features that suggest the concurrence of two immune-mediated liver diseases. Usually there is a predominant disease, such as autoimmune hepatitis, primary biliary cholangitis (PBC), or primary sclerosing cholangitis (PSC), and coincidental background features of another immune-mediated liver disease. Autoimmune hepatitis has the least disease-specific diagnostic features, and it is the most common component of the overlap syndromes. PBC and PSC have the most disease-specific diagnostic features, and an overlap syndrome with concurrent findings of PBC and PSC is rare. The overlap syndromes are probably variant forms of classical immune-mediated liver disease in which atypical laboratory, histological, or serological findings complicate the diagnosis. They could also a be transition stage in the evolution of classical disease, two classical diseases occurring in the same individual, or separate pathological entities with their own distinctive pathogenic mechanisms and clinical outcomes. The overlap syndromes occur in 3–17 % of patients with autoimmune

A.J. Czaja, M.D. (✉)
Division of Gastroenterology and Hepatology, Mayo Clinic College of Medicine,
200 First Street S.W., Rochester, MN 55905, USA
e-mail: czaja.albert@mayo.edu

© Springer International Publishing Switzerland 2017
K. Saeian, R. Shaker (eds.), *Liver Disorders*,
DOI 10.1007/978-3-319-30103-7_18

liver disease, and they almost always include features of autoimmune hepatitis either as the predominant or secondary component. The overlap syndromes are mainly clinical descriptions that have not been formally endorsed as separate pathological entities, and their major clinical relevance is that they respond variably to conventional treatments. The International Autoimmune Hepatitis Group has proposed that patients be categorized by their predominant disease and that those with overlapping features not be considered as separate entities.

2. How are overlap syndromes treated?

Management guidelines promulgated by the American Association for the Study of Liver Diseases (AASLD) and the European Association for the Study of the Liver (EASL) have recommended combination therapy with corticosteroids in combination with low-dose ursodeoxycholic acid (UDCA) (typically, 13–15 mg/kg daily). These recommendations are not strongly evidenced based, and treatments can be tailored to suit the predominant disease component and the individual treatment response. Patients with autoimmune hepatitis and background features of PBC who have serum levels of alkaline phosphatase ≤2-fold the upper limit of the normal range (UNL) may respond to conventional corticosteroid therapy, and patients with predominant features of PBC with weak or transient features of autoimmune hepatitis may respond to therapy with UDCA (13–15 mg/kg daily). Patients with 2 of 3 features of autoimmune hepatitis (serum alanine aminotransferase level ≥5-fold ULN, immunoglobulin G level ≥2-fold ULN or positive test for smooth muscle antibodies, and histological features of moderate to severe interface hepatitis) and 2 of 3 features of PBC (serum alkaline phosphatase level ≥2-fold ULN or γ-glutamyl transpeptidase level ≥5-fold ULN, positive test for AMA, and histological evidence of florid duct lesions) are candidates for combination therapy. Patients with features of autoimmune hepatitis and PSC are candidates for a treatment trial with corticosteroids in combination with UDCA (13–15 mg daily), recognizing that no treatment regimen has been consistently effective in this syndrome. Liver transplantation should be considered in patients who have or develop features of liver failure.

3. How will I do?

Treatment response is variable in part because of the empiric nature of the treatment and the absence of an established therapy for PSC. The severity of the cholestatic components, as reflected in the serum alkaline phosphatase and γ-glutamyl transpeptidase levels, histological findings of bile duct injury or loss, and the presence or absence of PSC, influence the responsiveness to treatment. Patients with autoimmune hepatitis, antimitochondrial antibodies, and histological evidence of isolated lymphoid, pleomorphic, or destructive cholangitis respond as well to conventional corticosteroid therapy as patients with classical autoimmune hepatitis if they have a serum alkaline phosphatase level ≤2-fold ULN. Clinical, laboratory, and histological features improve to normal or near-normal in 81 %, and disease progression (treatment failure) occurs in 14 %. Patients with more pronounced features of PBC, including serum alkaline phosphatase level >2-fold ULN or γ-glutamyl transpeptidase level ≥5-fold ULN and florid duct lesions on tissue examination, respond more frequently to combination therapy with corticosteroids and low-dose UDCA than treatment with corticosteroids or UDCA alone. Most patients have significant improvements in the serum levels of alkaline phosphatase, γ-glutamyl transpeptidase, and alanine aminotransferase (ALT) levels, and progressive hepatic fibrosis is prevented. Combination therapy has been effective in 20–100 % of patients with overlapping features of autoimmune hepatitis and PSC, and the variability of response probably reflects the severity of the cholestatic components. Median graft (10 years) and patient (11 years) survivals after liver transplantation for an overlap syndrome are similar to those of patients transplanted for a single immune-mediated liver disease, but the frequency of recurrent disease is greater (5 years, 53 %; 10 years, 69 %).

Background

Early diagnostic criteria for autoimmune hepatitis emphasized its inflammatory nature [1], and diagnostic algorithms were refined to strengthen the distinction between autoimmune hepatitis and the cholestatic diseases of primary biliary cholangitis (PBC) and primary sclerosing cholangitis (PSC) [2–6]. The subsequent codification of diagnostic criteria for autoimmune hepatitis [4, 7, 8], PBC [9], and PSC [10, 11] characterized the classical phenotypes, and diseases with mixed inflammatory and cholestatic features became more difficult to accommodate within the nomenclature [12–14]. Designations emerged to distinguish the syndromes with mixed inflammatory and cholestatic features from the classical phenotypes, and the concept of an overlap syndrome evolved [12, 15–27].

The diagnostic scoring systems for autoimmune hepatitis that had been developed mainly to ensure homogenous patient populations in clinical trials [4, 6] were applied in efforts to identify and quantify the autoimmune hepatitis component of a mixed syndrome [28–32], and other scoring systems emerged to grade the cholestatic component [33]. Empiric treatment strategies were promulgated, and outcomes that supported or dismissed empiric treatments varied in part because of the lack of established diagnostic criteria for the overlap syndromes and the heterogeneity of the treatment algorithms that were applied [16, 32, 34–48].

The absence of rigorous diagnostic and therapeutic guidelines and the burgeoning clinical experiences with the hybrid syndromes prompted the International Autoimmune Hepatitis Group (IAIHG) to issue a position statement which encouraged the designation of the mixed syndromes by their predominant component without reference to their atypical ("overlapping") features [49]. The IAIHG also cautioned against the misapplication of its diagnostic scoring systems for the diagnosis of these syndromes, and it projected that the performance of well-designed controlled clinical trials to resolve treatment issues was unlikely [49]. The American Association for the Study of Liver Diseases (AASLD) [10] and the European

Association for the Study of the Liver (EASL) [10, 11] endorsed treatment regimens based mainly on the combination of immunosuppressive medications with ursodeoxycholic acid (UDCA), but the clinical evidence for these recommendations was recognized as weak [25, 49].

The overlap syndromes of autoimmune hepatitis, PBC, and PSC continue to present diagnostic and therapeutic problems, and their major clinical relevance is their variable response to treatments conventionally used for the classical phenotypes [16, 46]. Therapies are empiric; regimens are individualized; and outcomes are uncertain [22–27].

Diagnosis

The overlap syndromes should be considered when features are recognized in otherwise classical autoimmune hepatitis, PBC, or PBC that are inconsistent with the conventional presentation [12, 24, 50]. These features commonly indicate excessive inflammatory activity in a mainly cholestatic disease (PBC or PSC) or unusual cholestasis in a mainly inflammatory disease (autoimmune hepatitis). The unusual inflammatory or cholestatic features may be recognized at presentation or develop later [36, 47, 51–55], and an overlap syndrome should be considered in all patients who fail to respond to conventional therapy for the classical disease [16, 24, 56]. Endoscopic or magnetic resonance cholangiography is warranted in patients with autoimmune hepatitis and concurrent inflammatory bowel disease, cholestatic laboratory features, histological evidence of bile duct injury or loss in the absence of AMA-positivity, or steroid-refractory liver disease [22, 24, 56, 57]. Hepatic fibrosis can distort the intrahepatic bile ducts and mistakenly suggest PSC by cholangiography, and focal bile duct strictures and dilations are required to confirm its presence [58, 59].

Autoimmune Hepatitis and PBC

The diagnosis of an overlap syndrome between autoimmune hepatitis and PBC requires predominant features of autoimmune hepatitis and findings suggestive of PBC, including antimitochondrial antibodies (AMA), elevated serum alkaline phosphatase and γ-glutamyl transpeptidase (GGT) levels, and histological findings of bile duct injury or loss [24–27] (Table 18.1). Patients with predominant features of PBC may have coincidental features of autoimmune hepatitis, including antinuclear antibodies (ANA), smooth muscle antibodies (SMA), atypically high serum levels of aspartate aminotransferase (AST), alanine aminotransferase (ALT) and immunoglobulin G (IgG), and histological findings of interface hepatitis [37, 41, 60, 61]. The designation of an overlap syndrome between autoimmune hepatitis and PBC is an insufficient descriptor of the clinical phenotype, and the distinction between

Table 18.1 Diagnostic features of the overlap syndromes

Overlap syndrome	Diagnostic features
AIH>PBC	Typical AIH with prominent interface hepatitis [16, 37, 60, 61]
	Serum AP level <2-fold ULN [16, 94]
	Serum IgG level above ULN [61]
	AMA present [16, 94]
	Mild cholangitis, isolated destructive lesions, or rare ductopenia [66, 96]
AIH=PBC	Equally weighted features of AIH and PBC (Paris criteria) [35, 49]
	2 of 3 features of AIH [35]:
	Serum ALT ≥5-fold ULN
	IgG level ≥2-fold ULN or presence of SMA
	Moderate-severe interface hepatitis
	2 of 3 features of PBC [35]:
	Serum AP level ≥2-fold ULN or GGT level ≥5-fold ULN
	AMA present
	Florid duct lesions (destructive cholangitis)
	Sensitivity, 92 %; specificity, 97 % (against clinical judgment) [62]
	EASL requires interface hepatitis in all patients [11, 49]
PBC>AIH	Predominant features of PBC [41]
	Mild or transient inflammatory features of AIH [41]
	Outside Paris criteria [63]
AIH−PSC	Features of autoimmune hepatitis [16]
	AMA absent [16]
	Serum AP and GGT levels frequently increased [16, 65]
	Bile duct injury or loss by histological examination [66]
	Focal bile duct strictures and dilations by ERC or MRC [16, 58, 59, 65]
	Concurrent ulcerative colitis commonly present [16, 56, 65, 68]
AIH−Cholestasis	Predominant features of AIH [16, 74]
	Serum AP and/or GGT levels above ULN [16, 74]
	AMA absent [16, 74, 82]
	Bile duct injury or loss by histological examination [69–73]
	Normal ERC or MRC [16, 74]
	May represent AMA-negative PBC or small duct PSC [77–82]

AIH autoimmune hepatitis, *ALT* alanine aminotransferase, *AMA* antimitochondrial antibodies, *AP* alkaline phosphatase, *ERC* endoscopic retrograde cholangiography, *GGT* gamma glutamyl transferase, IgG immunoglobulin G, *MRC* magnetic resonance cholangiography, *PBC* primary biliary cholangitis, *PSC* primary sclerosing cholangitis, *ULN* upper limit of the normal range

Numbers in brackets are references

autoimmune hepatitis with features of PBC and PBC with features of autoimmune hepatitis should be made to ensure an accurate diagnosis and appropriate management strategy [24, 49].

The "Paris criteria" provide a uniform diagnostic approach, and they define an overlap syndrome in which the features of autoimmune hepatitis and PBC are equally weighted [35, 49, 62] (Table 18.1). Three hallmark features of autoimmune hepatitis (serum ALT level ≥5 times the upper limit of the normal range [ULN], IgG level ≥twice ULN or positive test for SMA, and histological findings of moderate to severe interface hepatitis) must be present with three hallmark features of PBC (serum alkaline phosphatase level ≥twice ULN or GGT ≥5 times ULN, positive test for AMA, and histological evidence of florid duct lesions) [35, 49]. The sensitivity and specificity of the "Paris criteria" for the overlap syndrome of autoimmune hepatitis and PBC are 92 % and 97 %, respectively, using clinical judgment as the gold standard for diagnosis [62]. EASL has supported these diagnostic recommendations with the stipulation that interface hepatitis must be present in all patients with this overlap syndrome [11, 49].

Not captured by the "Paris criteria" are patients with predominant features of autoimmune hepatitis who have AMA and histological findings of bile duct injury or loss but less pronounced manifestations of cholestasis (serum alkaline phosphatase level <twice ULN and GGT level <5-fold ULN) [16] (Table 18.1). Similarly, patients with predominant features of PBC who have less-pronounced manifestations of liver inflammation (serum ALT level <5-fold ULN and IgG level <twice ULN) can be overlooked [41, 63]. Clinical judgment remains the gold standard for the diagnosis of the overlap syndromes, and patients with mixed features cannot be excluded from the diagnosis by arbitrarily set criteria [24, 26]. In one study, the "Paris criteria" identified the overlap syndrome in only 1 % of patients with PBC, whereas criteria that included patients with less-pronounced mixed features and responsiveness to corticosteroids increased the yield almost threefold [63].

Autoimmune Hepatitis and PSC

The diagnosis of an overlap syndrome between autoimmune hepatitis and PSC requires predominant features of autoimmune hepatitis, absence of AMA, and cholangiographic evidence of focal bile duct strictures and dilations [24–26, 57] (Table 18.1). Concurrent ulcerative colitis is commonly present [16, 56]; serum alkaline phosphatase and GGT levels are usually increased [64, 65]; and histological examination frequently discloses bile duct injury or loss [66]. Children with autoimmune hepatitis and cholangiographic changes of bile duct injury have been designated as having "autoimmune sclerosing cholangitis" [65, 67]. Female gender (55–74 %) and concurrent inflammatory bowel disease (44–75 %) are common in children with the overlap syndrome between autoimmune hepatitis and PSC [68], but these features are not requisites for the diagnosis [65]. Patients with predominant features of PSC and secondary findings of autoimmune hepatitis should be distinguished from those mainly with features of autoimmune hepatitis as they may respond differently to treatment [36, 42, 56].

Autoimmune Hepatitis and Cholestasis

Patients with predominant features of autoimmune hepatitis, elevated serum alkaline phosphatase and GGT levels, histological findings of bile duct injury or loss, absence of AMA, and normal cholangiograms have a cholestatic syndrome which is unclassifiable [24, 26]. These patients have been designated as having "autoimmune cholangitis" [69–77], but they probably constitute an overlap syndrome with AMA-negative PBC or small duct PSC [77–82] (Table 18.1). This category is still poorly defined, and patients with unclassified cholestasis should be separated from the overlap syndromes with mixed features compatible with classical diseases [24].

PBC and PSC

Patients with classical laboratory and histological features of PBC may have cholangiographic changes of PSC, and these mixed features have justified the designation of an overlap syndrome between PBC and PSC [83–85] (Table 18.1). Eight patients with the overlap syndrome of PSC and PBC have been reported in 6 clinical studies [83–88]. The frequency of this syndrome is estimated to be 0.7 % in a cohort of 261 patients with autoimmune liver disease followed for as long as 20 years [84]. The inflammatory manifestations of autoimmune hepatitis are not disease-specific [4, 7], whereas the serological (AMA) and histological (destructive cholangitis) features of PBC [9, 89] and the cholangiographic changes of PSC (focal biliary strictures and dilations) [10] are disease-specific. The low frequency of concurrent disease-specific findings for PBC and PSC suggests that these overlap syndromes are mainly inflammatory variants of PBC and PSC rather than two superimposed diseases [24].

Frequency

The frequency of the overlap syndromes varies in accordance with the diagnostic criteria that are applied and the patient cohort that is investigated [24]. The frequency of patients with predominantly autoimmune hepatitis, AMA, and histological features of bile duct injury or loss is 7 % [16]. The frequency of patients with predominantly PBC and features of autoimmune hepatitis is 3–13 % [16, 35, 63, 90, 91]. Cholangiographic changes of PSC occur in 2–11 % of patients with classical autoimmune hepatitis [16, 56, 58, 59, 92], and findings compatible with autoimmune hepatitis are present in 2–33 % of patients with classical PSC [3, 17, 40, 42, 51]. The wide range of occurrence and the occasionally high reported frequencies of this overlap syndrome probably reflect the frequency that nonspecific inflammatory changes reminiscent of autoimmune hepatitis can occur in PSC. Autoimmune hepatitis has unclassifiable cholestatic changes in 5–11 % [16, 26, 82]. The overall frequency of the overlap syndromes in cohorts of patients with autoimmune liver disease is estimated to be 14–20 % [16, 25, 40, 45, 90, 93].

Pathogenic Possibilities

The overlap syndromes have not been validated as distinct pathological entities, and they may simply be clinical descriptors that accommodate variant presentations of the classical diseases [18, 49]. The serum levels of AST, ALT, and IgG that are truly incompatible with the diagnosis of PBC, and the serum levels of alkaline phosphatase and GGT that are truly incompatible with the diagnosis of autoimmune hepatitis are uncertain [14, 94]. Similarly, the degrees of interface hepatitis and bile duct injury that confidently differentiate autoimmune hepatitis from PBC or PSC are unclear [76, 95–97]. The boundary between hepatitic PBC or PSC and cholestatic autoimmune hepatitis is poorly drawn [14, 37], and the overlap syndromes may constitute a diagnostic category that accommodates these uncertainties [24, 26].

The overlap syndromes could be transitional stages in the evolution of the classical disease [24, 26]. Early stages of PBC or PSC may lack disease-specific laboratory and histological findings [92], and the histological findings of early stage PBC and PSC may resemble those of autoimmune hepatitis [66]. Features of autoimmune hepatitis may coexist with features of PBC and small duct PSC during the evolution of each cholestatic disease [74, 76], and these transitions may explain the reported sequences of autoimmune hepatitis transitioning to PBC [55, 98], PBC transitioning to autoimmune hepatitis [53, 54, 98], and PSC emerging in autoimmune hepatitis [52]. Alternatively, each classical autoimmune liver disease may have shared pathogenic mechanisms that can produce similar manifestations or unmask neo-antigens that redirect the autoreactive response to secondary antigenic targets that are less typical of the primary disease [99, 100]. In this context, the overlap syndromes could be part of a continuous spectrum of immune-mediated injury involving liver and non-liver tissues [101]. The emergence of features of autoimmune hepatitis in 2.5 % of patients with PBC and the development of PBC in 1.2 % of patients with autoimmune hepatitis after a mean observation interval of 6.5 years (range, 1–14 years) support this hypothesis [98].

The overlap syndromes could be two autoimmune liver diseases that occur simultaneously in the same individual [18, 24]. HLA DRB1*04 is a genetic susceptibility factor for autoimmune hepatitis, and it occurs more frequently in patients with autoimmune hepatitis or PBC than in patients with PSC [99]. In contrast, patients with autoimmune hepatitis or PSC have a higher frequency of HLA DRB1*03 than patients with PBC [99]. These findings suggest that genetic factors may be shared and contribute to the clustering of certain autoimmune liver diseases. Furthermore, the concurrence of certain highly specific features of one disease (destructive cholangitis or focal biliary strictures and dilations) in another disease is difficult to accept as within a single diagnostic boundary [18, 95]. Certain protective genetic factors might also contribute to the rarity of an overlap syndrome between PBC and PSC [99].

The overlap syndromes could be independent pathological entities with their own distinctive pathogenic mechanisms and clinical phenotype [24]. This highly theoretical possibility is based on the presumption that diverse antigens can trigger autoreactive responses in genetically predisposed individuals that have targets within the liver and biliary system [102–104]. Patients with autoimmune hepatitis and mixed connective tissue disease are characterized by a high proportion of T cells that are positive for interferon-gamma (IFN-γ) and by a severe impairment of immune suppressor function [105]. These findings suggest that patients with overlap syndromes have immune reactivity that is poorly regulated and shewed along a cytokine pathway that favors the emergence of tissue-infiltrating cytotoxic T cells [105]. This mechanism may promote the emergence of multiple immune-mediated diseases or define a separate pathological entity. The possibility of a separate disease entity characterized by its own antigenic trigger, genetic predisposition, immunological defects, clinical presentation, and outcome are justifications for the continued separation and study of these diseases.

Management Strategies and Results

The overlap syndromes do not have therapies that have been rigorously evaluated by clinical trial [22, 24] (Fig. 18.1). The treatment regimens that have been promulgated have been based on weak clinical evidence [9–11], and management strategies must be individualized and directed by the predominant manifestations of the disease [38, 49]. The degree of cholestasis as reflected in the laboratory findings (serum alkaline phosphatase and GGT levels), histological features (destructive cholangitis and bile duct loss), and radiographic images (focal biliary strictures and dilations) is probably the principal factor associated with outcome [16, 35, 56, 94, 106].

Autoimmune Hepatitis-PBC Overlap

Patients with predominant features of autoimmune hepatitis and secondary features of PBC manifested mainly by AMA, serum alkaline phosphatase level <twice ULN, and histological findings of isolated bile duct injury or loss respond as well to corticosteroid therapy as patients with classical autoimmune hepatitis [16, 38] (Fig. 18.1).

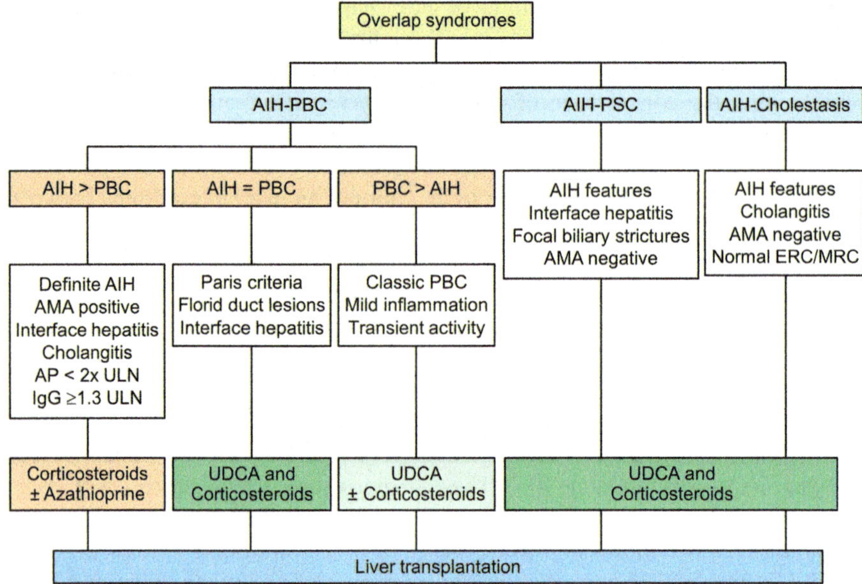

Fig. 18.1 Treatment algorithm for the overlap syndromes. All treatments are empiric and directed by the predominant features of the mixed syndrome. Patients with predominant features of autoimmune hepatitis (AIH) and secondary features of primary biliary cholangitis (PBC) that are outside the Paris criteria (AIH>PBC) are characterized by antimitochondrial antibodies (AMA) and serum alkaline phosphatase (AP) levels less than (<) twofold the upper limit of the normal range (ULN). These patients are frequently corticosteroid responsive, especially if serum immunoglobulin G (IgG) levels are 1.3-fold ULN or greater, and they can be managed with conventional corticosteroid regimens with or without (±) azathioprine. Patients that satisfy the Paris criteria have equally weighted features of AIH and PBC (AIH=PBC), and therapy with low-dose ursodeoxycholic acid (UDCA) in combination with corticosteroids has been recommended. Patients with predominant features of PBC and mild or transient inflammatory changes reminiscent of AIH (PBC>AIH) can be treated with UDCA alone or in combination with corticosteroids. Patients with AIH and cholangiographic features of focal biliary strictures and dilations (AIH-PSC) warrant a treatment trial with UDCA in combination with corticosteroids. Patients with AIH and a cholestatic syndrome that could be associated with AMA-negative PBC or small duct PSC are characterized by the absence of AMA and normal endoscopic retrograde cholangiography (ERC) or magnetic resonance cholangiography (MRC). These patients are also candidates for combination therapy with UDCA and corticosteroids. Salvage therapies with calcineurin inhibitors and mycophenolate mofetil have not been rigorously evaluated, and the emergence of features of liver failure warrant liver transplantation

Eighty-one percent improve to normal or near-normal liver tests and liver tissue with conventional corticosteroid treatment, and the frequency of treatment failure is similar to that of treated patients with classical autoimmune hepatitis (14 % versus 9 %) [16]. The frequency of improvement during corticosteroid therapy is 72–77 % in patients with serum IgG levels ≥1.3-fold ULN [61], definite autoimmune hepatitis by the simplified scoring system of the IAIHG [61], or histological activity scores that exceed activity scores for cholangitis [60]. These experiences indicate that the degree of inflammatory activity typical of autoimmune hepatitis is a key

Table 18.2 Management strategies for overlap syndromes

Overlap syndrome	Management strategy
AIH>PBC (outside Paris criteria)	Conventional corticosteroid therapy for classical AIH [7, 107]:
	Induction phase: prednisone or prednisolone, 30 mg daily × 1 week, 20 mg daily × 1 week, 15 mg daily × 2 weeks, and azathioprine, 50 mg daily
	Maintenance phase: prednisone or prednisolone, 10 mg daily, and azathioprine, 50 mg daily. Treatment until resolution of laboratory tests and liver tissue
	Monotherapy with prednisone or prednisolone for azathioprine intolerance or severe cytopenia requires doubling of steroid dose [7, 107]
	European preference is to administer prednisolone (up to 1 mg/kg daily) in combination with azathioprine (1–2 mg/kg daily) with gradual reduction in prednisolone dose over 2–3 months to 10 mg daily [8]
AIH=PBC (Paris criteria satisfied)	Combination therapy: UDCA, 13–15 mg/kg daily, and prednisone or prednisolone, 30–60 mg daily alone or in combination with azathioprine, 50–150 mg daily. Individualize steroid and azathioprine doses to response [11, 35, 49, 108].
	Salvage therapies (limited experience):
	Cyclosporine, 5–6 mg/kg daily; tacrolimus, 4–8 mg daily; mycophenolate mofetil, 2 g daily [108]
	Liver transplantation [122]
PBC>AIH (outside Paris criteria)	UDCA, 13–15 mg/kg daily alone or in combination with conventional corticosteroid regimen depending on severity of inflammatory activity [41, 108]
AIH–PSC	Combination therapy (preferred): UDCA, 13–15 mg/kg daily, prednisone or prednisolone, 10–15 mg daily, and azathioprine, 50–75 mg daily [10, 11, 42, 49]
	Salvage therapy: prednisolone or prednisone, 8.75–30 mg daily, and mycophenolate mofetil, 2 g daily (selected adults; limited study) [120], liver transplantation [122]
AIH–Cholestasis	Combination therapy (preferred): UDCA, 13–15 mg daily, prednisone or prednisolone, 10 mg daily, and azathioprine, 50 mg daily [32]
	Prednisone or prednisolone, 10–20 mg daily, with or without azathioprine, 50 mg daily, or UDCA, 13–15 mg/kg daily alone depending on predominant component [16, 69, 70, 72, 74, 78]

AIH autoimmune hepatitis, *PBC* primary biliary cholangitis, *PSC* primary sclerosing cholangitis, *UDCA* ursodeoxycholic acid

Numbers in brackets are references

consideration when deciding to treat with corticosteroids in patients with PBC. Prednisone in combination with azathioprine is the preferred treatment of classical autoimmune hepatitis [107], and it is the regimen that can be applied to those patients with strong features of autoimmune hepatitis and weak manifestations of PBC (Table 18.2).

Patients that satisfy the "Paris criteria" with equally weighted features of autoimmune hepatitis and PBC uniformly experience statistically significant improvements in serum alkaline phosphatase, GGT, and ALT levels when treated with corticosteroids in combination with UDCA, and the frequencies of response have been superior to those of patients treated with UDCA or corticosteroids alone [35] (Fig. 18.1). These findings have been supported by a retrospective analysis involving 88 patients who satisfied the "Paris criteria" from seven centers in five countries [108]. Therapy with UDCA (13–15 mg/kg daily) was ineffective in 37 %, and the lack of response was associated with severe interface hepatitis on histological examination. In contrast, 73 % of patients who were previously untreated or unresponsive to UDCA improved on combination therapy with UDCA and prednisone (30–60 mg daily) alone or in combination with azathioprine (50–150 mg daily) [108] (Table 18.2). Combination therapy has also been effective in another study involving eight patients who had initially failed monotherapy with UDCA. Laboratory tests improved in six patients and fibrosis did not progress during a mean observation interval of 7.5 years [43]. The combination regimen of corticosteroids and UDCA has been endorsed by EASL for the overlap syndrome of autoimmune hepatitis and PBC, and this recommendation has been based mainly on experiences with patients satisfying the Paris criteria [11, 49].

Patients with PBC who were identified retrospectively as having features of autoimmune hepatitis have also responded to UDCA alone (13–15 mg/kg daily), and the frequency of response has been similar to that of patients without these features [41] (Fig. 18.1). Furthermore, the manifestations of autoimmune hepatitis have been transient in some placebo-treated individuals [41]. The autoimmune hepatitis component in these patients may have constituted a self-limited inflammatory response rather than a sustained and important driver of disease activity. UDCA (13–15 mg/ kg daily) is a treatment option in those patients with predominant features of PBC and mild inflammatory or transient changes reminiscent of autoimmune hepatitis [41] (Table 18.2). In these patients, the severity of interface hepatitis on histological examination may be the critical determinant of when to add corticosteroids to the regimen with UDCA [108].

Salvage therapies with cyclosporine (5–6 mg/kg daily), tacrolimus (4–8 mg daily), mycophenolate mofetil (2 g daily) have been administered to 13 patients who failed to improve during initial therapy (Table 18.2), and 54 % responded by attaining complete or partial responses, including 3 of 5 patients treated with cyclosporine, one patient treated with cyclosporine and mycophenolate mofetil, 3 of 4 patients treated with tacrolimus, and three patients treated with mycophenolate mofetil [108]. Nonsteroidal immunosuppressive medications are considerations in the refractory patient, recognizing the empiric and limited nature of this rescue strategy.

Budesonide (3 mg thrice daily) has been used successfully in combination with UDCA in some patients with classical PBC [109, 110], but its use in the overlap syndrome between PBC and autoimmune hepatitis has been sparse and disappointing [48] (Table 18.2). Corticosteroid-induced side effects are possible in patients with cirrhosis probably because of decreased first-pass hepatic clearance of the drug and increased systemic bio-availability [48, 109, 111]. Therapy with budesonide has not been formally endorsed in the management of the overlap syndromes.

Autoimmune Hepatitis-PSC Overlap

Corticosteroids alone [16, 36, 51, 112] or in combination with UDCA [42, 47] have been the principal treatments of the overlap syndrome between autoimmune hepatitis and PSC [49]. Conventional corticosteroid regimens have induced laboratory and histological improvement in 20–100 % of patients, albeit the number of individuals in these reports has ranged from 5 to 16 [16, 36, 46, 51, 56, 112] (Table 18.2). Corticosteroid therapy has also had uncertain effects on survival. Death from liver failure or requirement for liver transplantation has occurred more frequently in patients with overlapping features of autoimmune hepatitis and PSC than in similarly treated patients with classical autoimmune hepatitis (33 % versus 8 %) [16]. Survival has also been lower in patients treated mainly with corticosteroids than in patients with classical autoimmune hepatitis (hazard ratio, 2.08) and patients with autoimmune hepatitis and PBC (hazard ratio, 2.14) [46]. The principal factors contributing to the variable corticosteroid responses are unclear, but they may relate to the degree of cholestasis and the intensity of the histological features of interface hepatitis. Patients with PSC who have responded to corticosteroid therapy have been characterized by higher serum levels of ALT and bilirubin and lower serum levels of alkaline phosphatase than nonresponders [112].

Prednisolone (or prednisone) in combination with UDCA has been the treatment recommended in the guidelines developed by EASL and AASLD [10, 11, 49], and currently this combination regimen is the preferred management strategy (Fig. 18.1). Prednisolone (initial dose, 0.5 mg/kg daily, tapered to 10–15 mg daily) in conjunction with azathioprine (50–75 mg daily) and UDCA (15–20 mg/kg daily) improved laboratory tests and survival in seven patients compared to 34 patients with classical PSC who were treated with UDCA alone [42, 49] (Table 18.2). Corticosteroid regimens that commonly included UDCA also decreased laboratory abnormalities in 23 of 27 children with autoimmune hepatitis and autoimmune sclerosing cholangitis (83 %) and improved histological findings in 17 (63 %) [49, 65, 113].

Laboratory improvement during combination therapy has not eliminated disease progression, and cirrhosis developed in 75 % of treated adults during a median observation period of 12 years [47]. Biliary changes also worsened in treated children with this overlap syndrome; transplant-free survival was reduced; and recurrent disease after liver transplantation was common [113, 114]. Furthermore, high-dose UDCA (28–30 mg/kg daily) in patients with classical PSC has been associated with an increased frequency of adverse events (63 % versus 37 %), including death and requirement for liver transplantation, compared to treatment with placebo [115]. Hepatic toxicity, possibly associated with the generation of lithocholic acid, may have contributed to these results [116], and empiric therapy with corticosteroids and UDCA in this population must be properly dosed (13–15 mg/kg daily) and carefully monitored (Table 18.2).

The experience with calcineurin inhibitors has been limited (two patients) [49, 117, 118]; therapy with UDCA alone has been poor [118]; and studies with mycophenolate mofetil have been small and variable [119, 120] (Table 18.2). Mycophenolate mofetil has not been effective in children with autoimmune hepatitis and sclerosing cholangitis [119], but it has reduced the serum AST or ALT level to less than twice ULN in 4 of 7 adults aged ≥20 years (57%) and normalized these tests in 1 of 7 patients (14%) [120]. These findings suggest that mycophenolate mofetil (1–2 g daily), administered with prednisolone or prednisone (median dose, 8.75–30 mg daily) in conjunction with azathioprine (median dose, 75–100 mg daily), may be effective in highly selected adults [120].

Autoimmune Hepatitis-Cholestasis

Patients with features of autoimmune hepatitis and cholestasis of undetermined cause ("autoimmune cholangitis") constitute a diagnostic category that probably includes patients with AMA-negative PBC and small duct PSC (Fig. 18.1). This heterogeneous group has been managed empirically with corticosteroids alone [16, 69, 70, 74], UDCA alone [72, 74, 78], or corticosteroids in combination with UDCA [32]. Combination therapy with prednisone or prednisolone (10 mg daily), azathioprine (50 mg daily), and UDCA (13–15 mg/kg daily) is the preferred treatment mainly because of potential effects on both the inflammatory and cholestatic components of the syndrome and disappointing outcomes with the monotherapies (Table 18.2).

Corticosteroids alone induced laboratory and histological improvement in three patients, but the histological improvements were restricted to the inflammatory manifestations and not the bile duct changes [69]. Seven corticosteroid-treated patients failed to improve in another study, and the disease progressed during an observation period of 1–5 years [70]. Similarly, only 1 of 8 corticosteroid-treated patients (12%) improved laboratory and histological findings after a mean treatment interval of 16±1 months, and two patients worsened during therapy (25%) [74].

Treatment with UDCA induced clinical improvement in all six treated patients described in two studies [72, 78], and outcomes were similar to those of patients with classical AMA-positive PBC in one of these studies [78]. In contrast, a study in which the cholestatic patients were identified within a cohort of patients with autoimmune hepatitis found that only 1 of 8 patients (12%) treated with UDCA improved during 4±2 months of therapy [74]. These findings underscored the importance of the predominant disease (PBC versus autoimmune hepatitis) in affecting the treatment strategy and outcome.

Treatment with corticosteroids and UDCA has been directed mainly at patients with autoimmune hepatitis and cholestatic changes consistent with AMA-negative PBC ("autoimmune cholangitis") [32]. These patients have had histological features of destructive cholangitis, ductopenia, ductular hyperplasia, and fibrosis more commonly than patients with the overlap syndrome of autoimmune hepatitis and AMA-positive PBC [121]. Complete laboratory resolution has been possible more frequently (90% versus 50%) and liver failure has occurred less often (10% versus 50%) in these patients than in those with classical AMA-positive PBC [32]. High scores by the comprehensive scoring system of the IAIHG [4] has characterized the patients responsive to combination therapy, and these findings suggest that the strength of the component resembling autoimmune hepatitis is a major determinant of a corticosteroid response [32].

The overlap syndrome of autoimmune hepatitis and "autoimmune cholangitis" is infrequent, and its preferred treatment has not been endorsed by a liver society. The combination regimen of UDCA (13–15 mg/kg daily) in combination with prednisone or prednisolone (maintenance dose, 10 mg daily) and azathioprine (50 mg daily) treats both the inflammatory and cholestatic components, and this choice is supported by its successful use in limited clinical experiences and the inconsistent outcomes associated with monotherapies (Table 18.2).

PBC-PSC Overlap

Ursodeoxycholic acid has been the principal agent used in the management of the eight patients reported with the overlap syndrome of PSC and PBC [83–88]. Dosing regimens have varied from a fixed dose (750 mg daily) [83, 84] to a weight-based dose (10 mg/kg daily increased to 15 mg/kg daily if histological progression) [88]. Prednisolone, 40 mg daily tapered to 5 mg daily, and azathioprine, 150 mg daily tapered to 100 mg daily, has been used in a patient who had features of autoimmune hepatitis in addition to those of PBC and PSC [84], and triple therapy with prednisolone, azathioprine, and ursodeoxycholic acid (doses unreported) has also been used in a patient with concurrent rheumatoid arthritis [85]. Monoclonal antibodies to tumor necrosis factor-alpha (adalimumab) was combined with ursodeoxycholic acid in one patient with concurrent rheumatoid arthritis [88]. Liver tests improved or normalized in most patients; features of persistent cholestasis could be stabilized long-term; and no patients died or required liver transplantation during observation intervals ranging from 3 to 17 years. Cholangitis recurred in two patients with large duct PSC, and progression to cirrhosis occurred in one patient.

Overview

The overlap syndromes of autoimmune hepatitis are mixed clinical phenotypes that must be recognized and treated as diseases that are commonly unresponsive to conventional therapies [12, 16, 24, 25, 27]. Patients with PBC or PSC may have with laboratory and histological manifestations of liver inflammation reminiscent of autoimmune hepatitis [35, 36, 65], and patients with autoimmune hepatitis may have secondary features of PBC or PSC [16] or a cholestatic component ("autoimmune cholangitis") that suggests AMA-negative PBC or small duct PSC [74]. Rarely, patients may have features of PBC and PSC or features of PBC, PSC, and autoimmune hepatitis [84]. The overlap syndromes lack codified diagnostic criteria.

The Paris criteria define the overlap syndrome between PBC and autoimmune hepatitis by equally weighting features of each disease, and it is the only objective diagnostic guideline [35, 62] (Table 18.1).

Management strategies have not been subjected to rigorous clinical trial. The predominance and severity of the inflammatory and cholestatic components affect the clinical presentation, outcome, and treatment of each syndrome [56, 94, 108]. All management strategies are empiric, based on limited clinical experiences, and variably effective. Monotherapy with corticosteroids (prednisone or prednisolone with or without azathioprine) can be considered in selected patients with predominant features of autoimmune hepatitis and cholestatic findings of PBC that are outside the Paris criteria [16]. Monotherapy with UDCA can be considered in selected patients with predominant features of PBC and mild or transient liver inflammation that are outside the Paris criteria [41]. Combination therapy with corticosteroids and UDCA is a blanket approach that can be applied to all syndromes [10, 11, 49], and it has been endorsed by the liver societies for the overlap syndrome between autoimmune hepatitis and PBC and autoimmune hepatitis and PSC [10, 11, 49]. It is also appropriate for patients with autoimmune hepatitis and a cholestatic phenotype consistent with AMA-negative PBC or small duct PSC [32].

Liver transplantation is an effective salvage therapy for patients with overlap syndromes that progress to liver failure. The median graft (10.2 ± 2.2 years versus 15 ± 0.7 years, $P=0.9$) and patient (11.2 ± 1.1 years versus 16.1 ± 0.7 years, $P=0.6$) survivals are similar to those of individuals without overlapping features [122]. Autoimmune liver disease recurs more commonly at 5 years (53% versus 17%, $P=0.001$) and 10 years (69% versus 29%, $P=0.001$) after transplantation than in patients without overlapping features, but this difference has not affected overall survival [122].

Acknowledgement This review did not receive financial support from a funding agency or institution, and Albert J. Czaja, MD has no conflict of interests to declare.

References

1. Johnson PJ, McFarlane IG. Meeting report: International Autoimmune Hepatitis Group. Hepatology. 1993;18:998–1005.
2. Czaja AJ, Carpenter HA. Validation of scoring system for diagnosis of autoimmune hepatitis. Dig Dis Sci. 1996;41:305–14.
3. Boberg KM, Fausa O, Haaland T, Holter E, Mellbye OJ, Spurkland A, et al. Features of autoimmune hepatitis in primary sclerosing cholangitis: an evaluation of 114 primary sclerosing cholangitis patients according to a scoring system for the diagnosis of autoimmune hepatitis. Hepatology. 1996;23:1369–76.
4. Alvarez F, Berg PA, Bianchi FB, Bianchi L, Burroughs AK, Cancado EL, et al. International Autoimmune Hepatitis Group Report: review of criteria for diagnosis of autoimmune hepatitis. J Hepatol. 1999;31:929–38.
5. Czaja AJ. Performance parameters of the diagnostic scoring systems for autoimmune hepatitis. Hepatology. 2008;48:1540–8.
6. Hennes EM, Zeniya M, Czaja AJ, Pares A, Dalekos GN, Krawitt EL, et al. Simplified criteria for the diagnosis of autoimmune hepatitis. Hepatology. 2008;48:169–76.

7. Manns MP, Czaja AJ, Gorham JD, Krawitt EL, Mieli-Vergani G, Vergani D, et al. Diagnosis and management of autoimmune hepatitis. Hepatology. 2010;51:2193–213.
8. Gleeson D, Heneghan MA. British Society of Gastroenterology (BSG) guidelines for management of autoimmune hepatitis. Gut. 2011;60:1611–29.
9. Lindor KD, Gershwin ME, Poupon R, Kaplan M, Bergasa NV, Heathcote EJ. AASLD Practice Guidelines. Primary biliary cirrhosis. Hepatology. 2009;50:291–308.
10. Chapman R, Fevery J, Kalloo A, Nagorney DM, Boberg KM, Shneider B, et al. Diagnosis and management of primary sclerosing cholangitis. Hepatology. 2010;51:660–78.
11. Beuers U, Boberg KM, Chapman RW, Chazouilleres O, Invernizzi P, Jones DEJ, et al. EASL Clinical Practice Guidelines: management of cholestatic liver diseases. J Hepatol. 2009;51:237–67.
12. Czaja AJ. The variant forms of autoimmune hepatitis. Ann Intern Med. 1996;125:588–98.
13. Heathcote J. Variant syndromes of autoimmune hepatitis. Clin Liver Dis. 2002;6:669–84.
14. Czaja AJ. Overlap syndrome of primary biliary cirrhosis and autoimmune hepatitis: a foray across diagnostic boundaries. J Hepatol. 2006;44:251–2.
15. Gohlke F, Lohse AW, Dienes HP, Lohr H, Marker-Hermann E, Gerken G, et al. Evidence for an overlap syndrome of autoimmune hepatitis and primary sclerosing cholangitis. J Hepatol. 1996;24:699–705.
16. Czaja AJ. Frequency and nature of the variant syndromes of autoimmune liver disease. Hepatology. 1998;28:360–5.
17. Dienes HP, Erberich H, Dries V, Schirmacher P, Lohse A. Autoimmune hepatitis and overlap syndromes. Clin Liver Dis. 2002;6:349–62. vi.
18. Poupon R. Autoimmune overlapping syndromes. Clin Liver Dis. 2003;7:865–78.
19. Beuers U, Rust C. Overlap syndromes. Semin Liver Dis. 2005;25:311–20.
20. Schramm C, Lohse AW. Overlap syndromes of cholestatic liver diseases and auto-immune hepatitis. Clin Rev Allergy Immunol. 2005;28:105–14.
21. Silveira MG, Lindor KD. Overlap syndromes with autoimmune hepatitis in chronic cholestatic liver diseases. Expert Rev Gastroenterol Hepatol. 2007;1:329–40.
22. Trivedi PJ, Hirschfield GM. Review article: overlap syndromes and autoimmune liver disease. Aliment Pharmacol Ther. 2012;36:517–33.
23. Mayo MJ. Cholestatic liver disease overlap syndromes. Clin Liver Dis. 2013;17:243–53.
24. Czaja AJ. The overlap syndromes of autoimmune hepatitis. Dig Dis Sci. 2013;58:326–43.
25. Czaja AJ. Diagnosis and management of the overlap syndromes of autoimmune hepatitis. Can J Gastroenterol. 2013;27:417–23.
26. Czaja AJ. Cholestatic phenotypes of autoimmune hepatitis. Clin Gastroenterol Hepatol. 2014;12:1430–8.
27. Czaja AJ. Overlap syndromes. Clin Liver Dis. 2014;3:2–5.
28. Talwalkar JA, Keach JC, Angulo P, Lindor KD. Overlap of autoimmune hepatitis and primary biliary cirrhosis: an evaluation of a modified scoring system. Am J Gastroenterol. 2002;97:1191–7.
29. Silveira MG, Talwalkar JA, Angulo P, Lindor KD. Overlap of autoimmune hepatitis and primary biliary cirrhosis: long-term outcomes. Am J Gastroenterol. 2007;102:1244–50.
30. Papamichalis PA, Zachou K, Koukoulis GK, Veloni A, Karacosta EG, Kypri L, et al. The revised international autoimmune hepatitis score in chronic liver diseases including autoimmune hepatitis/overlap syndromes and autoimmune hepatitis with concurrent other liver disorders. J Autoimmune Dis. 2007;4:3.
31. Neuhauser M, Bjornsson E, Treeprasertsuk S, Enders F, Silveira M, Talwalkar J, et al. Autoimmune hepatitis-PBC overlap syndrome: a simplified scoring system may assist in the diagnosis. Am J Gastroenterol. 2010;105:345–53.
32. Ozaslan E, Efe C, Akbulut S, Purnak T, Savas B, Erden E, et al. Therapy response and outcome of overlap syndromes: autoimmune hepatitis and primary biliary cirrhosis compared to autoimmune hepatitis and autoimmune cholangitis. Hepatogastroenterology. 2010;57:441–6.
33. Yamamoto K, Terada R, Okamoto R, Hiasa Y, Abe M, Onji M, et al. A scoring system for primary biliary cirrhosis and its application for variant forms of autoimmune liver disease. J Gastroenterol. 2003;38:52–9.

34. Duclos-Vallee JC, Hadengue A, Ganne-Carrie N, Robin E, Degott C, Erlinger S. Primary biliary cirrhosis-autoimmune hepatitis overlap syndrome. Corticoresistance and effective treatment by cyclosporine A. Dig Dis Sci. 1995;40:1069–73.
35. Chazouilleres O, Wendum D, Serfaty L, Montembault S, Rosmorduc O, Poupon R. Primary biliary cirrhosis-autoimmune hepatitis overlap syndrome: clinical features and response to therapy. Hepatology. 1998;28:296–301.
36. McNair AN, Moloney M, Portmann BC, Williams R, McFarlane IG. Autoimmune hepatitis overlapping with primary sclerosing cholangitis in five cases. Am J Gastroenterol. 1998;93:777–84.
37. Lohse AW, zum Buschenfelde KH, Franz B, Kanzler S, Gerken G, Dienes HP. Characterization of the overlap syndrome of primary biliary cirrhosis (PBC) and autoimmune hepatitis: evidence for it being a hepatitic form of PBC in genetically susceptible individuals. Hepatology. 1999;29:1078–84.
38. Ben-Ari Z, Czaja AJ. Autoimmune hepatitis and its variant syndromes. Gut. 2001;49:589–94.
39. Gunsar F, Akarca US, Ersoz G, Karasu Z, Yuce G, Batur Y. Clinical and biochemical features and therapy responses in primary biliary cirrhosis and primary biliary cirrhosis-autoimmune hepatitis overlap syndrome. Hepatogastroenterology. 2002;49:1195–200.
40. Muratori L, Cassani F, Pappas G, Guidi M, Mele L, Lorenza V, et al. The hepatitic/cholestatic "overlap" syndrome: an Italian experience. Autoimmunity. 2002;35:565–8.
41. Joshi S, Cauch-Dudek K, Wanless IR, Lindor KD, Jorgensen R, Batts K, et al. Primary biliary cirrhosis with additional features of autoimmune hepatitis: response to therapy with ursodeoxycholic acid. Hepatology. 2002;35:409–13.
42. Floreani A, Rizzotto ER, Ferrara F, Carderi I, Caroli D, Blasone L, et al. Clinical course and outcome of autoimmune hepatitis/primary sclerosing cholangitis overlap syndrome. Am J Gastroenterol. 2005;100:1516–22.
43. Chazouilleres O, Wendum D, Serfaty L, Rosmorduc O, Poupon R. Long term outcome and response to therapy of primary biliary cirrhosis-autoimmune hepatitis overlap syndrome. J Hepatol. 2006;44:400–6.
44. Renou C, Bourliere M, Martini F, Ouzan D, Penaranda G, Larroque O, et al. Primary biliary cirrhosis-autoimmune hepatitis overlap syndrome: complete biochemical and histological response to therapy with ursodesoxycholic acid. J Gastroenterol Hepatol. 2006;21:781–2.
45. Heurgue A, Vitry F, Diebold MD, Yaziji N, Bernard-Chabert B, Pennaforte JL, et al. Overlap syndrome of primary biliary cirrhosis and autoimmune hepatitis: a retrospective study of 115 cases of autoimmune liver disease. Gastroenterol Clin Biol. 2007;31:17–25.
46. Al-Chalabi T, Portmann BC, Bernal W, McFarlane IG, Heneghan MA. Autoimmune hepatitis overlap syndromes: an evaluation of treatment response, long-term outcome and survival. Aliment Pharmacol Ther. 2008;28:209–20.
47. Luth S, Kanzler S, Frenzel C, Kasper HU, Dienes HP, Schramm C, et al. Characteristics and long-term prognosis of the autoimmune hepatitis/primary sclerosing cholangitis overlap syndrome. J Clin Gastroenterol. 2009;43:75–80.
48. Efe C, Ozaslan E, Kav T, Purnak T, Shorbagi A, Ozkayar O, et al. Liver fibrosis may reduce the efficacy of budesonide in the treatment of autoimmune hepatitis and overlap syndrome. Autoimmun Rev. 2012;11:330–4.
49. Boberg KM, Chapman RW, Hirschfield GM, Lohse AW, Manns MP, Schrumpf E. Overlap syndromes: the International Autoimmune Hepatitis Group (IAIHG) position statement on a controversial issue. J Hepatol. 2011;54:374–85.
50. Czaja AJ. Variant forms of autoimmune hepatitis. Curr Gastroenterol Rep. 1999;1:63–70.
51. van Buuren HR, van Hoogstraten HJE, Terkivatan T, Schalm SW, Vleggaar FP. High prevalence of autoimmune hepatitis among patients with primary sclerosing cholangitis. J Hepatol. 2000;33:543–8.
52. Abdo AA, Bain VG, Kichian K, Lee SS. Evolution of autoimmune hepatitis to primary sclerosing cholangitis: a sequential syndrome. Hepatology. 2002;36:1393–9.
53. Poupon R, Chazouilleres O, Corpechot C, Chretien Y. Development of autoimmune hepatitis in patients with typical primary biliary cirrhosis. Hepatology. 2006;44:85–90.

54. Gossard AA, Lindor KD. Development of autoimmune hepatitis in primary biliary cirrhosis. Liver Int. 2007;27:1086–90.
55. Lindgren S, Glaumann H, Almer S, Bergquist A, Bjornsson E, Broome U, et al. Transitions between variant forms of primary biliary cirrhosis during long-term follow-up. Eur J Intern Med. 2009;20:398–402.
56. Perdigoto R, Carpenter HA, Czaja AJ. Frequency and significance of chronic ulcerative colitis in severe corticosteroid-treated autoimmune hepatitis. J Hepatol. 1992;14:325–31.
57. Trivedi PJ, Chapman RW. PSC, AIH and overlap syndrome in inflammatory bowel disease. Clin Rese Hepatol Gastroenterol. 2012;36:420–36.
58. Lewin M, Vilgrain V, Ozenne V, Lemoine M, Wendum D, Paradis V, et al. Prevalence of sclerosing cholangitis in adults with autoimmune hepatitis: a prospective magnetic resonance imaging and histological study. Hepatology. 2009;50:528–37.
59. Abdalian R, Dhar P, Jhaveri K, Haider M, Guindi M, Heathcote EJ. Prevalence of sclerosing cholangitis in adults with autoimmune hepatitis: evaluating the role of routine magnetic resonance imaging. Hepatology. 2008;47:949–57.
60. Tanaka A, Harada K, Ebinuma H, Komori A, Yokokawa J, Yoshizawa K, et al. Primary biliary cirrhosis - autoimmune hepatitis overlap syndrome: a rationale for corticosteroids use based on a nation-wide retrospective study in Japan. Hepatol Res. 2011;41:877–86.
61. Wang Q, Selmi C, Zhou X, Qiu D, Li Z, Miao Q, et al. Epigenetic considerations and the clinical reevaluation of the overlap syndrome between primary biliary cirrhosis and autoimmune hepatitis. J Autoimmun. 2013;41:140–5.
62. Kuiper EM, Zondervan PE, van Buuren HR. Paris criteria are effective in diagnosis of primary biliary cirrhosis and autoimmune hepatitis overlap syndrome. Clin Gastroenterol Hepatol. 2010;8:530–4.
63. Bonder A, Retana A, Winston DM, Leung J, Kaplan MM. Prevalence of primary biliary cirrhosis-autoimmune hepatitis overlap syndrome. Clin Gastroenterol Hepatol. 2011;9:609–12.
64. Balasubramaniam K, Wiesner RH, LaRusso NF. Primary sclerosing cholangitis with normal serum alkaline phosphatase activity. Gastroenterology. 1988;95:1395–8.
65. Gregorio GV, Portmann B, Karani J, Harrison P, Donaldson PT, Vergani D, et al. Autoimmune hepatitis/sclerosing cholangitis overlap syndrome in childhood: a 16-year prospective study. Hepatology. 2001;33:544–53.
66. Carpenter HA, Czaja AJ. The role of histologic evaluation in the diagnosis and management of autoimmune hepatitis and its variants. Clin Liver Dis. 2002;6:685–705.
67. Deneau M, Jensen MK, Holmen J, Williams MS, Book LS, Guthery SL. Primary sclerosing cholangitis, autoimmune hepatitis, and overlap in utah children: epidemiology and natural history. Hepatology. 2013;58:1392–400.
68. Rojas CP, Bodicharla R, Campuzano-Zuluaga G, Hernandez L, Rodriguez MM. Autoimmune hepatitis and primary sclerosing cholangitis in children and adolescents. Fetal Pediatr Pathol. 2014;33:202–9.
69. Ben-Ari Z, Dhillon AP, Sherlock S. Autoimmune cholangiopathy: part of the spectrum of autoimmune chronic active hepatitis. Hepatology. 1993;18:10–5.
70. Taylor SL, Dean PJ, Riely CA. Primary autoimmune cholangitis. An alternative to antimitochondrial antibody-negative primary biliary cirrhosis. Am J Surg Pathol. 1994;18:91–9.
71. Goodman ZD, McNally PR, Davis DR, Ishak KG. Autoimmune cholangitis: a variant of primary biliary cirrhosis. Clinicopathologic and serologic correlations in 200 cases. Dig Dis Sci. 1995;40:1232–42.
72. Omagari K, Ikuno N, Matsuo I, Shirono K, Hara K, Feeney SJ, et al. Autoimmune cholangitis syndrome with a bias towards primary biliary cirrhosis. Pathology. 1996;28:255–8.
73. Sherlock S. Ludwig Symposium on biliary disorders. Autoimmune cholangitis: a unique entity? Mayo Clin Proc. 1998;73:184–90.
74. Czaja AJ, Carpenter HA, Santrach PJ, Moore SB. Autoimmune cholangitis within the spectrum of autoimmune liver disease. Hepatology. 2000;31:1231–8.
75. Washington K. Autoimmune cholangitis: not just AMA-negative primary biliary cirrhosis. Adv Anat Pathol. 2002;9:244–50.

76. Czaja AJ, Muratori P, Muratori L, Carpenter HA, Bianchi FB. Diagnostic and therapeutic implications of bile duct injury in autoimmune hepatitis. Liver Int. 2004;24:322–9.
77. Vierling JM. Primary biliary cirrhosis and autoimmune cholangiopathy. Clin Liver Dis. 2004;8:177–94.
78. Lacerda MA, Ludwig J, Dickson ER, Jorgensen RA, Lindor KD. Antimitochondrial antibody-negative primary biliary cirrhosis. Am J Gastroenterol. 1995;90:247–9.
79. Nakanuma Y, Harada K, Kaji K, Terasaki S, Tsuneyama K, Moteki S, et al. Clinicopathological study of primary biliary cirrhosis negative for antimitochondrial antibodies. Liver. 1997;17:281–7.
80. Kim WR, Ludwig J, Lindor KD. Variant forms of cholestatic diseases involving small bile ducts in adults. Am J Gastroenterol. 2000;95:1130–8.
81. Angulo P, Maor-Kendler Y, Lindor KD. Small-duct primary sclerosing cholangitis: a long-term follow-up study. Hepatology. 2002;35:1494–500.
82. Muratori P, Muratori L, Gershwin ME, Czaja AJ, Pappas G, MacCariello S, et al. 'True' antimitochondrial antibody-negative primary biliary cirrhosis, low sensitivity of the routine assays, or both? Clin Exp Immunol. 2004;135:154–8.
83. Burak KW, Urbanski SJ, Swain MG. A case of coexisting primary biliary cirrhosis and primary sclerosing cholangitis: a new overlap of autoimmune liver diseases. Dig Dis Sci. 2001;46:2043–7.
84. Kingham JG, Abbasi A. Co-existence of primary biliary cirrhosis and primary sclerosing cholangitis: a rare overlap syndrome put in perspective. Eur J Gastroenterol Hepatol. 2005;17:1077–80.
85. Jeevagan A. Overlap of primary biliary cirrhosis and primary sclerosing cholangitis - a rare coincidence or a new syndrome. Int J Gen Med. 2010;3:143–6.
86. Rubel LR, Seeff LB, Patel V. Primary biliary cirrhosis-primary sclerosing cholangitis overlap syndrome. Arch Pathol Lab Med. 1984;108:360–1.
87. Oliveira EM, Oliveira PM, Becker V, Dellavance A, Andrade LE, Lanzoni V, et al. Overlapping of primary biliary cirrhosis and small duct primary sclerosing cholangitis: first case report. J Clin Med Res. 2012;4:429–33.
88. Floreani A, Motta R, Cazzagon N, Franceschet I, Roncalli M, Del Ross T, et al. The overlap syndrome between primary biliary cirrhosis and primary sclerosing cholangitis. Dig Liver Dis. 2015;47:432–5.
89. Czaja AJ. Performance parameters of the conventional serological markers for autoimmune hepatitis. Dig Dis Sci. 2011;56:545–54.
90. Gheorghe L, Iacob S, Gheorghe C, Iacob R, Simionov I, Vadan R, et al. Frequency and predictive factors for overlap syndrome between autoimmune hepatitis and primary cholestatic liver disease. Eur J Gastroenterol Hepatol. 2004;16:585–92.
91. Zhao P, Han Y. Low incidence of positive smooth muscle antibody and high incidence of isolated IgM elevation in Chinese patients with autoimmune hepatitis and primary biliary cirrhosis overlap syndrome: a retrospective study. BMC Gastroenterol. 2012;12:1.
92. Hunter M, Loughrey MB, Gray M, Ellis P, McDougall N, Callender M. Evaluating distinctive features for early diagnosis of primary sclerosing cholangitis overlap syndrome in adults with autoimmune hepatitis. Ulster Med J. 2011;80:15–8.
93. Arulprakash S, Sasi AD, Bala MR, Pugazhendhi T, Kumar SJ. Overlap syndrome: autoimmune hepatitis with primary biliary cirrhosis. J Assoc Physicians India. 2010;58:455–6.
94. Kenny RP, Czaja AJ, Ludwig J, Dickson ER. Frequency and significance of antimitochondrial antibodies in severe chronic active hepatitis. Dig Dis Sci. 1986;31:705–11.
95. Czaja AJ, Carpenter HA. Sensitivity, specificity, and predictability of biopsy interpretations in chronic hepatitis. Gastroenterology. 1993;105:1824–32.
96. Ludwig J, Czaja AJ, Dickson ER, LaRusso NF, Wiesner RH. Manifestations of nonsuppurative cholangitis in chronic hepatobiliary diseases: morphologic spectrum, clinical correlations and terminology. Liver. 1984;4:105–16.
97. Czaja AJ, Carpenter HA. Autoimmune hepatitis with incidental histologic features of bile duct injury. Hepatology. 2001;34:659–65.

98. Efe C, Ozaslan E, Heurgue-Berlot A, Kav T, Masi C, Purnak T, et al. Sequential presentation of primary biliary cirrhosis and autoimmune hepatitis. Eur J Gastroenterol Hepatol. 2014;26:532–7.
99. Czaja AJ, Santrach PJ, Breanndan Moore S. Shared genetic risk factors in autoimmune liver disease. Dig Dis Sci. 2001;46:140–7.
100. Rosen A, Casciola-Rosen L. Autoantigens in systemic autoimmunity: critical partner in pathogenesis. J Intern Med. 2009;265:625–31.
101. Floreani A, Franceschet I, Cazzagon N. Primary biliary cirrhosis: overlaps with other autoimmune disorders. Semin Liver Dis. 2014;34:352–60.
102. Doherty DG, Penzotti JE, Koelle DM, Kwok WW, Lybrand TP, Masewicz S, et al. Structural basis of specificity and degeneracy of T cell recognition: pluriallelic restriction of T cell responses to a peptide antigen involves both specific and promiscuous interactions between the T cell receptor, peptide, and HLA-DR. J Immunol. 1998;161:3527–35.
103. Czaja AJ, Doherty DG, Donaldson PT. Genetic bases of autoimmune hepatitis. Dig Dis Sci. 2002;47:2139–50.
104. Czaja AJ. Genetic factors affecting the occurrence, clinical phenotype, and outcome of autoimmune hepatitis. Clin Gastroenterol Hepatol. 2008;6:379–88.
105. Longhi MS, Ma Y, Grant CR, Samyn M, Gordon P, Mieli-Vergani G, et al. T-regs in autoimmune hepatitis-systemic lupus erythematosus/mixed connective tissue disease overlap syndrome are functionally defective and display a Th1 cytokine profile. J Autoimmun. 2013;41:146–51.
106. Geubel AP, Baggenstoss AH, Summerskill WH. Responses to treatment can differentiate chronic active liver disease with cholangitic features from the primary biliary cirrhosis syndrome. Gastroenterology. 1976;71:444–9.
107. Czaja AJ. Current and prospective pharmacotherapy for autoimmune hepatitis. Expert Opin Pharmacother. 2014;15:1715–36.
108. Ozaslan E, Efe C, Heurgue-Berlot A, Kav T, Masi C, Purnak T, et al. Factors associated with response to therapy and outcome of patients with primary biliary cirrhosis with features of autoimmune hepatitis. Clin Gastroenterol Hepatol. 2014;12:863–9.
109. Hempfling W, Grunhage F, Dilger K, Reichel C, Beuers U, Sauerbruch T. Pharmacokinetics and pharmacodynamic action of budesonide in early- and late-stage primary biliary cirrhosis. Hepatology. 2003;38:196–202.
110. Leuschner M, Maier KP, Schlichting J, Strahl S, Herrmann G, Dahm HH, et al. Oral budesonide and ursodeoxycholic acid for treatment of primary biliary cirrhosis: results of a prospective double-blind trial. Gastroenterology. 1999;117:918–25.
111. Geier A, Gartung C, Dietrich CG, Wasmuth HE, Reinartz P, Matern S. Side effects of budesonide in liver cirrhosis due to chronic autoimmune hepatitis: influence of hepatic metabolism versus portosystemic shunts on a patient complicated with HCC. World J Gastroenterol. 2003;9:2681–5.
112. Boberg KM, Egeland T, Schrumpf E. Long-term effect of corticosteroid treatment in primary sclerosing cholangitis patients. Scand J Gastroenterol. 2003;38:991–5.
113. Mieli-Vergani G, Vergani D. Autoimmune hepatitis in children: what is different from adult AIH? Semin Liver Dis. 2009;29:297–306.
114. Mieli-Vergani G, Vergani D. Autoimmune liver diseases in children - what is different from adulthood? Best Pract Res Clin Gastroenterol. 2011;25:783–95.
115. Lindor KD, Kowdley KV, Luketic VA, Harrison ME, McCashland T, Befeler AS, et al. High-dose ursodeoxycholic acid for the treatment of primary sclerosing cholangitis. Hepatology. 2009;50:808–14.
116. Sinakos E, Marschall HU, Kowdley KV, Befeler A, Keach J, Lindor K. Bile acid changes after high-dose ursodeoxycholic acid treatment in primary sclerosing cholangitis: relation to disease progression. Hepatology. 2010;52:197–203.
117. Lawrence SP, Sherman KE, Lawson JM, Goodman ZD. A 39 year old man with chronic hepatitis. Semin Liver Dis. 1994;14:97–105.
118. Olsson R, Glaumann H, Almer S, Broome U, Lebrun B, Bergquist A, et al. High prevalence of small duct primary sclerosing cholangitis among patients with overlapping autoimmune hepatitis and primary sclerosing cholangitis. Eur J Intern Med. 2009;20:190–6.

119. Aw MM, Dhawan A, Samyn M, Bargiota A, Mieli-Vergani G. Mycophenolate mofetil as rescue treatment for autoimmune liver disease in children: a 5-year follow-up. J Hepatol. 2009;51:156–60.
120. Baven-Pronk AM, Coenraad MJ, van Buuren HR, de Man RA, van Erpecum KJ, Lamers MM, et al. The role of mycophenolate mofetil in the management of autoimmune hepatitis and overlap syndromes. Aliment Pharmacol Ther. 2011;34:335–43.
121. Alric L, Thebault S, Selves J, Peron JM, Mejdoubi S, Fortenfant F, et al. Characterization of overlap syndrome between primary biliary cirrhosis and autoimmune hepatitis according to antimitochondrial antibodies status. Gastroenterol Clin Biol. 2007;31:11–6.
122. Bhanji RA, Mason AL, Girgis S, Montano-Loza AJ. Liver transplantation for overlap syndromes of autoimmune liver diseases. Liver Int. 2013;33:210–9.

Chapter 19
Metabolic and Genetic Liver Diseases: Alpha-1 Anti-trypsin Deficiency

Helen S. Te

Patient-Level Questions

1. What is alpha-1 antitrypsin (AAT) deficiency?

   Alpha-1 antitrypsin is a glycoprotein produced in the liver and works by preventing neutrophil proteases from destroying host tissues during inflammation. A hereditary mutation in the gene that codes for this protein leads to the production of a modified AAT protein, which folds in a way that prevents its secretion from the liver cell. Therefore, the abnormal AAT protein accumulates in the liver cell, leading to cell injury and eventually, severe scarring or cirrhosis. In addition, the absence of AAT protein in the lung leads to the absence of protection against the digestive actions of enzymes such as neutrophil elastase and proteinase 3 on the tissue structure of the lung, resulting in the premature development of emphysema.

2. What can be done about it?

   Lung disease from AATD can be treated with intravenous replacement with the protein, leading to improvement in lung function. Unfortunately, liver disease from AATD still has no direct treatment available, other than supportive measures to prevent or treat complications of cirrhosis. In those who have cirrhosis with complications, liver transplantation may be necessary. Currently, many investigators are actively studying various strategies geared towards removal or prevention of accumulation of the mutant AAT protein in the liver.

3. Is the rest of my family at risk?

   By virtue of its hereditary nature, the disease may affect more than one member of the family. However, the severity of the disease and clinical manifestations vary greatly amongst individuals with the same genetic mutations, suggesting

H.S. Te, M.D. (✉)
Center for Liver Diseases, University of Chicago Medicine, Chicago, IL, USA
e-mail: hte@medicine.bsd.uchicago.edu

© Springer International Publishing Switzerland 2017
K. Saeian, R. Shaker (eds.), *Liver Disorders*,
DOI 10.1007/978-3-319-30103-7_19

that other genetic modifiers and environmental factors may affect the clinical presentation of the disease. It would be prudent to screen family members for the disease to provide early detection and possible intervention and monitoring, if the disease is clinically significant.

4. Why do some patients with AATD manifest only lung disease, whereas others manifest only liver disease?

The peak ages for the diagnosis of liver and lung disease in AATD differ, with liver disorders usually detected during childhood or old age, whereas lung disease develops in middle age. This may give the impression that the presence of one organ involvement excludes the other, although the risk of lung and liver disease indeed seems to be quite independent of each other.

Lung disease in AATD results from deficiency of the AAT protein in the lungs, whereas liver disease results from the accumulation of the mutant protein in the liver cell, leading to liver injury and fibrosis. The involvement of one organ rather than the other may also be partially explained by the various genetic mutations that lead to AATD. Some cases of AATD involve the production of abnormal AAT proteins which predisposes to liver disease and in severe cases, lung disease, whereas other cases involve a decreased or complete absence of production of the AAT protein in the liver which can cause lung disease but not liver disease. However, even in the homozygous AATD, the clinical manifestation of the genetic mutation is highly variable, and the natural history is influenced by other genetic and environmental modifiers.

5. Are there things that I should avoid because of my diagnosis of AATD?

The development and severity of emphysema in AATD is significantly increased up to 1000-fold by cigarette smoking, so one must avoid smoking, pollution, or occupational exposure to inhaled substances that are toxic to the lungs in the setting of AATD. In terms of liver disease, there is no evidence to indicate that alcohol use exacerbates the progression of the liver disease. However, it would be prudent to avoid excessive alcohol intake, given a theoretical risk of an additive injury on top of the AATD that may cause a more rapid progression of the liver disease. An increase in the production of the mutant Z protein has been demonstrated with the use of nonsteroidal anti-inflammatory drugs (NSAIDS) in animal models of AAT liver disease, so it would also be prudent to avoid the use of NSAIDS in this patient population.

Introduction

First described by Laurell and Erikson in 1963, alpha-1 antitrypsin deficiency (AATD) was noted as an absent alpha-1 band on protein electrophoresis of the serum of a patient with a lung disorder [1]. Alpha-1 antitrypsin (AAT) is a serum glycoprotein synthesized by the liver and secreted into the blood. It can inhibit trypsin in vitro, but it physiologically functions to inhibit neutrophil elastase and several related neutrophil serine proteases released during inflammation, and prevent them from destroying structural host tissues. As such, its production is regulated by inflammation, with serum levels rising three to five times during the host response to inflammation [2]. The normal allele of the AAT gene (SERPINA1-serpin peptidase inhibitor, clade A (alpha-1 antiproteinase, antitrypsin), member 1) on chromosome 14 is the M gene, which produces the M protein and normal serum levels of AAT. Mutations in the AAT gene may present as one of over 100 variant alleles, but majority of patients with liver disease from AATD have a Glu342Lys substitution in both genes and are Pi*ZZ homozygotes (also known as ZZ; Pi :protease inhibitor). About 0.05 % of the United States population is homozygous for the Z allele, whereas 2 % of the population is heterozygous [3].

The mutant Z gene drives the production of a mutant Z protein which folds abnormally, impeding its secretion from the endoplasmic reticulum (ER) of the hepatocyte. Its accumulation in the hepatocyte ER leads to hepatocyte injury, inflammation, fibrosis, and in some patients, cirrhosis of the liver [4]. In addition, failure to excrete the protein from the liver leads to a deficiency state in the lung, with Pi*ZZ homozygotes having serum levels of only 10–15 % of normal ranges [2]. This translates to disinhibited connective tissue breakdown by the neutrophil proteases in the lung, resulting in premature emphysema [5]. Heterozygote carriers of a Z allele combined with a normal M gene, Pi*MZ, are generally healthy but appear to be more susceptible to liver disease in the presence of another injurious agent to the hepatocyte. The S variant, causing the Glu288Val substitution in the AAT gene, is common in North American and Western European populations particularly in Spain and Portugal. It may cause significant lung disease or liver disease when it is present in combination with the Z allele (Pi*SZ), but not when present in homozygous form Pi*SS [3]. Other rare mutations can yield a protein with a normal M migration on electrophoresis (M Duarte and M malton alleles), but when present in the heterozygous state with a Z allele, the protein may accumulate in the ER of the hepatocyte and cause liver disease. Such mutations can be detected by a profoundly low AAT level in peripheral blood that is below that expected for a Pi*MZ phenotype (Table 19.1) [6, 7]. The presence of null genes or other unusual alleles that do not direct the synthesis of a protein product that accumulates in the ER of the liver

Table 19.1 Clinical phenotype in alpha-1 antitrypsin deficiency

Phenotype	Alpha-1 antirtypsin serum level (% of normal) [36]	Risk of emphysema	Risk of liver disease
Pi*ZZ	12–15 %	High	High
Pi*MZ	69–85 %	Minimally increased	Slightly increased
Pi*SZ	33–39 %	Slightly increased	Increased
Pi*SS	67–75 %	Minimally increased	Slightly increased
Pi*null-null	0	High	None
Pi*Z-Null	0–0.5 %	High	Increased
Pi*MM	100 %	Normal	Normal

will not cause liver disease, but null genes with resulting undetectable serum AAT level will almost certainly result in lung disease.

Alpha-1 antitrypsin deficiency is the most common hereditary neonatal liver disease. It can lead to cirrhosis and hepatocellular carcinoma in some adults [8]. Although the classical Pi*ZZ form of AAT is found in 1 in 1600 to 1 in 2000 live births in most populations [9], prospective screening studies in Sweden report that only about 10 % of affected individuals develop clinically significant liver disease by the time they reach the fourth decade of life [10, 11], suggesting that other genetic and/or environmental factors may play a role in the phenotypic expression of the disease.

Pathophysiology of the AAT ZZ Liver Disease

The mutant Z protein is transcribed and translated in the hepatocyte, then transported into the endoplasmic reticulum, where it undergoes folding into its final conformation in preparation for secretion. Unfortunately, the mutant protein folds inefficiently due to the amino acid substitution. Its abnormal configuration impairs its secretion from the ER, and these proteins are directed mostly into a variety of proteolytic pathways referred to as "ER-associated degradation (ERAD)," but some survive and take various conformations, including the linkage of large groups of Z protein "polymers" by noncovalent bonds that allow them to become visible on light microscopy as "globules" [12]. Although the actual degradation mechanism remains to be elucidated, calnexin, and ER manosidase have been identified to be possible points of control [13]. Pi*ZZ homozygous patients with less efficient ERAD mechanisms are more susceptible to development of liver disease than those with more efficient mechanisms [14]. Autophagy is another important proteolytic pathway that is upregulated by the accumulation of Z protein polymers, leading to the degradation of abnormal proteins by specialized vacuoles. Increasing autophagy in animal models has led to a reduction in the accumulation of the Z protein polymers and consequent liver injury [15, 16]. Hepatocytes with large burden of polymerized Z proteins undergo apoptosis, initiating a chronic process of cell injury that leads to cell death, fibrosis, and eventually in some individuals, cirrhosis. However, it is well recognized that individuals with the same Pi*ZZ genotype demonstrate variable extents of clinical liver injury, invoking the probable roles of environmental and genetic modifiers that alter the rate and severity of the clinical manifestation of the disease.

Clinical Presentation and Natural History

As is seen in other liver diseases that affect neonates, persistent jaundice is the most common presenting symptom at 4–8 weeks of age in those who manifest the disease. Accompanying symptoms may include poor feeding, poor weight gain, and pruritus. Some babies may have hepatomegaly, and the laboratory derangements may demonstrate either a hepatitis picture with elevated serum transaminases, or cholestasis with elevated alkaline phosphatase [17]. Occasionally, neonates present with bleeding from the gastrointestinal tract or from the umbilical stump, or easy bruising [18].

Liver disease from AATD may be diagnosed later in childhood, presenting with asymptomatic hepatomegaly or elevated transaminases, or with jaundice that may occur during the course of an unrelated illness. It can also remain further undetected until the adolescence or adulthood, where it can present with complications of cirrhosis and portal hypertension, such as splenomegaly and hypersplenism, gastrointestinal bleeding from varices, ascites, or hepatic encephalopathy [17]. The diagnosis should be considered in adults who present with chronic liver disease or cirrhosis of unknown etiology.

The natural history of liver disease due to AATD is remarkably variable. Most infants that manifested jaundice early in life recover and become asymptomatic by age 1 year, despite the few who would require liver transplantation. Majority of these children will remain without symptoms as they grow older. In the only prospective study of AATD diagnosed by screening 200,000 neonates in Sweden in the 1970s, 127 infants were diagnosed with the classic form of AATD. Eleven percent of these infants had prolonged jaundice, 6 % had hepatomegaly with or without elevated serum transaminases, and approximately 43 % had elevated serum transaminases alone. Five of the twenty neonates with clinical evidence of liver disease died of cirrhosis in early childhood. Follow-up of the remaining population at age 18 years showed that only 12 % of the ZZ phenotype had elevated serum transaminases, although there were no clinical signs of liver disease, while 10 % of the SZ phenotype had similar findings. Therefore, although 17 % of the population had clinical evidence of liver disease in the first 18 years of life, almost 90 % of those who reached adulthood had normal liver enzymes, although biopsies were not performed to confirm the absence of liver injury [11].

Lung destruction in the form of emphysema caused by AATD usually manifests later in the third decade. The incidence of liver disease in patients who were diagnosed with emphysema from AATD is not clearly defined, although one small series reported elevated liver chemistry tests in 50 % [19].

Diagnosis

The diagnosis of AATD should be considered in an individual who presents with symptoms of chronic liver disease or demonstrates elevated liver chemistry tests, particularly those who do not have an obvious etiology. The disease is characterized by the presence of altered AAT proteins that accumulates in the liver, such that circulating serum AAT levels are expected to be low and the serum AAT phenotype determination by isoelectric-focusing electrophoresis would reveal the altered

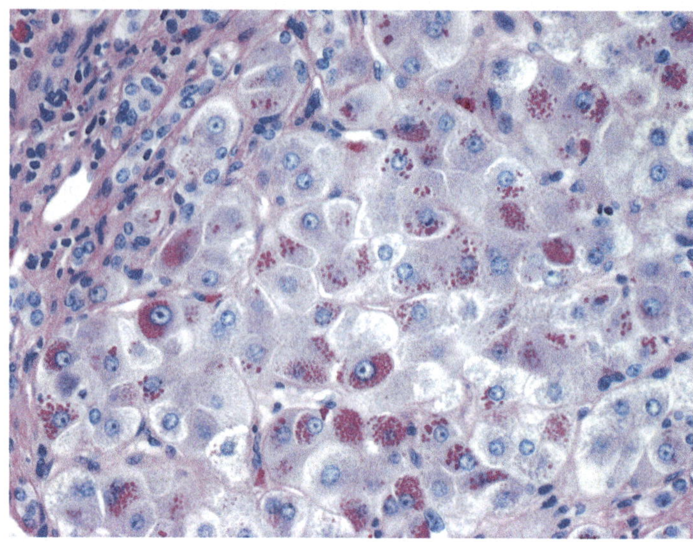

Fig. 19.1 Liver histology from a patient with ZZ alpha-1 antitrypsin deficiency, demonstrating eosinophilic periodic acid-Schiff-positive, diastase-resistant globules in the cytoplasm of the hepatocytes (Courtesy of John Hart, MD)

protein type. While screening for the disease is typically performed with the AAT level measurement, it is important to remember that these levels may be falsely elevated to normal or near-normal ranges in affected patients by a concomitant inflammatory host response. On the other hand, patients with advanced cirrhosis and compromised synthetic function of the liver may have low serum protein levels, including AAT levels. Therefore, both serum concentrations and phenotype determination should be obtained when the diagnosis is seriously considered.

Histologically, accumulation of the abnormal AAT molecules in the liver is represented by the presence of periodic acid-Schiff-positive, diastase-resistant globules in the endoplasmic reticulum of hepatocytes (Fig. 19.1). These inclusions are eosinophilic, round to oval, 1–40 μm in diameter located prominently in periportal hepatocytes, and less so in Kupffer cells and biliary epithelial cells [20]. However, it is important to note that the globules are not present in all hepatocytes, or can be small or "dust-like" in small infants, or totally absent in neonatal livers [21].

The lung manifestation of AATD is rarely seen in childhood or adolescence, but becomes more common when the individual reaches the mid to late 30 years of life. The development and severity of emphysema in AATD is significantly increased up to 1000-fold by cigarette smoking [22]. Alpha-1 antitrypsin deficiency has been associated with vasculitic diseases [23], and the closest association has been demonstrated in a genome-wide sequence analysis that demonstrated the association of anti-proteinase 3 antineutrophil cytoplasmic antibody (ANCA) with the gene encoding AAT (SERPINA1) [24]. It also has been associated with panniculitis, which can respond to augmentation therapy [25, 26].

Management

Whereas the management of lung disease from AATD focuses mostly on avoidance of smoking and pollution and augmentation therapy, these strategies do not have any impact on the liver. Referral to a pulmonologist to evaluate and manage any lung manifestation would be important, as regular monitoring of lung function would be essential as the risk of emphysema increases with age. Avoidance of first-hand or second-hand smoking as well as pollution must be stressed [27]. Augmentation therapy or exogenous AAT replacement, if indicated, can benefit lung disease.

Currently, the management of liver disease due to AATD consists mainly of supportive measures, as there is no available specific therapy targeted to the liver. The use of long-term ursodiol in children with milder liver disease from AAT has been associated with improvement in liver chemistry tests, but a true benefit on histologic disease or the natural history of the disease remains to be seen [28]. When cirrhosis of the liver is suspected or established, screening for hepatocellular carcinoma and for esophageal varices should be performed, and preventive measures against some complications such as variceal bleeding or malnutrition can be instituted. In the setting of advanced fibrosis or cirrhosis, abstinence from alcohol is necessary to avoid a more rapid decompensation. When hepatic decompensation or hepatocellular carcinoma has developed, liver transplantation may be necessary. Liver transplantation in children and adults is associated with excellent survival rates of 90 and 83 % in 5 years, respectively [29]. Animal models of AAT liver disease have demonstrated a unique toxicity of nonsteroidal anti-inflammatory drugs to the Pi*ZZ liver by increasing the production of the mutant Z protein [30], so it would be prudent to avoid the use of NSAIDS in this patient population.

Various directed therapies are currently under investigation for AATD. Similar to other genetic diseases, gene therapy for AAT have been demonstrated to succeed in mouse models, including one model where inhibition of the synthesis of the mutant Z protein by 80 % and generation of the normal M AAT protein were achieved with an exogenous mRNA incorporated into recombinant adeno-associated virus vectors, allowing prevention of liver disease and lung disease at the same time [31]. This therapy appears promising with its dual benefits, provided its efficacy can be duplicated in humans and safety concerns can be overcome. The use of stem cells as a delivery tool has also been explored in mouse models, where gene transfer via lentivirally transduced hematopoietic stem cells has led to sustained human AAT expression [32]. Induced pluripotent stem cells (IPSC) have been used to correct the point mutation in individuals with AATD, and these corrected IPSC's can differentiate into hepatocyte-like cells in vitro with demonstrated ability to function when transplanted into the liver of a mouse [33].

Studies on small molecules that may alter the folding process of the Z protein to prevent retention or polymerization and allow secretion or degradation have also been undertaken. A drug called 4-phenylbutyrate was able to increase the secretion of the mutant Z protein in cell culture and animal models [34], but unfortunately did not show this benefit in humans [35]. Other drugs that have been studied in animal models include rapamycin and carbamazepine, which are aimed at inducing autophagic degration of the mutant Z protein in the endoplasmic reticulum and preventing its accumulation. These interventions have led to reduced fibrosis and reduced levels of markers of liver injury [16, 28]. Known toxicities from these drugs in humans are a significant concern, however, so a clinical trial of carbamazepine to treat AATD in humans is currently being conducted at doses that are much lower than those given to animal models. At the present time, use of carbamazepine and rapamycin in AATD remain experimental.

Conclusions

Homozygous AATD is a common metabolic liver disease that affects children and adults with a highly variable penetrance and natural history that are influenced by other genetic and environmental modifiers. Accumulation of the mutant Z protein in the hepatocyte ER activates an intracellular injury cascade of cell injury that leads to apoptotic cell death, fibrosis, and eventually in some individuals, cirrhosis. Currently, there is no specific treatment for liver disease from AATD other than supportive measures, and liver transplantation if indicated, but promising avenues utilizing gene therapy, stem cell transplantation, and stimulation of autophagy are currently under active investigation.

References

1. Laurell C, Eriksson S. The electrophoretic alpha 1 globulin pattern of serum in alpha 1 antitrypsin deficiency. Scan J Clin Lab Invest. 1963;15:132–40.
2. Perlmutter DH. Alpha-1 antitrypsin deficiency. In: Suchy F, Sokol R, Balisteri W, editors. Liver disease in children. 3rd ed. Philadelphia: Lippincott Williams & Wilkins; 2007.
3. Nelson DR, Teckman J, Di Bisceglie AM, Brenner DA. Diagnosis and management of patients with alpha1-antitrypsin (A1AT) deficiency. Clin Gastroenterol Hepatol. 2012;10(6):575–80.
4. Lindblad D, Blomenkamp K, Teckman J. Alpha-1-antitrypsin mutant Z protein content in individual hepatocytes correlates with cell death in a mouse model. Hepatology. 2007;46(4):1228–35.
5. Eriksson S. Discovery of alpha 1-antitrypsin deficiency. Lung. 1990;168(Suppl):523–9.
6. Lomas DA, Elliott PR, Sidhar SK, Foreman RC, Finch JT, Cox DW, et al. alpha 1-Antitrypsin Mmalton (Phe52-deleted) forms loop-sheet polymers in vivo. Evidence for the C sheet mechanism of polymerization. J Biol Chem. 1995;270(28):16864–70.
7. Lomas DA, Finch JT, Seyama K, Nukiwa T, Carrell RW. Alpha 1-antitrypsin Siiyama (Ser53 → Phe). Further evidence for intracellular loop-sheet polymerization. J Biol Chem. 1993;268(21):15333–5.
8. Eriksson S, Carlson J, Velez R. Risk of cirrhosis and primary liver cancer in alpha 1-antitrypsin deficiency. N Engl J Med. 1986;314(12):736–9.
9. Sveger T. The natural history of liver disease in alpha 1-antitrypsin deficient children. Acta Paediatr Scand. 1988;77(6):847–51.
10. Sveger T. Liver disease in alpha1-antitrypsin deficiency detected by screening of 200,000 infants. N Engl J Med. 1976;294(24):1316–21.
11. Sveger T, Eriksson S. The liver in adolescents with alpha 1-antitrypsin deficiency. Hepatology. 1995;22(2):514–7.

12. Lomas DA, Mahadeva R. Alpha1-antitrypsin polymerization and the serpinopathies: pathobiology and prospects for therapy. J Clin Invest. 2002;110(11):1585–90.
13. Qu D, Teckman JH, Omura S, Perlmutter DH. Degradation of a mutant secretory protein, alpha1-antitrypsin Z, in the endoplasmic reticulum requires proteasome activity. J Biol Chem. 1996;271(37):22791–5.
14. Wu Y, Whitman I, Molmenti E, Moore K, Hippenmeyer P, Perlmutter DH. A lag in intracellular degradation of mutant alpha 1-antitrypsin correlates with the liver disease phenotype in homozygous PiZZ alpha 1-antitrypsin deficiency. Proc Natl Acad Sci U S A. 1994;91(19):9014–8.
15. Hidvegi T, Ewing M, Hale P, Dippold C, Beckett C, Kemp C, et al. An autophagy-enhancing drug promotes degradation of mutant alpha1-antitrypsin Z and reduces hepatic fibrosis. Science. 2010;329(5988):229–32.
16. Kaushal S, Annamali M, Blomenkamp K, Rudnick D, Halloran D, Brunt EM, et al. Rapamycin reduces intrahepatic alpha-1-antitrypsin mutant Z protein polymers and liver injury in a mouse model. Exp Biol Med. 2010;235(6):700–9.
17. Perlmutter DH. Alpha-1-antitrypsin deficiency: diagnosis and treatment. Clin Liver Dis. 2004;8(4):839–59. viii–ix.
18. Hope PL, Hall MA, Millward-Sadler GH, Normand IC. Alpha-1-antitrypsin deficiency presenting as a bleeding diathesis in the newborn. Arch Dis Child. 1982;57(1):68–70.
19. von Schonfeld J, Breuer N, Zotz R, Liedmann H, Wencker M, Beste M, et al. Liver function in patients with pulmonary emphysema due to severe alpha-1-antitrypsin deficiency (Pi ZZ). Digestion. 1996;57(3):165–9.
20. Yunis EJ, Agostini Jr RM, Glew RH. Fine structural observations of the liver in alpha-1-antitrypsin deficiency. Am J Pathol. 1976;82(2):265–86.
21. Teckman JH, Jain A. Advances in alpha-1-antitrypsin deficiency liver disease. Curr Gastroenterol Rep. 2014;16(1):367.
22. Silverman EK, Sandhaus RA. Clinical practice. Alpha1-antitrypsin deficiency. N Engl J Med. 2009;360(26):2749–57.
23. Morris H, Morgan MD, Wood AM, Smith SW, Ekeowa UI, Herrmann K, et al. ANCA-associated vasculitis is linked to carriage of the Z allele of alpha(1) antitrypsin and its polymers. Ann Rheum Dis. 2011;70(10):1851–6.
24. Lyons PA, Rayner TF, Trivedi S, Holle JU, Watts RA, Jayne DR, et al. Genetically distinct subsets within ANCA-associated vasculitis. N Engl J Med. 2012;367(3):214–23.
25. Lyon MJ. Metabolic panniculitis: alpha-1 antitrypsin deficiency panniculitis and pancreatic panniculitis. Dermatol Ther. 2010;23(4):368–74.
26. Valverde R, Rosales B, Ortiz-de Frutos FJ, Rodriguez-Peralto JL, Ortiz-Romero PL. Alpha-1-antitrypsin deficiency panniculitis. Dermatol Clin. 2008;26(4):447–51. vi.
27. Turner AM. Alpha-1 antitrypsin deficiency: new developments in augmentation and other therapies. BioDrugs. 2013;27(6):547–58.
28. Lykavieris P, Ducot B, Lachaux A, Dabadie A, Broue P, Sarles J, et al. Liver disease associated with ZZ alpha1-antitrypsin deficiency and ursodeoxycholic acid therapy in children. J Pediatr Gastroenterol Nutr. 2008;47(5):623–9.
29. Kemmer N, Kaiser T, Zacharias V, Neff GW. Alpha-1-antitrypsin deficiency: outcomes after liver transplantation. Transplant Proc. 2008;40(5):1492–4.
30. Rudnick DA, Shikapwashya O, Blomenkamp K, Teckman JH. Indomethacin increases liver damage in a murine model of liver injury from alpha-1-antitrypsin deficiency. Hepatology. 2006;44(4):976–82.
31. Mueller C, Tang Q, Gruntman A, Blomenkamp K, Teckman J, Song L, et al. Sustained miRNA-mediated knockdown of mutant AAT with simultaneous augmentation of wild-type AAT has minimal effect on global liver miRNA profiles. Mol Ther. 2012;20(3):590–600.
32. Wilson AA, Kwok LW, Hovav AH, Ohle SJ, Little FF, Fine A, et al. Sustained expression of alpha1-antitrypsin after transplantation of manipulated hematopoietic stem cells. Am J Respir Cell Mol Biol. 2008;39(2):133–41.

33. Yusa K, Rashid ST, Strick-Marchand H, Varela I, Liu PQ, Paschon DE, et al. Targeted gene correction of alpha1-antitrypsin deficiency in induced pluripotent stem cells. Nature. 2011;478(7369):391–4.
34. Burrows JA, Willis LK, Perlmutter DH. Chemical chaperones mediate increased secretion of mutant alpha 1-antitrypsin (alpha 1-AT) Z: a potential pharmacological strategy for prevention of liver injury and emphysema in alpha 1-AT deficiency. Proc Natl Acad Sci U S A. 2000;97(4):1796–801.
35. Teckman JH. Lack of effect of oral 4-phenylbutyrate on serum alpha-1-antitrypsin in patients with alpha-1-antitrypsin deficiency: a preliminary study. J Pediatr Gastroenterol Nutr. 2004;39(1):34–7.
36. Wise RA. Alpha-1 antitrypsin deficiency. In: Porter R, editor. Merck manual of diagnosis and therapy. Whitehouse Station, NJ: Merck Sharp & Dohme Corp, a subsidiary of Merck & Co, Inc.; 2014 [updated June 2014; cited 2015 January 2, 2015]. http://www.merckmanuals.com/professional/pulmonary_disorders/chronic_obstructive_pulmonary_disease_and_related_disorders/alpha-1_antitrypsin_deficiency.html. Accessed 2 Jan 2015.

Chapter 20
Metabolic and Genetic Liver Diseases: Hemochromatosis

Matthew J. Stotts and Bruce R. Bacon

1. *What are the most common symptoms of patients with hereditary hemochromatosis?*

   Currently, the majority of patients with hereditary hemochromatosis (HH) are identified through routine screening laboratory tests, or through screening family members of a patient with the disease. Patients identified in this manner usually have no symptoms or physical examination findings.

   When symptoms do occur, they are typically nonspecific and include fatigue and lethargy. Eventually, patients may develop more organ-specific symptoms or signs—such as joint pains and "bronzed" or grayish skin pigmentation—as well as symptoms related to HH complications such as chronic liver disease, congestive heart failure, and diabetes.

2. *How is the diagnosis of hemochromatosis made?*

   Patients with abnormal iron studies or liver function tests, symptoms or signs of hemochromatosis, or with a positive family history should be evaluated for the possible diagnosis of hemochromatosis.

   Initial evaluation should include serum iron, total iron-binding capacity (TIBC, or transferrin), and serum ferritin. The transferrin saturation (TS) should be calculated from the ratio of iron to TIBC. If the TS is greater than 45 % or if the serum ferritin is elevated, the diagnosis should be strongly considered and HFE mutation analysis should be performed.

   If a patient is homozygous for the C282Y allele or a compound heterozygote (C282Y/H63D) with abnormal iron studies as described above, they are consid-

M.J. Stotts, M.D. (✉)
Banner Health, Greeley, Colorado, St. Louis, MO, USA
e-mail: mstotts@slu.edu

B.R. Bacon, M.D.
Division of Gastroenterology & Hepatology, St. Louis University,
3635 Vista Avenue, Saint Louis, MO 63110, USA
e-mail: baconbr@slu.edu

© Springer International Publishing Switzerland 2017
K. Saeian, R. Shaker (eds.), *Liver Disorders,*
DOI 10.1007/978-3-319-30103-7_20

ered to have HH. For compound heterozygotes, other etiologies of liver disease should be additionally considered.

3. *What is the role of magnetic resonance imaging (MRI) in the diagnosis and management of hemochromatosis?*

   Given that the diagnosis of HH can be made based on serum iron studies and genetic testing, noninvasive assessment of hepatic iron concentration (HIC) is unlikely to aid in the diagnosis or management of these patients. When secondary causes of iron overload are present, however, ferritin is not a reliable predictor of total body iron stores. In this setting, a noninvasive and reliable measurement of HIC makes MRI an attractive modality, as it could aid in assessing the degree of iron overload in addition to monitoring iron stores with appropriate treatment.

   The use of MRI to assess HIC is currently limited to use in a few centers with special interest, as the diagnostic accuracy remains unclear. A recent rigorous meta-analysis noted substantial heterogeneity among the available literature, with studies using different MRI sequences and different thresholds for positivity [1]. More studies will need to be performed to make any firm conclusions regarding the use of MRI to measure HIC. A specific MRI protocol called FerriScan may have increased utility in this situation [2].

4. *What is the treatment for a patient with hereditary hemochromatosis?*

   The treatment of HH is relatively straightforward and requires serial phlebotomy to deplete excess iron stores. Once the serum ferritin is <50 µg/L and the transferrin saturation is <50 %, the majority of excessive iron stores have been depleted. At this point, most patients can begin a regimen of maintenance phlebotomy, typically 1 unit every 2–3 months.

   With treatment, patients typically have less fatigue and less abdominal pain. Liver enzymes and cardiac function may improve, and glucose intolerance may become more easily managed. Advanced cirrhosis, hypogonadism, and arthropathy typically do not improve with phlebotomy.

5. *What is the prognosis?*

   Patients diagnosed and treated before developing cirrhosis should expect a normal life span. Among patients not diagnosed and treated early, common causes of death include complications of chronic liver disease and the development of hepatocellular carcinoma.

6. *Should the family members of patients with hemochromatosis be screened?*

   Once a patient with hemochromatosis is identified, all first-degree relatives should be offered screening. This is done by obtaining both HFE mutation analysis (for C282Y and H63D mutations) and tests for transferrin saturation and ferritin simultaneously. If a relative is found to be a C282Y homozygote or a compound heterozygote (C282Y/H63D) and has abnormally elevated iron studies, they have the diagnosis of HH.

Introduction

Hereditary hemochromatosis (HH) refers to a group of iron metabolism disorders that can result in chronic deposition of iron into tissues. Left untreated, this relatively common disorder can result in life-threatening complications — including the development of cirrhosis, hepatocellular carcinoma, diabetes, and heart disease.

The principal underlying abnormality of the HFE gene was first described in 1996, identified as a missense mutation leading to a tyrosine for cysteine substitution at amino acid position 282 of the HFE protein [3]. Patients who are homozygous for this defect, known as C282Y, account for approximately 80–85 % of HH patients [4]. Two other regularly identified mutations of the HFE gene, H63D, and S65C, are generally not associated with iron overload unless they are a compound heterozygote with a C282Y mutation. Other inherited iron overload syndromes may occur independently of the HFE gene; these are thought to result from mutations of genes coding for iron regulatory proteins, namely hepcidin, hemojuvelin, transferrin receptor 2, and ferroportin [5]. These underlying mutations result in increased and inappropriate intestinal iron absorption, resulting from low expression of the iron-regulatory protein hepcidin [6, 7].

As iron is deposited into tissue, it interacts with oxygen to produce superoxide and hydroxyl radicals that can damage critical cell components. Long-standing iron overload can result in end-organ consequences. With early diagnosis and appropriate treatment, however, patients with HH can expect to have a normal lifespan and effectively halt disease progression [8].

Classification of Hemochromatosis: Primary Versus Secondary Iron Overload Syndromes

The classification of iron overload is typically divided into three groups: those with inherited causes (primary or hereditary hemochromatosis), those with various causes of secondary iron overload, and those with parenteral iron overload.

Of the primary form (HH), approximately 85–90 % of patients are homozygous for C282Y. A minority of patients are compound heterozygotes (meaning one allele has C282Y and one has either H63D or S65C). The remaining hereditary forms likely involve mutations in other genes of iron homeostasis.

Secondary iron overload occurs when the intestine absorbs excessive amounts of iron, caused by some other stimulus. Examples include various forms of anemia due to ineffective erythropoiesis (such as thalassemia, aplastic anemia, and some patients with sickle cell anemia), chronic liver disease, and, more rarely, an excessive intake of medicinal iron.

In instances of parenteral iron overload, patients receive excessive iron as either red blood cell transfusions or as parenteral iron. Over time, these patients can become significantly iron overloaded.

Epidemiology

Hereditary hemochromatosis is considered the most common known genetic disorder identified in Caucasians. It is inherited in an autosomal recessive fashion. The C282Y allele likely originated in Northern Europe — it is very common among descendants of the Celtic population. Prospective population studies show that one in eight people with European heritage are heterozygous for the trait and roughly one in 200–220 are homozygous [5, 9, 10]. It is important to note that only homozygotes (and occasionally C282Y/H63D compound heterozygotes) are at risk for developing serious iron overload, whereas heterozygotes have near normal iron metabolism and do not develop the disease.

The disease's clinical penetrance is variable, with studies indicating that approximately 70 % of C282Y homozygotes develop evidence of iron overload, of which fewer than 10 % develop severe iron overload accompanied by organ damage [11, 12]. In this setting, the European Association for the Study of the Liver (EASL) recognizes different stages of HH. Stage 1 refers to the "genetic susceptibility" for the disorder without increased iron stores, Stage 2 refers to those with evidence of iron overload without tissue or organ damage, and Stage 3 refers to those with iron overload who have developed tissue and organ damage [13].

Pathophysiology

The underlying pathophysiologic mechanisms of HH fall into the following four main categories: increased absorption of dietary iron, decreased expression of hepcidin (the iron-regulatory hormone), altered function of the HFE protein, and iron-induced tissue injury and fibrogenesis.

Increased Intestinal Iron Absorption: The earliest association between the HFE protein and iron metabolism occurred when the HFE protein (along with β2-microglobulin) was discovered to form a complex with the transferrin receptor-1 (TfR1) [14]. This association was observed in duodenal crypt enterocytes, which are considered to be the predominant sites of iron absorption in the intestine. This prompted a number of studies examining the effect of the HFE protein on iron uptake. This so-called crypt cell hypothesis is now regarded as less essential in the development of iron overload since hepcidin emerged as a key regulator in iron metabolism.

Hepcidin: Considered the principal iron-regulatory hormone, hepcidin is expressed predominantly in hepatocytes [15]. It is then secreted into the circulation, where it binds to ferroportin in macrophages and ferroportin on the basolateral surface of enterocytes. The ferroportin is then internalized and degraded, thereby inhibiting iron export [16].

By way of this process, hepcidin prevents iron absorption. Excess iron and inflammation induces hepcidin expression, resulting in decreased iron absorption and decreased iron release from macrophages [15]. Iron deficiency decreases hepcidin expression, resulting in increased iron absorption. Patients with mutations of the genes for HFE, hemojuvelin, hepcidin, or TfR2 will have inappropriate iron absorption as a result of decreased hepcidin expression [15].

HFE protein: The HFE gene encodes a 343-amino acid protein that consists of a large extracellular domain, a single transmembrane domain, and a short cytoplasmic tail [3]. The extracellular domain consists of three loops (α_1, α_2, α_3) with intramolecular disulfide bonds within the α_2 and α_3 loops. Its structure is similar to other major histocompatibility complex (MHC) class I proteins, although evidence indicates that it does not participate in antigen presentation [17].

The major mutation of HH, the C282Y mutation, is a missense mutation that results in a substitution of tyrosine for cysteine at amino acid position 282, abolishing the disulfide bond in the α_3 loop [3]. This subsequently interferes with the interaction of the HFE protein and β_2-microglobulin, resulting in decreased presentation to the cell surface and increased rates of degradation.

The major mechanism by which HFE influences iron-dependent regulation of hepcidin remains uncertain. HFE can bind to both TfR2 and the classic transferrin receptor, TfR1 [18, 19]. Additionally, both HFE and TfR2 may interact with HJV, suggesting that an HFE and TfR2 complex may regulate BMP6 signaling [20]. It has been proposed that the complex of HFE acts as an iron sensor at the cell membrane of the hepatocyte [19]. As transferrin saturation (TS) increases, the HFE protein is displaced from TfR1, making it available to bind to TfR2. The complex of HFE and TfR2 has been postulated to influence hepcidin expression [21].

Iron-Induced Liver Damage: Experimental iron overload in the liver has been shown to cause iron-dependent oxidative damage and associated impairment of membrane-dependent function of mitochondria, microsomes, and lysosomes [22, 23]. One hypothesis is that hepatocyte iron-induced lipid peroxidation causes hepatocellular injury and death. Byproducts then activate Kupffer cells, which produce profibrogenic cytokines and stimulate hepatic stellate cells to increase collagen synthesis and hepatic fibrinogenesis [24].

Clinical Features

The clinical course of HH involves progressive iron accumulation over decades. The first biochemical abnormality seen is elevated transferrin saturation (TS), with a subsequent rise of ferritin that occurs with a progressive increase in iron stores. Patients may develop nonspecific symptoms that commonly include weakness or lethargy, right upper quadrant abdominal pain, arthralgias (typically of the second and third metacarpophalangeal joints), chondrocalcinosis, impotence, and decreased libido. They may also develop porphyria cutanea tarda, a blistering skin rash that occurs in sun-exposed areas. With progressive disease, iron deposition in the pancreas leads to loss of beta cell function and the development of diabetes mellitus. Cardiomyopathy can develop. Cirrhosis can develop insidiously, often with normal or minimally elevated transaminases. The classic description of "bronze diabetes" refers to the bronzed or slate-gray skin changes, which requires careful clinical observation.

It is important to note the variable penetrance of the disease for those patients with HH, as not all patients with the genetic abnormality will go on to develop disease. In large population studies, approximately 70% of patients who are homozygous for C282Y have been shown to have an elevated ferritin, of whom only a small percentage develop the clinical consequences of iron storage disease [9, 11, 12]. In addition, older case series, wherein patients were diagnosed based on symptoms or examination findings, have shown that men typically presented 10 years earlier and ten times more frequently than women [5]. This difference is likely due to women experiencing progressive iron losses from menstruation and iron loss during pregnancy.

Over the last several decades, a notable transition has occurred in the presentation of patients with hemochromatosis. In case series from the 1950s to the 1980s, most patients identified had the classic signs and symptoms as described above [25–27]. Through the 1990s, however, patients with HH were identified increasingly by abnormal iron studies on routine labs or through family screening. In this setting, approximately 75% of those identified did not exhibit any symptoms or manifestations of advanced disease [28, 29].

Diagnosis

Persons should undergo evaluation for the diagnosis of HH if they have a family history of HH, suspected symptoms or organ involvement, or abnormal laboratory or radiographic findings suggestive of iron overload. All patients with abnormal liver function should have iron studies at some point in their evaluation [5].

The diagnosis of HH is based on documentation of increased iron stores, namely an elevation in serum ferritin, in addition to genotypic evidence of being homozygous for C282Y or a compound heterozygote for C282Y/H63D.

The diagnostic approach for HH is shown in Fig. 20.1, adapted from the guidelines of the American Association for the Study of Liver Diseases (AASLD) [5]. While patients with first degree relatives should be screened with both iron studies and HFE genotype (see below), the recommended algorithm for both symptomatic and asymptomatic patients is to first obtain *both* a serum transferrin saturation and ferritin level. Transferrin saturation (TS) is calculated as follows:

$$\text{Transferrin Saturation} = (\text{Iron / TIBC}) \times 100\%$$

The recommended cutoff for TS is 45%—higher values are considered abnormal and warrant further evaluation. Note that abnormal TS is often the earliest phenotypic manifestation of HFE-related HH.

While serum ferritin has less variability than TS, ferritin is often falsely positive in multiple inflammatory conditions. These include necroinflammatory liver

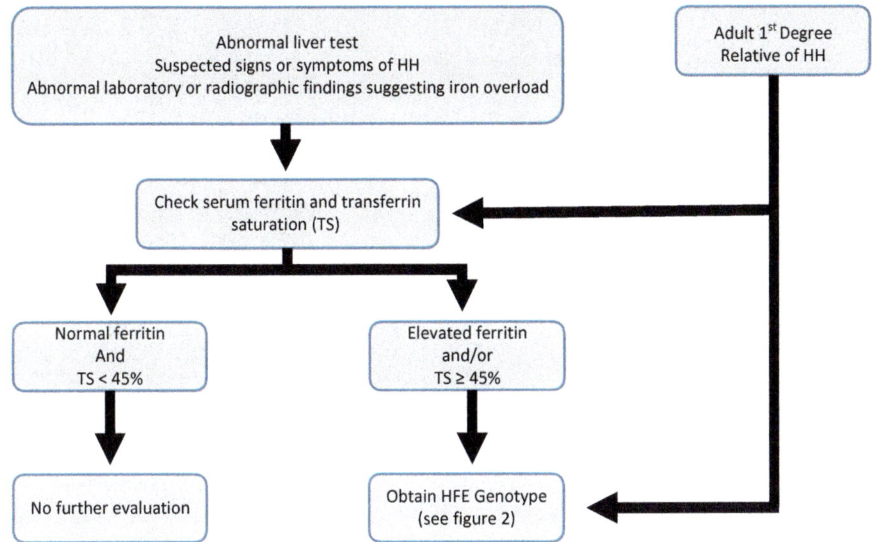

Fig. 20.1 Clinical algorithm for the evaluation of possible HFE-related hereditary hemochromatosis

diseases such as alcoholic liver disease, chronic hepatitis B and C, and nonalcoholic fatty liver disease (NAFLD). In this setting, ferritin is considered a nonspecific finding. In the absence of inflammation, however, serum ferritin concentration provides a valuable correlation with the degree of total body iron stores. In the HEIRS study (HEmochromatosis and IRon overload Screening) of 99,711 North American participants, serum ferritin levels were found to be elevated in 57 % of female and 88 % of males who were C282Y homozygotes [9]. In addition, serum ferritin levels have been shown to predict advanced fibrosis and cirrhosis in patients with HH (see below).

If both the ferritin level is normal and the transferrin saturation is less than 45 %, no further evaluation is required. Evidence for this includes a study of young patients under the age of 35, where this combination of laboratory findings had a negative predictive value of 97 % for excluding iron overload [30].

If either test is abnormal (TS ≥ 45 % or ferritin > the upper limit of normal), further workup with HFE mutation analysis should be performed.

Once HFE genotyping is performed, it is important to know how to interpret the results (see Fig. 20.2). If the patient is found homozygous for C282Y, they have hereditary hemochromatosis and should be managed accordingly. If they are compound heterozygotes (C282Y/H63D), they may have iron overload, but other causes of their symptoms or laboratory abnormalities should be considered. Liver biopsy may be useful (see below). If the patient is found to be non-C282Y or a C282Y heterozygote, they are not at risk for significant iron overload.

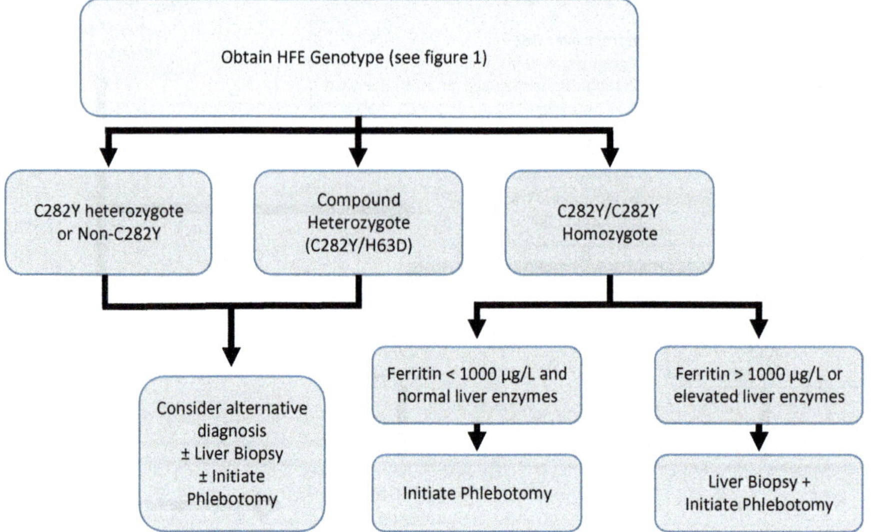

Fig. 20.2 Clinical algorithm for the evaluation of possible HFE-related hereditary hemochromatosis in patients with abnormal iron studies or a pertinent family history (see Fig. 20.1)

The Role of Liver Biopsy

With readily available genetic testing of the HFE gene, liver biopsy has become less important in the diagnosis of HH. Its primary role is to establish the presence of advanced fibrosis or cirrhosis, in addition to assisting when the diagnosis is unclear.

For patients with a known diagnosis of HH, the decision to perform a liver biopsy can be made based on laboratory parameters. If a patient is found to be C282Y homozygous or C282Y/H63D compound heterozygous with a ferritin level lower than 1000 µg/L and normal liver tests, they can be managed with phlebotomy without performing a liver biopsy. A ferritin of <1000 µg/L has been found to be an accurate predictor for the *absence* of cirrhosis [31, 32]. In a study of 670 asymptomatic C282Y homozygotes, 350 patients with an elevated serum ferritin (with a cutoff of 500 µg/L) or abnormal liver tests or hepatomegaly underwent a liver biopsy [32]. Cirrhosis was discovered in 5.6 % of males and 1.9 % of females. In this study, ferritin >1000 µg/L had 100 % sensitivity and 70 % specificity for identifying cirrhosis; specifically, no subject with a ferritin of <1000 µg/L had cirrhosis. Fewer than 2 % of C282Y homozygotes with a ferritin of <1000 µg/L at the time of diagnosis have cirrhosis or fibrosis in the absence of other risk factors [31, 33]. It should be noted, however, that alcohol changes the risk of developing cirrhosis. A study has shown that large amounts of alcohol consumption of greater than 60 g of alcohol a day noted that >60 % of patients with HH had cirrhosis, compared to <7 % of those who consumed less [34].

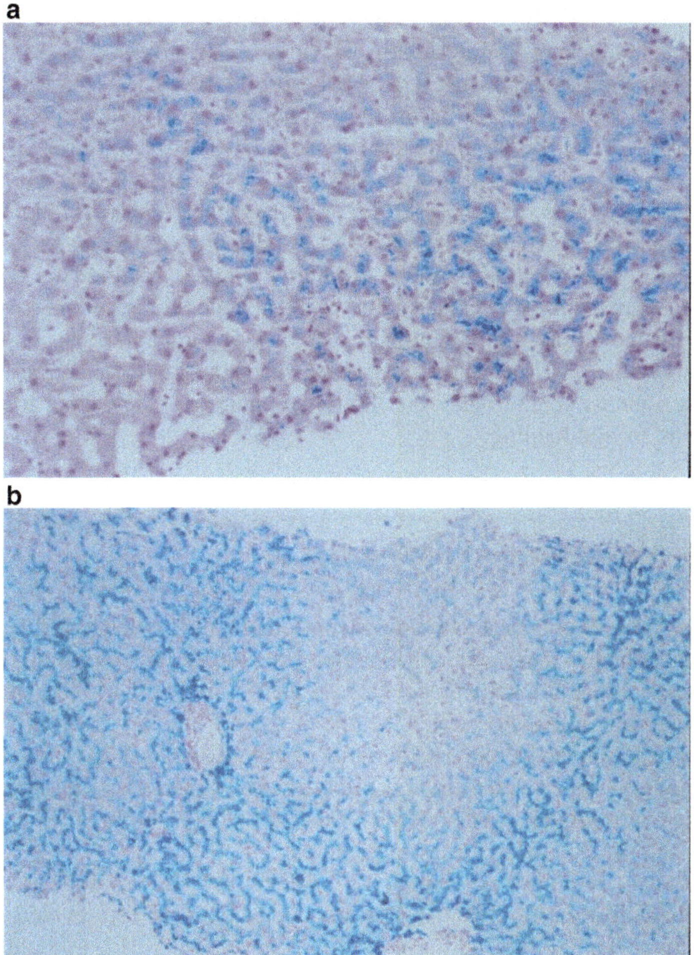

Fig. 20.3 Histology of HFE-related hereditary hemochromatosis. (**a**) This liver biopsy sample was obtained from a 53-year-old C282Y homozygous female who presented with a ferritin level of 1873 ng/mL and a transferrin saturation of 61 %. With Perls' Prussian blue staining, iron deposition is seen in perisinusoidal hepatocytes. (**b**) In this specimen taken from another patient with HFE-related hereditary hemochromatosis, iron deposition is seen much greater in the periportal zone (acinar zone 1) than in the centrilobular zone (acinar zone 3)

If the diagnosis is in question—and especially if the patient is not homozygous for C282Y—a liver biopsy should be considered to evaluate for other causes of liver disease.

When performed, a liver biopsy should include Perls' Prussian blue stains for the evaluation of hepatic iron stores (see Fig. 20.3). In addition, a portion of the liver can be obtained for the measurement of hepatic iron concentration (HIC). A hepatic iron index (HII) can be obtained which measures the rate of hepatic iron accretion; this is calculated by dividing the HIC (in μmol/g) by the patient's age in years, based on the concept that homozygotes would continue to absorb excess dietary iron throughout a lifetime. This is no longer routinely used but is useful in certain scenarios.

The AASLD recommends performing a biopsy in patients who are homozygous for C282Y or compound heterozygotes if liver enzymes (ALT, AST) are elevated or if the serum ferritin is >1000 μg/L. In patients with non-HFE-related HH, biopsy may provide diagnostic information, given that many patients with other liver diseases (such as ALD, NAFLD, chronic viral hepatitis) can have abnormal serum iron studies. When secondary iron overload occurs with other liver diseases, iron deposition is usually mild and generally occurs in perisinusoidal lining cells (Kupffer cells) and hepatocytes in a panlobular distribution [35]. In patients with non-HFE-related HH, data on hepatic iron concentration is useful, along with histopathologic iron staining, to determine the degree and cellular distribution of iron loading.

Clinical Management: Phlebotomy

While there has never been a randomized controlled trial of phlebotomy in the treatment of HH, evidence exists that the initiation of phlebotomy prior to the development of cirrhosis significantly reduces the associated morbidity and mortality [8]. A prospective study has demonstrated that the prognosis and development of complications depends on the amount and duration of iron excess, and that early diagnosis and treatment prior to the development of cirrhosis or diabetes could increase survival of patients with HH to that of the normal population [8]. In this setting, phlebotomy is considered the mainstay of treatment.

The decision to initiate phlebotomy in a patient with HH is based on the known survival benefit of early diagnosis and treatment. Patients with evidence of end organ damage (including abnormal liver tests) due to iron overload should undergo treatment. Considering asymptomatic patients who are homozygous for C282Y with an elevated ferritin and normal liver tests is more difficult given limited longitudinal data. However, because phlebotomy is easy and safe, in addition to the societal benefit of blood donation, current guidelines favor the initiation of prophylactic phlebotomy in these patients. Patients without iron overload (e.g. those with the genetic susceptibility but with a normal ferritin level) would be unlikely to benefit from therapy.

In addition to preventing progression of disease, clinical symptoms likely to be improved by phlebotomy include malaise, fatigue, skin pigmentation, and, if diabetic, insulin requirements. Symptoms less responsive to phlebotomy include arthropathy and testicular atrophy. Patients with established cirrhosis should not expect reversal, although reversal of hepatic fibrosis can be seen. Patients with established cirrhosis will continue to have an increased risk of the development of hepatocellular carcinoma despite depletion of iron stores and should continue to be screened.

Consensus guidelines from the American Association for the Study of Liver Disease (AASLD) provide recommendations for phlebotomy in these patients, with the goal of reducing total body iron stores while avoiding development of anemia of blood loss or eventual iron-deficiency [5]. Most patients in this setting are able to tolerate the removal of 1 unit of blood per week—younger patients can potentially tolerate 2 units a week. Each unit of blood contains an estimated 200–250 mg of iron. While a normal individual's total body iron averages 3–4 g, patients with hemochromatosis can have total body stores of greater than 20 g of iron. In this context, phlebotomy may require 2–3 years to adequately reduce stores. Each phlebotomy should be preceded by the measurement of a hemoglobin or hematocrit to ensure that these are not reduced by more than 20 % of the starting baseline values. In addition, serum ferritin levels should be measured after every 10–12 phlebotomies (roughly once every 3 months) in the initial stages of treatment. Once this value falls to 50–100 µg/L, the clinician can be confident that excess iron stores have been mobilized and depleted. To prevent the development of iron deficiency, serum ferritin levels may need to be followed closely as phlebotomy approaches these goal values.

Once the serum ferritin is at goal, patients should be monitored for iron reaccumulation with a target goal of a ferritin of 50–100 µg/L. Initially, checking ferritin levels every 3 months is useful for monitoring for the presence of excess iron. Most patients will require maintenance phlebotomy of 1 unit every 2–3 months, though this rate varies as some patients may not require maintenance phlebotomy, while others may require it monthly.

Vitamin C supplementation should be avoided in patients undergoing phlebotomy because it is known to accelerate the mobilization of iron to a level that may saturate the circulating transferrin and result in an increase in free radical activity [36]. This may be associated with an increased risk of sudden cardiac death in patients with advanced disease. No dietary adjustments are necessary, however.

Iron chelators are not recommended unless phlebotomy is contraindicated, as with instances of patients with severe anemias or dyserythropoeitic syndromes. Table 20.1 summarizes treatment strategies for patients with hemochromatosis.

Blood removed by phlebotomy from patients with hereditary hemochromatosis has been deemed safe for donation by the American Red Cross and the US Food and Drug Administration [37].

Clinical Management: Hepatocellular Cancer Screening

Hepatocellular carcinoma has long been associated with HH and is a major life-threatening complication that can develop [27]. The relative risk for the development of HCC is approximately 20, with an annual incidence of 3–4 %. This increased risk may be due to iron overload promoting hepatic carcinogenesis via free radicals. Theoretically, this risk would be decreased by reducing iron stores via phlebotomy. However, the risk of HCC is *not* eliminated by phlebotomy in HH patients with cirrhosis.

Table 20.1 Recommended treatment strategy of patients with hemochromatosis

Treatment of hereditary hemochromatosis
One phlebotomy (removal of 500 mL blood) weekly or biweekly
Check hemoglobin/hematocrit prior to each phlebotomy
Allow no more than a 20 % decrease from baseline
Check serum ferritin every 10–12 phlebotomies
Stop frequent phlebotomy when serum ferritin reaches 50–100 μg/L
Avoid vitamin C supplements

Note: patients with secondary iron overload due to dyserythropoiesis may require iron chelators

Given this risk, HH patients with cirrhosis should undergo screening for HCC at 6 month intervals as per AASLD guidelines [38]. Ultrasonography is the most widely used test for surveillance and is in line with current recommendations. AFP (serum alpha-fetoprotein) is an inadequate screening test and is not recommended [38].

Clinical Management: Transplant Considerations

With the development of decompensated cirrhosis or early-stage HCC, liver transplantation can be life-saving. In the past, the survival of patients with hemochromatosis was lower than that of patients undergoing liver transplantation for other causes, with deaths usually occurring in the perioperative period and related to infectious or cardiac conditions [39–41]. These complications may have been secondary to inadequate removal of excess iron stores prior to performing liver transplantation. Survival after liver transplantation is currently comparable to that of other patients [42].

Family Screening

Once a patient with hereditary hemochromatosis is identified, screening should be offered to screen all first-degree relatives [5]. For ease of testing, HFE mutation analysis (to obtain the genotype) in addition to iron studies (ferritin and transferrin saturation, to obtain the phenotype) should be performed simultaneously. This will allow for the detection of early disease and prevention of complications.

For children of an identified homozygous patient, HFE testing of the other parent can be useful. If the other parent has normal HFE testing, the child will be an obligate heterozygote and will not need further workup as they are not at risk for iron overload. However, if the other parent is a C282Y heterozygote, their offspring have a 50 % chance of being homozygous.

C282Y heterozygotes and H63D heterozygotes are not at risk of developing iron overload and should be reassured accordingly. Occasionally, H63D homozygotes can develop mild iron overload—though this is not thought to be clinically significant [43].

C282Y homozygotes or compound heterozygotes with an increased serum ferritin should be initiated with therapeutic phlebotomy. Those with normal ferritin should be followed with yearly iron studies.

General Population Screening

Given the low clinical penetrance of the disease in addition to existing economic models, screening of the average risk general population is not recommended [5].

Future trends: Since the discovery of the HFE gene in 1996, there have been major advances in the understanding of the mechanisms that control iron regulation and absorption. Recognizing that early treatment will prevent the manifestations of HH, ongoing studies should be performed to assess the cost-effectiveness of targeted screening.

References

1. Sarigianni M, Liakos A, Vlachaki E, Paschos P, Athanasiadou E, Montori VM, et al. Accuracy of magnetic resonance imaging in diagnosis of liver iron overload: a systemic review and meta-analysis. Clin Gastroenterol Hepatol. 2015;13(1):55–63.
2. Bacon BR. Measurement of hepatic iron concentration. Clin Gastroenterol Hepatol. 2014; 13(1):64–65.
3. Feder JN, Gnirke A, Thomas W, Tsuchihashi Z, Ruddy DA, Basava A, et al. A novel MHC class I-like gene is mutated in patients with hereditary haemochromatosis. Nat Genet. 1996;13(4):399–408.
4. European Association for the Study of the Liver. EASL clinical practice guidelines for HFE hemochromatosis. J Hepatol. 2010;53(1):3–22.
5. Bacon BR, Adams PC, Kowdley KV, Powell LW, Tavill AS. Diagnosis and management of hemochromatosis: 2011 practice guideline by the American Association for the Study of Liver Diseases. Hepatology. 2011;54(1):328–43.
6. Adams PC, Barton JC. Haemochromatosis. Lancet. 2007;370(9602):1855–60.
7. Pietrangelo A. Hereditary hemochromatosis: a new look at an old disease. N Engl J Med. 2004;350(23):2383–97.
8. Niederau C, Fischer R, Purschel A, Stremmel W, Haussinger D, Strohmeyer G. Long-term survival in patients with hereditary hemochromatosis. Gastroenterology. 1996;110(4):1107–19.
9. Adams PC, Reboussin DM, Barton JC, McLaren CE, Eckfeldt JH, McLaren GD, et al. Hemochromatosis and iron-overload screening in a racially diverse population. N Engl J Med. 2005;352(17):1769–78.
10. Phatak PD, Bonkovsky HL, Kowdley KV. Hereditary hemochromatosis: time for targeted screening. Ann Intern Med. 2008;149(4):270–2.
11. Allen KJ, Gurrin LC, Constantine CC, Osborne NJ, Delatycki MB, Nicoll AJ, et al. Iron-overload-related disease in HFE hereditary hemochromatosis. N Engl J Med. 2008;358(3):221–30.

12. Beutler E, Felitti VJ, Koziol JA, Ho NJ, Gelbart T. Penetrance of 845 G→A (C282Y) HFE hereditary hemochromatosis mutation in the USA. Lancet. 2002;359(9302):211–8.
13. Adams P, Brissot P, Powell LW. EASL international consensus conference on haemochromatosis. J Hepatol. 2000;33(3):485–504.
14. Fleming RE, Britton RS, Waheed A, Sly WS, Bacon BR. Pathogenesis of hereditary hemochromatosis. Clin Liver Dis. 2004;8(4):755–73.
15. Nemeth E, Ganz T. The role of hepcidin in iron metabolism. Acta Haematol. 2009;122(2–3):78–86.
16. Nemeth E, Tuttle MS, Powelson J, Vaughn MB, Donovan A, Ward DM, et al. Hepcidin regulates cellular efflux by binding to ferroportin and inducing its internalization. Science. 2004;306(5704):2090–3.
17. Fleming RE, Britton RS. Iron imports. VI. HFE and regulation of intestinal iron absorption. Am J Physiol Gastrointest Liver Physiol. 2006;290(4):G590–4.
18. Waheed A, Parkkila S, Saarnio J, Fleming RE, Zhou XY, Tomatsu S, et al. Association of HFE protein with transferrin receptor in crypt enterocytes of human duodenum. Proc Natl Acad Sci U S A. 1999;96(4):1579–84.
19. Goswami T, Andrews NC. Hereditary hemochromatosis protein, HFE, interaction with transferrin receptor 2 suggests a molecular mechanism for mammalian iron sensing. J Biol Chem. 2006;281(39):28494–8.
20. Ganz T. Iron homeostasis: fitting the puzzle pieces together. Cell Metab. 2008;7(4):288–90.
21. Fleming RE, Bacon BR. Orchestration of iron homeostasis. N Engl J Med. 2005;352(17):1741–4.
22. Bacon BR, Tavill AS, Brittenham GM, Park CH, Recknagel RO. Hepatic lipid peroxidation in vivo in rats with chronic iron overload. J Clin Invest. 1983;71(3):429–39.
23. Bacon BR, Britton RS. The pathology of hepatic iron overload: a free radical-mediated process? Hepatology. 1990;11(1):127–37.
24. Philippe MA, Ruddell RG, Ramm GA. Role of iron in hepatic fibrosis: one piece in the puzzle. World J Gastroenterol. 2007;13(35):4746–54.
25. Edwards CQ, Cartwright GE, Skolnick MH, Amos DB. Homozygosity for hemochromatosis: clinical manifestations. Ann Intern Med. 1980;93(4):519–25.
26. Milder MS, Cook JD, Stray S, Finch CA. Idiopathic hemochromatosis, an interim report. Medicine (Baltimore). 1980;59(1):34–49.
27. Niederau C, Fischer R, Sonnenberg A, Stremmel W, Trampisch HJ, Strohmeyer G. Survival and causes of death in cirrhotic and in noncirrhotic patients with primary hemochromatosis. N Engl J Med. 1985;313(20):1256–62.
28. Adams PC, Kertesz AE, Valberg LS. Clinical presentation of hemochromatosis: a changing scene. Am J Med. 1991;90(4):445–9.
29. Bacon BR, Sadiq SA. Hereditary hemochromatosis: presentation and diagnosis in the 1990s. Am J Gastroenterol. 1997;92(5):784–9.
30. Bassett ML, Halliday JW, Ferris RA, Powell LW. Diagnosis of hemochromatosis in young subjects: predictive accuracy of biochemical screening tests. Gastroenterology. 1984;87(3):628–33.
31. Morrison ED, Brandhagen DJ, Phatak PD, Barton JC, Krawitt EL, El-Seraq HB, et al. Serum ferritin level predicts advanced hepatic fibrosis among U.S. patients with phenotypic hemochromatosis. Ann Intern Med. 2003;138(8):627–33.
32. Powell LW, Dixon JL, Ramm GA, Purdie DM, Lincoln DJ, Anderson GJ, et al. Screening for hemochromatosis in asymptomatic subjects with or without a family history. Arch Intern Med. 2006;166(3):294–301.
33. Bacon BR, Olynyk JK, Brunt EM, Britton RS, Wolff RK. HFE genotype in patients with hemochromatosis and other liver diseases. Ann Intern Med. 1999;130(12):953–62.
34. Fletcher LM, Dixon JL, Purdie DM, Powell LW, Crawford DH. Excess alcohol greatly increases the prevalence of cirrhosis in hereditary hemochromatosis. Gastroenterology. 2002;122(2):281–9.
35. Brunt EM. Pathology of hepatic iron overload. Semin Liver Dis. 2005;25(4):392–401.
36. Lynch SR, Cook JD. Interaction of vitamin C and iron. Ann N Y Acad Sci. 1980;355:32–44.
37. Brittenham GM, Klein HG, Kushner JP, Ajioka RS. Preserving the national blood supply. Hematol Am Soc Hematol Educ Program. 2001;1:422–32.
38. Bruix J, Sherman M. Management of hepatocellular carcinoma. Hepatology. 2005;42(5):1208–36.

39. Ashrafian H. Hepcidin: the missing link between hemochromatosis and infections. Infect Immun. 2003;71(12):6693–700.
40. Poulos JE, Bacon BR. Liver transplantation for hereditary hemochromatosis. Dig Dis. 1996;14(5):316–22.
41. Farrell FJ, Nguyen M, Woodley S, Imperial JC, Garcia-Kennedy R, Man K, et al. Outcome of liver transplantation in patients with hemochromatosis. Hepatology. 1994;20(2):404–10.
42. Yu L, Ioannou GN. Survival of liver transplant recipients with hemochromatosis in the United States. Gastroenterology. 2007;133(2):489–95.
43. Gochee PA, Powell LW, Cullen DJ, Du Sart D, Rossi E, Olynyk JK. A population-based study of the biochemical and clinical expression of the H63D hemochromatosis mutation. Gastroenterology. 2002;122(3):646–51.

Chapter 21
Metabolic and Genetic Liver Diseases: Wilson's Disease

Syed Rahman and Kia Saeian

Patients' Questions

1. Question 1: How did I get Wilson's disease and are my siblings and/or children also going to get it?

   Patient level answer: Wilson's disease is passed on by a mutation in a gene. Genes come in pairs, with one gene in each pair coming from a parent. This genetic disorder is an autosomal recessive disorder, in which both genes in a pair need to be abnormal for the disease to be present, meaning that you need to inherit two abnormal genes from each of your parents. Please refer to Table 21.1 for a detailed explanation of genetic transmission based on individual scenarios. Of note, a carrier does not have the disease, but can pass genes to their children.
2. Question 2: How does my diet and intake of different foods affect the accumulation of copper in my liver and other organs?

   Patient level answer: Foods are absorbed, along with their respective copper content, in the intestines. Patients with Wilson's disease have impaired copper excretion, leading to unhealthy copper concentrations in the body. Patients with the disease, therefore, should generally avoid foods with high copper concentrations. Foods that should be avoided include shellfish, nuts, chocolate, mushrooms, and organ meats. Patients need to keep in mind environmental exposures, such as copper pipes, containers, or cookware, which may increase copper levels in foods and drinks.
3. Question 3: Besides changing my diet, how can my Wilson's disease be treated?

   Patient level answer: Wilson's disease can be treated with medications, including D-penicillamine, trientine, and zinc. D-penicillamine promotes urinary copper excretion with an extensive side effect profile complicated by skin, bone

S. Rahman, M.D. (✉) • K. Saeian, M.D., M.Sc., Epi (✉)
Division of Gastroenterology and Hepatology, Department of Medicine, Medical College of Wisconsin, 9200 W. Wisconsin Avenue, Milwaukee, WI 53226, USA
e-mail: srahman@mcw.edu; ksaeian@mcw.edu

© Springer International Publishing Switzerland 2017
K. Saeian, R. Shaker (eds.), *Liver Disorders*,
DOI 10.1007/978-3-319-30103-7_21

Table 21.1 Autosomal recessive inheritance in Wilson's disease from parents to children

Scenario (If the parents…)	Transmission (….then the children)
If both parents have the disease…	…then all children will have the disease
If one parent has the disease and one parent is a carrier…	…then there is a 50 % chance that the child will have the disease and a 50 % chance that the child will be a carrier
If only one parent has the disease…	…then all children will be carriers
If both parents are carriers…	…then there is a 25 % chance that the child will have the disease, a 50 % chance that the child will be a carrier, and a 25 % chance that the child will not have the disease or be a carrier
If only one parent is a carrier…	…then there is a 50 % chance that the child will be a carrier and a 50 % chance that the child will not have the disease or be a carrier
If neither parent has the disease and is not a carrier….	….then none of the children will have the disease or be a carrier

marrow, liver, and kidney problems. Trientine also promotes urinary copper excretion, albeit with less potency, but also with fewer side effects. Zinc interferes with the absorption of copper from the intestines; however, the most problematic side effect is gastric irritation. Lastly, antioxidants, specifically vitamin E, may serve as adjunctive therapy.

4. Question 4: What can I expect and do I necessarily need a liver transplant down the line?

   Patient level answer: Wilson's disease is present on a spectrum from patients who do not have symptoms to patients afflicted with hematological, ocular, hepatic, neurological, and/or psychiatric symptoms. Potential complications of Wilson's disease include, but are not limited to, neurological disabilities, hemolytic anemia, scarring of the liver or cirrhosis, and, occasionally, cancer. Liver transplant is necessary when medications fail or liver disease has progressed to liver failure.

Background

Wilson's disease (WD), or hepatolenticular degeneration, is an inherited autosomal recessive disease initially described by Samuel Alexander Kinnier Wilson in 1912, who initially described some of its protean neurological manifestations [1]. It is caused by a gene mutation on chromosome 13q 14.3 or ATP7B gene encoding a copper-transporting P-type ATPase. The gene is expressed in hepatocytes and functions in the transmembrane transport of copper [2–4]. To identify and manage WD, a rudimentary understanding of copper metabolism is necessary. Copper is initially absorbed via enterocytes in the duodenum and proximal jejunum, transported through the portal circulation bound to albumin, and is eventually delivered to the liver. In the liver, copper is intracellularly bound to the protein metallothionein.

Any excess copper acts as a substrate for ATPase, with two major cellular functions: to incorporate copper into ceruloplasmin and to permit copper excretion via the biliary system. Ceruloplasmin not bound to copper is called apoceruloplasmin.

The prevalence of WD is 3–30 in one million individuals [5]. WD is generally diagnosed in patients between the ages of 3 and 35 years, although it can be diagnosed at any age. Clinicians should consider WD when confronting unexplained liver disease, elevated serum aminotransferase, or clinical features of chronic liver disease, particularly, but not necessarily, when concomitant neurological signs and symptoms are present [6]. Although there is no gold standard, a number of clinical and biochemical parameters define WD. A high index of suspicion and appropriate interpretation of the testing is required for early recognition and treatment.

As no single test or finding defines WD, the clinician often uses the preponderance of the evidence to make the diagnosis. The overlap of serological or histological features with other disorders adds complexity to the diagnosis. For instance, serum immunoglobulins and autoantibodies classically seen in autoimmune hepatitis may be present in WD, as may plasma cells on histological evaluation from a liver biopsy. More importantly, patients with presumed autoimmune hepatitis refractory to corticosteroid therapy should be assessed for WD.

Clinical Manifestations

Dysfunction in copper metabolism consequently results in toxic copper accumulation in the blood, cornea, brain, and liver. This translates to a spectrum of expression ranging from completely asymptomatic to symptomatic, classically resulting in hepatic and neurological sequelae. The variable and at times incomplete penetrance of the WD gene is responsible for the range of presentation, including its hepatic, neurological, psychiatric, hematological, gastrointestinal, endocrinological, renal, cardiac, skeletal, and ocular symptoms (Fig. 21.1). Notably, neurological symptoms should prompt a neurological evaluation and radiographic imaging of the brain, preferably via magnetic resonance imaging (MRI). Specifically, proton-density MRI sequences remain sensitive in displaying the extent of neuropathology [7]. Histologically, astrocytes are increased within the gray matter associated with swollen glia, liquefaction, and spongiform degeneration. Clinically, in a case series of 25 patients with WD, 11 of the 25 patients, or 44 %, presented with neurological symptoms [8]. Specifically, movement abnormalities are categorized as akinetic–rigid syndromes, similar to Parkinson's disease, pseudosclerosis dominated by tremor, ataxia, and dystonic syndrome [9]. Behavioral and psychiatric symptoms, particularly in children, consist of personality changes and unstable behavior resulting in deteriorating school performance. In reference to hematological symptoms, Coombs-negative hemolytic anemia is often neglected as a presenting symptom in WD. Marked hemolysis is often associated with severe liver disease. Clinicians should also be aware of ocular signs and symptoms, in particular Kayser–Fleischer rings (Fig. 21.2) and sunflower cataracts caused by copper deposition on Descemet's membrane in the cornea and lens respectively, necessitating a slit lamp examination [10, 11]. Up to 95 % of patients with neuropsychiatric

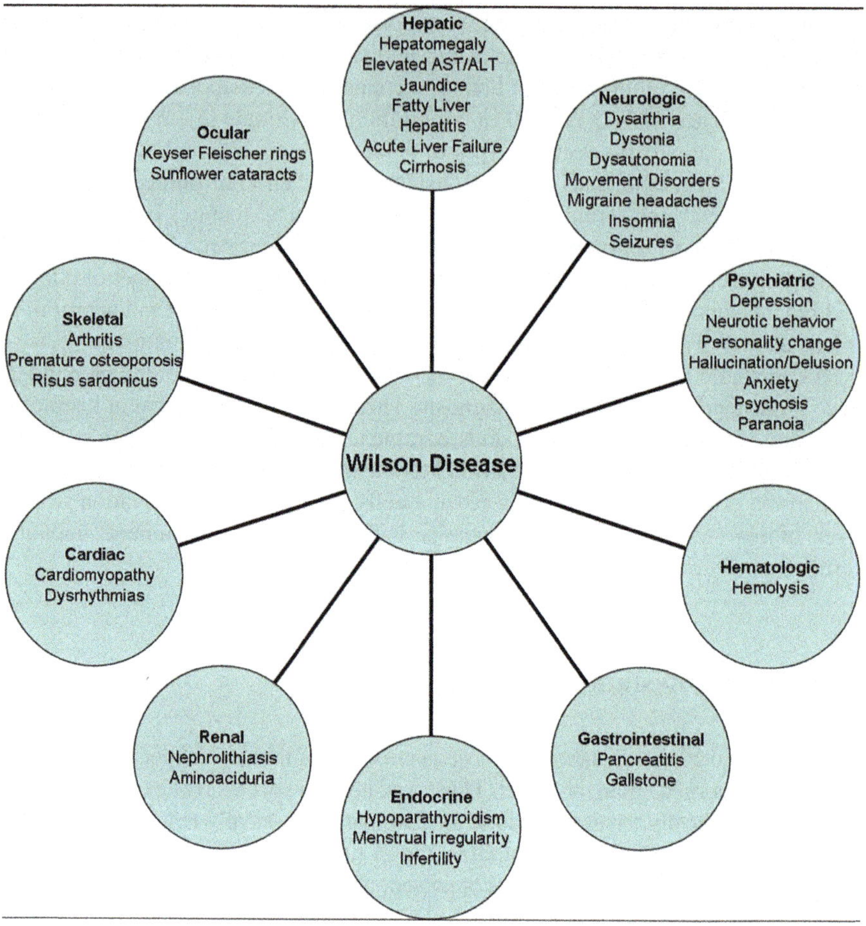

Fig. 21.1 Signs and Symptoms in Wilson's disease

Fig. 21.2 Kayser–Fleischer ring. Printed with permission of British Journal of Ophthalmology

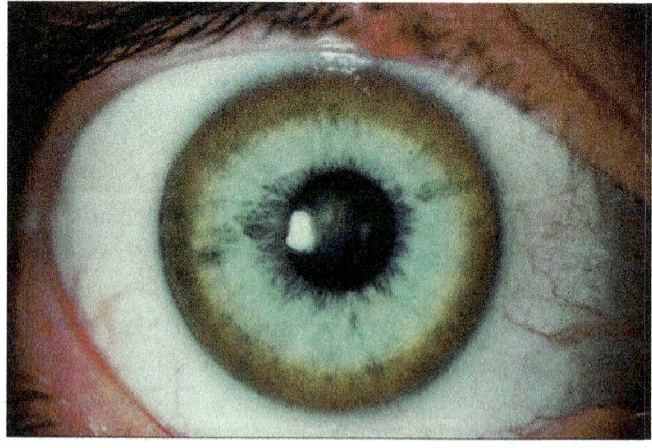

Table 21.2 Characteristic clinical findings in fulminant hepatic failure [13–19]

Clinical findings
Coombs-negative hemolytic anemia with features of acute intravascular hemolysis
Coagulopathy nonresponsive to parenteral vitamin K
Rapid progression to renal failure
Serum aminotransferases (<2,000 IU/L)
Normal or subnormal serum alkaline phosphatase (<40 IU/L) with an alkaline phosphatase to total bilirubin ratio of less than 4 [23]
Female:male ratio 2:1

symptoms have Kayser–Fleischer rings, whereas they are less often encountered in those with a hepatic presentation. In a case series of 30 patients with WD, 14 out of 22 or 63 % of patients without fulminant hepatic failure (FHF) and 6 out of 8 patients or 75 % of patients with FHF presented with Kayser–Fleischer rings [12]. At the same time, the absence of Kayser–Fleischer rings does not exclude the diagnosis of WD and other cholestatic liver diseases (which may also result in excessive copper accumulation due to decreased biliary excretion) have been associated with the development of Kayser–Fleischer rings.

The natural history of WD is variable, with the most worrisome complication being FHF. It is important to recognize characteristic clinical findings in FHF (Table 21.2) [13–19]. Predominantly in young females (the female:male ratio is 4:1), FHF, if untreated, carries an almost 95 % risk of mortality [20]. Traditionally, a ratio of serum alkaline phosphatase to total bilirubin <1 has been believed to have 86 % sensitivity and 50 % specificity for a diagnosis of fulminant WD [21, 22], a more recent study by Korman et al. [23] reporting that an alkaline phosphatase to total bilirubin ratio of less than 4 yielded 94 % sensitivity and 96 % specificity for FHF due to WD. Thus, a proportionately low alkaline phosphatase level should be a clue to the clinician with regard to WD, particularly in the patient with FHF. A prognostic scoring system for WD (Table 21.3) was developed by Nazer et al. [24] with score of 7 and above suggestive of high mortality in a combined pediatric and adult WD population and subsequently, a modified version based on bilirubin, aspartate aminotransferase, albumin, white cell count, and international normalized ratio was prospectively validated in a pediatric population (Table 21.4). Based on the new index, a score greater than 11 predicts a high risk of mortality, a requisite for liver transplantation with sensitivity 93 %, specificity 97 %, positive predictive value 92 %, and negative predictive value 97 % [25]. Patients with advanced fibrosis and cirrhosis are susceptible to complications associated with cirrhosis, which are detailed elsewhere in this text. Although copper chelation therapy does not necessarily lead to regression of advanced fibrosis, disease stabilization with chelation therapy is the rule in those without a fulminant presentation, although a proportion of patients, 15–20 %, experience a worsening of their neurological symptoms with chelation. Lastly, in a retrospective case series of 363 patients with WD, the frequency of malignancy was 0, 4.2, 5.3, and 15 % in the <10 years age group, 10–19 years, 20–29 years, and 30–39 years respectively. In general, malignancy, and particularly hepatocellular carcinoma, is an uncommon complication of WD isolated to those with cirrhosis, who should be screened on a regular basis [26].

Table 21.3 Prognostic index according to Nazer et al. [24]

Score	Serum bilirubin (μmol/L)	Serum aspartate (IU/L)	Prolongation in prothrombin time (s)
0	<100	<100	<4
1	100–150	100–150	4–8
2	151–200	151–200	9–12
3	201–300	201–300	13–20
4	>300	>300	>30

Table 21.4 New Wilson Index for predicting mortality [25]

Score	Bilirubin (μmol/L)	International normalized ratio	Aspartate (IU/L)	White cell count (10^9/L)	Albumin (g/L)
0	0–100	0–1.29	0–100	0–6.7	>45
1	101–150	1.3–1.6	101–150	6.8–8.3	34–44
2	151–200	1.7–1.9	151–300	8.4–10.3	25–33
3	201–300	2.0–2.4	301–400	10.4–15.3	1–24
4	>301	>2.5	>401	>15.4	<20

Diagnosis

When the diagnosis of WD is suspected, initial testing should be pursued with serum ceruloplasmin, 24-h urinary copper excretion, and slit-lamp examination to assess for Kayser–Fleischer rings. When warranted based on this initial testing, further testing, including the serum free copper concentration, hepatic copper concentration based on biopsy, the D-penicillamine challenge test, and genetic testing are options that can be considered (Table 21.5) [13].

Ceruloplasmin

An extremely low serum ceruloplasmin level <50 mg/L is highly suspicious for WD, but a serum ceruloplasmin within the normal range does not exclude the diagnosis, especially as ceruloplasmin is an acute phase reactant and ongoing inflammation may result in an "elevation" to within the normal range [13]. In a prospective study using serum ceruloplasmin as a screening test for WD of 2,867 patients tested, only 17 had a ceruloplasmin level <20 mg/L, and only 1 of these was confirmed to have WD, proving that subnormal ceruloplasmin has a low positive predictive value [27]. Disorders resulting in protein loss, such as nephrotic syndrome and poor protein synthesis, such as end-stage liver disease, may also result in low ceruloplasmin levels in the absence of WD.

Table 21.5 Standard laboratory tests used to diagnose Wilson's disease

Laboratory test	Normal value	Diagnostic value	Notes
Serum copper concentration	<150 µg/L	>200 µg/L	Most useful during follow-up and to assess response
Ceruloplasmin level	200–400 mg/L	<200 mg/L	<200 mg/L in 1 % of controls and 10 % in carriers and known copper deficiency
Hepatic copper concentration	<40–50 µg/g	>250 µg/g	<250 µg/g in 20 % of patients with Wilson's disease
24 h urinary copper concentration	<40 µg/24 h	>100 µg/24 h	High urinary copper levels may be found in various chronic liver diseases
D-penicillamine challenge		>1600 µg/24 h	Test by 500 mg of D-penicillamine at baseline and then again at 12 h
Genetic testing			Negative result does not exclude a diagnosis

24-h Urinary Copper Excretion

The 24-h urinary copper excretion measurement should be elevated (>100 µg/day) in patients with WD, but care must be taken to ascertain adequate urine collection (the volume and urine creatinine can confirm adequacy). Care must also be taken to avoid contamination, as actions as simple as rinsing the container with tap water can potentially falsely elevate the copper concentration. In patients with renal insufficiency or failure, this test is unfortunately not reliable. Measurement of urinary copper excretion after a challenge by two doses of D-penicillamine (e.g., 500 mg) 12 h apart, followed by a 24-h urine collection, has been validated in the pediatric population as a sensitive diagnostic test, but because of the lack of validation in adults and variable dosing regimens reported, this test is not typically used in adult patients.

The findings of low serum ceruloplasmin, high 24-h urinary copper excretion, and Kayser–Fleischer rings essentially point to a diagnosis of WD, but if there is a discrepancy amongst these findings, further testing, particularly liver biopsy with hepatic parenchymal copper quantitation and genetic testing, should be pursued.

Liver Biopsy and Hepatic Copper Quantitation

Measurement of the hepatic parenchymal copper concentration is a reliable method for the diagnosis of WD. Care must be taken to obtain an adequate sample (preferably > 1 cm in length), to use copper-free containers, and to ship the sample dry for processing. Hepatic copper concentration of > 250 µg/g of dry weight is essentially diagnostic of WD, with levels of <40–50 µg/g of dry weight essentially eliminating

WD as the etiology. Further testing may be required in those with intermediate hepatic copper concentrations. Histochemical stains, such as rhodamine or orcein, may detect copper overload, but are often insufficient, particularly in younger individuals as they only detect lysosomal deposition of copper, which is a later phenomenon, thus missing the predominant cytoplasmic copper bound to metallothionein. Histologically, hepatic copper deposition in WD progresses from diffuse cytoplasmic accumulation, to steatosis, to steatohepatitis, and eventually, to cirrhosis. Initially, early accumulation of copper results in glycogenated nuclei, microvesicular, and macrovesicular steatosis [28]. Subsequently, progression is characterized histologically by periportal inflammation, including plasma cells, mononuclear cellular infiltrates, erosion of the limiting plate, lobular necrosis, and bridging fibrosis [29, 30]. Mallory bodies are also observed in 50 % of biopsy specimens [31]. If FHF develops, it is characterized by parenchymal apoptosis and necrosis in the setting of cirrhosis [32]. Ultrasound abnormalities demonstrate enlargement and separation of the mitochondrial inner and outer membranes, increased density and granularity of the matrix, and the occurrence of large vacuoles pathognomonic of WD [33]. As a clinical pearl, clinicians should be wary that WD may histologically resemble nonalcoholic fatty liver disease, nonalcoholic steatohepatitis, or autoimmune hepatitis.

Serum Free Copper Concentration

The measurement of serum copper includes measurement of copper bound to ceruloplasmin, thus depending on the ceruloplasmin concentration. The total serum copper measurement may have a range of values in WD [9]. A more reliable measure is that of the serum free or nonceruloplasmin bound copper concentration, which can be calculated by subtracting ceruloplasmin-bound copper ($3.15 \times$ ceruloplasmin in mg/L equals the amount of ceruloplasmin-bound copper in µg/L) from the total serum copper concentration (in µg/L; serum copper in µmol/L $\times 63.5$ equals serum copper in µg/L) [34]. A number of other conditions, including cholestatic liver diseases, can have an impact on the measurement of this level, but a value >200 µg/L is suggestive of WD. Most clinicians do not use this test in the diagnostic algorithm, but rather as a measure to assess the efficacy of treatment.

Genetic Testing

Genetic tests can directly examine disease-specific ATP7B gene mutations on both alleles of chromosome 13. Specifically, molecular diagnostic studies can be used for the screening of first-degree relatives in newly diagnosed patients with WD, to classify patterns of either haplotypes or DNA polymorphisms with regard to the ATP7B gene. A diagnostic scoring system was proposed for WD based on clinical and laboratory parameters: >4, certain of WD; 2–3 likely WD; and 0–1 unlikely WD (Table 21.6). In addition, a phenotypic classification was developed distinguishing WD based on hepatic and neurological presentations (Table 21.7) [35].

Table 21.6 A scoring system for the diagnosis of Wilson's disease [35]

Score category	Score
Symptoms	
Kayser–Fleischer rings (slit-lamp examination)	
Present	2
Absent	0
Neuropsychiatric symptoms suggestive of Wilson's disease (on typical brain MRI)	
Present	2
Absent	0
Coombs-negative hemolytic anemia (positive high serum copper)	
Present	1
Absent	0
Laboratory tests	
Urinary copper (in the absence of acute hepatitis)	
Normal	0
1–2× ULN	1
>2× ULN	2
Normal, but >5× ULN 1 day after challenge with 2× 0.5 g D-penicillamine	2
Liver copper quantitation	
Normal	-1
Up to 5× ULN	1
>5× ULN	2
Rhodamine-positive hepatocytes (only if quantitative copper measurement is not available)	
Present	0
Absent	1
Serum ceruloplasmin (nephelometric assay, normal: >20 mg/day	
Normal	0
10–20	1
<10	2
Mutation analysis	
Disease causing mutations on both chromosomes	4
Disease causing mutations on one chromosome	1
No disease causing mutation detected	0

ULN upper limit of normal

Treatment

Treatment for WD is based on clinical, laboratory, or histological evidence of disease; neurological or hepatic involvement; and being asymptomatic or symptomatic at presentation. In the absence of FHF, initial treatment should be started early and involve chelating agents (D-penicillamine and trientine). Zinc is mainly used for maintenance treatment, with the exception of neuropsychiatric symptoms necessitating zinc as first-line therapy. Medications are tailored on an individual basis taking into consideration clinical response and side effect profiles (Table 21.8) [13]. Owing

Table 21.7 Phenotypic classification of Wilson's disease [35]

Hepatic presentation
The definition of hepatic presentation requires the exclusion of neurological symptoms by a detailed clinical neurological examination at the time of diagnosis
H1: Acute hepatic Wilson's disease
Acutely occurring jaundice in a previously apparently healthy subject, either due to a hepatitis-like illness or Coombs-negative hemolytic disease, or a combination of both. May progress to liver failure necessitating emergency liver transplantation
H2: Chronic hepatic Wilson's disease
Any type of chronic liver disease, with or without symptoms. May lead to or even present as decompensated cirrhosis. Diagnosis is based on standard biochemical, and/or radiological, or biopsy evidence
Neurological presentation
Patients in whom neurological and/or psychiatric symptoms are present at diagnosis
N1: Associated with symptomatic liver disease
Usually patients have cirrhosis at the time of the diagnosis of neurological Wilson's disease. Chronic liver disease may predate the occurrence of neurological symptoms by many years or may be diagnosed during the diagnostic workup in a neurologically symptomatic patient
N2: Not associated with symptomatic liver disease
Documentation of the absence of marked liver disease (fibrosis/steatosis may be present any time); requires a liver biopsy
NX: Presence or absence of liver disease not investigated

to an initial rise in serum free copper, a small proportion of patients experience neurological deterioration with initiation of therapy. Based on the side effect profile, it is now our practice to consider trientine more often initially. Ultimately, for patients with refractory WD or those with FHF, liver transplantation is the only viable treatment option, although the neurological and psychiatric complications may not respond to this intervention. These complications may also present an obstacle to adherence to the post-transplantation regimen. Overall, patient survival rates at 6 and 12 months and 5 and 10 years after liver transplantation are 89.1, 89.1, 75.6 and 58.8 % respectively [36]. Ammonium tetrathiomolybdate, currently not commercially available, is a promising agent that prevents intestinal absorption and cellular uptake of copper by forming a complex with it. Although considered experimental, it has been effective in limited studies and is particularly intriguing as it may preclude neurological deterioration with the onset of therapy, likely by avoiding an initial increase in serum free copper.

Pregnant patients with WD who are stable on a treatment regimen should be maintained on therapy, although breast feeding should be interrupted because of concern regarding precipitating FHF. Of note, zinc and trientine are the safest drugs for pregnant patients with WD [37]. Clinicians should ensure compliance, understandably given the severe nature of WD, by measuring at least annual 24-h urinary copper excretion and serum free copper. On treatment, 24-h urinary copper excretion should rise up to 200–500 µg/24 h (either of the chelating agents) or to 50–125 µg/24 h on zinc. Alternatively, serum free copper should be approximately

Table 21.8 Treatment for Wilson's disease

Therapy	Mechanism of action	Side effects	Notes
D-Penicillamine	Promotes urinary copper excretion	Hypersensitivity reaction, nephrotoxicity, lupus-like reaction, Goodpasture syndrome, bone marrow toxicity, myasthenia gravis, polymyositis	Induce vitamin B6 deficiency requiring supplementation Urine protein excretion should be monitored on therapy.
Trientine	Promotes urinary copper excretion	Lupus-like syndrome, sideroblastic anemia	
Zinc	Inhibits copper absorption	Gastric irritation	Mainly used as first-line therapy in asymptomatic patients or as maintenance therapy.
Tetrathiomolybdate	Inhibits copper absorption and cellular uptake	Bone marrow toxicity, hepatotoxicity	Not commercially available. May prevent neurological deterioration.
Antioxidants			Adjunctive therapy.
Dietary restrictions	Decrease copper absorption		Avoid foods rich in copper (examples include chocolate, liver, nuts, mushrooms, and shellfish).
Liver transplantation			Typically reserved for fulminant hepatic failure or decompensated cirrhotics.

100 μg/L on treatment [6]. Treatment is life-long unless a liver transplant is performed. Interestingly, Kayser–Fleischer rings may become less prominent or disappear with chelation therapy.

Conclusion

Future trends in the field focus on better and more reliable diagnostic measures, hepatocyte transplantation, and gene therapy offering new diagnostic options and potential cures. Currently, only preclinical data on animal models exist on the latter providing a proof of concept. Further advances in immune tolerance, safe methods for selective proliferation in hepatocyte transplanted cells, and the utilization of alternative vectors or even non-viral-based gene methods to ensure gene expression are needed [38]. Alternatively, research into early diagnostic markers along with new methods of ascertaining compliance will continue to help clinicians to diagnose and treat patients afflicted with WD.

References

1. Wilson SAK. Progressive lenticular degeneration: a familial nervous disease associated with cirrhosis of the liver. Brain. 1912;34:295–509.
2. Bull PC, Thomas GR, Rommens JM, Forbes JR, Cox DW. The Wilson disease gene is a putative copper transporting P-type ATPase similar to the Menkes gene. Nat Genet. 1993;5:327–37.
3. Tanzi RE, Petrukhin K, Chernov I, Pellequer JL, Wasco W, Ross B, et al. The Wilson disease gene is a copper transporting ATPase with homology to the Menkes disease gene. Nat Genet. 1993;5:344–50.
4. Yamaguchi Y, Heiny ME, Gitlin JD. Isolation and characterization of a human liver cDNA as a candidate gene for Wilson disease. Biochem Biophys Res Commun. 1993;197:271–7.
5. Frydman M. Genetic aspects of Wilson's disease. J Gastroenterol Hepatol. 1990;5:483–90.
6. Medici V, Rossaro L, Sturniolo GC. Wilson disease – a practical approach to diagnosis, treatment and follow-up. Dig Liver Dis. 2007;39:601–9.
7. Page RA, Davie CA, MacManus D, et al. Clinical correlation of brain MRI and MRS abnormalities in patients with Wilson disease. Neurology. 2004;63:638–43.
8. Walshe JM. Wilson's disease. The presenting symptoms. Arch Dis Child. 1962;37:253–6.
9. Ferenci P, Czlonkowska A, Stremmel W, Houwen R, Rosenberg W, Schilsky M. EASL clinical practice guidelines: Wilson's disease. J Hepatology. 2012;56:671–85.
10. Wiebers DO, Hollenhorst RW, Goldstein NP. The ophthalmologic manifestations of Wilson's disease. Mayo Clin Proc. 1977;52:409–16.
11. Cairns JE, Williams HP, Walshe JM. "Sunflower cataract" in Wilson's disease. BMJ. 1969;3:95–6.
12. Gow PJ, Smallwood RA, Angus PW, Smith AL, Wall AJ, Sewell RB. Diagnosis of Wilson's disease: an experience over three decades. Gut. 2000;46:415–9.
13. Roberts EA, Schilsky ML. Diagnosis and treatment of Wilson disease: an update. Hepatology. 2008;47(6):2089–111.
14. Roche-Sicot J, Benhamou JP. Acute intravascular hemolysis and acute liver failure associated as a first manifestation of Wilson's disease. Ann Intern Med. 1977;86:301–3.
15. Hamlyn AN, Gollan JL, Douglas AP, Sherlock S. Fulminant Wilson's disease with haemolysis and renal failure: copper studies and assessment of dialysis regimens. Br Med J. 1977;2:660–2.
16. McCullough AJ, Fleming CR, Thistle JL, Baldus WP, Ludwig J, McCall JT, et al. Diagnosis of Wilson's disease presenting as fulminant hepatic failure. Gastroenterology. 1983;84:161–7.
17. Rector Jr WG, Uchida T, Kanel GC, Redeker AG, Reynolds TB. Fulminant hepatic and renal failure complicating Wilson's disease. Liver. 1984;4:341–7.
18. Enomoto K, Ishibashi H, Irie K, Okumura Y, Nomura H, Fukushima M, et al. Fulminant hepatic failure without evidence of cirrhosis in a case of Wilson's disease. Jpn J Med. 1989;28:80–4.
19. Ferlan-Marolt V, Stepec S. Fulminant Wilsonian hepatitis unmasked by disease progression: report of a case and review of the literature. Dig Dis Sci. 1999;44:1054–8.
20. Walshe JM. The liver in Wilson's disease. In: Schiff L, Schiff ER, editors. Diseases of the liver. 6th ed. Philadelphia: Lippincott; 1987. p. 1037–50.
21. Tissieres P, Chevret L, Debray D, Devictor D. Fulminant Wilson's disease in children: appraisal of a critical diagnosis. Pediatr Crit Care Med. 2003;4:338–43.
22. Sallie R, Katsiyiannakis L, Baldwin D, et al. Failure of simple biochemical indexes to reliably differentiate fulminant Wilson's disease from other causes of fulminant liver failure. Hepatology. 1992;16:1206–11.
23. Korman JD, Volenber I, Balko J, et al. Screening for Wilson disease in acute liver failure: a comparison of currently available diagnostic tests. Hepatology. 2008;48(4):1167–74.
24. Nazer H, Ede RJ, Mowat AP, Williams R. Wilson's disease: clinical presentation and use of prognostic index. Gut. 1986;27:1377–81.
25. Dhawan A, Taylor RM, Cheeseman P, De Silva P, Katsiyiannakis L, Mieli-Vergani G. Wilson's disease in children: 37-year experience and revised King's score for liver transplantation. Liver Transplant. 2005;11:441–8.

26. Walshe JM, Waldenstrom E, Sams V, Nordlinder H, Westermark K. Abdominal malignancies in patients with Wilson's disease. QJM. 2003;96:657–62.
27. Cauza E, Maier-Dobersberger T, Polli C, Kaserer K, Kramer L, Ferenci P. Screening for Wilson's disease in patients with liver diseases by serum ceruloplasmin. J Hepatology. 1997;27:358–62.
28. Alt ER, Sternlieb I, Goldfischer S. The cytopathology of metal overload. Int Rev Exp Pathol. 1990;31:165–88.
29. Sternlieb I. Mitochondrial and fatty changes in hepatocytes of patients with Wilson's disease. Gastroenterology. 1968;55:354–67.
30. Schilsky ML, Scheinberg IH, Sternlieb I. Prognosis of Wilsonian chronic active hepatitis. Gastroenterology. 1991;100:762–7.
31. Muller T, Langner C, Fuchsbichler A, et al. Immunohistochemical analysis of Mallory bodies in Wilsonian and non-Wilsonian hepatic copper toxicosis. Hepatology. 2004;39:963–9.
32. Strand S, Hofmann WJ, Grambihler A, et al. Hepatic failure and liver cell damage in acute Wilson's disease involve CD95 (APO-1/Fas) mediated apoptosis. Nat Med. 1998;4:588–93.
33. Ala A, Walker AP, Askhan K, Dooley JS, Schilsky ML. Wilson's disease. Lancet. 2007;369:397–408.
34. Danks DM. Disorders of copper transport. In: Scriver CR, Beaudet AL, Sly WS, Valle D, editors. The metabolic basis of inherited disease. New York: McGraw-Hill; 1995. p. 4125.
35. Ferenci P, Caca K, Loudianos G, Mieli-Vergani G, Tanner S, Sternlieb I, et al. Diagnosis and phenotypic classification of Wilson disease. Liver Int. 2003;23:139–42.
36. Medici V, Mirante VG, Fassati LR, Pompili M, Forti D, Del Gaudio M, et al. Liver transplantation for Wilson's disease: the burden of neuropsychiatric disorders. Liver Transplant. 2005;11:1056–63.
37. Devesa R, Alvarez A, de las Heras G, de Miguel JR. Wilson's disease treated with trientine during pregnancy. J Pediatr Gastroenterol Nutrition. 1995;20:102–3.
38. Schilsky ML. Wilson disease: new insights into pathogenesis, diagnosis, and future therapy. Curr Gastroenterol Rep. 2005;7:26–31.

Chapter 22
Metabolic and Genetic Liver Diseases: Glycogen Storage Diseases

Grzegorz W. Telega

Question 1. Why do we think of glycogen storage disease?

(a) Low glucose.

Glycogen is a form of glucose storage. The body produces glycogen from the excess of glucose that is present inside the cells. Glycogen allows glucose storage, while limiting oncotic pressure from concentrated glucose. Glycogen is formed from several hundreds of glucose molecules bound by 1–6 and 1–4 (branching) bonds. Glycogen is stored in many tissues, most prominently in muscles and in the liver. Only the liver, however, is able to release glucose from glycogen into the circulation. Other tissues can break down glycogen to glucose 6-phosphate, which enters the glycolysis pathway and is used for energy production inside the cell.

A common feature of glycogen storage disorders (GSD) is the inefficient release of glucose from glycogen stores; this can lead to hypoglycemia at the time of starvation. As brain energy metabolism depends heavily on the availability of glucose, severe hypoglycemia can lead to metabolic strokes, irreversible brain damage, and death. The duration of starvation, the rate of glucose utilization (which is increased in febrile illness), and the type of GSD determine the severity of hypoglycemia. Hypoglycemia tends to be more severe in GSD type Ia, less severe in types VI and IX, and there is generally no hypoglycemia in type V and type VII GSD.

G.W. Telega, M.D., M.S. (✉)
Department of Pediatric Gastroenterology, Hepatology, and Nutrition,
Medical College of Wisconsin, Milwaukee, WI 53201, USA
e-mail: gtelega@mcw.edu

© Springer International Publishing Switzerland 2017
K. Saeian, R. Shaker (eds.), *Liver Disorders*,
DOI 10.1007/978-3-319-30103-7_22

Hypoglycemia may manifest as lethargy, a change in mental status, seizures, focal neurological symptoms, tremors, irritability, and excessive frequency of feedings. Hypoglycemia causes an increase in the levels of triglycerides, lactic acid, ketones, and uric acid, which can be detected even after hypoglycemia is corrected. These laboratory abnormalities support any suspicion of GSD, if hypoglycemia has not been directly documented [1–3].

(b) Large liver.

In GSD, glycogen cannot be properly metabolized, which leads to an accumulation of glycogen inside the cells. As the liver is the main storage site of glycogen, liver size is increased in most types of glycogen storage disorders (with the exception of types II, V, and VII).

Despite its enlarged size in GSD, the liver is generally not fibrotic and the hepatomegaly may be missed on casual physical examination. When GSD is suspected, special attention should be given to palpation and percussion of the liver. Ultrasound can provide supportive evidence for hepatomegaly. Typically, there is no jaundice and aminotransferase levels are normal or only mildly elevated [1–3].

Only in GSD type IV and in adults with type III can liver fibrosis develop. In these patients, splenomegaly may be present as a result of portal hypertension.

(c) Weak muscles.

Skeletal muscle involvement is a feature of some forms of GSD (types II, III, V, VII, and IX). Muscle involvement is a dominant presentation in GSD types II, V, and VII; thus, these patients are rarely referred to the hepatologist. Myopathy usually involves both skeletal and cardiac muscle. In GSD type IX hepatomegaly can be associated with mild muscle involvement [1, 2, 4].

(d) Multiple hepatic adenomata.

The diagnosis of GSD should be considered in patients who are found to have multiple hepatic adenomata, which do carry a small risk for transformation into hepatocellular carcinoma.

Question 2. How is the diagnosis of GSD made?

(a) Genetic testing.

Direct genetic testing is available for most types of glycogen storage disease. The clinician should choose appropriate testing based on the observed clinical pattern, as many types of GSD have specific clinical features. Tables 22.1 and 22.2 provide clinical vignettes and corresponding genes and enzymes specific to the GSD type.

(b) Liver biopsy.

Liver biopsy can be used when genetic testing is equivocal or inconsistent with the clinical picture. Biopsy allows for the direct

Table 22.1 Types of glycogen storage disease (GSD)

Type	Enzyme	Clinical features
Ia	Glucose 6-phosphatase	Presentation in early infancy, severe hypoglycemia, hepatomegaly, unable to tolerate starvation [3, 5]
Ib	Glucose-6-phosphate specific transporter deficiency	Presentation in early infancy, severe hypoglycemia, hepatomegaly, unable to tolerate starvation, neutropenia, frequent infections, enterocolitis (IBD-like symptoms), renal involvement [4, 5]
II	Lysosomal acid alpha-1,4-glucosidase	Currently classified as lysosomal storage disease. Onset in early infancy, muscle weakness, cardiomyopathy, abnormal brain myelination, no hypoglycemia, no hepatomegaly [1, 7]
III	Debranching enzyme deficiency	Presentation in infancy, usually (>85 % of cases type IIIa) combined liver and skeletal muscle involvement, liver only (type IIIb 15 %), cardiomyopathy, lactic acidosis and hyperuricemia are less severe than in GSD type I [4, 6]
IV	Branching enzyme deficiency	Presentation in late infancy, poor growth, mild hypoglycemia, hepatosplenomegaly, progressive liver fibrosis and portal hypertension, muscle involvement, broad spectrum of severity [1, 7]
V	Muscle phosphorylase deficiency	Myopathy, exercise intolerance, rhabdomyolysis, no hypoglycemia, no liver involvement [1, 7]
VI	Liver phosphorylase deficiency	Presentation in childhood, mild hypoglycemia, hepatomegaly [2, 8]
VII	Muscle phosphofructokinase deficiency	Myopathy, exercise intolerance, no hypoglycemia, no liver involvement, mild hemolytic anemia [1, 7]
IX	Phosphorylase kinase deficiency	presentation in childhood, mild hypoglycemia, hepatomegaly, mild myopathy [1, 2, 7, 8]

IBS irritable bowel syndrome

Table 22.2 Genetic factors in the various types of GSD [1–3]

Type	Gene	Location	Inheritance
Ia	G6PC	17q21.31	Recessive
Ib	SLC37A4	11q23.3	Recessive
II	GAA	17q25.3	Recessive
III	AGL	1p21.2	Recessive
IV	GBE1	3p12.2	Recessive
V	PYGM	11q13.1	Recessive
VI	PYGL	14q22.1	Recessive
VII	PFKM	12q13.11	Recessive
IX	PHKA2	Xp22.13	X-linked
	PHKB	16q12.1	Recessive
	PHKG1	7p11.2	Recessive
	PHKG2	16p11.2	Recessive

testing of glycogen content, and the measurement of enzyme activity in glycogen synthesis and degradation pathways (Table 22.1).

Additionally, liver biopsy can suggest alternative diagnoses in the investigation of the hepatomegaly without hepatitis (lysosomal storage, peroxisomal, mitochondrial, beta oxidation disorders, lymphomas). Liver biopsy can provide an estimate of the degree of fibrosis in GSD types III and IV, and can serve as a supplemental study in the evaluation of adenomas when radiological investigation is equivocal.

While performing a liver biopsy the clinician needs to pay attention to appropriate test selection based on the clinical pattern observed. Samples for enzymatic studies need to be flash-frozen and shipped to the reference laboratory according to specifications [1–3].

Question 3. How do you get GSD?

- Genetics of glycogen storage disease.

  Most glycogen storage disorders are autosomal recessive. The patient has mutations of both copies of the specific gene for a given GSD type. The exception is GSD type IX, which has complex genetics consisting of both autosomal recessive and X-linked forms. The complex genetics of type IX GSD stems from the fact that the enzyme is a complex protein consisting of 16 subunits encoded by four separate genes. (Table 22.2) [1–3].

Question 4. What is the danger of doing nothing?

(a) Risk of hypoglycemia.

  - Mortality.

    Episodes of severe hypoglycemia can lead to life-threatening brain injury. The maintenance of normoglycemia through the ingestion of uncooked corn starch, and/or continuous enteral feeds drastically improve survival.

  - Brain damage.

    Severe hypoglycemia can result in brain injury, which can be irreversible and could accumulate over the course of the disease. The prevention of hypoglycemia is essential to avoid brain damage.

(b) Other complications.

  - Adenomas frequently develop in patients who survive to adolescence or adulthood. Adenomas are most common in GSD types Ia and Ib, but they have been described in other forms of GSD involving the liver. They present as hypervascular lesions with a small risk of malignant transformation and are mainly confined to adults.

- Abnormal growth and short stature are common in most forms of GSD.
- Hyperlipidemia is a compensatory response to insufficient glucose supply.
- Gout can be a consequence of long-lasting hyperuricemia resulting from the increased production and decreased renal clearance of uric acid.
- Osteoporosis.
- Liver fibrosis is a feature of GSD type IV and to a lesser degree type III. Hepatocyte damage results from the abnormal molecular structure of glycogen.
- Renal disease is a feature of GSD type Ib.
- Myopathies are a feature of GSD types II, III, V, VII, and to a lesser degree IX. Muscle weakness is progressive and can involve both skeletal and cardiac muscle.

Question 5. How can we manage the disease?

(a) Dietary management: the goal of dietary management is the maintenance of euglycemia. This requires a constant supply of dietary carbohydrates, which can be achieved by frequent meals containing uncooked cornstarch. The benefit of uncooked cornstarch is that its digestion inside the gastrointestinal tract is slow enough that it can provide a stable carbohydrate supply for a few hours. The disadvantage of cornstarch is its poor palatability, which leads to the need for enteral access (nasogastric or gastrostomy tube) in most patients. The alternative to cornstarch is a continuous enteral feeding regimen with an adequate carbohydrate supply. As the diet requires a high carbohydrate supply, it frequently leads to protein, essential fatty acids or vitamin deficiencies. The clinician needs to closely monitor the patient's nutritional status. Milder forms of GSD (types VI, IX) may only require uncooked cornstarch meals at night-time [6, 7]. Whenever patients with GSD are in a catabolic state (infection, gastroenteritis, nil by mouth for procedures) they need to be closely monitored for hypoglycemia and may require intravenous glucose infusion.

(b) Liver transplantation may be indicated for patients with liver adenomas and those with poor metabolic control. A liver transplant normalizes glucose control, improves growth, and eliminates the need for a special diet. It will not change myopathies in GSD types II, V, and VII and is not indicated in those conditions. Liver transplantation will not correct neutropenia and renal involvement in GSD type Ib, but it does improve the overall phenotype [8].

6. What about other children and… grandchildren?

- Genetic counseling is indicated for all patients with GSD. Most forms of GSD are recessive; thus, parents are faced with an approximately 25 % risk of another child having GSD. A genetic counselor can explain to the family the testing available and provide advice regarding procreative choices.

References

1. Bao Y et al. Hepatic and neuromuscular forms of glycogen storage disease type IV caused by mutations in the same glycogen-branching enzyme gene. J Clin Invest. 1996;97(4):941–8.
2. Roscher A et al. The natural history of glycogen storage disease types VI and IX: long-term outcome from the largest metabolic center in Canada. Mol Genet Metab. 2014;113(3):171–6.
3. Ullrich K, Smit GP. Clinical aspects of glycogen storage disease type I: summary of the discussions. Eur J Pediatr. 1993;152 Suppl 1:87–8.
4. Coleman RA et al. Glycogen debranching enzyme deficiency: long-term study of serum enzyme activities and clinical features. J Inherit Metab Dis. 1992;15(6):869–81.
5. Smit GP. The long-term outcome of patients with glycogen storage disease type Ia. Eur J Pediatr. 1993;152 Suppl 1:S52–5.
6. Chen YT, Cornblath M, Sidbury JB. Cornstarch therapy in type I glycogen-storage disease. N Engl J Med. 1984;310(3):171–5.
7. Greene HL et al. Continuous nocturnal intragastric feeding for management of type 1 glycogen-storage disease. N Engl J Med. 1976;294(8):423–5.
8. Faivre L et al. Long-term outcome of liver transplantation in patients with glycogen storage disease type Ia. J Inherit Metab Dis. 1999;22(6):723–32.

Chapter 23
Metabolic and Genetic Liver Diseases: Urea Cycle Defects

Grzegorz W. Telega

Question 1. Why do we think of urea cycle defects?

(a) Change in mental status.

The urea cycle is a series of enzymatic reactions converting highly toxic ammonia into less toxic urea. Ammonia is a ubiquitous byproduct of amino acid metabolism. The urea cycle takes place exclusively in the liver. Although ammonia can be toxic to all tissues, the brain is the most prominent target of ammonia toxicity. Acute encephalopathy is associated with astrocyte swelling without axonal damage. Patients present with a change in mental status or ataxia. Severe or prolonged hyperammonemia ultimately leads to progressive irreversible changes in the brain characterized by cortical and brain stem gliosis and neuronal atrophy. Encephalopathy is the main cause of mortality and morbidity in urea cycle defects [1, 2].

As the most common and severe form of urea cycle defect – ornithine transcarbamylase (OTC) deficiency – is X linked, males are at a higher risk of acute presentation. The most dramatic presentation of OTC deficiency would be a male newborn without any apparent obstetric risk who does well for the first few hours of life, but then develops lethargy, hypothermia, and apnea in the first 24–28 h of life. Although most male patients present in the newborn period, late presentation can occur. Heterozygote females with OTC deficiency and less severe forms of urea cycle defects

G.W. Telega, M.D., M.S. (✉)
Department of Pediatric Gastroenterology, Hepatology, and Nutrition,
Medical College of Wisconsin, Milwaukee, WI 53201, USA
e-mail: gtelega@mcw.edu

© Springer International Publishing Switzerland 2017
K. Saeian, R. Shaker (eds.), *Liver Disorders*,
DOI 10.1007/978-3-319-30103-7_23

"

(carbamyl phosphate synthetase deficiency, argininosuccinate synthetase deficiency, argininosuccinate lyase deficiency, and arginase deficiency) frequently have a history of episodic changes in mental status associated with a high protein intake and may present in adulthood [1, 2].

Respiratory alkalosis can be early sign of encephalopathy. This distinguishes urea cycle defects from organic acidurias, where hyperammonemia is accompanied by acidosis and ketosis. Valproic acid is known to cause episodes of hyperammonemia and metabolic decompensation in patients with mild forms of OTC deficiency. Family history may provide clues to the diagnosis.

(b) High ammonia.

Hyperammonemia is the cardinal metabolic abnormality of urea cycle defects. Levels of ammonia can fluctuate depending on dietary protein intake and the presence of a catabolic state.

(c) Liver dysfunction.

Ornithine transcarbamylase (OTC) deficiency is associated with liver dysfunction which occasionally leads to a misdiagnosis of liver failure.

Question 2. How do we make the diagnosis?

(a) Laboratory workup.

Any patient presenting with acute onset or progressive encephalopathy in the absence of obvious intoxication or portal hypertension should undergo ammonia measurement.

Once hyperammonemia has been documented, the clinical focus should be on the rapid correction of ammonia levels and the prevention of permanent brain damage. Diagnosis of a specific defect, although important, should not delay therapy.

An organic acid profile may suggest a specific condition; diagnosis can be confirmed by genetic testing or by measurement of specific enzyme activity at liver biopsy.

(b) Genetic testing.

Genetic tests are available for each specific disorder as a diagnostic tool, but can also be used for the prenatal diagnosis or detection of heterozygote carriers. Tables 23.1 and 23.2 provide clinical vignettes and the corresponding genes and enzymes of specific disorders.

3. How did I get it?

(a) Genetics of urea cycle defects.

Ornithine transcarbamylase, the most common urea cycle defect is X-linked, although heterozygote females can experience mild encephalopathy with high-protein meals. Other urea cycle defects are autosomal recessive [3].

Table 23.1   Clinical features of urea cycle defects

Enzyme	Typical clinical features
Ornithine transcarbamylase	Severe encephalopathy with onset at between 24 and 48 h of life in male homozygotes. Mild recurrent encephalopathy after protein-rich meals in female heterozygotes. Mild liver dysfunction [1, 3]
Carbamyl phosphate synthetase	Early onset: in the first month of life, lethargy, coma Late onset: coma induced by pregnancy or valproic acid, rarely focal strokes [1, 2]
Citrullinemia type I Argininosuccinic acid synthetase	Pediatric onset: vomiting, failure to thrive, hepatomegaly, developmental delay, protein avoidance, lethargy. Adult onset: insomnia, sleep reversal, nocturnal sweats and terrors, recurrent vomiting (especially at night), diarrhea, tremors, episodes of confusion after meals, lethargy, convulsions, delusions and hallucinations, and brief episodes of coma [1, 2]
Argininosuccinate lyase	Vomiting, feeding lethargy in the first few days of life, subsequently developmental delays and infection-induced episodes of hyperammonemia. Mild liver fibrosis [1, 2]
Arginase	Onset in childhood, developmental delay, seizures, lethargy after high-protein meals [1, 2]

Table 23.2   Genes involved in specific disorders [2, 3]

Disease	Gene	Location	Inheritance
Ornithine transcarbamylase deficiency	OTC	Xp11.4	X-linked
Carbamyl phosphate synthetase deficiency	CPS1	2q34	Recessive
Argininosuccinic acid synthetase citrulinemia type I	ASS1	9q34.11	Recessive
Argininosuccinate lyase deficiency	ASL	7q11.21	Recessive
Arginase deficiency	ARG1	6q23.2	Recessive

(b) Metabolic changes in urea cycle defects.

The most typical metabolic feature of urea cycle defects is the presence of severe hyperammonemia in the absence of acidosis. Plasma glutamine levels are frequently elevated. Elevated citrulline is characteristic of citrullinemia type I (very high levels) and argininosuccinate lyase deficiency (moderate elevation). High urinary orotic acid levels are characteristic of ornithine transcarbamylase deficiency [2].

Question 4. What is the danger of doing nothing?

(a) Risk of hyperammonemia.

(b) Mortality.

Severe forms of urea cycle defect are universally lethal without treatment (males with OTC deficiency). Milder forms of urea cycle defects can lead to progressive brain damage and subsequent mortality related to neurological complications [1].

(c) Brain damage.

Every episode of symptomatic hyperammonemia has the potential to cause brain damage. The main goal of therapy is to reduce the frequency and severity of hyperammonemia episodes. Brain damage is preventable in most patients with early diagnosis and proper management [1].

(d) Other complications.

Liver dysfunction (elevated aminotransferases, hyperbilirubinemia, mild coagulopathy) may be present in urea cycle defects, particularly in OTC deficiency. The level of dysfunction is not typically a serious concern in itself. Its significance is related to the fact that liver dysfunction can misdirect the evaluation of hyperammonemia to the workup of liver failure and delay the diagnosis and treatment of urea cycle defects [1].

Question 5. How can we manage the disease?

(a) Dietary management.

Goal of therapy is to provide sufficient supply of protein and energy to prevent activation of protein catabolism, gluconeogenesis and ammonia production. Diet should be carefully monitored as excess of protein can also lead to hyperammonemia.

Management of urea cycle defects revolves around nitrogen metabolism. Clinician should monitor nitrogen intake (protein, amino acids), nitrogen retention (appropriate growth) and nitrogen excretion (ammonia, glutamine). A positive nitrogen balance will result in hyperammonemia by inducing catabolism of amino acids. Negative nitrogen balance will lead to protein breakdown, gluconeogenesis and ammonia production. Although protein restriction is necessary it is essential that well balanced mixture of amino acids, including essential amino acids is provided [4].

Dietary management can fail in severe forms of urea cycle defects since hyperammonemia can be triggered by infections. Rhabdomyolysis leading to ammonia production can be directly caused by viral infections or can be a result of gluconeogenesis activated by increased energy requirements [4].

(b) Treatment.

Treatment of acute hyperammonemia is necessary in situations when dietary management fails to prevent hyperammonemia. Arginine can be used to increase renal ammonia excretion by the formation of argininosuccinic acid. This is particularly effective in argininosuccinate lyase deficiency, where the excretion of argininosuccinic acid is limited by the availability of arginine. Sodium benzoate and phenylacetate can serve as ammonia scavengers and are effective in reducing ammonia levels in OTC and CPS deficiency [4].

(c) Liver transplant.

Liver transplantation is curative in urea cycle defects and is indicated in severe forms of disease where dietary management is not likely to prevent brain damage over a prolonged period of time. Liver transplant survival in urea cycle defects is no different than in other indications for liver transplantation [1].

Question 6. What about other children and… grandchildren?

- Genetic counseling should be offered for all families affected by urea cycle defects, as early diagnosis and management can prevent permanent brain damage. Genetic testing can identify asymptomatic carriers and is available for pre-natal diagnosis [1].

References

1. Batshaw ML, Tuchman M, Summar M, Seminara J, Members of the Urea Cycle Disorders Consortium. A longitudinal study of urea cycle disorders. Mol Genet Metab. 2014;113:127–30.
2. Testai FD, Gorelick PB. Inherited metabolic disorders and stroke. II. Homocystinuria, organic acidurias, and urea cycle disorders. Arch Neurol. 2010;67:148–53.
3. Tuchman M, Jaleel N, Morizono H, Sheehy L, Lynch MG. Mutations and polymorphisms in the human ornithine transcarbamylase gene. Hum Mutat. 2002;19:93–107.
4. Brusilow SW, Danney M, Waber LJ, Batshaw M, Burton B, Levitsky L, et al. Treatment of episodic hyperammonemia in children with inborn errors of urea synthesis. N Eng J Med. 1984;310:1630–4.

Chapter 24
Metabolic and Genetic Liver Diseases: Porphyrias

Grzegorz W. Telega

Porphyrias are diverse disorders related to abnormal heme production. Heme is an iron-containing molecule involved in oxygen transport (hemoglobin) and the function of oxidative enzymes (cytochrome P450 complex, catalase, mitochondrial cytochromes). Bone marrow and liver are the main sites of heme production; thus, the symptomatology of porphyrias involves liver and erythroid cells. Accumulation of porphyrins (intermediate products in heme production) can be neurotoxic, leading to peripheral neuropathies. Other porphyrins lead to severe photosensitivity and skin injury.

The complexity of enzyme regulation makes symptoms highly sensitive to environmental (alcohol, lead, drugs, diet, infections) and endogenous (hormones, hemochromatosis) factors. In some patients, symptoms of porphyria can be induced without apparent genetic mutation. The most common example is sporadic porphyria cutaena tarda, where uroporphyrinogen decarboxylase can be inhibited by an excess of hepatic iron, estrogen administration, pregnancy, alcohol intake, hepatitis C or HIV infection [1].

Question 1. Why do we think of it?

> (a) Acute porphyrias.
> Symptoms of acute (hepatic) porphyrias are typically triggered by increased demands for hepatic heme production, which can be induced by exposure to toxins, estrogen hormones, or infections.

G.W. Telega, M.D., M.S. (✉)
Department of Pediatric Gastroenterology, Hepatology, and Nutrition,
Medical College of Wisconsin, Milwaukee, WI 53201, USA
e-mail: gtelega@mcw.edu

© Springer International Publishing Switzerland 2017
K. Saeian, R. Shaker (eds.), *Liver Disorders*,
DOI 10.1007/978-3-319-30103-7_24

- Abdominal pain.
  Abdominal pain is usually episodic, evolving over a few hours to days. Episodes of pain almost always start after puberty and are more common in girls than in boys. Pain is poorly localized, frequently associated with vomiting, constipation, and ileus. Abdominal pain can be associated with increased adrenergic activity (tachycardia, hypertension, pallor, sweating), dysuria, and urinary retention. The mechanism of abdominal pain is poorly understood, but it appears to be neurological (small fiber neuropathy) rather than inflammatory in nature. Tenderness, leukocytosis, and fever are absent or mild. Although symptoms are not specific, the presence of a recurrent pattern, particularly in association with neuropathy and dark urine should suggest porphyria.
- Neuropathy.
  Neuropathy is common, but does not occur in all patients with porphyria, even when abdominal symptoms are severe. Peripheral neuropathy is primarily a motor neuropathy. Symptoms usually start as a proximal weakness of the extremities. Deep tendon reflexes are diminished, although they may be normal in the early stages. Neuropathy is the result of axonal degeneration rather than demyelination. Cranial nerves, particularly VII and X, can be affected [2].
- Central nervous system involvement.
  Psychiatric symptoms, such as anxiety, insomnia, depression, and suicidal ideation, are common. Seizures, disorientation, hallucinations, optic neuropathy, cortical blindness, bulbar paralysis, and death have been described. Syndrome of inappropriate antidiuretic hormone secretion with resulting hyponatremia is common in acute attacks [2].

(b) Cutaneous presentation.

Cutaneous presentation related to photosensitivity is a feature in most types of porphyria (congenital erythropoietic porphyria [CEP], porphyria cutanea tarda [PCT], hereditary coproporphyria [HCP], variegate porphyria [VP]). Skin friability, blistering, hypo- and hyperpigmentation develop in the areas exposed to sun [1, 3].

(c) Hepatic changes in porphyrias.

Elevated aminotransferases have been reported in porphyrias (especially PCT and erythropoietic protoporphyria [EPP]). Fibrosis and cirrhosis have been described. In EPP, some patients progressed to acute liver failure. Microscopic evaluation of liver biopsy tissue rarely shows significant abnormalities. Most characteristic is red fluorescence of the liver tissue upon exposure to ultraviolet light. The risk for hepatocellular carcinoma is increased (PCT, acute intermittent porphyria [AIP], HCP, VP) [2, 3].

Table 24.1 Clinical features of porphyrias

Type	Enzyme	Clinical features
5-aminolevulinic acid dehydratase porphyria	5-aminolevulinic acid dehydratase	Rare, primarily neurological symptoms, no photosensitivity [2]
Acute intermittent porphyria	Porphobilinogen deaminase	The most common acute form of porphyria. Intermittent neurological symptoms (up to 80 % of carriers are asymptomatic), no photosensitivity. Symptoms usually after puberty, more prevalent in females than in males [2]
Congenital erythropoietic porphyria	Uroporphyrinogen III synthetase	Anemia and photosensitivity. Extremely variable severity ranging from fetal hydrops to mild photosensitivity in adults. Hypertrichosis [1]
Porphyria cutanea tarda	Uroporphyrinogen decarboxylase	Anemia and photosensitivity. Sporadic cases are common. Photosensitivity is severe, presenting in the first year of life in familial cases. Symptoms respond to phlebotomy and low-dose chloroquine and hydroxychloroquine. Associated with alcohol use and chronic hepatitis C [1]
Hereditary coproporphyria	Coproporphyrinogen oxidase	Intermittent neurological symptoms, mild photosensitivity
Variegate porphyria	Protoporphyrinogen oxidase (PPO)	Intermittent neurological symptoms, mild to moderate photosensitivity [2–6]
Erythropoietic protoporphyria	Ferrochelatase	Acute blistering photosensitivity, liver failure, motor neuropathy [2, 4]

Question 2. How do we make the diagnosis?

    (a) Laboratory evaluation.

Initial screening for porphyrias should include urinary porphyrin precursors (5-aminolevulinic acid and porphobilinogen) and plasma porphyrins for cutaneous porphyrias. 5-Aminolevulinic acid dehydratase level can be measured in erythrocytes.

Specific enzyme activity can be measured on liver biopsy in hepatic forms of porphyria. This can be used in patients who are suspected to have the sporadic form of porphyria or when genetic testing is not diagnostic.

    (b) Genetic testing.

The clinician should select appropriate genetic testing based on clinical symptomatology and screening tests. Tables 24.1 and 24.2 provide clinical vignettes and corresponding genes and specific enzymes. Genetic testing is available for diagnosis, the identification of asymptomatic carriers, and prenatal diagnosis.

Table 24.2 Genes involved in porphyria [1, 3, 6]

Disease	Classification	Gene	Location	Inheritance
5-aminolevulinic acid dehydratase porphyria	Hepatic	ALAD	9q32	Recessive
Acute intermittent porphyria	Hepatic	HMBS	11q23.3	Dominant
Congenital erythropoietic porphyria	Erythropoietic	UROS	10q26.1–q26.2	Recessive
Porphyria cutanea tarda	Hepatic	UROD	1p34.1	Type 1 sporadic Type 2 – dominant
Hereditary coproporphyria	Hepatic	CPOX	3q11.2–q12.1	Dominant
Variegate porphyria	Hepatic	PPOX	1q23.3	Dominant
Erythropoietic protoporphyria	Erythropoietic	FECH	18q21.31	Dominant

3. How did I get it?

   (a) Genetics of porphyrias.
       Most porphyrias are autosomal dominant, although rare recessive disorders (ALAD deficiency porphyria [ADP], CEP) have been described. Sporadic forms, where symptoms are induced by a combination of external and endogenous factors rather than gene mutation, are common in patients with symptoms of PCT, with the adult population reported to have an association with alcohol use and chronic hepatitis C. "Dual porphyrias," where a single patient has mutations in two separate genes in the heme synthesis pathway, have also been described [1].

4. What is the danger of doing nothing?

   (a) Mortality.
       Historically, prognosis in acute neurovisceral porphyria has been poor, with mortality approaching 80 % in some reports. Recent experience shows that with proper diagnosis, efforts to prevent acute attacks, and supportive care during the attacks, mortality can be reduced to less than 6 %. Up to 75 % of patients diagnosed with AIP and VP report "leading a normal life" [3].

   (b) Seizures.
       Seizures may be the result of the direct toxicity of porphyrins, but are most often associated with hyponatremia. Many anti-epileptic medications can induce heme synthesis and precipitate acute attacks of porphyria.

   (c) Neuropathy.
       After an acute attack has been successfully treated, neurological symptoms improve within a few days. A severe attack can lead to prolonged (years) or permanent neuropathy. Recovery from recurrent attacks is usually more prolonged than from the initial attack [2].

(d) Gastrointestinal symptoms.

After an acute attack, abdominal pain improves within a few hours. Patients with known acute porphyrias face the danger of misdiagnosis of acute abdominal disorders (appendicitis, pancreatitis, gallstones), which can be misrepresented as acute porphyria.

(e) Photosensitivity and skin disease.

Photosensitivity is a feature of most types of porphyria (CEP, PCT, HCP, VP). Skin lesions (friability, blistering, hypo- and hyperpigmentation) develop in the areas of direct sun exposure. Recurrent exposure leads to scarring and supra-infections, which result in deformities of the digits, eyelids, ears, nose, and face, and can cause severe disability. Involvement of the cornea can lead to blindness. Brown/red discoloration of the teeth can result from porphyrin deposition.

(f) Hematological abnormalities.

Hemolysis is a frequent feature of CEP and EPP. Anisocytosis, reticulocytosis, polychromasia, and unconjugated hyperbilirubinemia are frequent features. Secondary splenomegaly and hyersplenism can develop.

Question 5. How can we manage the disease?

Treatment depends on the accurate diagnosis of porphyria.

(a) Avoidance of precipitating drugs.

Most common groups of medications that are unsafe in acute porphyria include:

Angiotensin-converting-enzyme inhibitors

Antibiotics (dapsone, rifampin, sulfonamides)

Anti-diabetic (chlorpropamide, sulfonylurea derivatives)

Anti-epileptics (barbiturates, carbamazepine, felbamate, lamotrigine, mephenytoin, valproic acid)

Antifungals (griseofulvin, ketoconazole)

Calcium channel blockers

Ergot preparations

Hormonal therapy (danazol, progestins)

Hypnotic/sedative (glutethimide, meprobamate, methyprylon)

Muscle relaxants (cadisoprodol)

Non-steroidal anti-inflammatory drugs (diclofenac, phenylbutazone)

Others (metoclopramide)

Many other medications could potentially induce attacks of acute porphyria; thus, all medications should be checked for effects on cytochrome P450 and the heme production pathway, and for clinical reports of porphyria attacks [1, 2]. Patients should avoid smoking and alcohol intake.

(b) Skin protection.

In porphyrias associated with photosensitivity (CEP, PCT, HCP, and VP) skin should be protected from direct sun exposure at all times. After inadvertent exposure, special efforts should be focused on the prevention of the skin infections, which should be aggressively treated with antibiotics [1].

(c) Dietary management.

Glucose administration improves symptoms in acute porphyrias (AIP, HCP, VP). Owing to the risk of hyponatremia, electrolytes should be closely monitored, particularly when infusing a large volume of glucose-based intravenous solutions.

Special attention to adequate carbohydrate intake should be paid during infections, surgeries, and other serious illnesses, as acute porphyria attacks are more likely to occur under such circumstances. Adequate (but not excessive) iron intake can alleviate the course of acute porphyria [2].

(d) Transfusions.

Transfusions can be effective in the treatment of erythropoietic forms of porphyria (CEP). Transfusions downregulate heme synthesis and the production of porphyrins, leading as a consequence to a reduction in photosensitivity.

(e) Phlebotomy.

Phlebotomy is effective and results in remission of PCT, but not VP. It is most commonly used in combination with low-dose chloroquine. The mechanism of the effect of phlebotomy is likely related to a reduction in hepatic iron deposits that upregulates uroporphyrinogen decarboxylase activity [1, 4].

(f) Medications.

Intravenous heme arginate, heme albumin or hematin can be used in the treatment of acute porphyria attacks (AIP, HCP, VP) [2]. Chloroquine and hydroxychloroquine can be effective in the management of PCT [1]. Oral charcoal can increase the excretion of porphyrins in CEP, beta carotene improves sun tolerance, and cholestyramine can improve protoporphyrin excretion in EPP.

(g) Liver and bone marrow transplant.

Bone marrow transplantation is curative in erythropoietic porphyrias (CEP, EPP). Patients with severe forms of the disease can qualify for bone marrow transplantation.

Liver transplantation is curative in hepatic forms of porphyria; it may be indicated in severe forms of acute intermittent porphyria [5].

Question 6. What about other children and… grandchildren?

Genetic counseling is indicated in all familial forms of porphyria. Genetic testing is available for diagnosis, the identification of asymptomatic carriers, and for prenatal diagnosis.

References

1. De Verneuil H, Sassa S, Kappas A. Effects of polychlorinated biphenyl compounds, 2,3,7,8-te trachlorodibenzo-p-dioxin, phenobarbital and iron on hepatic uroporphyrinogen decarboxylase. Implications for the pathogenesis of porphyria. Biochem J. 1983;214(1):145–51.
2. Lambrecht RW, Thapar M, Bonkovsky HL. Genetic aspects of porphyria cutanea tarda. Semin Liver Dis. 2007;27(1):99–108.
3. Soonawalla ZF et al. Liver transplantation as a cure for acute intermittent porphyria. Lancet. 2004;363(9410):705–6.
4. Becker DM, Kramer S. The neurological manifestations of porphyria: a review. Medicine (Baltimore). 1977;56(5):411–23.
5. Epstein JH, Redeker AG. Porphyria cutanea tarda. A study of the effect of phlebotomy. N Engl J Med. 1968;279(24):1301–4.
6. Fromke VL et al. Porphyria variegata. Study of a large kindred in the United States. Am J Med. 1978;65(1):80–8.

Chapter 25
Drug-Induced Liver Injury

Raj Vuppalanchi

Question 1: Doc, what caused my liver problem if all my blood tests came back negative?

Patient Level Answer: Since test results for other causes of acute liver injury such as hepatitis A, B, or C and autoimmune hepatitis were negative and imaging including ultrasound or CT scan did not reveal any blockage by gall stones or problems with gallbladder or pancreas, we need to suspect drug-induced liver injury (DILI) as a potential cause keeping in mind that it is primarily a diagnosis of exclusion. Let us review your recent medication history including your herbal and dietary supplement (HDS) usage to see if there is any temporal association between exposure to those agents and onset of your liver injury.

Question 2: What do you mean by drug-induced liver injury? I did not take any Tylenol (acetaminophen)!

Patient Level Answer: Although liver injury from accidental or intentional overdose of acetaminophen is the most familiar scenario, there are many other drugs or HDS that can cause DILI due to rare and unpredictable hepatotoxic injury. One recent study showed antibiotics, antidepressants, and HDS products as commonly implicated agents for DILI.

Question 3: How do you make a diagnosis of DILI?

Patient Level Answer: DILI cannot be diagnosed simply by blood chemistries alone, or by liver biopsy or imaging studies. Although it is a diagnosis of exclusion, it requires pertinent clinical information and careful medication and HDS usage history to find a temporal association between the implicated agent and

R. Vuppalanchi, M.D. (✉)
Division of Gastroenterology and Hepatology, Indiana University School of Medicine, 702 Rotary Building, Suite 225, Indianapolis, IN 46202, USA
e-mail: rvuppala@iu.edu

onset of liver injury. It is important to identify the offending agent to avoid inadvertent re-exposure.

Question 4: Will my liver recover? Will I develop cirrhosis or need a liver transplant?

Patient Level Answer: The majority of DILI cases improve with discontinuation of the offending agent, and liver-related deaths are infrequent at less than 5%. In the rare case when liver injury is severe, individuals may develop acute liver failure and require evaluation for liver transplantation. In certain instances of liver injury from dietary supplements containing anabolic steroids, the jaundice is pronounced and recovery is very slow.

Introduction

Drugs that enter the systemic circulation undergo biotransformation in the liver to more water soluble forms for eventual elimination through bile or urine. The central role of the liver in the process of metabolism and detoxification, unfortunately, places it at a disproportionate risk for drug-induced injury. Individuals with liver injury resulting from damage to hepatocytes (hepatocellular) or biliary tree (cholestatic) or both (cholestatic hepatitis or mixed) develop asymptomatic abnormalities in liver tests or develop symptoms such as upper abdominal pain, jaundice, acholic stools, dark urine or other constitutional symptoms [1, 2]. Drug-induced liver injury (DILI) can mimic almost all known liver diseases and diagnosis can be difficult due to a lack of established biomarkers and varied clinical presentation [3–5]. Clinical judgment, often by exclusion of competing etiology, is probably the most frequent method used to identify a case of DILI. In clinical trials, modified Hy's law, i.e., ALT elevation >3 times upper limit of normal (ULN) with total bilirubin >2 times ULN is used as a surrogate for a drug likely to cause severe DILI (fatal or requiring transplant) [6]. Valid methods for accurate diagnosis, phenotyping with prediction of severity and outcome of DILI are lacking and are a significant unmet need [7, 8].

DILI may be broadly classified as intrinsic, that is predictable and dose dependent, or idiosyncratic hepatotoxicity that is rare and not necessarily dose dependent [9]. Intrinsic liver injury is often reproducible with characteristic histologic change affecting a particular zone of the liver lobule and is usually testable in animal models. Very few drugs causing intrinsic hepatotoxicity remain on the market since these compounds are excluded from moving forward in the preclinical phase of drug development. Agents that cause intrinsic DILI are further subclassified as either direct, in which the agent itself is a poison or indirect, in which the agent is metabolized reproducibly to a toxic substance. Examples of direct hepatotoxins include carbon tetrachloride or the herbicide Paraquat. Acetaminophen (paracetamol, *N*-acetyl-*p*-aminophenol or APAP) is a classic example of an indirect intrinsic hepatotoxin.

Intrinsic DILI

Drugs that cause dose-dependent hepatotoxicity are usually legacy drugs and have been in use for several decades prior to the current liver safety assessment for new drugs by Food and Drug Administration [10]. One such classic example is acetaminophen (paracetamol, *N*-acetyl-*p*-aminophenol or APAP). It first became available in the United States in 1955 when phenacetin was removed from the market in the early 1950s due to nephrotoxicity associated with chronic use. Soon after the recognition of Reye syndrome with aspirin [11], APAP became the drug of choice for the treatment of fever and pain in the US and around the world. The toxicity of APAP was initially reported by Thomson and Prescott in 1966, following ingestion of large doses of the drug in two patients [12]. These patients developed severe hepatotoxicity with characteristic histologic appearance of hepatocellular necrosis in the centrilobular areas of the liver resulting in death within 3 days of ingestion [12]. Prior to the late 1990s, APAP was not widely recognized as a cause of acute liver failure (ALF) in the United States and did not appear in the transplant databases until that time. In 2005, Larson et al. reported that APAP accounted for 42 % of all cases of ALF enrolled across several transplant centers participating in the Acute Liver Failure Study Group [13]. The annual percentage of APAP-related ALF during the study rose from 28 % in 1998 to 51 % in 2003. Unintentional (chronic therapeutic usage) and intentional overdoses equally accounted for these cases. In the unintentional group, it was recognized that up to 40 % took two or more acetaminophen preparations simultaneously, and up to 60 % use APAP in combination with narcotics [13]. It was also recognized that APAP contributed to ALF in children with recent data suggesting that it is responsible for 14–25 % of cases [14, 15]. One major regulatory event that occurred recently was reduction in the unit of APAP from 500 to 325 mg in combination-opioid products (http://www. fda.gov/NewsEvents/Newsroom/PressAnnouncements/ucm239894.htm). APAP is currently found in more than 600 different over-the-counter and prescription medicines including pain relievers, fever reducers, sleep aids, and numerous cough, cold, and flu medicines. Concerns related to unintentional overdose have resulted in increased scrutiny from Regulatory agencies leading to the recent initiative such as "know your dosage" campaign (http://www.knowyourdose.org/).

Susceptibility profile for APAP hepatotoxicity is of interest as some patients may be more prone than others to the adverse event. These risk factors could be genetic or nongenetic host-related factors such as chronic alcoholism causing induction of CYP2E1 or malnutrition associated with glutathione (GSH) deficiency. The toxicity of acetaminophen is dose related and occurs because of the generation of a toxic intermediate metabolite, NAPQI by hepatic cytochrome P450 2E1 (CYP2E1). Although this toxic metabolite is generated with the consumption of therapeutic doses of acetaminophen; it is rapidly detoxified by conjugation with GSH. In humans with chronic alcoholism, there is a several-fold induction of hepatic CYP2E1 activity that lasts up to 48 h from the time of the last drink. Coupled with hepatic depletion of GSH because of malnutrition and starvation, patients with alcoholism might be predisposed to APAP toxicity at therapeutic doses. Existing data suggest that these patients might be sensitive to acetaminophen at therapeutic doses, but findings from systematic studies are unavailable. Kuffner et al., administered 4 g of APAP or placebo for 3 days to patients with alcoholism who had entered a detoxification center and showed no significant difference in liver tests between the placebo and APAP groups [16]. Although the authors concluded that it was safe to administer the maximum recommended daily dose of APAP to newly-abstinent patients with alcoholism for up to 3 days, it is very likely that in real-life individuals may take APAP over prolonged periods while continuing to consume alcohol [17].

Some studies have also reported increased risk of APAP hepatotoxicity in patients receiving the antiepileptic drugs phenobarbital and phenytoin likely related to decreased glucuronidation from inhibition of UDP-glucuronosyltransferases [18]. Investigations of genotypic variants of GST and UGT, however, failed to confer a phenotypic susceptibility to APAP toxicity [19]. There has been some concern about obesity and associated nonalcoholic fatty liver disease (NAFLD) as a risk factor for APAP hepatotoxicity based on animal studies [20]. Unfortunately, these studies did not unequivocally establish the mechanism(s) whereby NAFLD could favor APAP hepatotoxicity, although some investigations suggested that preexistent induction of CYP2E1 could play a significant role by increasing the generation of NAPQI, the toxic metabolite of APAP. Moreover, preexistent mitochondrial dysfunction associated with NAFLD could also be involved. In contrast, some investigations suggested that factors that could reduce the risk and severity of APAP hepatotoxicity in obesity and NAFLD include higher hepatic APAP glucuronidation, reduced CYP3A4 activity, and increased volume of body distribution. Thus, the occurrence and the outcome of APAP-induced liver injury in an obese individual with NAFLD might depend on a delicate balance between metabolic factors that can be protective and others that favor large hepatic levels of NAPQI [20]. Currently, there does not appear to be a clear signal with regard to BMI and risk of APAP hepatotoxicity.

Traditionally, toxicity has been defined as a single acute ingestion of APAP of greater than 150 mg/kg in children and greater than 10 g in adults [21]. Definitions of chronic toxicity, or multiple time point ingestions, vary but daily use of more than 90 mg/kg in children and more than 4 g/day in adults is considered toxic. The diagnosis of APAP toxicity for patients that present for medical evaluation in the first 24 h with clear histories of APAP ingestion is relatively straightforward. The Rumack-Matthew nomogram (http://www.tylenolprofessional.com/assets/Nomogram.pdf) was created as a risk stratification tool for patients presenting for medical evaluation following acute single-dose ingestions of APAP [22]. The nomogram defines an APAP concentration of greater than 150 µg/mL obtained 4 h after the overdose as the threshold level of toxicity that indicates the need for treatment [22]. However, alternative clinical scenarios such as staggered or chronic ingestions of APAP and ingestions in individuals with increased CYP2E1 from alcoholism are not accounted for this nomogram [23]. Rarely, chronic ingestion has been attributed to result in progressive liver disease and cirrhosis but this phenomenon has not been well documented. Additional discussion about treatment aspects is beyond the scope of this chapter and is the subject of a recent review and position statement from American Association for Study of Liver Disease [24, 25].

Idiosyncratic DILI

Idiosyncratic DILI is a heterogeneous and rare entity caused by multitude of prescription or herbal and dietary supplements with a varied presentation, ranging from asymptomatic liver test abnormalities to fatal liver failure [2, 26]. It is primarily a diagnosis of exclusion and thus prone to misdiagnosis both in clinical practice and in clinical trial setting [27]. Idiosyncratic DILI from any one drug is not only rare, but a largely unpredictable event causing hepatic damage at therapeutic concentrations and causing nonzonal necrosis. One population-based study from Iceland suggested an incidence of 19 cases per 100,000 inhabitants per year [28]. The incidence is more prevalent with certain agents such as amoxicillin-clavulanic acid (~1 in 2300 users), diclofenac, azathioprine, infliximab and nitrofurantoin [28].

Mechanisms of injury are usually immunogenic or host susceptibility from genetic or acquired inability to detoxify hepatotoxic drug intermediates [29]. Therefore, it has been difficult to systematically investigate the prevalence and risk factors for developing idiosyncratic DILI [30, 31]. The international consensus meeting on DILI held in 1989 recommended that in the absence of a liver biopsy DILI should be defined as ALT or conjugated bilirubin >2-fold increase over the upper limit of normal (ULN) or a combined increase of AST, alkaline phosphatase or bilirubin provided one of them is twofold above ULN [32]. Although the European investigators continue to adopt this definition (e.g., Spanish DILI network investigators), the US DILI Network (DILIN) investigators viewed this definition as far too inclusive and felt it cannot discriminate DILI from fluctuations in liver biochemistries that are known to occur in individuals with underlying fatty liver (seen in up to 30 % US adults). The criteria for enrollment into DILIN was therefore more restrictive and set at AST or ALT at >5 times ULN or alkaline phosphatase (Alk P) >2 times ULN on two consecutive occasions or Bilirubin >2.5 mg/dl along with elevated AST or ALT or Alk P or INR >1.5 along with elevated AST or ALT or Alk P.

Clinical Features and Natural History

Acute DILI has been traditionally characterized into hepatocellular, cholestatic and mixed (hepatocellular and cholestatic) patterns based on "*R*" ratio calculated using the formula of (ALT/ULN)/(AlkP/ULN) from the blood test results at the time of initial presentation. *R* ratios of >5 are defined as hepatocellular, <2 as cholestatic, and between 2 and 5 as a mixed pattern of enzymes. If the ALT value is >2 times ULN and the AlkP is normal, the pattern is considered hepatocellular, and an *R* ratio need not be calculated. Similarly, if the AlkP value is >2 times ULN but the ALT is normal, the pattern is considered cholestatic, and an *R* ratio need not be calculated. This biochemical pattern of liver injury in part forms the basis for the so-called signature pattern of DILI caused by a specific compound (e.g., amoxicillin-clavulanic acid causes cholestatic liver injury, isoniazid (INH) causes hepatocellular liver injury). Interestingly, recent data from the DILIN suggest that such a signature is neither sensitive nor specific. Furthermore, there appears to be no significant correlation between biochemical pattern of liver injury and liver histology in patients with DILI [33]. Chronic DILI is currently defined as evidence of persistent laboratory, radiological, or pathological abnormalities 6 months after DILI onset. Data from the DILIN study show that up to 7 % of children and 14 % of adults developed chronic DILI and liver biopsies in these individuals often reveal evidence of chronic hepatitis or bile duct injury [2, 34].

There are a plethora of presentations for idiosyncratic DILI. Clinical scenarios may range from asymptomatic liver enzyme abnormalities to symptoms that could be general (fatigue, itching, pain etc.), immuno-allergic (fever, rash, peripheral or tissue eosinophilia), vascular (nodular regenerative hyperplasia) or severe with jaundice, coagulopathy, ascites sometimes progressing to fulminant hepatic failure. However, in real life, patients with these symptoms come to the attention of the health care provider at variable time points and careful history taking is essential to determine the chronology of events leading to the presenting symptoms. The clinical phenotype with characteristic histologic features from example agents is summarized in Table 25.1.

Diagnosis of DILI

Making a diagnosis of DILI is often very challenging due to varied presentations in varied clinical scenarios with reliable diagnostic tests. One of the commonly used instruments in the clinical trials and by regulatory authorities is the Roussel Uclaf Causality Assessment Method (RUCAM). It is a structured means of assigning points for temporal association, clinical, biochemical, serologic and radiological features. The overall score ranges from −9 to +14 with a higher score associated with a higher likelihood of DILI from the implicated agent. In the real world, however, first and foremost in the diagnosis of DILI, is to entertain the possibility of DILI in any patient with unexplained liver injury. Clinical judgment, often by exclusion of competing etiology, is probably the most frequent method used to identify a case of DILI (Fig. 25.1). In judging the likelihood of DILI from an implicated agent, a process called causality assessment primarily based on six features are crucial for a definitive diagnosis.

Table 25.1 Plethora of clinical presentations with characteristic histologic features from example agents

Phenotype	Histological features	Example agents
Acute fatty liver with lactic acidosis	Microvesicular hepatic steatosis ± other tissue involvement	Didanosine, Fialuridine, Valproate
Acute hepatic necrosis	Collapse and necrosis of liver parenchyma	Isoniazid, Niacin
Autoimmune-like hepatitis	Plasma cells and interface hepatitis with detectable autoantibodies	Nitrofurantoin, Minocycline
Bland cholestasis	Balloon hepatocytes with minimal inflammation	Anabolic steroids
Cholestatic hepatitis	Balloon hepatocytes with inflammation, predominance of serum alkaline phosphate elevation (phenytoin, amoxicillin-clavulanic acid)	Phenytoin, Augmentin
Fibrosis/cirrhosis	Hepatic collagenization with minimal inflammation	Methotrexate, Amiodarone
Immunoallergic hepatitis	Eosinophilic infiltrate	Trimethoprim-sulfamethoxazole
Nodular regeneration	Micro- or macroscopic liver nodules	Azathioprine, Oxaliplatin, TDM1
Nonalcoholic fatty liver	Macro- and microsteatosis, hepatocyte ballooning and periportal inflammation	Tamoxifen
Sinusoidal obstruction syndrome	Inflammation with obliteration of central veins	Busulfan
Vanishing bile duct syndrome	Paucity of interlobular bile ducts	Sulfonamides, Beta-lactams

Modified from Hayashi et al. Seminar liver Disease 2014 [65]

- Latency: The duration between the exposure to the offending agent and the onset of liver injury is typically called the latency period and could be variable ranging from 5 days and up to 3 months. Drugs such as sulfonamides and macrolide antibiotics have short latency period of few days where as drugs such as INH, nitrofurantoin or amiodarone have long latency period of up to several months.
- Dechallenge: Improvement in liver tests is usually observed within a few days (acetaminophen) or few weeks (macrolide antibiotics or sulfonamides) of discontinuation of the offending agent. Certain drugs, however, cause persistent elevations in liver tests and often associated with bile duct damage or chronic hepatitis.
- Pattern of injury: Drugs often have a signature pattern in their clinical presentation. For example, anabolic steroids cause bland cholestasis, or amoxicillin-clavulanic acid (Augmentin) causes mixed pattern, or INH causes hepatocellular. A few drugs can cause immune-allergic hepatitis with features such a rash, facial edema, myalgia, arthralgia, eosinophilia and atypical lymphocytes. For example, allopurinol causes these symptoms with short latency. Telaprevir is another

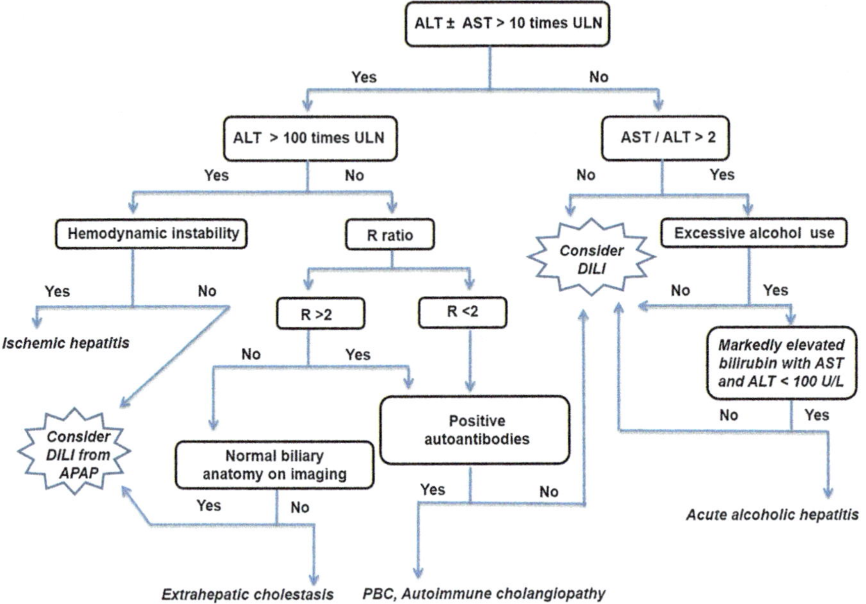

Fig. 25.1 Flow chart for evaluation of a case of apparent DILI. The diagnosis of DILI requires pertinent clinical information and adequate evaluation for exclusion of competing etiology

recent example of a drug that has been associated with Drug Rash Eosinophilia and Systemic Symptoms (DRESS).

- Exclusion of competing etiology: A careful history and work up for exclusion of competing etiology is crucial as DILI is primarily a diagnosis of exclusion. For exclusion of acute hepatitis C, the routinely ordered viral hepatitis panel that include hepatitis C antibody is inadequate since it takes approximately 4 weeks to develop positive antibodies. A hepatitis C virologic assay is necessary to exclude acute hepatitis C. A liver biopsy is not required to make a diagnosis of DILI. However, rarely a liver biopsy should be considered if autoimmune hepatitis remains a competing etiology or when liver enzymes fail to improve with discontinuation of the offending drug.

- Prior reports of the implicated agent: Some drugs are well known, well described, and well reported to cause DILI and have a characteristic signature with more than 50 cases including case series that have been described. Causality assessment of such cases in general is easier when adequate information is available. Alternatively, certain drugs despite extensive use have no evidence that they cause liver injury. Although single case reports may have been published, they are largely unconvincing. Implicating such an agent as the cause for DILI would raise concerns about concomitant drugs that could have been missed, or surreptitious use of herbal and dietary supplements often under the perception of being safe due to natural ingredients.

- Re-challenge: Although included in several causality instruments, a premeditated re-challenge with the suspected drug is not recommended. However, inadvertent re-challenge followed by a repeat liver injury is very convincing for DILI related to that drug.

LiverTox: A Clinical and Research Information Resource on DILI

A significant development in this field is LiverTox (livertox.nih.gov), a novel online resource with content developed by Liver Disease Branch of the National Institute of Diabetes and Digestive and Kidney Diseases (NIDDK) with help from National Library of Medicine. It is in the public domain and freely available to use. It includes a complete and accurate summary of clinical features, diagnosis, cause, frequency, patterns, and management of DILI associated with prescription and nonprescription drugs such as HDS. LiverTox is a single-destination shortest path for easy accesses to up-to-date, accurate, and comprehensive information for the health care provider facing challenging cases of apparent DILI. The RUCAM worksheet is also available through the LiverTox website (http://www.livertox.nih.gov/rucam.html).

Drug-Induced Autoimmune Hepatitis

Certain drugs can cause autoimmune hepatitis with presence of autoantibodies, hyper gammaglobulinemia, and characteristic liver histology similar to de novo autoimmune hepatitis [35]. Resolution of liver test abnormalities has also been reported with discontinuation of the offending drug but often in real world, steroids are initiated due to difficulty in differentiating from de novo autoimmune hepatitis (AIH). When liver tests improve with steroid therapy, consideration could be given for cessation of steroid therapy through a slow taper especially in drugs that have a definite association with AIH such as nitrofurantoin, minocycline, methylodopa, hydralazine, or halothane. Latency period with these agents is typically long and could be several months. For example, nitrofurantoin (Macrobid), characteristically causes a chronic hepatitis after many weeks, months or even years of therapy with some cases presenting with cirrhosis associated with serum antinuclear antibodies (ANA) [35].

Herbal and Dietary Supplement-Related Liver Injury

A dietary supplement is any product intended to supplement diet and may contain vitamins, minerals, herbs, amino acids or extracts thereof. Unlike most prescribed pharmaceuticals, attribution of DILI to herbal and dietary supplements (HDS) is confounded by product variability, complexity, and contamination or adulteration [36]. These factors notwithstanding, the problem of DILI attributable to HDS remains an important concern for Americans, as HDS are the second most common cause of DILI among enrollees into the DILIN. The widespread use of HDS, the current lack of regulation, and the uncertainty of the manufacturer or provider-initiated reporting of adverse events preclude an accurate estimation of the frequency of use and the scope of attributable hepatotoxicity. That said, approximately 15 % of the DILIN cohort have experienced liver injury caused by HDS [37]. In the recent report from DILIN, liver injury caused by HDS increased from 7 to 20 % ($P<0.001$) during the study period between 2004 and 2013 [37]. Bodybuilding HDS caused prolonged jaundice (median, 91 days) in young men, but did not result in any fatalities or liver transplantation. Non-bodybuilding HDS cases presented more with hepatocellular injury, predominantly in middle-aged women, and, more frequently, led to death or transplantation, compared to injury from conventional medications (13 % vs. 3 %; $P<0.05$) [37].

DILI in Patients with Disease State

Certain disease conditions may predispose individuals to DILI due to alterations in host immune function, drug metabolizing enzyme activity, lower serum albumin, glutathione reserve in the liver and overall ability to scavenge chemically reactive metabolites that can induce hepatotoxicity. One classic example is the increased incidence of trimethoprim–sulfamethoxazole hepatotoxicity (up to 20 %) in patients with acquired immune deficiency syndrome compared to the general population [38]. Another, well-known example is the increased incidence of DILI from antituberculosis treatment in patients who have advanced disease and lower pretreatment serum albumin (<3.5 g/dl) [39]. A recent study examined the association between on-treatment weight loss and risk of DILI from tuberculosis treatment and reported that weight loss of 2 kg or more within 4 weeks, concomitant hepatitis C, older age and multi-drug resistant TB were independently associated risk factors [40]. Among these, the strongest risk factor was on-treatment weight loss (OR 211, 95 % CI: 36–1232) [40]. Furthermore, patients with concomitant alcohol intake had threefold higher odds of developing hepatotoxicity [39]. Alcohol consumption is one of the criteria in the RUCAM causality assessment instrument [32] although the risk of liver injury has only been reported in select medications such as INH, methotrexate or halothane [41]. Chronic alcohol abuse might increase the hepatotoxicity of antituberculosis treatment through the induction of hepatic CYP2E1 [42, 43]. It has been suggested that alcoholism in conjunction with patient's poor nutritional status may result in poor glutathione reserve and increased risk of DILI [17, 43].

Obesity, diabetes, and hepatic steatosis result in a chronic oxidant stress and mitochondrial dysfunction [44], which may enhance the toxicity of drugs that target mitochondria, e.g., acetaminophen [45]. However, concern related to baseline liver test abnormalities from underlying nonalcoholic fatty liver disease (NAFLD) or chronic hepatitis C and risk of hepatotoxicity especially with drugs such as statins and thiazolidinediones (rosiglitazone and pioglitazone) did not really pan out and currently liver safety iof these agents in patients with underlying chronic liver disease is much less of an issue [46–50]. Minor fluctuations in aminotransferases upon initiating statin therapy are not uncommon but serious hepatotoxicity is quite rare and even when happens, it is almost universally reversible upon prompt recognition and withdrawal of the offending agent [46, 51]. Rare cases of statin-induced autoimmune hepatitis have been reported and in such cases immunosuppressive therapy may be necessary until sustained biochemical improved is achieved [52]. Recommendations of the Liver Expert Panel to the National Lipid Association on Statin Safety states that current evidence supports the use of statins to treat hyperlipidemia in patients with nonalcoholic fatty liver disease and nonalcoholic steatohepatitis [53].

Treatment of DILI

The mainstay of treatment for DILI is prompt recognition, discontinuation, and avoiding reexposure to the offending agent. The recovery period is varied with relatively rapid improvement unless there is bile duct damage or drug-induced AIH. A low-fat diet is generally recommended in those with jaundice and anti-pruritic agents such a doxepin or hydroxyzine are prescribed to alleviate symptoms of itching. For some specific drugs, however, there are specific therapies available. These include *N*-actyl cysteine (NAC or mucomyst) for acetaminophen poisoning, intravenous L-carnitine for valproate toxicity, cholestyramine for leflunomide (Arava), and steroid or immunosuppressant therapy for drug-induced AIH. Close follow-up until a 50 % improvement in ALT or AlkP with subsequent follow-up to document normalization of liver test abnormalities is required to ensure that the patient has not progressed to chronic DILI. We generally recommend follow up until normalization of liver test abnormalities and then discharge from our clinic. Consideration should be given for referral of the patient with apparent DILI to one of the DILIN centers (https://dilin.dcri.duke.edu/).

Total Parenteral Nutrition-Related Liver Injury

Parenteral nutrition-associated liver disease (PNALD) is characterized by elevated liver tests, hepatic steatosis and progressive hepatic fibrosis that could evolve into a life-threatening disease with high mortality and morbidity [54]. It is estimated that up 40 % of patients receiving long-term total parenteral nutrition (TPN) develop PNALD [55]. Progression to cirrhosis and portal hypertension occurs rarely but appears to be more common in infants and neonates than in adults [55]. Although the exact pathogenesis is unclear and probably multifactorial, there is accumulating evidence over the past few decades that the lipid component of TPN is the most probable cause of PNALD. Both animal and human research during the past decade has implicated phytosterols and ω-6 (n–6) fatty acids as the most likely components in the current lipid formulations as primary reasons for PNALD [56–58].

PNALD should be suspected in all patients receiving TPN in the hospital or at home. Pattern of injury is often mixed pattern or cholestatic and competing etiologies such as extra-hepatic causes of cholestasis and DILI should be excluded. In most cases, elevated liver tests are observed after the first 2 weeks of TPN, although some patients may develop abnormalities several months later [55, 59]. Histologic examinations reveal mild to moderate cholestasis with minimal inflammation or necrosis and no evidence of fat accumulation [60]. With continued TPN and enteral fasting, severe cholestasis is associated with bile duct regeneration, portal inflammation, and fibrosis with cirrhosis developing within months [55, 60].

Vital information with regard to treatment aspect of PNALD comes from the pediatric world. Several nonrandomized human trials provide substantial data to the beneficial effects of ω-3-rich fatty acids in the treatment of PNALD [61–63]. Recent data suggest marked improvement in survival when PNALD is recognized at early stages and treated with lipid emulsions that contain fish oil rather than plant-based lipid emulsions [62–64]. Unfortunately, in the United States, only plant-based lipid emulsions are currently approved for use, with fish oil based lipid emulsions available only through compassionate-use program.

In summary, DILI is a diagnosis of exclusion and should be considered during evaluation of every case of unexplained liver injury. Our knowledge about PNALD is evolving and we certainly hope that formulations with fish oil based lipid emulsions are available in the US sooner than later.

References

1. Zimmerman HJ. The spectrum of hepatotoxicity. Perspect Biol Med. 1968;12:135–61.
2. Chalasani N, Fontana RJ, Bonkovsky HL, et al. Causes, clinical features, and outcomes from a prospective study of drug-induced liver injury in the United States. Gastroenterology. 2008;135:1924–34. 1934.e1–4.
3. Davern TJ, Chalasani N. Drug-induced liver injury in clinical trials: as rare as hens' teeth. Am J Gastroenterol. 2009;104:1159–61.
4. Rockey DC, Seeff LB, Rochon J, et al. Causality assessment in drug-induced liver injury using a structured expert opinion process: comparison to the Roussel-Uclaf causality assessment method. Hepatology. 2010;51:2117–26.
5. Garcia-Cortes M, Stephens C, Lucena MI, et al. Causality assessment methods in drug induced liver injury: strengths and weaknesses. J Hepatol. 2011;55:683–91.
6. Temple R. Hy's law: predicting serious hepatotoxicity. Pharmacoepidemiol Drug Saf. 2006;15:241–3.
7. Grant LM, Rockey DC. Drug-induced liver injury. Curr Opin Gastroenterol. 2012;28:198.
8. Lozano-Lanagran M, Robles M, Lucena MI, et al. Hepatotoxicity in 2011--advancing resolutely. Rev Esp Enferm Dig. 2011;103:472–9.
9. Senior JR. What is idiosyncratic hepatotoxicity? What is it not? Hepatology. 2008;47:1813–5.

10. Senior JR. Evolution of the Food and Drug Administration approach to liver safety assessment for new drugs: current status and challenges. Drug Saf. 2014;37 Suppl 1:S9–17.
11. Sillanpaa M, Makela AL, Koivikko A. Acute liver failure and encephalopathy (Reye's syndrome?) during salicylate therapy. Acta Paediatr Scand. 1975;64:877–80.
12. Thomson JS, Prescott LF. Liver damage and impaired glucose tolerance after paracetamol overdosage. Br Med J. 1966;2:506–7.
13. Larson AM, Polson J, Fontana RJ, et al. Acetaminophen-induced acute liver failure: results of a United States multicenter, prospective study. Hepatology. 2005;42:1364–72.
14. Bower WA, Johns M, Margolis HS, et al. Population-based surveillance for acute liver failure. Am J Gastroenterol. 2007;102:2459–63.
15. Squires Jr RH, Shneider BL, Bucuvalas J, et al. Acute liver failure in children: the first 348 patients in the pediatric acute liver failure study group. J Pediatr. 2006;148:652–8.
16. Kuffner EK, Green JL, Bogdan GM, et al. The effect of acetaminophen (four grams a day for three consecutive days) on hepatic tests in alcoholic patients--a multicenter randomized study. BMC Med. 2007;5:13.
17. Vuppalanchi R. How safe is acetaminophen for the treatment of pain and fever in newly-abstinent patients with alcoholism? Nat Clin Pract Gastroenterol Hepatol. 2008;5:134–5.
18. Pirotte JH. Apparent potentiation of hepatotoxicity from small doses of acetaminophen by phenobarbital. Ann Intern Med. 1984;101:403.
19. Court MH, Duan SX, von Moltke LL, et al. Interindividual variability in acetaminophen glucuronidation by human liver microsomes: identification of relevant acetaminophen UDP-glucuronosyltransferase isoforms. J Pharmacol Exp Ther. 2001;299:998–1006.
20. Michaut A, Moreau C, Robin MA, et al. Acetaminophen-induced liver injury in obesity and nonalcoholic fatty liver disease. Liver Int. 2014;34:e171–9.
21. Whitcomb DC, Block GD. Association of acetaminophen hepatotoxicity with fasting and ethanol use. JAMA. 1994;272:1845–50.
22. Rumack BH, Peterson RC, Koch GG, et al. Acetaminophen overdose. 662 cases with evaluation of oral acetylcysteine treatment. Arch Intern Med. 1981;141:380–5.
23. Manchanda A, Cameron C, Robinson G. Beware of paracetamol use in alcohol abusers: a potential cause of acute liver injury. N Z Med J. 2013;126:80–4.
24. Polson J, Lee WM. AASLD position paper: the management of acute liver failure. Hepatology. 2005;41:1179–97.
25. Stravitz RT, Kramer AH, Davern T, et al. Intensive care of patients with acute liver failure: recommendations of the U.S. Acute Liver Failure Study Group. Crit Care Med. 2007;35:2498–508.
26. Ostapowicz G, Fontana RJ, Schiodt FV, et al. Results of a prospective study of acute liver failure at 17 tertiary care centers in the United States. Ann Intern Med. 2002;137:947–54.
27. Shapiro MA, Lewis JH. Causality assessment of drug-induced hepatotoxicity: promises and pitfalls. Clin Liver Dis. 2007;11:477–505. v.
28. Bjornsson ES, Bergmann OM, Bjornsson HK, et al. Incidence, presentation, and outcomes in patients with drug-induced liver injury in the general population of Iceland. Gastroenterology. 2013;144:1419–25. 1425.e1–3; quiz e19–20.
29. Gandolfi AJ, Brown BR. Hypoxia and halothane hepatotoxicity. Anesth Analg. 1983;62:859–61.
30. Bell LN, Chalasani N. Epidemiology of idiosyncratic drug-induced liver injury. Semin Liver Dis. 2009;29:337–47.
31. Chalasani N, Bjornsson E. Risk factors for idiosyncratic drug-induced liver injury. Gastroenterology. 2010;138:2246–59.
32. Benichou C. Criteria of drug-induced liver disorders. Report of an international consensus meeting. J Hepatol. 1990;11:272–6.
33. DE Kleiner CN, Conjeevaram HS, Bonkovsky H, Russo M, Davern T, McHutchison JG, et al. Relationship of biochemical variables to histologic findings and the pathological pattern of injury among cases identified in the NIH DILIN Study. Gastroenterology. 2007;132:M1775.

34. Molleston JP, Fontana RJ, Lopez MJ, et al. Characteristics of idiosyncratic drug-induced liver injury in children: results from the DILIN prospective study. J Pediatr Gastroenterol Nutr. 2011;53:182–9.
35. Czaja AJ. Drug-induced autoimmune-like hepatitis. Dig Dis Sci. 2011;56:958–76.
36. Seeff LB, Bonkovsky H, Navarro VJ, Wang G. Herbal products and the liver - a review of adverse effects and mechanisms. Gastroenterology. 2015;148:517.
37. Navarro VJ, Barnhart H, Bonkovsky HL, et al. Liver injury from herbals and dietary supplements in the U.S. Drug-Induced Liver Injury Network. Hepatology. 2014;60:1399.
38. Small CB, Harris CA, Friedland GH, et al. The treatment of Pneumocystis carinii pneumonia in the acquired immunodeficiency syndrome. Arch Intern Med. 1985;145:837–40.
39. Sharma SK, Balamurugan A, Saha PK, et al. Evaluation of clinical and immunogenetic risk factors for the development of hepatotoxicity during antituberculosis treatment. Am J Respir Crit Care Med. 2002;166:916–9.
40. Warmelink I, ten Hacken NH, van der Werf TS, et al. Weight loss during tuberculosis treatment is an important risk factor for drug-induced hepatotoxicity. Br J Nutr. 2011;105:400–8.
41. Zimmerman HJ. Drug-induced liver disease. Clin Liver Dis. 2000;4:73–96. vi.
42. Liu LG, Yan H, Yao P, et al. CYP2E1-dependent hepatotoxicity and oxidative damage after ethanol administration in human primary hepatocytes. World J Gastroenterol. 2005;11:4530–5.
43. Cederbaum AI. Role of CYP2E1 in ethanol-induced oxidant stress, fatty liver and hepatotoxicity. Dig Dis. 2010;28:802–11.
44. Pessayre D, Fromenty B, Mansouri A. Mitochondrial injury in steatohepatitis. Eur J Gastroenterol Hepatol. 2004;16:1095–105.
45. Pessayre D, Fromenty B, Berson A, et al. Central role of mitochondria in drug-induced liver injury. Drug Metab Rev. 2012;44:34–87.
46. Chalasani N. Statins and hepatotoxicity: focus on patients with fatty liver. Hepatology. 2005;41:690–5.
47. Vuppalanchi R, Teal E, Chalasani N. Patients with elevated baseline liver enzymes do not have higher frequency of hepatotoxicity from lovastatin than those with normal baseline liver enzymes. Am J Med Sci. 2005;329:62–5.
48. Chalasani N, Teal E, Hall SD. Effect of rosiglitazone on serum liver biochemistries in diabetic patients with normal and elevated baseline liver enzymes. Am J Gastroenterol. 2005;100:1317–21.
49. Tandra S, Vuppalanchi R. Use of statins in patients with liver disease. Curr Treat Options Cardiovasc Med. 2009;11:272–8.
50. Khorashadi S, Hasson NK, Cheung RC. Incidence of statin hepatotoxicity in patients with hepatitis C. Clin Gastroenterol Hepatol. 2006;4:902–7. quiz 806.
51. Chalasani N, Aljadhey H, Kesterson J, et al. Patients with elevated liver enzymes are not at higher risk for statin hepatotoxicity. Gastroenterology. 2004;126:1287–92.
52. Russo MW, Hoofnagle JH, Gu J, et al. Spectrum of statin hepatotoxicity: experience of the drug-induced liver injury network. Hepatology. 2014;60:679–86.
53. McKenney JM, Davidson MH, Jacobson TA, et al. Final conclusions and recommendations of the National Lipid Association Statin Safety Assessment Task Force. Am J Cardiol. 2006;97:89C–94.
54. Squires RH, Duggan C, Teitelbaum DH, et al. Natural history of pediatric intestinal failure: initial report from the Pediatric Intestinal Failure Consortium. J Pediatr. 2012;161:723–8.e2.
55. Chan S, McCowen KC, Bistrian BR, et al. Incidence, prognosis, and etiology of end-stage liver disease in patients receiving home total parenteral nutrition. Surgery. 1999;126:28–34.
56. Carter BA, Taylor OA, Prendergast DR, et al. Stigmasterol, a soy lipid-derived phytosterol, is an antagonist of the bile acid nuclear receptor FXR. Pediatr Res. 2007;62:301–6.
57. Mayer K, Fegbeutel C, Hattar K, et al. Omega-3 vs. omega-6 lipid emulsions exert differential influence on neutrophils in septic shock patients: impact on plasma fatty acids and lipid mediator generation. Intensive Care Med. 2003;29:1472–81.
58. Meisel JA, Le HD, de Meijer VE, et al. Comparison of 5 intravenous lipid emulsions and their effects on hepatic steatosis in a murine model. J Pediatr Surg. 2011;46:666–73.

59. Chung C, Buchman AL. Postoperative jaundice and total parenteral nutrition-associated hepatic dysfunction. Clin Liver Dis. 2002;6:1067–84.
60. Mullick FG, Moran CA, Ishak KG. Total parenteral nutrition: a histopathologic analysis of the liver changes in 20 children. Mod Pathol. 1994;7:190–4.
61. Le HD, de Meijer VE, Zurakowski D, et al. Parenteral fish oil as monotherapy improves lipid profiles in children with parenteral nutrition-associated liver disease. JPEN J Parenter Enteral Nutr. 2010;34:477–84.
62. Premkumar MH, Carter BA, Hawthorne KM, et al. High rates of resolution of cholestasis in parenteral nutrition-associated liver disease with fish oil-based lipid emulsion monotherapy. J Pediatr. 2013;162:793–8.e1.
63. Premkumar MH, Carter BA, Hawthorne KM, et al. Fish oil-based lipid emulsions in the treatment of parenteral nutrition-associated liver disease: an ongoing positive experience. Adv Nutr. 2014;5:65–70.
64. Lam HS, Tam YH, Poon TC, et al. A double-blind randomised controlled trial of fish oil-based versus soy-based lipid preparations in the treatment of infants with parenteral nutrition-associated cholestasis. Neonatology. 2014;105:290–6.
65. Hayashi PH, Fontana RJ. Clinical features, diagnosis, and natural history of drug-induced liver injury. Semin Liver Dis. 2014;34:134–44.

Chapter 26
Miscellaneous Disorders: Pregnancy-Associated Liver Disorders, Vascular Disorders, Granulomatous Diseases, and Amyloidosis

Eric F. Martin

This chapter discusses miscellaneous hepatic disorders including pregnancy-associated liver disorders, vascular disorders of the liver, granulomatous diseases of the liver, and hepatic amyloidosis. This chapter reviews the normal physiologically adaptive changes that occur during pregnancy and the subsequent changes in the liver biochemical profile. Liver diseases unique to pregnancy are one of five liver disorders—hyperemesis gravidarium (HG), intrahepatic cholestasis of pregnancy (ICP), preeclampsia, HELLP syndrome, and acute fatty liver of pregnancy (AFLP). This chapter also discusses the epidemiology, pathogenesis, radiographic findings, diagnosis, and the treatment of various vascular disorders affecting the liver, namely portal vein thrombosis, Budd-Chiari syndrome, and sinusoidal occlusive syndrome. This chapter also reviews the incidence, etiology, and pertinent clinical and laboratory findings of various granulomatous liver diseases and explains the indications for treatment. This chapter concludes by explaining the etiologies, clinical and laboratory findings, management, and outcomes of hepatic amyloidosis.

Pregnancy-Associated Liver Disorders

1. Is it normal to have elevated liver enzymes during pregnancy?

    Due to the significant physiologic, hormonal, and metabolic changes that occur during pregnancy, alterations in the liver biochemical profile are expected and normal. However, abnormal liver tests which require further investigation occur in 3–5 % of all pregnancies. Abnormally elevated liver enzymes during pregnancy are either due to a specific set of diseases that are unique to pregnancy

E.F. Martin, M.D. (✉)
Division of Hepatology, Miami University Miller School of Medicine,
1500 NW 12th Ave., Miami, FL 33163, USA
e-mail: efm10@med.miami.edu

© Springer International Publishing Switzerland 2017
K. Saeian, R. Shaker (eds.), *Liver Disorders*,
DOI 10.1007/978-3-319-30103-7_26

(i.e. hyperemesis gravidarum, intrahepatic cholestasis of pregnancy, preeclampsia, HELLP syndrome, and acute fatty liver of pregnancy) or diseases that are not unique to pregnancy.
2. What imaging studies are safe for the baby?

Ultrasonography remains the safest technique to visualize the liver during pregnancy. If additional imaging is needed, magnetic resonance imaging (MRI) is considered safe during pregnancy; however, gadolinium, which is the intravenous (IV) contrast most commonly used with MRI, should be avoided. Gadolinium-based contrast has been shown to cross the blood–placenta barrier after IV administration. The effects on the exposed fetus are unknown.

Normal Physiological and Hormonal Changes in Pregnancy

Throughout pregnancy, the body undergoes a multitude of physiologically adaptive changes that affect all organ systems including the liver. The subsequent changes in the liver biochemical profile, therefore, are normal and expected in pregnancy (Table 26.1). Any changes in the liver biochemical profile should be interpreted in this context. However, 3–5 % of all pregnancies are complicated by liver disorders [1]. The recognition of liver disease during pregnancy is imperative as early diagnosis may improve maternal and fetal outcomes.

Plasma volume increases by approximately 50 % during pregnancy; however, the blood flow to the liver remains constant. In addition to a rise in maternal heart

Table 26.1 Biochemical changes during normal pregnancy

Test	Change from nonpregnant state
Bilirubin (total)	Unchanged (or slightly decreased)
Aminotransferases (AST, ALT)	Unchanged
Alkaline phosphatase	Increases 2–4 fold
Albumin	Decreases
Prothrombin time	Unchanged
Fibrinogen	Increases by 50 %
Globulin	Increases in α and β globulins, decreases in γ globulin
Alpha-fetoprotein	Increases
White blood cell count	Increases
Platelets	Unchanged
Ceruloplasmin	Increases
Cholesterol	Increases twofold
Triglycerides	Increases
Hemoglobin	Decreases (from second trimester)
Cell volume	Decreases
Uric acid	Decreases

rate and cardiac output, there is also a decrease in blood pressure and systemic vascular resistance (SVR). These changes may mimic the physiologic changes seen in patients with decompensated chronic liver disease. Spider angiomata and palmar erythema, which are also seen in those with chronic liver disease, are the result of increased serum estrogen levels and are normal findings in pregnancy and usually resolve after delivery.

During a normal pregnancy, alkaline phosphatase levels are elevated due to increased placental isoenzyme activity and serum albumin concentrations fall due to the expansion in plasma volume [2–4]. Serum aminotransferase concentrations (aspartate aminotransferase [AST] and alanine aminotransferase [ALT]), total bilirubin, and γ-glutamyl transpeptidase (GGT) remain normal throughout pregnancy or are marginally reduced due to hemodilution [2, 3]. Therefore, any elevations of AST, ALT, and serum bilirubin are considered pathologic and require further investigation.

Ultrasonography remains the safest modality to visualize the liver during pregnancy. If additional detailed imaging is needed, MRI without contrast is safe during pregnancy with no harmful effects towards the developing fetus [5, 6]. However, gadolinium-enhanced MRI should be avoided due to the transplacental transfer of gadolinium, whose effects on the fetus are largely unknown [7].

Classification of Liver Diseases in Pregnancy

Liver diseases in pregnancy are broadly categorized as diseases that are unique to pregnancy and those that are not (Table 26.2). Most liver dysfunction that occurs during pregnancy is directly related to the pregnant state and is due to one of five liver diseases unique to pregnancy—hyperemesis gravidarum (HG), intrahepatic cholestasis of pregnancy (ICP), preeclampsia, HELLP syndrome, and acute fatty liver of pregnancy (AFLP). Liver diseases that are not related to pregnancy are further categorized upon the presence or absence of preexisting liver disease (Table 26.2).

Table 26.2 Classification of liver disease in pregnancy

	Diseases not unique to pregnancy	
Diseases unique to pregnancy	Preexisitng liver diseases	Liver disease coincident with pregnancy
Hyperemesis gravidarum (HG)	Chronic hepatitis B and C	Viral hepatitis
Intrahepatic cholestasis of pregnancy (ICP)	Cirrhosis and portal hypertension	Biliary disease
Acute fatty liver of pregnancy (AFLP)	Autoimmune liver disease	Budd-Chiari syndrome
Preeclampsia and eclampsia	Wilson disease	Drug-induced liver injury (DILI)
HELLP syndrome		Liver transplantation

HELLP hemolysis, elevated liver enzymes, and low platelets

Table 26.3 Characteristic timing of liver diseases unique to pregnancy

Liver disease	Trimester
Hyperemesis gravidarum (HG)	1, 2
Intrahepatic cholestasis of pregnancy (ICP)	1[a], 2, 3
Pre-eclampsia	2, 3
HEELP	2, 3
Acute fatty liver of pregnancy (AFLP)	2, 3

HEELP hemolysis, elevated liver enzymes, and low platelets

[a]Rare case reports of ICP developing as early as gestational week 6–10

Liver Diseases Unique to Pregnancy

Gestational age at the time of onset of signs and symptoms is critical in determining the etiology of liver disease as each condition has a characteristic timing of onset (Table 26.3).

Hyperemesis Gravidarum

Definition and Diagnosis

Nausea and vomiting of pregnancy (NVP), which is often referred to as "morning sickness," is common and affects nearly 80 % of pregnant women [8, 9]. Hyperemesis gravidarum (HG), which represents a severe end of the spectrum of NVP, occurs in only 0.3–2.0 % of all pregnancies [10, 11]. The diagnosis of HG is clinical and is supported by intractable vomiting resulting in dehydration, electrolyte imbalance, muscle wasting, ketosis, and weight loss of more than 5 % body weight. Symptoms related to HG may manifest as early as week 4 of pregnancy and typically subside by 18–20 weeks of gestation [12].

Etiology

The exact cause of HG remains unclear; however, immunological, hormonal, and psychological factors likely play a role. Risk factors for HG include elevated body-mass index (BMI), hyperthyroidism, underlying psychiatric illness, molar pregnancy, preexisting diabetes mellitus, and multiple pregnancies [13, 14].

Serum aminotransferases are elevated in nearly 50 % of patients diagnosed with HG, the levels of which may rise to more than 20 times the upper limit of normal [14, 15]. Hyperbilirubinemia is uncommon in HG but if present rarely exceeds 4 mg/dL. The degree of elevation in liver biochemical tests correlates with the severity of symptoms. The elevated liver tests quickly normalize upon resolution of vomiting.

Pathology

Given the typical clinical manifestations of HG, a diagnostic liver biopsy is seldom needed. If performed, majority of liver biopsies are normal or with nonspecific findings demonstrating cholestasis with mild centrilobular necrosis [16].

Treatment

The first-line approach to mild presentations of HG typically includes avoidance of environmental triggers with bowel rest followed by reintroduction of small and frequent meals and anti-histamines. Thiamine (vitamin B1) supplement is recommended to prevent Wernicke encephalopathy, especially in women with a protracted course of emesis. Hospitalization is often necessary for more severe presentations and may require intravenous rehydration, nutritional support, and antiemetic therapy. Treatment of HG using intravenous corticosteroids remains controversial and typically reserved for severe refractory cases.

Outcomes and Recurrence

Infants of mothers with HG may be born prematurely, be small for gestational age and have significantly lower birth weights than infants born to mothers without HG [17, 18]. There are no clear associations with HG and congenital anomalies or perinatal death. If untreated, there are reports of consequences related to micronutritent deficiency, namely Wernicke encephalopathy and malnutrition, namely poor wound healing, muscle wasting, and immunosuppression [19, 20].

HG often recurs in subsequent pregnancies. There is a 15 % increased risk of HG in the second pregnancy in women with a history of HG compared to only 0.7 % increased risk in women without previous HG [21].

Intrahepatic Cholestasis of Pregnancy

Introduction and Epidemiology

Intrahepatic cholestasis of pregnancy (ICP) is characterized by pruritus and an elevation in serum bile acid concentrations. While ICP typically occurs during the second or third trimester, rare cases developing as early at 6–10 weeks have been reported [22–24]. The prevalence of ICP has significant geographic variation. The highest prevalence rates of ICP were previously reported in Bolivia and Chile with a prevalence from 11.8 to 27.6% [25, 26]. The prevalence in the US is estimated at 0.3–5.6% [27, 28].

Pathogenesis

The exact cause of ICP is largely unknown but recent epidemiologic and clinical studies suggest that hormonal, genetic, and environmental factors are likely involved [29].

Estrogen and progesterone directly inhibit the bile salt export pump and induce cholestasis. Serum concentrations of estrogen during pregnancy peak in the third trimester, which correlate with the onset of ICP. Genetic variants in genes encoding for several hepatobiliary transporters were discovered in patients with ICP that likely explain familial cases and the higher incidence in certain ethnic groups. The multidrug resistance 3 (MDR3) protein, which serves as the transporter for phosphotidylcholine across the canalicular membrane into bile, is associated with ICP. Specifically several mutations in the *ABCB4* gene that encodes MDR3 have been identified in patients with ICP. Mutations in the *ABCB4* gene leads to loss of function of MDR3, which results in elevated serum bile acids without phospholipids leading to injury of the canalicular membrane and cholestasis [30, 31]. The incidence of *ABCB4* gene mutations in Caucasian patients diagnosed with ICP is estimated at 16% [32].

Clinical Manifestations and Laboratory Findings

The onset of ICP is typically preceded by the development of pruritus. Pruritus predominates on the palms and soles of the feet, but may be generalized and become intolerable. Pruritus is typically worse at night and often disrupts sleep. Pruritus usually resolves within a few days after delivery. Jaundice, which typically presents after the onset of pruritus, develops in less than 20% of patients [33]. Women with ICP may develop diarrhea and steatorrhea due to severe cholestasis requiring fat soluble vitamin supplementation.

The laboratory hallmark of ICP is elevated serum total bile acid concentrations, which may be the first or only laboratory abnormality [34]. Total and direct bilirubin along with 5' nucleotidase may also be elevated. Total bilirubin levels rarely exceed 10 mg/dL. Alkaline phosphatase is also elevated, but is not specific for cholestasis during pregnancy due to expression of placental alkaline phosphatase isoenzyme. On the other hand, serum levels of gamma glutamyl transpeptidase (GGT) are often normal or only slightly elevated in ICP, which is atypical in cholestatic liver disease as GGT levels typically parallel other cholestatic markers. Elevated GGT levels may indicate MDR3 mutation or underlying liver disease unrelated to pregnancy. Serum aminotransferase levels may at times exceed 1000 U/L, which should also prompt distinction from concurrent viral hepatitis. The prothrombin time (PT) is usually normal, but it may become prolonged due to vitamin K deficiency in the setting of severe cholestasis with jaundice or recent use of bile acid sequestrants, namely cholestyramine, rather than intrinsic liver dysfunction. For this reason, vitamin K should be administered prior to delivery to prevent postpartum hemorrhage.

Diagnosis

The diagnosis of ICP is based upon the presence of pruritus with elevated total serum bile acid concentrations and/or aminotransferases in the absence of diseases that may produce similar clinical and laboratory findings. A fasting serum bile acid concentration >10 µmol/L is considered diagnostic [35].

Pathology

Given the characteristic clinical and laboratory findings in ICP, liver biopsy is rarely needed to confirm the diagnosis. When performed, histopathology is characterized by cholestasis in the absence of inflammation or necrosis. The portal tracts are unaffected [36].

Medical Management

Ursodeoxycholic acid (ursodiol) is the first-line treatment of ICP and should be given from time of diagnosis until delivery. Ursodiol (10–15 mg/kg/day) provides relief from pruritus, improves liver biochemical tests and is well tolerated by mother and fetus [37]. As in other chronic cholestatic liver diseases, ursodiol, which is a hydrophilic bile acid, may provide some degree of cytoprotection against the hepatotoxic effects of the hydrophobic bile acids. In addition, ursodiol increases bile flow, decreases plasma bile acid and sulphated progesterone metabolite concentrations, increases bile sale export pump expression, and restores proper transport of bile across the placenta, which is impaired in ICP [38, 39].

There are no clear guidelines regarding the optimal time for delivery in patients with ICP [40]. In severe cases of ICP, current consensus opinion supports the practice of induction of labor between 36 and 38 weeks gestation to allow for fetal lung maturity and minimize incidence of intrauterine fetal demise (IUFD) that is associated with ICP [40].

Maternal and Fetal Outcomes

Overall, the maternal prognosis in ICP is good. Pruritus typically disappears within a few days after delivery and is accompanied by normalization of total serum bile acid concentrations and other liver biochemical markers. Recurrent cholestasis occurs in up to 70 % of subsequent pregnancies with variable degrees of severity. In two recent longitudinal population-based cohort studies from Sweden and Finland, women with a history of ICP had a significantly increased risk for developing hepatobiliary disease, namely hepatitis C virus (HCV), fibrosis, cirrhosis, gallstones disease, cholangitis, nonalcoholic pancreatitis, and nonalcoholic liver cirrhosis including cases of PBC cirrhosis [41, 42].

In contrast to a more favorable maternal prognosis, ICP carries significant fetal risk. Fetal complications correlate with serum bile acid concentrations, with a negligible risk if levels remain <40 µmol/L [35, 43]. The main complications of ICP include prematurity and IUFD, which has an estimated incidence between 1 and 2 % [44, 45].

Preeclampsia and HELLP Syndrome

Definition and Epidemiology

Preeclampsia is a common complication of pregnancy with an incidence of 2–7 % in healthy nulliparous women [46]. It is characterized by new onset hypertension and either proteinuria or end-organ dysfunction after 20 weeks of gestation [47]. Preeclampsia itself typically does not have liver involvement; however, if present signifies severe disease. Multiple risk factors for the development of preeclampsia include a personal or family history of preeclampsia, presence of antiphospholipid antibodies, preexisting diabetes mellitus, pre-pregnancy body mass index (BMI) >35 kg/m^2, nulliparity, a twin pregnancy, and maternal age ≥ 40 years [48].

HELLP syndrome represents a severe form of preeclampsia and occurs in up to 0.8 % of all pregnancies and 10–20 % of women with severe preeclampsia. HELLP syndrome is characterized by hemolysis (H), elevated liver enzymes (EL), and low platelets (LP). In contrast to preeclampsia, nulliparity is not a risk factor for HELLP syndrome as at least 50 % of patients with HELLP syndrome are multiparous [49].

Pathogenesis

The exact pathophysiology of HELLP syndrome is unknown, but proposed mechanisms include aberrant placental development and function with subsequent vascular remodeling and uteroplacental ischemia. The ensuing thrombotic microangiopathy leads to microangiopathic hemolytic anemia and liver damage.

Clinical Presentation

The clinical presentation of HELLP syndrome varies. The most common symptom is epigastric or right upper quadrant abdominal pain, which is often associated with nausea, vomiting, and malaise. Mistaking these nonspecific symptoms for a viral illness is an unfortunate error that may result in significant maternal morbidity or mortality because severe right upper quadrant pain may suggest imminent hepatic rupture [50].

Table 26.4 Diagnostic criteria for HELLP syndrome

Tennessee classification	Mississippi classifications
Complete syndrome	Class 1: platelets $\leq 50 \times 10^9$/L
Platelets $\leq 100 \times 10^9$/L	1. AST or ALT ≥ 70 U/L
AST ≥ 70 U/L	2. LDH ≥ 600 U/L
LDH ≥ 600 U/L	Class 2: platelets $\leq 100 \times 10^9$/L
Incomplete syndrome	1. $>50 \times 10^9$/L
Any 1 or 2 of the above	2. AST or ALT ≥ 70 U/L
	3. LDH ≥ 600 U/L
	Class 3: platelets $\leq 150 \times 10^9$/L
	1. $\geq 100 \times 10^9$/L
	2. AST or ALT ≥ 40 U/L
	3. LDH ≥ 600 U/L

The majority of cases present between 28 and 36 weeks of gestation. However, postpartum HELLP may occur in up to 30 % of cases, most of which present within 48 h of delivery with some as far out as 7 days after delivery [51].

Diagnosis

The diagnosis of HELLP syndrome relies on the abnormalities comprising its name—hemolysis (microangiopathic hemolytic anemia with schistocytes), elevated liver enzymes, and low platelet count. Elevated serum aminotransferases are seen in up to 10 % of pregnant women with severe preeclampsia, but the frequency and severity of which is much higher in HELLP syndrome than in severe preeclampsia [52]. Serum aminotransferases in HELLP are often >500 U/L. Classification systems for the diagnosis of HELLP have been developed and include the Tennessee [49, 53] and Mississippi [52] classifications (Table 26.4).

The differential diagnosis for a clinical presentation similar to that of HELLP syndrome includes acute viral hepatitis, hemolytic uremic syndrome (HUS), thrombotic thrombocytopenic purpura (TTP), antiphospholipid syndrome, acute appendicitis, gallbladder disease, lupus flare, and AFLP.

Pathology

Liver biopsy remains a high-risk procedure due to thrombocytopenia. When performed, biopsy demonstrates findings typical of preeclamptic livers, which include periportal hemorrhage and fibrin deposition. Moderate amount of lobular macrovesicular steatosis may be present, which is in contrast to the centrizonal microvesicular steatosis that is typical of AFLP [54].

Management

Bed rest and control of hypertension is imperative for all patients with preeclampsia/HELLP. In addition, all women with severe preeclampsia/HELLP should receive intravenous magnesium sulfate to prevent cerebral changes and eclamptic seizures. Urgent delivery is indicated if HELLP syndrome develops after 34 weeks of gestation, or earlier in the setting of multiorgan dysfunction, renal failure, DIC, liver infarction or hemorrhage, suspected abruptio placentae, or fetal distress. Although corticosteroids have been shown to significantly improve platelet counts, their use did not reduce the risk of severe maternal morbidity, maternal death, or perinatal/infant death [55]. Plasma exchange therapy has been used successfully in patients with severe HELLP syndrome with organ failure or refractory disease resulting in significant improvement in abnormal laboratory values, shorter ICU stay, and improved mortality rates [56, 57].

Outcomes and Prognosis

A variety of maternal and fetal morbidities are associated with HELLP syndrome. The risk of serious morbidity correlates with the severity of maternal symptoms and laboratory abnormalities [58]. Maternal signs and symptoms typically improve within 48 h of delivery; however, a protracted course may ensue. Maternal complications include retinal detachment, DIC, abruptio placentae, acute kidney injury, pulmonary edema, subcapsular liver hematoma, and hepatic rupture [51]. Various surgical and interventional radiologic procedures have been described for the management of hepatic rupture, namely hepatic artery ligation, hepatic packing or lobectomy, arterial embolization, and liver transplantation.

Prematurity is common and results in 70 % of births [59]. Overall perinatal mortality is 7–20 %. The commonest causes of perinatal death include prematurity, intrauterine growth retardation, and abruptio placentae [60]. The recurrence rate of HELLP is low at 2–6 % [51, 61, 62].

Acute Fatty Liver of Pregnancy

Definition and Epidemiology

Acute fatty liver of pregnancy (AFLP) is a rare but potentially fatal complication that occurs in the third trimester. AFLP is rare with an estimated incidence of 1 in 7000 to 1 in 20,000 pregnancies [63, 64]. It is characterized by microvesicular fatty infiltration of hepatocytes. It was first described in 1934 as "acute yellow atrophy of the liver" and at the time was thought to be universally fatal [65]. Fortunately, early diagnosis and prompt delivery have dramatically improved the prognosis [66].

Pathogenesis

There is a strong association between AFLP and fetal deficiency of mitochondrial long-chain 3-hydroxyacyl CoA dehydrogenase (LCHAD), which is an inherited defect in mitochondrial β-oxidation of fatty acids [67]. LCHAD is part of the mitochondrial trifunctional protein (MTP), which is a complex mitochondrial enzyme alpha subunit. Several mutations have been observed in the gene coding for LCHAD in families with a child with LCHAD deficiency whose mothers developed AFLD [67]. *G1528C* is the most common mutation associated with LCHAD deficiency. Fetal LCHAD deficiency results in accumulation of hepatotoxic fetal fatty acids to which the mother is exposed via maternal–fetal circulation. These hepatotoxic metabolites deposit in the maternal liver and cause liver injury. LCHAD-deficient fetuses were found in approximately 20 % of women who developed AFLP [68]. On the other hand, an LCHAD-deficient fetus was associated with a 79 % chance of developing either ALFP or HELLP [67]. Most LCHAD-deficient newborns present with a metabolic crisis within the first year of life while others may suffer a sudden and unexpected death as early as a few months of age [69]. Therefore, screening the offspring of women who develop AFLP as early as possible after delivery can be lifesaving [69, 70]. Identifying LCHAD-deficient newborns early is particularly important as treatment with dietary modifications can dramatically reduce morbidity and mortality.

Clinical and Laboratory Findings

AFLP typically occurs in the third trimester. The initial manifestations of AFLP are nonspecific and often include nausea or vomiting, epigastric or right upper quadrant pain, headache, fatigue, anorexia, and jaundice. Hypertension, edema, and ascites may also be present as nearly 50 % of patients with AFLP have associated preeclampsia [71]. Serum aminotransferase levels are elevated with levels typically ≤500 IU/mL. The bilirubin level is almost always elevated. In severe cases, progression may be rapid within hours to days with progression to hepatic failure, renal failure, and severe coagulopathy with hemorrhage leading to death of the mother and fetus [72].

Diagnosis

The diagnosis of AFLP is generally a clinical diagnosis based on the presentation in relation to gestational age and compatible laboratory and radiographic findings. However, there is often a large clinical overlap between AFLP and HELLP that may make it difficult to differentiate between the two. Evidence of hepatic dysfunction such as encephalopathy or hypoglycemia in the setting of coagulopathy is more indicative of AFLP.

Liver biopsy is diagnostic for AFLP showing characteristic microvesicular hepatic steatosis [73]. The fat droplets are small and surround centrally located

Table 26.5 Swansea criteria for diagnosis of AFL

Six or more of the following features in the absence of another explanation	
Vomiting	Leukocytosis ($>11 \times 10^6$/L)
Abdominal pain	Ascites or bright liver on ultrasound
Polydipsia/polyuria	Transaminemia (AST or ALT >42 IU/mL)
Encephalopathy	Hyperammonia (>47 µmol/L)
Hyperbilirubinemia (>14 µmol/L)	Renal insufficiency (serum Cr >150 µmol/L)
Hypoglycemia	Coagulopathy (PT > 14 or APTT > 34)
Hyperuricemia (>340 µmol/L)	Microvesicular steatosis on liver biopsy

AST aspartate aminotransferase, *ALT* alanine aminotransferase, *Cr* creatinine, *PT* prothrombin time, *APTT*-activated partial thromboplastin time

nuclei, which give the cytoplasm a distinctive foamy appearance. The vacuolated hepatocytes stain red with use of an oil red O stain. These histologic changes disappear within days to weeks after delivery without persistent injury. The Swansea diagnostic criteria have been proposed as an alternative to liver biopsy for the diagnosis of AFLP (Table 26.5) [1].

Management

AFLP does not typically resolve before delivery and is considered an obstetric emergency. If delivery is delayed catastrophic complications may develop, namely hemorrhage or intrauterine death. Therefore, treatment includes a combination of maternal stabilization and prompt delivery of the fetus, regardless of gestational age.

Maternal and Fetal Outcome

Liver biochemical and coagulation profiles usually normalize within 7–10 days after delivery [74]. Although most patients recover with no significant clinical sequelae, substantial morbidity and mortality can occur [74]. The maternal mortality rates for AFLP are estimated at 1.8–4.0 % with stillbirth rates as high as 12 % [64, 74]. Some patients with severe AFLP that persisted after delivery were successfully treated with liver transplantation [64, 75, 76] including a case report of a successful auxiliary liver transplant [77]. AFLP can recur in subsequent pregnancies even if the workup for the LCHAD mutation is negative; however, the exact risk in unknown.

Vascular Disorders

1. Do all patients diagnosed with portal vein thrombosis need anticoagulation? If so, for how long?

Anticoagulation for portal vein thrombosis (PVT) depends largely on the time interval since the blood clot was formed because the indication and duration of anticoagulation is different for acute PVT compared to chronic PVT. The goal of treatment of acute PVT is to recanalize or reopen the obstructed veins, which will prevent congestion of venous blood in the intestines that could cause intestinal infarction and portal hypertension. Therefore, anticoagulation should be given for at least 3 months to all patients with acute PVT to allow for recanalization of the obstructed veins or longer in causes when acute PVT is associated with permanent thrombotic risk factors that are not otherwise correctable. On the other hand, the goal of treatment of chronic PVT with anticoagulation is to prevent recurrent-thrombosis. Long-term anticoagulation is generally given to all patients with chronic PVT without cirrhosis that have an identifiable, uncorrected risk factor for venous thrombosis as long as there is no major contraindication.

Portal Vein Thrombosis

Portal vein thrombosis (PVT) refers to obstruction of the portal vein (PV) or its branches due to thrombosis or to invasion or constriction by a malignant tumor. The prevalence of PVT in population based autopsy studies was nearly 1 % [78, 79]. From a clinical prospective, PVT is subdivided into acute and chronic. Although acute and chronic PVT represent successive stages of the same disease and share similar causes, their respective management is different. In addition to the stage at which the PVT is recognized, management is also based on the presence or absence of cirrhosis (Portal vein thrombosis in cirrhosis is discussed separately in Chap. 10).

Causes of Portal Vein Thrombosis

Numerous local and systemic risk factors are associated with the development of PVT (Table 26.6). Malignant tumor invasion of the PV and cirrhosis are the most common local risk factors for PVT [80–82]. An inherited or acquired prothrombotic condition is a common risk factor for the development of PVT, regardless of the presence of a local risk factor (Table 26.7) [81, 83–96]. In young adults without malignancy or cirrhosis, PVT is commonly the presenting manifestation of an underlying myeloproliferative disease, namely polycythemia vera or essential thrombocytosis [90, 97].

Acute Portal Vein Thrombosis

Acute PVT refers to the sudden formation of a thrombus within the main PV and/or its branches or involves a variable portion of the mesenteric veins and/or splenic vein. Occlusion can be partial or complete.

Table 26.6 Local risk factors for portal vein thrombosis

Malignancy	Injury to the portal venous system
Any abdominal organ	Splenectomy
Cirrhosis	Colectomy, Gastrectomy
Focal inflammatory lesions	Cholecystectomy
Neonatal	Liver transplantation
Neonatal omphalitis	Abdominal trauma
Umbilical vein catheterization	Surgical portosystemic shunting, TIPS
Diverticulitis, Appendicitis	
Pancreatitis	
Duodenal ulcer	
Cholecystitis	
Tuberculous lymphadenitis	
Inflammatory bowel disease	
Cytomegalovirus hepatitis	

Table 26.7 Prevalence of acquired and inherited risk factors for acute PVT and BCS

Risk factor	Acute PVT (%)	BCS (%)
Myeloproliferative disorders	21–40	40–50
Antiphospholipid antibody syndrome	6–19	4–25
Parosysmal nocturnal hemoglobinuria	0–2	0–19
Factor V Leiden mutation	3–32	6–32
Prothrombin gene (Factor II) mutation	14–40	3–7
Protein C deficiency	0–26	4–30
Protein S deficiency	2–30	3–20
Antithrombin III deficiency	0–26	0–23
Hyperhomocysteinemia	11–22	22–37
Recent pregnancy	1–40	6–12
Recent contraceptive use	12–44	6–60
Systemic disease[a]	4	23
>1 risk factor	52	46
Local factor (Table 26.6)	21	6

[a]Including connective tissue disease, IBD, Behcet disease, and HIV

Clinical and Laboratory Features

The presentation of acute PVT usually includes acute onset abdominal pain. Rebound tenderness and guarding may be present in the setting of an inflammatory focus as cause for the PVT or when PVT is complicated by intestinal infarction. Although partial thrombosis is often associated with fewer symptoms, rapid and complete obstruction of the portal or mesenteric veins may cause intestinal congestion resulting in severe continuous colicky abdominal pain and diarrhea. Although a transient, moderate increase in serum aminotransferases may be seen in patients with acute PVT, liver function is preserved on account of increased hepatic arterial blood flow that compensates for the decreased portal venous inflow as well as collateral circulation that quickly develops from preexisting veins in the porta hepatis [98].

In the absence of thrombus extension to mesenteric venous arches, all manifestations of acute PVT are reversible by way of recanalization or development of a cavernoma [99]. Intestinal infarction is the most dreaded complication of acute PVT and has been reported in 2–28 % of cases [99–102]. Intestinal infarction occurs after thrombosis extends to the mesenteric veins causing intestinal congestion, ischemia, and eventually infarction. Clinical features suggestive of transmural intestinal ischemia include persistent severe abdominal pain lasting more than 5–7 days, bloody diarrhea, ascites, or multiorgan failure with metabolic acidosis [103, 104]. Intestinal infarction carries a mortality rate of 20–60 % with significant morbidity due to extensive intestinal resection or post-ischemic intestinal stenosis [105–109].

A thrombus may become infected resulting in acute septic PVT, which is referred to as acute pylephlebitis [110]. Blood cultures often grow *Bacteroides* species with radiographic evidence of multiple, small liver abscesses. Acute septic PVT is almost always associated with an abdominal infection [99, 110, 111].

Radiographic Features and Diagnosis

Sonographic findings of acute PVT include hyperechoic material in the vessel lumen with distension of the PV and its tributaries with Doppler imaging demonstrating absent flow in part or all of the lumen [112]. A CT or MRI can provide additional information regarding the extent of the thrombus, dating of the thrombus, presence of a local factor, or intestinal congestion and/or ischemia [113]. Thinning of the intestinal wall or lack of mucosal enhancement of a thickened intestinal wall after intravenous contrast is suggestive of intestinal infarction [114].

Treatment

The goal of treatment of acute PVT is to allow recanalization of the obstructed veins and prevent portal hypertension and intestinal infarction. Immediate initiation of systemic anticoagulation therapy is generally recommended for acute PVT [109, 115]. Although anticoagulation therapy is of proven benefit in patients with acute DVT [116], there are no controlled studies of anticoagulation therapy in patients with acute PVT. As such, DVT data are extrapolated to patients with acute PVT. However, pooled data from retrospective surveys showed that when started immediately, 6 months of anticoagulation resulted in complete recanalization in 50 %, partial recanalization in 40 %, and no recanalization in 10 % of patients [99]. In the case of pylephlebitis, antibiotics alone may result in recanalization [111, 117].

The optimal duration of anticoagulation for acute PVT is unknown. An international panel of experts recommend that in patients with acute PVT, anticoagulation be given for at least 3 months, while indefinite anticoagulation be given for those with chronic prothrombotic conditions [99]. The published data on other treatment modalities (transjugular intrahepatic portosystemic shunt [TIPS], thrombolysis, or surgical thrombectomy) in the management of acute PVT is limited [118, 119].

Chronic Portal Vein Thrombus

In patients with chronic PVT, the obstructed portal vein becomes replaced by a network of portoportal collaterals that bypass the obstructed venous segment. Collectively, these collaterals are referred to as a portal cavernoma. These enlarged portoportal collaterals can cause compression and deformation of the biliary lumen, termed portal cholangiopathy or portal biliopathy [120, 121]. In adults, chronic extrahepatic PVT is often complicated by recurrent gastrointestinal bleeding related to portal hypertension and hepatic encephalopathy due to extensive portosystemic shunting [101, 102, 122]. However, gastrointestinal bleeding is usually better tolerated than other causes of portal hypertension due to younger age of patients and preserved liver function.

Radiographic Findings and Diagnosis

A diagnosis of chronic PVT with cavernous transformation is often made by abdominal ultrasound, CT, or MRI that demonstrates serpiginous structures while the main portal vain and/or its main branches are not visible.

Treatment

Treatment for chronic PVT is divided into three approaches—prevention and treatment of gastrointestinal bleeding, prevention of recurrent thrombosis, and treatment of portal cholangiopathy. Endoscopic screening for gastroesophageal varices with beta-adrenergic blockers and/or endoscopic variceal ligation should be performed for patients with portal cavernoma as is the practice for patients with cirrhosis [108, 123]. Currently, there are no consensus guidelines for permanent anticoagulation in the setting of chronic PVT. As such, management should be developed on a case-by-case basis with consideration of the thrombotic potential of the underlying condition, the extension of the thrombus, and the increased risk of portal hypertensive bleeding. Retrospective studies including patients with acute and chronic PVT showed that anticoagulation therapy significantly decreased the risk of recurrent thrombosis without increasing the risk of gastrointestinal bleeding [101]. However, on account of the paucity of data, expert opinion recommends anticoagulation therapy for patients with chronic PVT only in those with a documented permanent prothrombotic condition [108]. Endoscopic or percutaneous therapies may be used for symptomatic management of portal cholangiopathy. Biliary surgery without portal decompression is extremely hazardous and best avoided.

Outcomes

The prognosis of patients who are anticoagulated for chronic PVT is good with a 5-year mortality from intestinal infarction or gastrointestinal bleeding of less than 5% [101].

Budd-Chiari Syndrome

Definition and Etiology

Budd-Chiari syndrome (BCS) describes hepatic venous outflow tract obstruction independent of the level or mechanism of obstruction [115, 124]. Cardiac and pericardial diseases as well as sinusoidal obstruction syndrome are generally excluded from this definition. BCS is typically caused by thrombosis of the hepatic vein (HV) or the terminal portion of the inferior vena cava (IVC). BCS is a rare disorder with an estimated incidence of 0.2–0.8 per million per year [125–128]. Pure IVC or IVC/HV obstruction predominates in Asia, whereas pure HV obstruction predominates in Western countries [128]. BCS is divided into "primary" BCS when related to a primary venous disease (i.e. thrombosis or phlebitis) and "secondary" BCS when related to compression, thrombosis, and/or invasion by a lesion originating outside the veins (Table 26.8).

Similar to PVT, BCS is strongly associated with prothrombotic conditions (Table 26.7). Myeloproliferative neoplasms, antiphospholipid syndrome, and oral contraceptive use are among the most common risk factors for BCS. More than 1 thrombotic risk factor may be present in 25–46% of cases [90, 129]. Thus, routine screening for all thrombotic risk factors is recommended in patients diagnosed with BCS.

Clinical and Laboratory Features

The clinical presentation of BCS is variable and depends largely on the extent and rate of outflow obstruction, as well as the development of collaterals [130]. The clinical presentation ranges from asymptomatic to fulminant hepatic failure, or to

Table 26.8 Inherited and acquired risk factors for Budd-Chiari syndrome

Primary	Secondary
Myeloproliferative disorders	Hepatocellular carcinoma
Polycythemia vera	Renal cell carcinoma
Essential thrombocytosis	Adrenal adenocarcinoma
Chronic myelogenous leukemia	Primary hepatic hemangiosarcoma
Inherited thrombophilia	Epitheloid hemangioendothelioma
Antiphospholipid antibody syndrome	Sarcoma of the IVC
Parosysmal nocturnal hemoglobinuria	Right atrial myxoma
Factor V Leiden mutation	Alveolar hydatid disease
Prothrombin gene mutation	Cysts (parasitic/nonparasitic)
Protein C deficiency	Abscess
Protein S deficiency	Large FNH
Antithrombin III deficiency	Hepatic resection or transplantation
Factor II mutation	Blunt abdominal trauma
Hyperhomocysteinemia	Pancreatitis
Methylene-tetrahydrofolate reductase mutation	
Acquired disorders	
Pregnancy	
Oral contraceptives	
Systemic disease	
Inflammatory bowel disease	
Behcet disease	
Human immunodeficiency virus	
Sarcoidosis	
Idiopathic	

cirrhosis with complications of portal hypertension [129, 131]. Nearly 20 % of BCS cases are asymptomatic [132]. Common signs and symptoms include abdominal pain, fevers, ascites, lower extremity edema, gastrointestinal bleeding, and hepatic encephalopathy [126, 133]. Dilated truncal subcutaneous veins are highly specific for IVC obstruction. Liver biochemical profile may be normal or increased. The protein level in ascitic fluid is variable, though ascites protein >2.5 g/dL with a serum-ascites albumin concentration gradient ≥1.1 g/dL is suggestive of BCS or cardiac/pericardial disease. The disease onset may be insidious or rapid. Given these nonspecific clinical and laboratory signs, BCS should be considered in all patients with acute or chronic liver disease [109, 115].

Radiographic Findings

Fluroscopic venography has long been the gold standard for evaluation of the HV. Fortunately, sonographic findings correlate well with venography [134–136] and pathologic examination [137]. Doppler ultrasound by an experienced examiner is often the most effective and reliable means of diagnosis [109]. MRI and CT can confirm the diagnosis if an experienced Doppler ultrasound examiner is not available. Caudate lobe hypertrophy is found in nearly 75 % of patients with BCS [80, 137]. This is due to separate venous drainage of the caudate lobe directly into the IVC that allows for sparing of the outflow with compensatory hypertrophy [138]. Thus, invasive procedures such as venography and liver biopsy are necessary only in patients when the diagnosis remains unclear after noninvasive radiographic procedures [109].

Histopathology

Sinusoidal dilation, congestion, and centrilobular fibrosis are characteristic histopathological features of BCS (Fig. 26.1) [139, 140]. Cirrhosis may ultimately be seen. In the most-advanced cases, thrombosis of intrahepatic portal veins may be seen with fibrous enlargement of the portal tract.

Management

The conventional management of BCS includes immediate anticoagulation, medical management of the complications of portal hypertension, and treatment of the underlying prothrombotic disease [141, 142]. Table 26.9 summarizes the algorithm for the treatment strategy of primary BCS [115, 124]. Similar to PVT, there are no prospective randomized controlled trials of anticoagulation in patients with BCS. For this reason, guidelines directing anticoagulation for patients with DVT are often extrapolated to patients with BCS, which support the use of indefinite systemic anticoagulation in patients who develop an

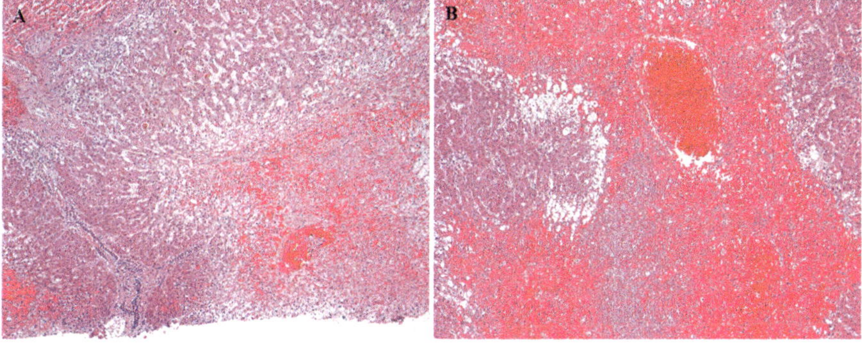

Fig. 26.1 Budd-Chiari syndrome. (**a**) Low magnification showing perivenular congestion and necrosis with intact perioportal parenchyma in a patient with Budd-Chiari syndrome (H&E). (**b**) Higher magnification demonstrates centrilobular hemorrhage and necrosis with an acute thrombus (H&E) (Courtesy of Monica T. Garcia-Buitrago, MD, University of Miami)

Table 26.9 Proposed algorithm for treatment of primary Budd-Chiari Syndrome

1. In all patients with primary BCS
– Anticoagulation as soon as diagnosis is established
– Treatment of underlying (hematologic) condition
– Symptomatic treatment of complications of portal hypertension
– Look for short-length stenosis of HV or IVC and perform angioplasty/stenting
2. Consider TIPS if patients are not suitable for or unresponsive to angioplasty/stenting
3. Consider liver transplantation in patients unresponsive to TIPS

idiopathic DVT with a permanent risk factor without definitive cure of the underlying thrombophilia [116]. Platelet count should be carefully monitored given the high incidence of heparin-induced thrombocytopenia in BCS patients [143, 144]. Oral contraceptives should be stopped. Percutaneous recanalization of the HV or ICV utilizing thrombolysis, angioplasty and/or stent should be considered in patients with short-length stenosis of main HV or IVC [145, 146]. TIPS has been successfully used in a subset of patients who did not respond to medical treatment or recanalization with excellent long-term survival [147]. Patients who develop cirrhosis from HV obstruction are less likely to respond to these measures and may need to be referred for LT.

Outcomes and Prognosis

The natural history of BCS is poorly understood. However, improvement in diagnostic and therapeutic strategies has resulted in 5-year survival rates approaching 90 % [129, 145, 146].

HCC is rare in BCS and is primarily seen in patients with long-standing disease, especially in those with obstruction of the suprahepatic IVC [89, 148–150]. Particularly challenging is differentiating HCC from benign macroregenerative nodules, which frequently develop in patients with well-controlled BCS [151]. Most of these nodules are benign and resemble focal nodular hyperplasia (FNH) on radiographic and pathologic examination.

Patients with splanchnic vein thrombosis and myeloproliferative disease are at increased risk of developing myelofibrosis or acute leukemia [97]. Therefore, despite adequate medical management, long-term prognosis may be threatened more by subsequent neoplastic disease than by liver failure. However, studies have shown that the slow course of myeloproliferative syndromes is not significantly affected by LT, and that LT is an acceptable option in these patients despite the potential negative long-term effects [152, 153].

Sinusoidal Obstruction Syndrome

Introduction

Sinusoidal obstruction syndrome (SOS), previously termed hepatic venooclusive disease (VOD), is characterized by hepatomegaly, right upper quadrant pain, jaundice, and ascites. The acute form of SOS occurs most commonly as a consequence of myeloablative regimens used in preparation for hematopoietic stem cell transplant (HSCT). These so-called conditioning regimens are combinations of high-dose chemotherapy drugs with or without total body irradiation (TBI). A chronic, more indolent form of SOS may develop following toxicity of pyrrolizidine alkaloids from plants that are often ingested in the form of herbal teas, hence the term Jamaican brush tea disease. SOS clinically resembles BCS; however, HV outflow obstruction in SOS is due to the occlusion of the terminal hepatic sinusoids and venules rather than the HV and/or IVC in BCS.

Pathogenesis

SOS begins with injury to the HV endothelium. Specific to HSCT, sinusoidal endothelial cells (ECs) become activated by the conditioning regimen, drugs used during the procedure (i.e. granulocyte colony stimulating factor or calcineurin inhibitors) [154, 155], and the complex process of engraftment [156]. Activation of sinusoidal ECs trigger multiple pro-inflammatory pathways that result in accumulation of cells and debris in the space of Disse, the perisinusoidal space located between the endothelium and the hepatocyte, resulting in narrowing of the hepatic sinusoids. The ECs become detached and embolize to the central area of the lobule where they cause a postsinusoidal outflow obstruction, namely SOS.

Epidemiology and Risk Factors

Including myeloablative conditioning regimens, multiple other risk factors for the development of SOS have been identified (Table 26.10). The reported incidence between HSCT units range from 0 to 50 % [157–162]. An incidence of SOS around 20–40 % is seen more consistently in those who receive more liver-toxic regimens, which has led many centers to abandon high-dose conditioning regimens in favor of the increasingly popular reduced-intensity conditioning regimens that carry little or no risk for SOS. The regimens known to cause the most liver injury are those that contain cyclophosphamide in combination with either busulfan or TBI (greater than 12 Gy), regimens that include N,N-bis(2-chloroethyl)-N-nitrosourea (BCNU) or multiple alkylating agents [109].

Table 26.10 Risk factors for sinusoidal obstruction syndrome

Patient factors	Disease factors	Transplant factors
Younger age (in children)	Advanced malignancy	Myeloablative conditioning
Older age (in adults)	Acute leukemia	Cyclophosphamide with busulfan
Poor performance status	Neuroblastoma	Cyclophosphamide with TBI
Preexisitng liver disease	Thalassemia major	Allogenic HSCT (greater than autologous)
HCV or HBV	Delayed platelet engraftment	Unrelated donor HSCT
Hepatic fibrosis	Presence of acute GVHD	Mismatched HSCT
Iron overload	Abdominal radiotherapy	Subsequent transplants
Positive CMV serology	Prior chemotherapy	Sirolimus GVHD prophylaxis
Prior fungal infection	6-mercaptopurine	Norethisterone use
HFE C282Y genotype	6-thioguanine	
Exposure to toxins	Actinomycin D	
Pyrrolizidine alkaloids	Azathioprine (Imuran)	
Herbal medications	Cytarabine	
	Cytosine arabinoside	
	Dacarbazine	
	Gemtuzumab ozogamicin (Mylotarg)	
	Melphalan (Alkeran)	
	Oxaliplatin (Eloxatin)	
	Urethane	

HCV hepatitis C virus, *HBV* hepatitis B virus, *CMV* cytomegalovirus, *GVHD* graft-versus-host-disease, *TBI* total body irradiation, *HSCT* hematopoietic stem cell transplantation

Clinical and Laboratory Findings

The clinical signs and symptoms of SOS include weight gain with or without ascites, right upper quadrant pain of liver origin, hepatomegaly, and jaundice [109]. Symptom onset is typically between 10 and 20 days after initiation of therapy using cyclophosphamide-containing regimens, but may be as late as 30 days after completing non-cyclophosphamide myeloablative therapy [162–164].

Diagnosis

Diagnostic criteria have been published to define SOS, which include the Seattle and Baltimore criteria (Table 26.11) [160, 162]. Most patients who receive liver-toxic conditioning regimens will develop some degree of sinusoidal injury, even in the absence of clinical signs and symptoms [165]. Confounding diagnoses that are

Table 26.11 Diagnostic criteria for SOS after hematopoietic stem cell transplantation

Seattle criteria	Baltimore criteria
2 or 3 of the following within 20 days of HSCT	Serum total bilirubin >2 mg/dL + ≥2 other criteria
• Serum total bilirubin >2 mg/dL	• Hepatomegaly (usually painful)
• Hepatomegaly or RUQ pain of liver origin	• >5 % weight gain
• >2 % weight gain due to fluid accumulation	• Ascites

also common in this population include sepsis-induced cholestasis, drug-induced cholestasis, fluid overload from renal failure or congestive heart failure, liver involvement of fungal or viral infections in the setting of immunosuppression, and (hyper)acute graft-versus-host disease (GVHD).

Radiographic evaluation may support the diagnosis of SOS but imaging itself is not diagnostic. Imaging is helpful to confirm the presence of hepatomegaly and ascites as well as rule out biliary obstruction. Sonographic findings that are suggestive of SOS include reversal of portal venous flow, attenuation of hepatic venous flow, gallbladder wall edema, and increased resistive indices to hepatic artery flow [166–168].

The current gold standard to confirm the diagnosis of SOS is transjugular liver biopsy with portal pressure measurements. Percutaneous approach for a liver biopsy is often contraindicated due to thrombocytopenia, coagulopathy, and ascites. Transvenous approach is preferred not only for liver biopsy but it also allows for measurement of hepatic venous pressure gradient (HVPG), which is particularly helpful in distinguishing SOS from GVHD. In HSCT patients, HVPG >10 mmHg has specificity greater than 90 % and positive predictive value greater than 85 % for the diagnosis of SOS [169].

Liver histology shows sinusoidal dilation and congestion around the central vein with central venous subendothelial edema and perivenular hepatic necrosis (Fig. 26.2). The portal tracts are typically normal without evidence of inflammation [113]. These histologic features also aid in differentiating SOS from GVHD. In GVHD, typical features include bile duct damage and apoptosis, which are absent in SOS. Likewise, centrizonal hepatocellular damage seen in SOS is not characteristic of GVHD.

Management

The most important approach to prevent SOS is avoidance of liver-toxic conditioning regimens in high-risk patients. Reduced-intensity regimens, which include fludarabine with low dose TBI or fludarabine with busulfan and antithymocyte globulin, are increasingly used to offset the high morbidity and mortality associated with high-dose myeloablative conditioning regimens. Switching fludarabine for cyclophosphamide results in a much lower incidence of SOS with improved transplant outcomes [170, 171].

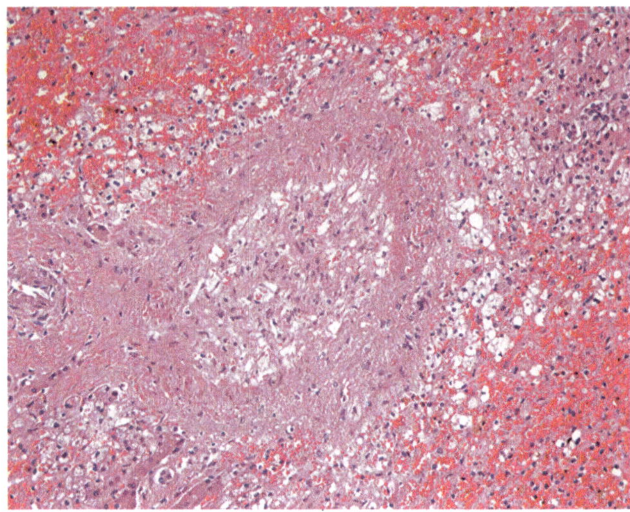

Fig. 26.2 Sinusoidal obstruction syndrome. Fibrous occlusion of a centrilobular vein in a patient with SOS (H&E) (Courtesy of Monica T. Garcia-Buitrago, MD, University of Miami)

Prophylactic Medical Therapy

The preventative effects of ursodiol, heparin, prostaglandin E1, and pentoxyfylline on SOS have been studied but with mixed results [172–176]. Defibrotide is arguably the drug with the most promise in the management of SOS by way of prophylaxis and treatment of established disease. It is a polydeoxyribonucleotide adenosine receptor agonist that possesses antithrombotic, anti-inflammatory, and anti-ischemic properties without significant systemic anticoagulation effects [177–181]. Prophylactic defibrotide was shown to decrease the incidence of SOS in children at high risk for SOS undergoing myeloablative allogeneic HSCT [182].

Medical Management of Established Disease

The management of SOS depends largely upon the severity of the disease. The severity of SOS on presentation is variable and is conventionally divided into mild, moderate, and severe disease based on serum total bilirubin and aminotransferases (AST and ALT), weight above baseline, renal function, and disease tempo (Table 26.12) [162]. Mild SOS by definition has a self-limiting course and does not require treatment. Moderate SOS requires analgesics and/or treatment of fluid excess, but resolves completely. Severe SOS is defined as disease that does not resolve by day 100 or results in death. Supportive care is the basis of management for all patients with SOS and includes maintenance of fluid and electrolyte balance, minimization of exposure to hepatotoxic agents, and pain control. Patients

Table 26.12 Proposed grading systems for severity of SOS

	Mild	Moderate	Severe
Total bilirubin (mg/dL)	<5.0	<5.1–8.0	>8.0
AST/ALT	<3 × normal	3–8 × normal	>8 × normal
Weight above baseline	<2 %	2–5 %	>5 %
Serum creatinine	Normal	<2 × normal	>2 × normal
Disease tempo	Slow	Moderate	Rapid

with mild to moderate SOS generally have good outcomes with supportive care, whereas severe SOS predicts poor outcomes and requires more aggressive therapy. Multiple pharmacologic agents for the treatment of severe SOS have been investigated. Of these, defibrotide has generated the best outcomes and is the preferred therapy for severe SOS. Defibrotide is currently an investigational agent that is available for the treatment of SOS through an Expanded Access Treatment IND Protocol [183]. Defibrotide was associated with a substantial decrease in 100-day mortality with a strong correlation between complete remission of SOS and survival [184]. Patients who fail defibrotide therapy may be considered for TIPS or LT [185–187]. However, SOS is most often a complication of the conditioning myeloablative regimen for HSCT for patients with hematologic malignancy, therefore, the underlying malignancy itself is often a contraindication to LT. Thus, LT may be considered only for those who underwent HSCT for a benign condition or in whom the underlying malignancy has a favorable prognosis after transplant.

Prognosis

Similar to the variable incidence rates of SOS, fatality rates vary depending on the diagnostic criteria used for SOS. Fatality rates following high-dose myeloablative conditioning regimens are 15–20 %.

Granulomatous Liver Disease

1. How common are hepatic granulomas?

   In autopsy studies, granulomas are found in up to 10 % of liver biopsies. However, an isolated granuloma found on a liver biopsy is not enough to diagnose granulomatous liver disease. Likewise, granulomas may be found in patients with known liver disease and may be an incidental finding with no association with clinical course or response to therapy. On the other hand, hepatic granulomas may serve as a clue for an underlying systemic disorder, the diagnosis of which will most often be made with a thorough history, physical exam, and laboratory testing.

2. Do all hepatic granulomas require treatment?

   Although the majority of hepatic granulomas that are found incidentally are asymptomatic, a thorough history, physical exam, and laboratory evaluation should be completed to identify the cause. Hepatic granulomas may not require treatment, especially if involvement is isolated to the liver. The goal of treating hepatic granulomas is predicated on treating the underlying disease.

Definition and Incidence

Granulomas are rounded aggregates of activated macrophages called epitheloid macrophages accompanied by a rim of $CD4^+$ helper T (T_H) lymphocytes and fibroblasts that develop over time within a host tissue, including the liver, as result of an immunologic response to exogenous and/or endogenous antigenic stimuli. They are often well circumscribed and separate from adjacent, uninvolved tissue. Granulomas may occur anywhere in the hepatic lobule in a variety of conditions. Their locations are often helpful in the differential diagnosis of specific disease processes. Granulomas are found in 4–10 % of needle liver biopsies [188].

Morphologic Types

Several types of granulomas are described in liver disease based on their histologic features and constituents (Table 26.13). These include necrotizing, non-necrotizing, fibrin-ring, and lipogranulomas.

Causes of Hepatic Granulomas

Many disease states are associated with hepatic granulomas, which include sarcoidosis, autoimmune, infectious diseases, drug, cancer, and idiopathic (Table 26.14). Hepatic granulomata may be seen in patients with established chronic liver disease and may not necessarily indicate the presence of a second disease process [189, 190]. Likewise, the presence of a single granuloma on liver biopsy may be an innocuous finding without any indication of underlying granulomatous liver disease [191].

Clinical and Laboratory Findings

The clinical manifestations of granulomatous liver disease depend largely on the underlying cause and its severity. Granulomas are typically asymptomatic though signs and symptoms may include abdominal pain, weight loss, fatigue, chills,

Table 26.13 Types of granuloma

Type	Histologic features	Examples
Necrotizing	Peripheral macrophages with or without giant cells	Tuberculosis
	Central necrosis	
Non-necrotizing	Cluster of macrophages with or without giant cells	Sarcoidosis
		Drugs
Lipogranuloma	Lipid vacuole(s) surrounded by macrophages and lymphocytes	Fatty liver
		Mineral oil
Fibrin-ring	Central lipid vacuole or empty space	Q fever
	Macrophages and lymphocytes	Allopurinol
	Ring of fibrin	Hodgkin's lymphoma

Table 26.14 Disease states involved in granulomatous disease

Sarcoidosis
Autoimmune
Infectious disease
Drugs
Cancer
Idiopathic

hepatosplenomegaly, lymphadenopathy, and fever. Although liver biochemical tests may be normal, the typical liver biochemical test pattern is that of infiltrative disease with elevated alkaline phosphatase levels and normal or mildly elevated serum aminotransferases and bilirubin. Peripheral eosinophilia may be present in drug- or parasite-related granulomatous disease.

Specific Types of Granulomatous Liver Disease

Sarcoidosis

Sarcoidosis is one of the most common causes of hepatic graulomata in the US [192]. Sarcoidosis is a systemic granulomatous disease of unknown etiology that is characterized by formation of non-necrotizing granulomas (Fig. 26.3). Sarcoidosis is more common in young African Americans, but it can affect people of any age, gender, and race [193, 194]. Although hepatic granulomata are present in 50–80 % of patients with sarcoidosis, symptomatic hepatic sarcoidosis occurs in only 5–15 % of patients with sarcoidosis [193, 195].

Typical laboratory findings include elevated alkaline phosphatase and GGT. Serum angiotensin-converting enzyme (ACE) levels are elevated in 75 % of patients with sarcoidosis due to secretion of ACE from epithelioid cells of

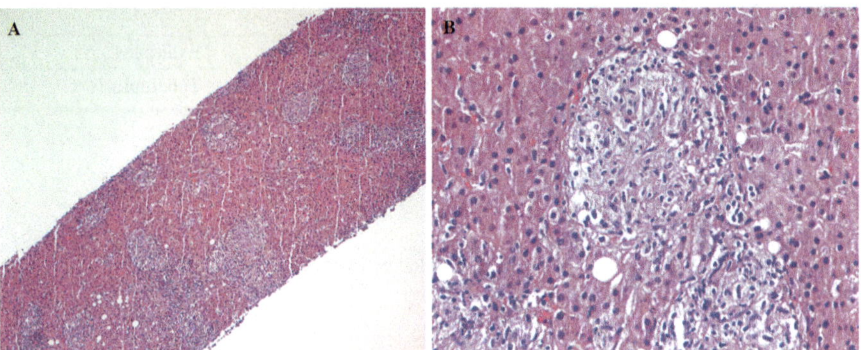

Fig. 26.3 Hepatic sarcoidosis. (**a**) Low power view of liver parenchyma with portal and periportal non-necrotizing granulomatous inflammation in a patient with sarcoidosis (H&E). (**b**) High power view of non-necrotizing granulomas consisting of compact aggregates of epithelioid histiocytes and a sparse rim of lymphocytes in a patient with sarcoidosis (H&E) (Courtesy of Monica T. Garcia-Buitrago, MD, University of Miami)

the hepatic granulomas. However, there are no pathognomonic laboratory or histopathologic findings that clearly establish the diagnosis of hepatic sarcoidosis. Therefore, a definitive diagnosis of sarcoidosis often involves identification of characteristic extrahepatic manifestations of sarcoidosis, namely pulmonary and dermatologic findings [196]. Because hepatic sarcoidosis typically has a benign course without a definitive diagnostic test, other causes of hepatic granulomatous disease must be ruled out before establishing a diagnosis of hepatic sarcoidosis.

Treatment of hepatic sarcoidosis is usually not recommended. A short course of corticosteroids may be considered in the setting of portal hypertension and cirrhosis; however, it is unclear if this is helpful as the endpoints of therapy or outcome measures are not clearly defined.

Autoimmune

PBC is another common cause of hepatic granulomata in the US. Hepatic granulomas are present in 25 % of patients with PBC [192]. In addition to elevated alkaline phosphatase, bilirubin, and GGT, anti-mitochondrial antibody (AMA) is positive in more than 90 % of patients with PBC often with an elevated serum immunoglobulin M (IgM) [197]. The histologic findings of PBC are similar to those in sarcoidosis with the exception that patients with PBC also have bile duct inflammation.

Treatment of PBC includes ursodiol 13–15 mg/kg/day [198]. Although ursodiol may slow the progression of disease, PBC may continue to progress and develop cirrhosis. Other autoimmune disease associated with hepatic granulomas include Crohn's disease and Wegener's granulomatosis (polyangiitis) [199, 200].

Table 26.15 Causes of hepatic granulomas

Infection		
	Viral	CMV
		Infectious mononucleosis
		HAV
		HCV
	Bacterial	Brucella
	Mycobacteria	*M. tuberculosis*
		M. aviam-intercellulare
	Rickettsiae	Q fever
	Fungi	Histoplasmosis
		Coccidioidomycosis
		Blastomycosis
	Protozoa	Toxoplasmosis
	Spirochetes	*T pallidum*
	Helminths	Schistomsomiasis
		Toxocara canis
		Fasciola hepatica
		Ascaris lumbricoides
Systemic disease		Systemic disease
		Crohn's disease
Drugs		Allopurinol
		Phenytoin
		Penicillin
Primary biliary cirrhosis		Early stages (most commonly)
Foreign bodies		Talc
		Suture
Neoplasms		Hodgkin's lymphoma

Infectious Diseases

Numerous infectious diseases are associated with the development of hepatic granulomatosis (Table 26.15).

Tuberculosis

Hepatic granulomas are found in nearly 20 % of patients with pulmonary tuberculosis, 75 % of patients with extrapulmonary tuberculosis, and more than 90 % of patients with miliary tuberculosis [201]. Systemic symptoms may include fevers, weight loss, anorexia, and night sweats.

Abnormal liver biochemical tests include elevated alkaline phosphatase and GGT with mildly elevated serum bilirubin. Hepatic granulomas are typically found in the portal tract and are most often necrotizing (Fig. 26.4). Rupture into the bile ducts may result in tuberculous cholangitis.

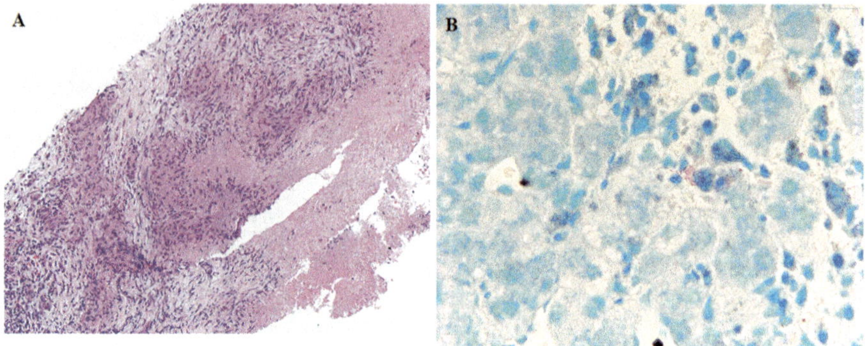

Fig. 26.4 Hepatic tuberculosis. (**a**) Necrotizing granulomatous inflammation from a case of mycobacterial infection in the liver (H&E). (**b**) Acid-fast stain of a hepatic granuloma showing few acid-fast bacilli (Ziehl-Neelsen×100) (Courtesy of Monica T. Garcia-Buitrago, MD, University of Miami)

Anti-tuberculosis medications should be promptly initiated once the diagnosis is confirmed. If the diagnosis of tuberculosis cannot be confidently ruled out, anti-tuberculous therapy should be considered prior to starting an empiric course of corticosteroids.

Mycobacterium avium-intracellulare complex (MAC) is associated with hepatic granulomatosis and may be seen in immunocompromised patients, such as those with HIV [202]. MAC should be considered in patients with cholestasis and fevers, especially if the patient is HIV positive and hepatic granulomas are seen on liver biopsy.

Histoplasmosis and coccidiodomycosis are among the most common fungal infections associated with hepatic granulomas in the US. Histoplasmosis should be considered in patients who live in the Southern or Central US, while coccidioido-mycosis should be considered in those who live in the Southwestern US. Less commonly, hepatic granulomatosis may also be seen in candidiasis, blastomycosis, or cryptococcosis.

Q fever results from infection with *Coxiella burnetti* (a rickettsial organism). Hepatic granulomas seen with Q fever are classically referred to as fibrin-ring granulomas, characterized by a fibrinoid necrotic ring surrounded by histiocytes and lymphocytes [203].

Advanced schistosomiasis results in dense portal fibrosis known as Symmer's clay pipestem fibrosis. Schistosome eggs reach the portal vein radicles where granulomas typically form with a characteristic peripheral rim of abundant eosinophils often with eggs detected within the granuloma.

Hepatic granulomas have been reported in patients with chronic HCV and HBV [204, 205]. Granulomas are typically small and non-necrotizing and may recur after LT if untreated.

Lipogranuloma

Lipogranulomas result from fatty liver or ingestion of mineral oil in the form of laxatives or food products. These granulomas are characterized by fat droplets surrounded by macrophages and lymphocytes. Lipogranulomas do not result in significant liver injury and are not of major clinical consequence.

Cancer

Hodgkin lymphoma is the most common malignancy associated with hepatic granulomatosis. Non-Hodgkins lymphoma and renal cell carcinoma are also associated with hepatic granulomatous disease [206, 207].

Drugs

Many drugs have been associated with hepatic granulomatosis (Table 26.16, Fig. 26.5). Drug-related granulomas generally resolve without significant clinical sequelae.

Foreign Body

Granulomas due to retained foreign body are typically comprised of macrophages forming giant cells. Common examples include talc from intravenous drug users and retained suture material [208].

Idiopathic

Idiophatic granulomatous hepatitis is often seen in patients with fever of unknown origin with no identifiable cause for the granulomas. Symptomatic idiopathic granulomatous hepatitis may be treated with an empiric course of corticosteroids.

Hepatic Amyloidosis

1. How common is hepatic amyloidosis and what are the common clinical and laboratory findings?

   According to several autopsy series, 56–95 % of patients with amyloidosis were found to have hepatic involvement. Nearly 50 % of these patients had signs or symptoms of hepatic involvement. Despite its relative high prevalence, clinical

Table 26.16 Drugs associated with granulomatous liver disease

Anti-Inflammatory	Cardiovascular
Aspirin	Chinidine
Dimethicone	Diltiazem
Gold	Disopyramide
Mesalamine	Hydralazine
Sulfasalazine	Metolazone
Phenazone	Phenprocoumon
Anti-Neoplastic	Prajmalium
Procarbazine	Procainamide
Antimicrobial	Quinidine
Amoxicillin-clavulanic acid	Tocainide
Cephalexin	Trichlormethiazide
Dapsone	Hydrochlorothiazide
Isoniazid	Neurologic
Mebendazole	Carbamazepine
Nitrofurantoin	Chlorpromazine
Oxacillin	Diazepam
Penicillin	Methyldopa
Sulfa antibiotics	Phenytoin
Biologic	Miscellaneous
Etanercept	Allopurinol
Pegylated interferon	Bacille Calmette-Guerin (BCG)
Herbal/Alternative	Contraceptives
Greeen juice	Feprazone
Seatone	Halothane
Hypoglycemic	Mineral oil
Glyburide	Papaverine
Chlorpropamide	Ranitidine
Rosiglitazone	Quinine
Tolbutamide	Propylthiouracil
	Saridon (Excedrin)

manifestations of hepatic amyloidosis are typically mild. The most common findings include hepatomegaly and elevated alkaline phosphatase levels.

2. Do I need a liver biopsy to diagnosis amyloidosis of my liver?

   The role for liver biopsy in diagnosing amyloidosis of the liver is controversial. Liver biopsy for presumed hepatic amyloidosis is considered high risk due to increased risk of bleeding and generally should be avoided. The diagnosis of amyloidosis may be made by performing a much less invasive biopsy of the rectum or abdominal fat.

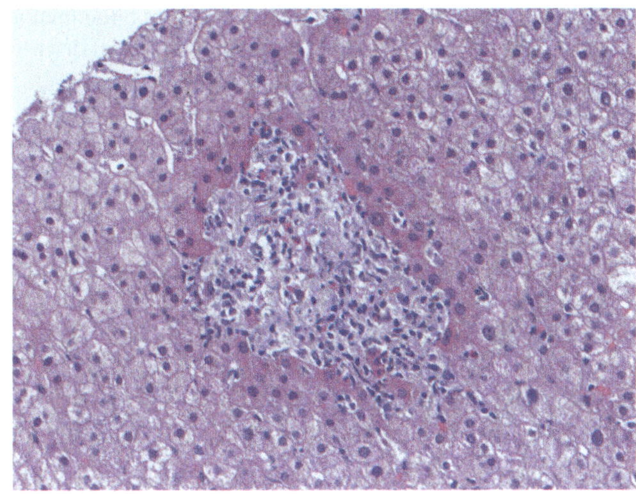

Fig. 26.5 Allopurinol-induced hepatic granuloma. Non-necrotizing granuloma with eosinophils from a case of allopurinol-induced granulomatous liver disease (H&E ×40) (Courtesy of Monica T. Garcia-Buitrago, MD, University of Miami)

Table 26.17 Classification of amyloidosis

Type	Fibril	Syndrome
AA	Serum amyloid A	Reactive amyloid (secondary)
		– Acquired (from chronic infections or inflammation)
		– Hereditary (Familial Mediterranean fever, FMF)
AL	Monoclonal immunoglobulin light chain	Primary amyloid
ATTR	Transthyretin (TTR)	Familal amyloidotic polyneuropathy (FAP)

Other types include $A\beta_2M$ (dialysis-associated amyloid), $A\beta$ (Alzheimer's disease), and A1APP (diabetes/insulinoma)

Introduction

Systemic amyloidosis is characterized by deposition of insoluble glycoprotein fibrils in the extracellular matrix and blood vessel walls. These deposits result in a wide range of clinical manifestations depending on their type, amount of deposition, and the organ in which they are deposited. Classification of amyloidosis is based on the protein involved (Table 26.17). Systemic amyloidosis is also classified as primary amyloidosis (AL) or secondary amyloidosis (AA). In AL, which accounts for 80 % of all cases, the amyloid consists of kappa or lamba immunoglobulin light chains that are produced by a monoclonal population of plasma cells. In AA, the amyloid is derived from serum amyloid A, which is an acute phase reactant that is secreted from the liver in response to chronic infections or inflammatory processes such as rheumatoid arthritis, osteomyelitis, inflammatory bowel disease, tuberculosis, leprosy, or lymphoma.

Familial Mediterranean fever (FMF) is an autosomal recessive disorder that is characterized by acute attacks of fever with sterile peritonitis, pleurisy or synovitis that predisposes to AL amyloidosis [209]. Although renal dysfunction is the most common manifestation of amyloidosis in FMF, the gastrointestinal tract, liver, and spleen may also be involved.

Familial amyloidotic polyneuropathy (FAP) is a variant of amyloidosis that is caused by deposition of variant transthyretin (TTR) [210]. Normal TTR is produced predominantly in the liver and transports vitamin A and thyroid hormones. FAP is characterized by progressive peripheral and autonomic neuropathy that develops due to accumulation of mutant TTR that is deposited in nerves, spleen, heart, eyes, thyroid, and adrenals. The liver is generally spared.

Clinical and Laboratory Findings

The clinical presentation of systemic amyloidosis is generally related to the organ in which the amyloid deposits and includes early satiety, intestinal malabsorption, nephrotic syndrome, heart failure, peripheral or autonomic neuropathy, dysgeusia, and carpal tunnel syndrome. Hepatic involvement may be seen in up to 90 % of patients with AL amyloidosis and 60 % of patients with AA amyloidosis [211–213]. Hepatic amyloidosis should be suspected in those with hepatomegaly in the setting of chronic infectious or inflammatory processes, particularly if it is associated with proteinuria or monoclonal gammopathy, involuntary weight loss, and unexplained elevation of alkaline phosphatase. Hepatomegaly, which is either due to passive congestion or infiltration, is present in 57–83 % of patients with hepatic amyloidosis. Although patients may develop ascites with hepatic amyloidosis, it is more likely due to concurrent heart failure or hypoalbuminemia. Patients may develop sinusoidal portal hypertension with gastrointestinal bleeding from esophageal varices [214, 215]. The most common biochemical abnormality is an elevated alkaline phosphatase, which may be >500 IU/mL with mildly elevated serum aminotransferases [216]. Serum albumin levels may also be low largely due to proteinuria, which may be in the nephrotic range in 30 % of patients.

Radiographic Findings

Ultrasonographic findings typically include heterogenous echogenicity [217]. Focal or diffuse parenchymal attenuation with or without extensive calcifications are often seen on CT scan. MRI demonstrates markedly increased signal intensity on T1-weighted images of the liver without significantly changed signal intensity on T2-weighted images.

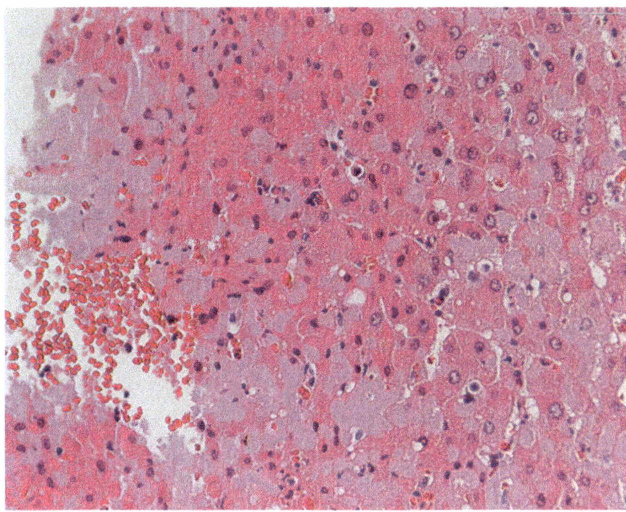

Fig. 26.6 Hepatic amyloidosis. Liver biopsy showing globular eosinophilic deposits of amyloid along the sinusoids in the space of Disse (H&E) (Courtesy of Monica T. Garcia-Buitrago, MD, University of Miami)

Histopathology

The role of liver biopsy in the diagnosis of hepatic amyloidosis remains controversial due to the increased risk of bleeding and/or hepatic rupture with reported rates of hemorrhage in 4–5% patients with hepatic amyloidosis [218]. However, these findings have not been consistently reproduced [195]. Although biopsy of the affected tissue is likely to be diagnostic, it is generally safer to sample other areas such as subcutaneous abdominal fat pad, rectal mucosa, and labial salivary gland. For these reasons, a liver biopsy is generally avoided. If liver biopsy is performed, characteristic findings on liver biopsy include amyloid fibril deposits in the vessel walls and/or hepatic sinusoids (Fig. 26.6). The amyloid fibrils stain with Congo red and appear as apple-green birefringence under polarized light.

Management

Management of AA amyloidosis is based on treating the underlying disease, which is associated with regression of signs and symptoms [219]. Treatment of AL amyloidosis remains more difficult. Variable degrees of regression of hepatic amyloidosis have been reported after cytotoxic chemotherapy [220].

LT is the definitive treatment for FAP. Because TTR is predominately produced in the liver, LT effectively suppresses the production of circulating mutant TTR and theoretically ceases the formation of amyloid and disease progression [221, 222].

Compared to 10-year survival rates of 56–62 % for untreated controls, 10-year survival rates after LT are 83–100 % [223, 224]. In addition, sequential liver transplantation, also known as domino liver transplantation (DLT), has been successfully utilized in the management of FAP. In DLT, the explanted liver from patients with FAP can be transplanted into selected patients, on the basis that these livers maintain normal structure and function apart from the production of variant TTR, which was removed only to arrest the accumulation of amyloid and clinical progression of polyneuropathy. Recipient selection is critical as recipients of FAP livers develop sensory neuropathy as early as 7–10 years after successful DLT [225–227].

Outcome

Prognosis varies according to the type of amyloidosis, the degree of organ involvement, and the response to therapy of the underlying disorder. The 5-year survival for AA amyloidosis with hepatic involvement is 43 % compared to 72 % for those without hepatic involvement. The prognosis for AL amyloidosis is generally poor with a mean survival of less than 2 years. Mortality is usually due to cardiac or renal disease and only rarely due to hepatic involvement. Patients with FAP have a more rapid progression of cardiac and neurologic disease with an average life expectancy of 9–13 years after onset of symptoms [210, 222].

Acknowledgement This review did not receive financial support from a funding agency or an institution.

Eric F. Martin, MD has no conflict of interests to declare.

References

1. Ch'ng CL, Morgan M, Hainsworth I, Kingham JG. Prospective study of liver dysfunction in pregnancy in Southwest Wales. Gut. 2002;51(6):876–80.
2. Bacq Y, Zarka O, Brechot JF, Mariotte N, Vol S, Tichet J, et al. Liver function tests in normal pregnancy: a prospective study of 103 pregnant women and 103 matched controls. Hepatology. 1996;23(5):1030–4.
3. Girling JC, Dow E, Smith JH. Liver function tests in pre-eclampsia: importance of comparison with a reference range derived for normal pregnancy. Br J Obstet Gynaecol. 1997;104(2):246–50.
4. Valenzuela GJ, Munson LA, Tarbaux NM, Farley JR. Time-dependent changes in bone, placental, intestinal, and hepatic alkaline phosphatase activities in serum during human pregnancy. Clin Chem. 1987;33(10):1801–6.
5. De Wilde JP, Rivers AW, Price DL. A review of the current use of magnetic resonance imaging in pregnancy and safety implications for the fetus. Prog Biophys Mol Biol. 2005;87(2-3):335–53.
6. Nagayama M, Watanabe Y, Okumura A, Amoh Y, Nakashita S, Dodo Y. Fast MR imaging in obstetrics. Radiographics. 2002;22(3):563–80. discussion 80–2.

7. Shellock FG, Kanal E. Safety of magnetic resonance imaging contrast agents. J Magn Reson Imaging. 1999;10(3):477–84.
8. Gadsby R, Barnie-Adshead AM, Jagger C. A prospective study of nausea and vomiting during pregnancy. Br J Gen Pract. 1993;43(371):245–8.
9. Lacroix R, Eason E, Melzack R. Nausea and vomiting during pregnancy: a prospective study of its frequency, intensity, and patterns of change. Am J Obstet Gynecol. 2000;182(4):931–7.
10. Fairweather DV. Nausea and vomiting during pregnancy. Obstet Gynecol Annu. 1978;7:91–105.
11. Kallen B. Hyperemesis during pregnancy and delivery outcome: a registry study. Eur J Obstet Gynecol Reprod Biol. 1987;26(4):291–302.
12. Jueckstock JK, Kaestner R, Mylonas I. Managing hyperemesis gravidarum: a multimodal challenge. BMC Med. 2010;8:46.
13. Fell DB, Dodds L, Joseph KS, Allen VM, Butler B. Risk factors for hyperemesis gravidarum requiring hospital admission during pregnancy. Obstet Gynecol. 2006;107(2 Pt 1):277–84.
14. Kuscu NK, Koyuncu F. Hyperemesis gravidarum: current concepts and management. Postgrad Med J. 2002;78(916):76–9.
15. Conchillo JM, Pijnenborg JM, Peeters P, Stockbrugger RW, Fevery J, Koek GH. Liver enzyme elevation induced by hyperemesis gravidarum: aetiology, diagnosis and treatment. Neth J Med. 2002;60(9):374–8.
16. Larrey D, Rueff B, Feldmann G, Degott C, Danan G, Benhamou JP. Recurrent jaundice caused by recurrent hyperemesis gravidarum. Gut. 1984;25(12):1414–5.
17. Gross S, Librach C, Cecutti A. Maternal weight loss associated with hyperemesis gravidarum: a predictor of fetal outcome. Am J Obstet Gynecol. 1989;160(4):906–9.
18. Veenendaal MV, van Abeelen AF, Painter RC, van der Post JA, Roseboom TJ. Consequences of hyperemesis gravidarum for offspring: a systematic review and meta-analysis. BJOG. 2011;118(11):1302–13.
19. Chiossi G, Neri I, Cavazzuti M, Basso G, Facchinetti F. Hyperemesis gravidarum complicated by Wernicke encephalopathy: background, case report, and review of the literature. Obstet Gynecol Surv. 2006;61(4):255–68.
20. van Stuijvenberg ME, Schabort I, Labadarios D, Nel JT. The nutritional status and treatment of patients with hyperemesis gravidarum. Am J Obstet Gynecol. 1995;172(5):1585–91.
21. Trogstad LI, Stoltenberg C, Magnus P, Skjaerven R, Irgens LM. Recurrence risk in hyperemesis gravidarum. BJOG. 2005;112(12):1641–5.
22. Bacq Y, Sentilhes L, Reyes HB, Glantz A, Kondrackiene J, Binder T, et al. Efficacy of ursodeoxycholic acid in treating intrahepatic cholestasis of pregnancy: a meta-analysis. Gastroenterology. 2012;143(6):1492–501.
23. Brites D, Rodrigues CM, Cardoso Mda C, Graca LM. Unusual case of severe cholestasis of pregnancy with early onset, improved by ursodeoxycholic acid administration. Eur J Obstet Gynecol Reprod Biol. 1998;76(2):165–8.
24. Fagan EA. Intrahepatic cholestasis of pregnancy. Clin Liver Dis. 1999;3(3):603–32.
25. Reyes H, Gonzalez MC, Ribalta J, Aburto H, Matus C, Schramm G, et al. Prevalence of intrahepatic cholestasis of pregnancy in Chile. Ann Intern Med. 1978;88(4):487–93.
26. Reyes H, Taboada G, Ribalta J. Prevalence of intrahepatic cholestasis of pregnancy in La Paz, Bolivia. J Chronic Dis. 1979;32(7):499–504.
27. Laifer SA, Stiller RJ, Siddiqui DS, Dunston-Boone G, Whetham JC. Ursodeoxycholic acid for the treatment of intrahepatic cholestasis of pregnancy. J Matern Fetal Med. 2001;10(2):131–5.
28. Lee RH, Goodwin TM, Greenspoon J, Incerpi M. The prevalence of intrahepatic cholestasis of pregnancy in a primarily Latina Los Angeles population. J Perinatol. 2006;26(9):527–32.
29. Arrese M, Macias RI, Briz O, Perez MJ, Marin JJ. Molecular pathogenesis of intrahepatic cholestasis of pregnancy. Expert Rev Mol Med. 2008;10:e9.
30. Keitel V, Vogt C, Haussinger D, Kubitz R. Combined mutations of canalicular transporter proteins cause severe intrahepatic cholestasis of pregnancy. Gastroenterology. 2006;131(2):624–9.

31. Oude Elferink RP, Paulusma CC. Function and pathophysiological importance of ABCB4 (MDR3 P-glycoprotein). Pflugers Arch. 2007;453(5):601–10.
32. Bacq Y, Gendrot C, Perrotin F, Lefrou L, Chretien S, Vie-Buret V, et al. ABCB4 gene mutations and single-nucleotide polymorphisms in women with intrahepatic cholestasis of pregnancy. J Med Genet. 2009;46(10):711–5.
33. Reyes H. The spectrum of liver and gastrointestinal disease seen in cholestasis of pregnancy. Gastroenterol Clin North Am. 1992;21(4):905–21.
34. Favre N, Abergel A, Blanc P, Sapin V, Roszyk L, Gallot D. Unusual presentation of severe intrahepatic cholestasis of pregnancy leading to fetal death. Obstet Gynecol. 2009;114(2 Pt 2):491–3.
35. Glantz A, Marschall HU, Mattsson LA. Intrahepatic cholestasis of pregnancy: relationships between bile acid levels and fetal complication rates. Hepatology. 2004;40(2):467–74.
36. Rolfes DB, Ishak KG. Liver disease in pregnancy. Histopathology. 1986;10(6):555–70.
37. Mazzella G, Rizzo N, Azzaroli F, Simoni P, Bovicelli L, Miracolo A, et al. Ursodeoxycholic acid administration in patients with cholestasis of pregnancy: effects on primary bile acids in babies and mothers. Hepatology. 2001;33(3):504–8.
38. Serrano MA, Brites D, Larena MG, Monte MJ, Bravo MP, Oliveira N, et al. Beneficial effect of ursodeoxycholic acid on alterations induced by cholestasis of pregnancy in bile acid transport across the human placenta. J Hepatol. 1998;28(5):829–39.
39. Marschall HU, Wagner M, Zollner G, Fickert P, Diczfalusy U, Gumhold J, et al. Complementary stimulation of hepatobiliary transport and detoxification systems by rifampicin and ursodeoxycholic acid in humans. Gastroenterology. 2005;129(2):476–85.
40. Mays JK. The active management of intrahepatic cholestasis of pregnancy. Curr Opin Obstet Gynecol. 2010;22(2):100–3.
41. Marschall HU, Wikstrom Shemer E, Ludvigsson JF, Stephansson O. Intrahepatic cholestasis of pregnancy and associated hepatobiliary disease: a population-based cohort study. Hepatology. 2013;58(4):1385–91.
42. Ropponen A, Sund R, Riikonen S, Ylikorkala O, Aittomaki K. Intrahepatic cholestasis of pregnancy as an indicator of liver and biliary diseases: a population-based study. Hepatology. 2006;43(4):723–8.
43. Glantz A, Marschall HU, Lammert F, Mattsson LA. Intrahepatic cholestasis of pregnancy: a randomized controlled trial comparing dexamethasone and ursodeoxycholic acid. Hepatology. 2005;42(6):1399–405.
44. European Association for the Study of the Liver. EASL Clinical Practice Guidelines: management of cholestatic liver diseases. J Hepatol. 2009;51(2):237–67.
45. Lee RH, Kwok KM, Ingles S, Wilson ML, Mullin P, Incerpi M, et al. Pregnancy outcomes during an era of aggressive management for intrahepatic cholestasis of pregnancy. Am J Perinatol. 2008;25(6):341–5.
46. Sibai B, Dekker G, Kupferminc M. Pre-eclampsia. Lancet. 2005;365(9461):785–99.
47. American College of Obstetricians and Gynecologists, Task Force on Hypertension in Pregnancy. Hypertension in pregnancy. Report of the American College of Obstetricians and Gynecologists' Task Force on Hypertension in Pregnancy. Obstet Gynecol. 2013;122(5):1122–31.
48. Duckitt K, Harrington D. Risk factors for pre-eclampsia at antenatal booking: systematic review of controlled studies. BMJ. 2005;330(7491):565.
49. Audibert F, Friedman SA, Frangieh AY, Sibai BM. Clinical utility of strict diagnostic criteria for the HELLP (hemolysis, elevated liver enzymes, and low platelets) syndrome. Am J Obstet Gynecol. 1996;175(2):460–4.
50. Isler CM, Rinehart BK, Terrone DA, Martin RW, Magann EF, Martin Jr JN. Maternal mortality associated with HELLP (hemolysis, elevated liver enzymes, and low platelets) syndrome. Am J Obstet Gynecol. 1999;181(4):924–8.
51. Sibai BM, Ramadan MK, Usta I, Salama M, Mercer BM, Friedman SA. Maternal morbidity and mortality in 442 pregnancies with hemolysis, elevated liver enzymes, and low platelets (HELLP syndrome). Am J Obstet Gynecol. 1993;169(4):1000–6.

52. Martin Jr JN, Rinehart BK, May WL, Magann EF, Terrone DA, Blake PG. The spectrum of severe preeclampsia: comparative analysis by HELLP (hemolysis, elevated liver enzyme levels, and low platelet count) syndrome classification. Am J Obstet Gynecol. 1999;180(6 Pt 1):1373–84.
53. Sibai BM. The HELLP syndrome (hemolysis, elevated liver enzymes, and low platelets): much ado about nothing? Am J Obstet Gynecol. 1990;162(2):311–6.
54. Barton JR, Riely CA, Adamec TA, Shanklin DR, Khoury AD, Sibai BM. Hepatic histopathologic condition does not correlate with laboratory abnormalities in HELLP syndrome (hemolysis, elevated liver enzymes, and low platelet count). Am J Obstet Gynecol. 1992;167(6):1538–43.
55. Woudstra DM, Chandra S, Hofmeyr GJ, Dowswell T. Corticosteroids for HELLP (hemolysis, elevated liver enzymes, low platelets) syndrome in pregnancy. Cochrane Database Syst Rev 2010; (9):CD008148.
56. Eser B, Guven M, Unal A, Coskun R, Altuntas F, Sungur M, et al. The role of plasma exchange in HELLP syndrome. Clin Appl Thromb Hemost. 2005;11(2):211–7.
57. Hartwell L, Ma T. Acute fatty liver of pregnancy treated with plasma exchange. Dig Dis Sci. 2014;59(9):2076–80.
58. Martin Jr JN, Rose CH, Briery CM. Understanding and managing HELLP syndrome: the integral role of aggressive glucocorticoids for mother and child. Am J Obstet Gynecol. 2006;195(4):914–34.
59. Abramovici D, Friedman SA, Mercer BM, Audibert F, Kao L, Sibai BM. Neonatal outcome in severe preeclampsia at 24 to 36 weeks' gestation: does the HELLP (hemolysis, elevated liver enzymes, and low platelet count) syndrome matter? Am J Obstet Gynecol. 1999;180(1 Pt 1):221–5.
60. Sibai BM. Diagnosis, controversies, and management of the syndrome of hemolysis, elevated liver enzymes, and low platelet count. Obstet Gynecol. 2004;103(5 Pt 1):981–91.
61. Chames MC, Haddad B, Barton JR, Livingston JC, Sibai BM. Subsequent pregnancy outcome in women with a history of HELLP syndrome at < or = 28 weeks of gestation. Am J Obstet Gynecol. 2003;188(6):1504–7. discussion 7–8.
62. van Pampus MG, Wolf H, Mayruhu G, Treffers PE, Bleker OP. Long-term follow-up in patients with a history of (H)ELLP syndrome. Hypertens Pregnancy. 2001;20(1):15–23.
63. Castro MA, Fassett MJ, Reynolds TB, Shaw KJ, Goodwin TM. Reversible peripartum liver failure: a new perspective on the diagnosis, treatment, and cause of acute fatty liver of pregnancy, based on 28 consecutive cases. Am J Obstet Gynecol. 1999;181(2):389–95.
64. Knight M, Nelson-Piercy C, Kurinczuk JJ, Spark P, Brocklehurst P, UKOS System. A prospective national study of acute fatty liver of pregnancy in the UK. Gut. 2008;57(7):951–6.
65. Sheehan HL. The pathology of acute yellow atrophy and delayed chloroform poisoning. J Obstet Gynaecol Br Emp. 1940;47:49–62.
66. Bacq Y, Riely CA. Acute fatty liver of pregnancy: the hepatologist's view. Gastroenterologist. 1993;1(4):257–64.
67. Ibdah JA, Bennett MJ, Rinaldo P, Zhao Y, Gibson B, Sims HF, et al. A fetal fatty-acid oxidation disorder as a cause of liver disease in pregnant women. N Engl J Med. 1999;340(22):1723–31.
68. Yang Z, Zhao Y, Bennett MJ, Strauss AW, Ibdah JA. Fetal genotypes and pregnancy outcomes in 35 families with mitochondrial trifunctional protein mutations. Am J Obstet Gynecol. 2002;187(3):715–20.
69. Ibdah JA. Role of genetic screening in identifying susceptibility to acute fatty liver of pregnancy. Nat Clin Pract Gastroenterol Hepatol. 2005;2(11):494–5.
70. Yang Z, Yamada J, Zhao Y, Strauss AW, Ibdah JA. Prospective screening for pediatric mitochondrial trifunctional protein defects in pregnancies complicated by liver disease. JAMA. 2002;288(17):2163–6.
71. Buytaert IM, Elewaut GP, Van Kets HE. Early occurrence of acute fatty liver in pregnancy. Am J Gastroenterol. 1996;91(3):603–4.

72. Hammoud GM, Ibjah JA. Preeclampsia-induced liver dysfunction, HELLP syndrome, and acute fatty liver of pregnancy. Clin Liver Dis. 2014;4(3):69–73.
73. Bacq Y. Acute fatty liver of pregnancy. Semin Perinatol. 1998;22(2):134–40.
74. Nelson DB, Yost NP, Cunningham FG. Acute fatty liver of pregnancy: clinical outcomes and expected duration of recovery. Am J Obstet Gynecol. 2013;209(5):456.e1–7.
75. Amon E, Allen SR, Petrie RH, Belew JE. Acute fatty liver of pregnancy associated with preeclampsia: management of hepatic failure with postpartum liver transplantation. Am J Perinatol. 1991;8(4):278–9.
76. Ockner SA, Brunt EM, Cohn SM, Krul ES, Hanto DW, Peters MG. Fulminant hepatic failure caused by acute fatty liver of pregnancy treated by orthotopic liver transplantation. Hepatology. 1990;11(1):59–64.
77. Franco J, Newcomer J, Adams M, Saeian K. Auxiliary liver transplant in acute fatty liver of pregnancy. Obstet Gynecol. 2000;95(6 Pt 2):1042.
78. Acosta S, Alhadad A, Verbaan H, Ogren M. The clinical importance in differentiating portal from mesenteric venous thrombosis. Int Angiol. 2011;30(1):71–8.
79. Rajani R, Bjornsson E, Bergquist A, Danielsson A, Gustavsson A, Grip O, et al. The epidemiology and clinical features of portal vein thrombosis: a multicentre study. Aliment Pharmacol Ther. 2010;32(9):1154–62.
80. Baert AL, Fevery J, Marchal G, Goddeeris P, Wilms G, Ponette E, et al. Early diagnosis of Budd-Chiari syndrome by computed tomography and ultrasonography: report of five cases. Gastroenterology. 1983;84(3):587–95.
81. Janssen HL, Meinardi JR, Vleggaar FP, van Uum SH, Haagsma EB, van Der Meer FJ, et al. Factor V Leiden mutation, prothrombin gene mutation, and deficiencies in coagulation inhibitors associated with Budd-Chiari syndrome and portal vein thrombosis: results of a case-control study. Blood. 2000;96(7):2364–8.
82. Ogren M, Bergqvist D, Bjorck M, Acosta S, Eriksson H, Sternby NH. Portal vein thrombosis: prevalence, patient characteristics and lifetime risk: a population study based on 23,796 consecutive autopsies. World J Gastroenterol. 2006;12(13):2115–9.
83. Ahuja V, Marwaha N, Chawla Y, Dilawari JB. Coagulation abnormalities in idiopathic portal venous thrombosis. J Gastroenterol Hepatol. 1999;14(12):1210–1.
84. Amitrano L, Brancaccio V, Guardascione MA, Margaglione M, Iannaccone L, Dandrea G, et al. High prevalence of thrombophilic genotypes in patients with acute mesenteric vein thrombosis. Am J Gastroenterol. 2001;96(1):146–9.
85. Bayraktar Y, Balkanci F, Bayraktar M, Calguneri M. Budd-Chiari syndrome: a common complication of Behcet's disease. Am J Gastroenterol. 1997;92(5):858–62.
86. Bhattacharyya M, Makharia G, Kannan M, Ahmed RP, Gupta PK, Saxena R. Inherited prothrombotic defects in Budd-Chiari syndrome and portal vein thrombosis: a study from North India. Am J Clin Pathol. 2004;121(6):844–7.
87. Chamouard P, Pencreach E, Maloisel F, Grunebaum L, Ardizzone JF, Meyer A, et al. Frequent factor II G20210A mutation in idiopathic portal vein thrombosis. Gastroenterology. 1999;116(1):144–8.
88. Dayal S, Pati HP, Pande GK, Sharma MP, Saraya AK. Multilineage hemopoietic stem cell defects in Budd Chiari syndrome. J Hepatol. 1997;26(2):293–7.
89. Deltenre P, Denninger MH, Hillaire S, Guillin MC, Casadevall N, Briere J, et al. Factor V Leiden related Budd-Chiari syndrome. Gut. 2001;48(2):264–8.
90. Denninger MH, Chait Y, Casadevall N, Hillaire S, Guillin MC, Bezeaud A, et al. Cause of portal or hepatic venous thrombosis in adults: the role of multiple concurrent factors. Hepatology. 2000;31(3):587–91.
91. Egesel T, Buyukasik Y, Dundar SV, Gurgey A, Kirazli S, Bayraktar Y. The role of natural anticoagulant deficiencies and factor V Leiden in the development of idiopathic portal vein thrombosis. J Clin Gastroenterol. 2000;30(1):66–71.
92. Hirshberg B, Shouval D, Fibach E, Friedman G, Ben-Yehuda D. Flow cytometric analysis of autonomous growth of erythroid precursors in liquid culture detects occult polycythemia vera in the Budd-Chiari syndrome. J Hepatol. 2000;32(4):574–8.

93. Mahmoud AE, Elias E, Beauchamp N, Wilde JT. Prevalence of the factor V Leiden mutation in hepatic and portal vein thrombosis. Gut. 1997;40(6):798–800.
94. Mohanty D, Shetty S, Ghosh K, Pawar A, Abraham P. Hereditary thrombophilia as a cause of Budd-Chiari syndrome: a study from Western India. Hepatology. 2001;34(4 Pt 1):666–70.
95. Primignani M, Barosi G, Bergamaschi G, Gianelli U, Fabris F, Reati R, et al. Role of the JAK2 mutation in the diagnosis of chronic myeloproliferative disorders in splanchnic vein thrombosis. Hepatology. 2006;44(6):1528–34.
96. Primignani M, Martinelli I, Bucciarelli P, Battaglioli T, Reati R, Fabris F, et al. Risk factors for thrombophilia in extrahepatic portal vein obstruction. Hepatology. 2005;41(3):603–8.
97. Chait Y, Condat B, Cazals-Hatem D, Rufat P, Atmani S, Chaoui D, et al. Relevance of the criteria commonly used to diagnose myeloproliferative disorder in patients with splanchnic vein thrombosis. Br J Haematol. 2005;129(4):553–60.
98. Valla DC, Condat B. Portal vein thrombosis in adults: pathophysiology, pathogenesis and management. J Hepatol. 2000;32(5):865–71.
99. Condat B, Pessione F, Helene Denninger M, Hillaire S, Valla D. Recent portal or mesenteric venous thrombosis: increased recognition and frequent recanalization on anticoagulant therapy. Hepatology. 2000;32(3):466–70.
100. Plessier A, Darwish-Murad S, Hernandez-Guerra M, Consigny Y, Fabris F, Trebicka J, et al. Acute portal vein thrombosis unrelated to cirrhosis: a prospective multicenter follow-up study. Hepatology. 2010;51(1):210–8.
101. Condat B, Pessione F, Hillaire S, Denninger MH, Guillin MC, Poliquin M, et al. Current outcome of portal vein thrombosis in adults: risk and benefit of anticoagulant therapy. Gastroenterology. 2001;120(2):490–7.
102. Amitrano L, Guardascione MA, Scaglione M, Pezzullo L, Sangiuliano N, Armellino MF, et al. Prognostic factors in noncirrhotic patients with splanchnic vein thromboses. Am J Gastroenterol. 2007;102(11):2464–70.
103. Clavien PA. Diagnosis and management of mesenteric infarction. Br J Surg. 1990;77(6):601–3.
104. Kumar S, Sarr MG, Kamath PS. Mesenteric venous thrombosis. N Engl J Med. 2001;345(23):1683–8.
105. Acosta S, Alhadad A, Svensson P, Ekberg O. Epidemiology, risk and prognostic factors in mesenteric venous thrombosis. Br J Surg. 2008;95(10):1245–51.
106. Brunaud L, Antunes L, Collinet-Adler S, Marchal F, Ayav A, Bresler L, et al. Acute mesenteric venous thrombosis: case for nonoperative management. J Vasc Surg. 2001;34(4):673–9.
107. Condat B, Valla D. Nonmalignant portal vein thrombosis in adults. Nat Clin Pract Gastroenterol Hepatol. 2006;3(9):505–15.
108. de Franchis R. Evolving consensus in portal hypertension. Report of the Baveno IV consensus workshop on methodology of diagnosis and therapy in portal hypertension. J Hepatol. 2005;43(1):167–76.
109. DeLeve LD, Valla DC, Garcia-Tsao G. American Association for the Study Liver D. Vascular disorders of the liver. Hepatology. 2009;49(5):1729–64.
110. Trum JW, Valla D, Cohen G, Degott C, Rueff B, Santoni P, et al. Bacteroides bacteremia of undetermined origin: strong association with portal vein thrombosis and cryptogenic pylephlebitis. Eur J Gasroenterol Hepatol. 1993;5(8):655–9.
111. Plemmons RM, Dooley DP, Longfield RN. Septic thrombophlebitis of the portal vein (pylephlebitis): diagnosis and management in the modern era. Clin Infect Dis. 1995;21(5):1114–20.
112. Van Gansbeke D, Avni EF, Delcour C, Engelholm L, Struyven J. Sonographic features of portal vein thrombosis. AJR Am J Roentgenol. 1985;144(4):749–52.
113. Plessier A, Rautou PE, Valla DC. Management of hepatic vascular diseases. J Hepatol. 2012;56 Suppl 1:S25–38.
114. Chou CK, Mak CW, Tzeng WS, Chang JM. CT of small bowel ischemia. Abdom Imaging. 2004;29(1):18–22.
115. de Franchis R, Baveno VF. Revising consensus in portal hypertension: report of the Baveno V consensus workshop on methodology of diagnosis and therapy in portal hypertension. J Hepatol. 2010;53(4):762–8.

116. Bates SM, Ginsberg JS. Clinical practice. Treatment of deep-vein thrombosis. N Engl J Med. 2004;351(3):268–77.
117. Baril N, Wren S, Radin R, Ralls P, Stain S. The role of anticoagulation in pylephlebitis. Am J Surg. 1996;172(5):449–52. discussion 52–3.
118. Hollingshead M, Burke CT, Mauro MA, Weeks SM, Dixon RG, Jaques PF. Transcatheter thrombolytic therapy for acute mesenteric and portal vein thrombosis. J Vasc Interv Radiol. 2005;16(5):651–61.
119. Malkowski P, Pawlak J, Michalowicz B, Szczerban J, Wroblewski T, Leowska E, et al. Thrombolytic treatment of portal thrombosis. Hepatogastroenterology. 2003;50(54):2098–100.
120. Dhiman RK, Behera A, Chawla YK, Dilawari JB, Suri S. Portal hypertensive biliopathy. Gut. 2007;56(7):1001–8.
121. Llop E, de Juan C, Seijo S, Garcia-Criado A, Abraldes JG, Bosch J, et al. Portal cholangiopathy: radiological classification and natural history. Gut. 2011;60(6):853–60.
122. Garcia-Pagan JC, Hernandez-Guerra M, Bosch J. Extrahepatic portal vein thrombosis. Semin Liver Dis. 2008;28(3):282–92.
123. Garcia-Tsao G, Sanyal AJ, Grace ND, Carey W. Practice Guidelines Committee of the American Association for the Study of Liver D, Practice Parameters Committee of the American College of G. Prevention and management of gastroesophageal varices and variceal hemorrhage in cirrhosis. Hepatology. 2007;46(3):922–38.
124. Janssen HL, Garcia-Pagan JC, Elias E, Mentha G, Hadengue A, Valla DC, et al. Budd-Chiari syndrome: a review by an expert panel. J Hepatol. 2003;38(3):364–71.
125. Almdal TP, Sorensen TI. Incidence of parenchymal liver diseases in Denmark, 1981 to 1985: analysis of hospitalization registry data. The Danish Association for the Study of the Liver. Hepatology. 1991;13(4):650–5.
126. Okuda H, Yamagata H, Obata H, Iwata H, Sasaki R, Imai F, et al. Epidemiological and clinical features of Budd-Chiari syndrome in Japan. J Hepatol. 1995;22(1):1–9.
127. Rajani R, Melin T, Bjornsson E, Broome U, Sangfelt P, Danielsson A, et al. Budd-Chiari syndrome in Sweden: epidemiology, clinical characteristics and survival - an 18-year experience. Liver Int. 2009;29(2):253–9.
128. Valla DC. Hepatic venous outflow tract obstruction etiopathogenesis: Asia versus the West. J Gastroenterol Hepatol. 2004;19:204–11.
129. Darwish Murad S, Plessier A, Hernandez-Guerra M, Fabris F, Eapen CE, Bahr MJ, et al. Etiology, management, and outcome of the Budd-Chiari syndrome. Ann Intern Med. 2009;151(3):167–75.
130. Valla DC. Hepatic vein thrombosis (Budd-Chiari syndrome). Semin Liver Dis. 2002;22(1):5–14.
131. Langlet P, Escolano S, Valla D, Coste-Zeitoun D, Denie C, Mallet A, et al. Clinicopathological forms and prognostic index in Budd-Chiari syndrome. J Hepatol. 2003;39(4):496–501.
132. Hadengue A, Poliquin M, Vilgrain V, Belghiti J, Degott C, Erlinger S, et al. The changing scene of hepatic vein thrombosis: recognition of asymptomatic cases. Gastroenterology. 1994;106(4):1042–7.
133. Dilawari JB, Bambery P, Chawla Y, Kaur U, Bhusnurmath SR, Malhotra HS, et al. Hepatic outflow obstruction (Budd-Chiari syndrome). Experience with 177 patients and a review of the literature. Medicine. 1994;73(1):21–36.
134. Chawla Y, Kumar S, Dhiman RK, Suri S, Dilawari JB. Duplex Doppler sonography in patients with Budd-Chiari syndrome. J Gastroenterol Hepatol. 1999;14(9):904–7.
135. Grant EG, Perrella R, Tessler FN, Lois J, Busuttil R. Budd-Chiari syndrome: the results of duplex and color Doppler imaging. AJR Am J Roentgenol. 1989;152(2):377–81.
136. Millener P, Grant EG, Rose S, Duerinckx A, Schiller VL, Tessler FN, et al. Color Doppler imaging findings in patients with Budd-Chiari syndrome: correlation with venographic findings. AJR Am J Roentgenol. 1993;161(2):307–12.
137. Miller WJ, Federle MP, Straub WH, Davis PL. Budd-Chiari syndrome: imaging with pathologic correlation. Abdom Imaging. 1993;18(4):329–35.
138. Parker RG. Occlusion of the hepatic veins in man. Medicine. 1959;38:369–402.

139. Ludwig J, Hashimoto E, McGill DB, van Heerden JA. Classification of hepatic venous outflow obstruction: ambiguous terminology of the Budd-Chiari syndrome. Mayo Clin Proc. 1990;65(1):51–5.
140. Tanaka M, Wanless IR. Pathology of the liver in Budd-Chiari syndrome: portal vein thrombosis and the histogenesis of veno-centric cirrhosis, veno-portal cirrhosis, and large regenerative nodules. Hepatology. 1998;27(2):488–96.
141. Valla DC. The diagnosis and management of the Budd-Chiari syndrome: consensus and controversies. Hepatology. 2003;38(4):793–803.
142. Zimmerman MA, Cameron AM, Ghobrial RM. Budd-Chiari syndrome. Clin Liver Dis. 2006;10(2):259–73. viii.
143. Plessier A, Sibert A, Consigny Y, Hakime A, Zappa M, Denninger MH, et al. Aiming at minimal invasiveness as a therapeutic strategy for Budd-Chiari syndrome. Hepatology. 2006;44(5):1308–16.
144. Randi ML, Tezza F, Scapin M, Duner E, Scarparo P, Scandellari R, et al. Heparin-induced thrombocytopenia in patients with Philadelphia-negative myeloproliferative disorders and unusual splanchnic or cerebral vein thrombosis. Acta Haematol. 2010;123(3):140–5.
145. Eapen CE, Velissaris D, Heydtmann M, Gunson B, Olliff S, Elias E. Favourable medium term outcome following hepatic vein recanalisation and/or transjugular intrahepatic portosystemic shunt for Budd Chiari syndrome. Gut. 2006;55(6):878–84.
146. Plessier A. Budd Chiari syndrome. Gastroenterol Clin Biol. 2006;30(10):1162–9.
147. Garcia-Pagan JC, Heydtmann M, Raffa S, Plessier A, Murad S, Fabris F, et al. TIPS for Budd-Chiari syndrome: long-term results and prognostics factors in 124 patients. Gastroenterology. 2008;135(3):808–15.
148. Havlioglu N, Brunt EM, Bacon BR. Budd-Chiari syndrome and hepatocellular carcinoma: a case report and review of the literature. Am J Gastroenterol. 2003;98(1):201–4.
149. Moucari R, Rautou PE, Cazals-Hatem D, Geara A, Bureau C, Consigny Y, et al. Hepatocellular carcinoma in Budd-Chiari syndrome: characteristics and risk factors. Gut. 2008;57(6):828–35.
150. Shin SH, Chung YH, Suh DD, Shin JW, Jang MK, Ryu SH, et al. Characteristic clinical features of hepatocellular carcinoma associated with Budd-Chiari syndrome: evidence of different carcinogenic process from hepatitis B virus-associated hepatocellular carcinoma. Eur J Gastroenterol Hepatol. 2004;16(3):319–24.
151. Cazals-Hatem D, Vilgrain V, Genin P, Denninger MH, Durand F, Belghiti J, et al. Arterial and portal circulation and parenchymal changes in Budd-Chiari syndrome: a study in 17 explanted livers. Hepatology. 2003;37(3):510–9.
152. Mentha G, Giostra E, Majno PE, Bechstein WO, Neuhaus P, O'Grady J, et al. Liver transplantation for Budd-Chiari syndrome: a European study on 248 patients from 51 centres. J Hepatol. 2006;44(3):520–8.
153. Srinivasan P, Rela M, Prachalias A, Muiesan P, Portmann B, Mufti GJ, et al. Liver transplantation for Budd-Chiari syndrome. Transplantation. 2002;73(6):973–7.
154. Fuste B, Mazzara R, Escolar G, Merino A, Ordinas A, Diaz-Ricart M. Granulocyte colony-stimulating factor increases expression of adhesion receptors on endothelial cells through activation of p38 MAPK. Haematologica. 2004;89(5):578–85.
155. Mercanoglu F, Turkmen A, Kocaman O, Pinarbasi B, Dursun M, Selcukbiricik F, et al. Endothelial dysfunction in renal transplant patients is closely related to serum cyclosporine levels. Transplant Proc. 2004;36(5):1357–60.
156. Carreras E, Diaz-Ricart M. The role of the endothelium in the short-term complications of hematopoietic SCT. Bone Marrow Transplant. 2011;46(12):1495–502.
157. Carreras E, Bertz H, Arcese W, Vernant JP, Tomas JF, Hagglund H, et al. Incidence and outcome of hepatic veno-occlusive disease after blood or marrow transplantation: a prospective cohort study of the European Group for Blood and Marrow Transplantation. European Group for Blood and Marrow Transplantation Chronic Leukemia Working Party. Blood. 1998;92(10):3599–604.
158. Ganem G, Saint-Marc Girardin MF, Kuentz M, Cordonnier C, Marinello G, Teboul C, et al. Venocclusive disease of the liver after allogeneic bone marrow transplantation in man. Int J Radiat Oncol Biol Phys. 1988;14(5):879–84.

159. Hasegawa S, Horibe K, Kawabe T, Kato K, Kojima S, Matsuyama T, et al. Veno-occlusive disease of the liver after allogeneic bone marrow transplantation in children with hematologic malignancies: incidence, onset time and risk factors. Bone Marrow Transplant. 1998;22(12):1191–7.

160. Jones RJ, Lee KS, Beschorner WE, Vogel VG, Grochow LB, Braine HG, et al. Venoocclusive disease of the liver following bone marrow transplantation. Transplantation. 1987;44(6):778–83.

161. McDermott WV, Stone MD, Bothe Jr A, Trey C. Budd-Chiari syndrome. Historical and clinical review with an analysis of surgical corrective procedures. Am J Surg. 1984;147(4):463–7.

162. McDonald GB, Hinds MS, Fisher LD, Schoch HG, Wolford JL, Banaji M, et al. Veno-occlusive disease of the liver and multiorgan failure after bone marrow transplantation: a cohort study of 355 patients. Ann Intern Med. 1993;118(4):255–67.

163. Carreras E, Rosinol L, Terol MJ, Alegre A, de Arriba F, Garcia-Larana J, et al. Veno-occlusive disease of the liver after high-dose cytoreductive therapy with busulfan and melphalan for autologous blood stem cell transplantation in multiple myeloma patients. Biol Blood Marrow Transplant. 2007;13(12):1448–54.

164. Lee JL, Gooley T, Bensinger W, Schiffman K, McDonald GB. Veno-occlusive disease of the liver after busulfan, melphalan, and thiotepa conditioning therapy: incidence, risk factors, and outcome. Biol Blood Marrow Transplant. 1999;5(5):306–15.

165. Shulman HM, Fisher LB, Schoch HG, Henne KW, McDonald GB. Veno-occlusive disease of the liver after marrow transplantation: histological correlates of clinical signs and symptoms. Hepatology. 1994;19(5):1171–81.

166. Hommeyer SC, Teefey SA, Jacobson AF, Higano CS, Bianco JA, Colacurcio CJ, et al. Venocclusive disease of the liver: prospective study of US evaluation. Radiology. 1992;184(3):683–6.

167. McCarville MB, Hoffer FA, Howard SC, Goloubeva O, Kauffman WM. Hepatic veno-occlusive disease in children undergoing bone-marrow transplantation: usefulness of sonographic findings. Pediatr Radiol. 2001;31(2):102–5.

168. Teefey SA, Brink JA, Borson RA, Middleton WD. Diagnosis of venoocclusive disease of the liver after bone marrow transplantation: value of duplex sonography. AJR Am J Roentgenol. 1995;164(6):1397–401.

169. Shulman HM, Gooley T, Dudley MD, Kofler T, Feldman R, Dwyer D, et al. Utility of transvenous liver biopsies and wedged hepatic venous pressure measurements in sixty marrow transplant recipients. Transplantation. 1995;59(7):1015–22.

170. Bornhauser M, Storer B, Slattery JT, Appelbaum FR, Deeg HJ, Hansen J, et al. Conditioning with fludarabine and targeted busulfan for transplantation of allogeneic hematopoietic stem cells. Blood. 2003;102(3):820–6.

171. DeLima M, Ghaddar H, Pierce S, Estey E. Treatment of newly-diagnosed acute myelogenous leukaemia in patients aged 80 years and above. Br J Haematol. 1996;93(1):89–95.

172. Attal M, Huguet F, Rubie H, Charlet JP, Schlaifer D, Huynh A, et al. Prevention of regimen-related toxicities after bone marrow transplantation by pentoxifylline: a prospective, randomized trial. Blood. 1993;82(3):732–6.

173. Dignan FL, Wynn RF, Hadzic N, Karani J, Quaglia A, Pagliuca A, et al. BCSH/BSBMT guideline: diagnosis and management of veno-occlusive disease (sinusoidal obstruction syndrome) following haematopoietic stem cell transplantation. Br J Haematol. 2013;163(4):444–57.

174. Imran H, Tleyjeh IM, Zirakzadeh A, Rodriguez V, Khan SP. Use of prophylactic anticoagulation and the risk of hepatic veno-occlusive disease in patients undergoing hematopoietic stem cell transplantation: a systematic review and meta-analysis. Bone Marrow Transplant. 2006;37(7):677–86.

175. Rosenthal J, Sender L, Secola R, Killen R, Millerick M, Murphy L, et al. Phase II trial of heparin prophylaxis for veno-occlusive disease of the liver in children undergoing bone marrow transplantation. Bone Marrow Transplant. 1996;18(1):185–91.

176. Tay J, Tinmouth A, Fergusson D, Huebsch L, Allan DS. Systematic review of controlled clinical trials on the use of ursodeoxycholic acid for the prevention of hepatic veno-occlusive

disease in hematopoietic stem cell transplantation. Biol Blood Marrow Transplant. 2007;13(2):206–17.

177. Bacher P, Kindel G, Walenga JM, Fareed J. Modulation of endothelial and platelet function by a polydeoxyribonucleotide derived drug "defibrotide". A dual mechanism in the control of vascular pathology. Thromb Res. 1993;70(4):343–8.

178. Benimetskaya L, Wu S, Voskresenskiy AM, Echart C, Zhou JF, Shin J, et al. Angiogenesis alteration by defibrotide: implications for its mechanism of action in severe hepatic veno-occlusive disease. Blood. 2008;112(10):4343–52.

179. Berti F, Rossoni G, Biasi G, Buschi A, Mandelli V, Tondo C. Defibrotide, by enhancing prostacyclin generation, prevents endothelin-1 induced contraction in human saphenous veins. Prostaglandins. 1990;40(4):337–50.

180. Evangelista V, Piccardoni P, de Gaetano G, Cerletti C. Defibrotide inhibits platelet activation by cathepsin G released from stimulated polymorphonuclear leukocytes. Thromb Haemost. 1992;67(6):660–4.

181. Zhou Q, Chu X, Ruan C. Defibrotide stimulates expression of thrombomodulin in human endothelial cells. Thromb Haemost. 1994;71(4):507–10.

182. Corbacioglu S, Cesaro S, Faraci M, Valteau-Couanet D, Gruhn B, Rovelli A, et al. Defibrotide for prophylaxis of hepatic veno-occlusive disease in paediatric haemopoietic stem-cell transplantation: an open-label, phase 3, randomised controlled trial. Lancet. 2012;379(9823):1301–9.

183. Available from: www.gentium.com.

184. Richardson P, Tomblyn M, Kernan N, Brochstein JA, Mineishi S, Termuhlen A. Defibrotide (DF) in the treatment of severe hepatic veno-occlusive disease (VOD) with multi-organ failure (MOF) following stem cell transplantation (SCT): results of a phase 3 study utilizing a historical control. Blood. 2009;114:272a.

185. Kim ID, Egawa H, Marui Y, Kaihara S, Haga H, Lin YW, et al. A successful liver transplantation for refractory hepatic veno-occlusive disease originating from cord blood transplantation. Am J Transplant. 2002;2(8):796–800.

186. Koenecke C, Kleine M, Schrem H, Krug U, Nashan B, Neipp M, et al. Sinusoidal obstruction syndrome of the liver after hematopoietic stem cell transplantation: decision making for orthotopic liver transplantation. Int J Hematol. 2006;83(3):271–4.

187. Mellgren K, Fasth A, Saalman R, Olausson M, Abrahamsson J. Liver transplantation after stem cell transplantation with the same living donor in a monozygotic twin with acute myeloid leukemia. Ann Hematol. 2005;84(11):755–7.

188. Kleiner DE. Granulomas in the liver. Semin Diagn Pathol. 2006;23(3-4):161–9.

189. Ozaras R, Tahan V, Mert A, Uraz S, Kanat M, Tabak F, et al. The prevalence of hepatic granulomas in chronic hepatitis C. J Clin Gastroenterol. 2004;38(5):449–52.

190. Tahan V, Ozaras R, Lacevic N, Ozden E, Yemisen M, Ozdogan O, et al. Prevalence of hepatic granulomas in chronic hepatitis B. Dig Dis Sci. 2004;49(10):1575–7.

191. Klatskin G, Yesner R. Hepatic manifestations of sarcoidosis and other granulomatous diseases; a study based on histological examination of tissue obtained by needle biopsy of the liver. Yale J Biol Med. 1950;23(3):207–48.

192. Drebber U, Kasper HU, Ratering J, Wedemeyer I, Schirmacher P, Dienes HP, et al. Hepatic granulomas: histological and molecular pathological approach to differential diagnosis--a study of 442 cases. Liver Int. 2008;28(6):828–34.

193. Ayyala US, Padilla ML. Diagnosis and treatment of hepatic sarcoidosis. Curr Treat Options Gastroenterol. 2006;9(6):475–83.

194. Rybicki BA, Iannuzzi MC. Epidemiology of sarcoidosis: recent advances and future prospects. Semin Respir Crit Care Med. 2007;28(1):22–35.

195. Ebert EC, Nagar M. Gastrointestinal manifestations of amyloidosis. Am J Gastroenterol. 2008;103(3):776–87.

196. Studdy PR, Bird R. Serum angiotensin converting enzyme in sarcoidosis--its value in present clinical practice. Ann Clin Biochem. 1989;26(Pt 1):13–8.

197. Kaplan MM, Gershwin ME. Primary biliary cirrhosis. N Engl J Med. 2005;353(12):1261–73.

198. Poupon RE, Poupon R, Balkau B. Ursodiol for the long-term treatment of primary biliary cirrhosis. The UDCA-PBC Study Group. N Engl J Med. 1994;330(19):1342–7.
199. Maurer LH, Hughes RW, Folley JH, Mosenthal WT. Granulomatous hepatitis associated with regional enteritis. Gastroenterology. 1967;53:301–5.
200. Holl-Ulrich K, Klass M. Wegener s granulomatosis with granulomatous liver involvement. Clin Exp Rheumatol. 2010;28(1 Suppl 57):88–9.
201. Alvarez SZ, Carpio R. Hepatobiliary tuberculosis. Dig Dis Sci. 1983;28(3):193–200.
202. Horsburgh Jr CR. Mycobacterium avium complex infection in the acquired immunodeficiency syndrome. N Engl J Med. 1991;324(19):1332–8.
203. Hofmann CE, Heaton Jr JW. Q fever hepatitis. Gastroenterology. 1982;83(2):474–9.
204. Emile JF, Sebagh M, Feray C, David F, Reynes M. The presence of epithelioid granulomas in hepatitis C virus-related cirrhosis. Hum Pathol. 1993;24(10):1095–7.
205. Kanno A, Murakami K. A transient emergence of hepatic granulomas in a patient with chronic hepatitis B. Tohoku J Exp Med. 1998;185(4):281–5.
206. Chagnac A, Gal R, Kimche D, Zevin D, Machtey I, Levi J. Liver granulomas: a possible paraneoplastic manifestation of hypernephroma. Am J Gastroenterol. 1985;80(12):989–92.
207. Kadin ME, Donaldson SS, Dorfman RF. Isolated granulomas in Hodgkin's disease. N Engl J Med. 1970;283(16):859–61.
208. Co DO, Hogan LH, Il-Kim S, Sandor M. T cell contributions to the different phases of granuloma formation. Immunol Lett. 2004;92(1-2):135–42.
209. Bodar EJ, Drenth JP, van der Meer JW, Simon A. Dysregulation of innate immunity: hereditary periodic fever syndromes. Br J Haematol. 2009;144(3):279–302.
210. Ando Y, Nakamura M, Araki S. Transthyretin-related familial amyloidotic polyneuropathy. Arch Neurol. 2005;62(7):1057–62.
211. Buck FS, Koss MN. Hepatic amyloidosis: morphologic differences between systemic AL and AA types. Hum Pathol. 1991;22(9):904–7.
212. Iwata T, Hoshii Y, Kawano H, Gondo T, Takahashi M, Ishihara T, et al. Hepatic amyloidosis in Japan: histological and morphometric analysis based on amyloid proteins. Hum Pathol. 1995;26(10):1148–53.
213. Levine RA. Amyloid disease of the liver. Correlation of clinical, functional and morphologic features in forty-seven patients. Am J Med. 1962;33:349–57.
214. Serra L, Poppi MC, Criscuolo M, Zandomeneghi R. Primary systemic amyloidosis with giant hepatomegaly and portal hypertension: a case report and a review of the literature. Ital J Gastroenterol. 1993;25(8):435–8.
215. Zeijen RN, Sels JP, Flendrig JA, Arends JW. Portal hypertension and intrahepatic cholestasis in hepatic amyloidosis. Neth J Med. 1991;38(5-6):257–61.
216. Park MA, Mueller PS, Kyle RA, Larson DR, Plevak MF, Gertz MA. Primary (AL) hepatic amyloidosis: clinical features and natural history in 98 patients. Medicine. 2003;82(5):291–8.
217. Kim SH, Han JK, Lee KH, Won HJ, Kim KW, Kim JS, et al. Abdominal amyloidosis: spectrum of radiological findings. Clin Radiol. 2003;58(8):610–20.
218. Harrison RF, Hawkins PN, Roche WR, MacMahon RF, Hubscher SG, Buckels JA. 'Fragile' liver and massive hepatic haemorrhage due to hereditary amyloidosis. Gut. 1996;38(1):151–2.
219. Kuroda T, Otaki Y, Sato H, Fujimura T, Nakatsue T, Murakami S, et al. A case of AA amyloidosis associated with rheumatoid arthritis effectively treated with Infliximab. Rheumatol Int. 2008;28(11):1155–9.
220. Farhangi M, Thakur VM, Durham JB. Objective response in amyloidosis treated with intermittent chemotherapy. South Med J. 1984;77(6):775–7.
221. Benson MD. Liver transplantation and transthyretin amyloidosis. Muscle Nerve. 2013;47(2):157–62.
222. Suhr OB, Herlenius G, Friman S, Ericzon BG. Liver transplantation for hereditary transthyretin amyloidosis. Liver Transpl. 2000;6(3):263–76.
223. Okamoto S, Wixner J, Obayashi K, Ando Y, Ericzon BG, Friman S, et al. Liver transplantation for familial amyloidotic polyneuropathy: impact on Swedish patients' survival. Liver Transpl. 2009;15(10):1229–35.

224. Yamashita T, Ando Y, Okamoto S, Misumi Y, Hirahara T, Ueda M, et al. Long-term survival after liver transplantation in patients with familial amyloid polyneuropathy. Neurology. 2012;78(9):637–43.
225. Barreiros AP, Geber C, Birklein F, Galle PR, Otto G. Clinical symptomatic de novo systemic transthyretin amyloidosis 9 years after domino liver transplantation. Liver Transpl. 2010;16(1):109.
226. Bolte FJ, Schmidt HH, Becker T, Braun F, Pascher A, Klempnauer J, et al. Evaluation of domino liver transplantations in Germany. Transpl Int. 2013;26(7):715–23.
227. Goto T, Yamashita T, Ueda M, Ohshima S, Yoneyama K, Nakamura M, et al. Iatrogenic amyloid neuropathy in a Japanese patient after sequential liver transplantation. Am J Transplant. 2006;6(10):2512–5.

Part III
Care of the Cirrhotic Patient

Chapter 27
Portal Hypertension

Douglas A. Simonetto and Vijay H. Shah

Commonly Encountered Patient Questions and Answers

1. What is portal hypertension and what causes it?

    Portal hypertension means elevated pressures in the vascular system responsible for draining the venous blood from the intestines, stomach, pancreas, and spleen into the liver. The most common cause of portal hypertension is cirrhosis ("scarring") of the liver, which in turn is a result of chronic injury or inflammation, such as alcohol abuse, viral hepatitis, fatty liver, etc. The cirrhotic liver becomes shrunken and hard from scarring, limiting the passage of the incoming venous blood thus resulting in portal hypertension. Other causes of portal hypertension include clotting of the veins draining in or out of the liver and uncommon conditions such as sarcoidosis, amyloidosis, lymphoma, etc. Occasionally, the cause of portal hypertension is not identified and called idiopathic noncirrhotic portal hypertension.

2. What are the consequences of portal hypertension?

    The most important consequence of portal hypertension is the formation of gastroesophageal varices. Given the increased pressures, the blood draining from the gastrointestinal tract tries to find an alternative route to bypass the stiff and shrunken liver (collaterals). One of these routes goes through small veins in the stomach and esophagus, turning them into large varicose veins filled with blood. The most dreadful complication of portal hypertension is rupture of these varicose veins, which may result in vomiting of blood in large volumes. This complication can be prevented with medications or endoscopic therapies. Another important consequence of portal hypertension is the development of hepatic encephalopathy. One important

D.A. Simonetto, M.D. • V.H. Shah, M.D. (✉)
Department of Gastroenterology and Hepatology, Mayo Clinic Hospital,
Guggenheim 10-21, 200 First ST SW, Rochester, MN 55905, USA
e-mail: shah.vijay@mayo.edu

© Springer International Publishing Switzerland 2017
K. Saeian, R. Shaker (eds.), *Liver Disorders*,
DOI 10.1007/978-3-319-30103-7_27

function of the liver is to clear toxins from the blood, absorbed in the intestines. However, the blood coming from the intestines, containing toxins, now is bypassing the liver through collaterals. These toxins then can reach the brain and lead to confusion, disorientation, daytime sleepiness and, when severe, even coma.

3. How do I know if I have portal hypertension?

There are invasive and noninvasive ways of diagnosing portal hypertension. The noninvasive methods are preferred given their safety and lower costs. Imaging tests, such as ultrasound of the abdomen, can reveal an enlarged spleen. This finding is very suggestive of portal hypertension as the spleen becomes engorged with extra blood that cannot be drained through the cirrhotic liver. Low platelet count is often noted on blood tests, as platelets are getting trapped on the now enlarged spleen. Measuring the stiffness of the liver or the spleen, with magnetic resonance or ultrasound can be used as well to help diagnose portal hypertension. An important test, not only helpful to diagnose portal hypertension, but to detect esophageal varices (varicose veins in the esophagus) is upper endoscopy. During this procedure, an endoscope (long slender instrument with a camera on the tip) is introduced through the mouth and driven down to the esophagus and stomach. The presence of esophageal varices confirms the diagnosis of portal hypertension and their finding is important so preventive measures can be instituted to avoid their rupture and bleeding. Finally, the most accurate way of diagnosing portal hypertension is by directly measuring the pressure in the veins inside and outside the liver. This test is not routinely used given its associated risks and cost; however it may be required in certain circumstances.

Introduction

Portal hypertension refers to a pathologic pressure elevation of the splanchnic veins draining to the liver and it is defined by an increase of the portal pressure gradient (difference in pressure between the portal vein and the inferior vena cava) above the normal range of 1–5 mmHg. Development of portal hypertension is one of the most important events in the progression of liver cirrhosis and it is a cause of significant morbidity and mortality in this population [1]. Complications directly related to portal hypertension include variceal bleeding, ascites, and hepatic encephalopathy, all of which will be reviewed in the following chapters. Therefore, assessment of portal hypertension is clinically important for risk stratification and patient management. This is an area of ongoing research as we attempt to identify less-invasive, inexpensive, and reproducible methods for diagnosis of portal hypertension. This chapter will focus on the pathophysiology, causes, and assessment of portal hypertension.

Pathophysiology

The primary factor in the development of portal hypertension is an increased resistance of portal venous flow. In cirrhosis, the most common cause of portal hypertension worldwide, the formation of fibrous tissue and regenerative nodules hinders the portal blood flow through the liver. Besides this structural factor, a dynamic and potentially reversible component was demonstrated in 1985 by Bhathal and Grossman [2]. In this study, the authors demonstrated that the use of nitroprusside was able to partially reduce the portal pressure. This dynamic component accounts for 30 % of the increased intrahepatic resistance in cirrhosis and it results from the contraction of activated hepatic stellate cells and myofibroblasts surrounding the hepatic sinusoids. This model allowed for the subsequent discovery of a number of vasoactive substances and drugs able to modify the intrahepatic vascular resistance. Disequilibrium between the production and response of vasoconstrictors (endothelins, thromboxanes, angiotensin II, etc.) and vasodilators (mainly, nitric oxide) was subsequently demonstrated (Fig. 27.1).

The second contributing factor to portal hypertension results from increased portal-collateral blood flow. The hyperdynamic circulatory state in cirrhosis was first described in 1953 by Abelmann and Kowaski [3]. They demonstrated that

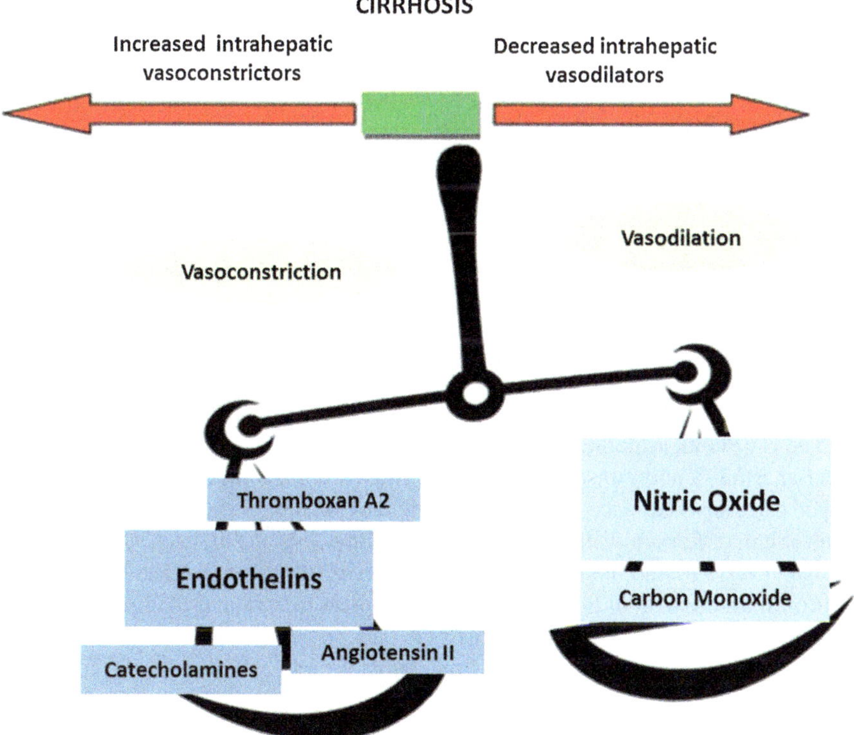

Fig. 27.1 Imbalance of vasoconstrictors and vasodilators in cirrhosis

patients with alcoholic cirrhosis presented with increased cardiac output and reduced peripheral vascular resistance. Vasodilation of the splanchnic circulation was later demonstrated and found to be a result of increased systemic levels of vasodilator substances and local hyporesponsiveness to vasoconstrictors. The increase of blood flow into the portal system is responsible for maintenance and further aggravation of portal hypertension.

Neoangiogenesis—formation of new blood vessels—, resultant of vascular endothelial growth factor (VEGF) release, also plays a major role in the development of a hyperkinetic state and the formation of porto-systemic collaterals. Unfortunately, these collaterals are not able to fully accommodate the excess flow or alleviate the portal pressure and they lead to one of the most dreaded complications of portal hypertension, the development of esophageal varices.

Assessment of Portal Hypertension

The direct measurement of portal pressure, which in normal individuals ranges from 7 to 12 mmHg [4], can be accomplished via transhepatic or transvenous catheterization of the portal vein. However these methods harbor a significant risk of complications, including intraperitoneal bleed, and are no longer performed, except in selected cases [5]. In recent years, many advances have been made in the assessment of portal hypertension with the goal of identifying less-invasive and reproducible diagnostic methods. Below we review the currently used methods and future directions.

Hepatic Venous Pressure Gradient

Portal hypertension can be accurately determined by the pressure gradient between the portal vein and the inferior vena cava, measured by the hepatic venous gradient pressure (HVPG). This gradient represents the actual liver portal perfusion pressure, which in normal individuals ranges from 1 to 5 mmHg [1].

The HVPG measurement is a safe and reproducible technique performed under local anesthesia and conscious sedation. Under fluoroscopic guidance a balloon-tipped catheter is advanced into the main right hepatic vein via the internal jugular, antecubital, or femoral vein. HVPG is then calculated as the difference between the wedged (WHVP) and the free (FHVP) hepatic venous pressures. The WHVP is an indirect measurement of the hepatic sinusoidal pressure which provides a good estimate of the portal vein pressure in cirrhotic patients [6–8]. The WHVP is obtained by inflating the balloon at the tip of the catheter and occluding the hepatic vein. FHVP is measured by maintaining the tip of the catheter floating freely in the hepatic vein, about 2–4 cm distal to the IVC.

Accuracy in HVPG measurement is extremely important and therefore several recommendations have been published to assure adequate measurements [9]. The operators should wait for stabilization of the venous pressures, at 60 s for WHVP and 20 s for FHVP. All measurements should be permanently recorded or printed to allow for later review of the tracings. Also important is to obtain at least duplicate and ideally triplicate measurements, to ensure accurate results. Significant variability is suggestive of errors.

As mentioned above, HVPG measurement is a safe procedure with no absolute contraindications. Caution should be exerted in patients with a history of cardiac arrhythmias when moving the catheter through the right atrium. Also, coagulopathies are common in cirrhotic patients and may require correction prior to the procedure according to individual center's guidelines. Allergy to iodine contrast is not a contraindication as CO_2 may be used or patients may be premedicated with systemic steroids. The risk of complications is small (<1 %) and are usually related to the venous puncture site. The use of ultrasound assistance helps to decrease the risk of complications [10].

HVPG is considered the gold standard test for diagnosis of portal hypertension. Recently, HVPG has been also utilized for prognostic evaluation, monitoring response to therapy and determining the etiology or classification of portal hypertension.

HVPG and Diagnosis of Portal Hypertension

As mentioned earlier, the HVPG in normal subjects ranges from 1 to 5 mmHg. HVPG values greater than 10 mmHg correspond to clinically significant portal hypertension, characterized by the development of esophageal varices and/or ascites. Values between 6 and 9 mmHg correspond to subclinical portal hypertension [11]. Unfortunately, HVPG is not widely available and therefore, it is not utilized routinely in most centers for the sole diagnosis of portal hypertension. The exception are patients undergoing a transjugular liver biopsy, where the HVPG can be easily obtained with little added cost or risks.

HVPG and Classification of Portal Hypertension

In addition to cirrhosis, portal hypertension can be caused by myriad conditions which can be classified according to their anatomical location: prehepatic, intrahepatic, or posthepatic (Table 27.1). Intrahepatic portal hypertension, most commonly caused by cirrhosis, presents with elevated HVPG, resultant of increased WHVP and normal FHVP. In prehepatic or presinusoidal portal hypertension both the WHVP and the FHVP are normal resulting in a normal HVPG. Whereas, in posthepatic portal hypertension, both the WHVP and FHVP are elevated.

Table 27.1 Hepatic venous pressure gradient in the classification of portal hypertension

Types of portal hypertension	Wedged (WHVP)	Free (FHVP)	Gradient (HVPG)
Prehepatic	Normal	Normal	Normal
Intrahepatic			
Pre-sinusoidal	Normal	Normal	Normal
Sinusoidal	Increased	Normal	Increased
Post-sinusoidal	Increased	Normal	Increased
Posthepatic	Increased	Increased	Normal

HVPG and Prognosis in Portal Hypertension

Several studies have correlated the HVPG values with different outcomes in portal hypertension secondary to cirrhosis. The development of gastroesophageal varices is noted when HVPG values are above 10 mmHg, whereas variceal bleeding typically ensues when HVPG is above 12 mmHg [12–14]. HVPG has also been shown to be a good predictor of survival, with values above 16 mmHg in alcoholic cirrhosis associated with increased mortality [15]. HVPG above 20 mmHg within 48 h of an acute variceal bleed episode was also associated with poor outcomes and low 1-year survival [16]. When adjusted by MELD score, presence of ascites, encephalopathy, and age, HVPG remained as an independent prognostic variable with an increased in mortality risk of 3 % for each 1 mmHg increase in the gradient [17]. HVPG has also been studied in preoperative risk assessment of hepatic decompensation in patients undergoing hepatoma resection. HVPG levels above 10 mmHg were associated with persistent decompensation 3 months after surgery [18].

Acute alcoholic hepatitis leads to a significant temporary rise in portal pressure, likely driven by a robust inflammatory response [19, 20]. HVPG values greater than 22 mmHg were independently associated with higher in-hospital mortality [21]. Finally, HVPG has also been found to be an independent predictor of the development of hepatocellular carcinoma, when values are above 10 mmHg [22].

HVPG and Treatment Response in Portal Hypertension

The use of pharmacological therapy to prevent recurrent variceal bleeding was first demonstrated in 1984 by Lebrec et al. [23]. They found that daily administration of propranolol, a nonselective beta-blocker, at doses reducing the heart rate by 25 %, was able to consistently decrease the HVPG values compared to placebo [24]. HVPG has since been used in clinical studies to assess the effects of vasoactive drugs in portal hypertension.

A clinically significant hemodynamic response has been defined by a reduction of HVPG by at least 20 % from baseline or to values below 12 mmHg. When at least one of these goals are achieved, either with pharmacological therapy [25]

or spontaneously [26], the risk of first or recurrent variceal bleed decreases to less than 10%, compared to 20–50% in nonresponders. In addition to variceal bleed prevention, studies have demonstrated a significant reduction in ascites and spontaneous bacterial peritonitis when these hemodynamic parameters are reached [27, 28]. Finally, the effect of hemodynamic response on improvement of survival has been well demonstrated and adjusted for improvement in liver function [27, 29, 30].

The timing and frequency of HVPG monitoring, however, has not been well established. Most studies have repeated HVPG measurement in 1–3 months after a bleeding episode, whereas the highest risk for rebleeding is within the first several days. Therefore a high proportion of patients (30–40%) had to be excluded from the studies due to early death or rebleeding. Also, repeated measurements of HVPG have been suggested not to be a cost-effective approach in clinical practice [31].

Endoscopic Assessment of Portal Hypertension

Given limited availability, cost and invasiveness of HVPG measurement, esophagogastroduodenoscopy (EGD) or upper endoscopy remains the most widely used test in clinical practice for assessment of portal hypertension and its complications, including esophageal varices, gastric varices, and portal hypertensive gastropathy (PHG). The role of endoscopy in the diagnosis and management of gastroesophageal varices will be reviewed in later chapters. At the present time, endoscopy is still recommended at diagnosis of cirrhosis although esophageal varices are present in only approximately 30–40% of patients with compensated cirrhosis [32]. In the future, less-invasive and inexpensive methods may become available and validated for assessment of portal hypertension and risk stratification. In that case, we may be able to determine which patients may benefit from endoscopic assessment of varices based on the presence and/or severity of portal hypertension.

Physical Examination

On first assessment of patients with chronic liver disease, the physical examination may provide diagnostic clues for the presence of portal hypertension and cirrhosis. The findings of splenomegaly, telangiectasias, abdominal wall varicosities (caput medusae), encephalopathy (e.g. asterixis), and ascites are highly specific (range 75–98%) but have low sensitivity (range 15–68%) for diagnosis of cirrhosis, especially in the compensated state [33]. The presence of telangiectasias or spider angiomata, in addition to laboratory parameters discussed below, was a fair predictor of the presence of esophageal varices in compensated cirrhosis [34].

Biochemical Parameters

Laboratory studies have been extensively investigated, either isolated or in combination with other parameters, in the assessment of portal hypertension and gastroesophageal varices. The combination of serum albumin, bilirubin, and INR, as used in the Child-Turcotte-Pugh score have been shown to correlate with HVPG levels greater than 20 mmHg [35]. A model combining serum albumin, ALT, and INR was able to predict the presence of clinically significant portal hypertension (HVPG > 10 mmHg) with 93 % sensitivity and 61 % specificity, and an area under the curve (AUC) of 0.952. Otherwise, thrombocytopenia (with platelet count less than 88,000) has been the only parameter most frequently associated with the presence of large esophageal or gastric varices [36]. Several different combinations of laboratory markers have been evaluated to determine the presence or stage of liver fibrosis. The aspartate aminotransferase/platelet ratio index (APRI), a well validated noninvasive tool for diagnosis of liver fibrosis/cirrhosis, has been recently tested in the assessment of clinically significant portal hypertension. APRI greater than 1.09 demonstrated 66 % sensitivity and 73 % specificity for predicting clinically significant portal hypertension (HVPG > 12 mmHg) and an area under the curve (AUC) of 0.716 [37].

Other fibrosis markers, including the presence of circulating endothelial cells (CEC) and CEC/platelet count index, have not been specifically evaluated in the assessment of portal hypertension however they may have a role also in this setting [38, 39]. Serum laminin levels have been shown to correlate well with HVPG values; however its diagnostic accuracy for HVPG greater than 12 mmHg was only 70 % [40]. Similar results have been obtained with measurement of serum hyaluronic acid levels [41].

FibroTest, a commercially available panel of biochemical markers of fibrosis, has also been shown to correlate well with HVPG [42]. However the area under the receiver operating characteristic curves (AUROC) for the diagnosis of severe portal hypertension (HVPG greater than 12 mmHg) was only 0.79, equivalent to that of platelet count and Child-Turcotte-Pugh score.

Abdominal Imaging

Imaging studies, such as ultrasound, magnetic resonance imaging, or computed tomography, are able to identify morphologic features of liver cirrhosis and signs of portal hypertension. While splenomegaly is a sensitive sign of portal hypertension, it markedly lacks specificity [34]. Contrastingly, the presence of portal-systemic collaterals, such as paraumbilical vein recanalization, spleno-renal collaterals, and dilated left short gastric veins, are virtually a 100 % specific for clinically significant portal hypertension, however their sensitivity is limited, especially in compensated cirrhosis [43, 44].

Liver Stiffness

Assessment of liver stiffness, mainly by transient elastography, has been demonstrated to correlate with the presence of portal hypertension [45]. Liver stiffness is mainly determined by the presence of fibrosis, which in turn leads to development of portal hypertension by increasing the intrahepatic resistance to portal blood flow. Recently, liver stiffness, measured by magnetic resonance elastography, has been directly correlated with elevated portal pressure, in the absence of fibrosis, in an animal model of posthepatic portal hypertension [46].

Transient elastography (TE) has been first demonstrated to correlate with HVPG in patients with viral hepatitic C recurrence post liver transplantation [47]. The AUROCs for the diagnosis of portal hypertension (HVPG > 6 mmHg) and clinically significant portal hypertension (HVPG > 12 mmHg) were 0.93 and 0.94, respectively. Interestingly, the correlation of liver stiffness and HVPG was only significant for values below 12 mmHg [48]. This suggests that further increase in portal pressure, becomes almost independent from fibrosis progression as assessed by liver stiffness. A recent meta-analysis including 18 studies and 3644 patients, demonstrated TE to be a good screening tool for diagnosis of clinically significant portal hypertension (HVPG > 10 mmHg) with 90 % sensitivity and 79 % specificity. The role of TE in diagnosis of esophageal varices, however, was not as promising with a sensitivity of 87 % but specificity of only 53 % [49]. Finally, TE cannot be obtained or provides unreliable results in 3–16 % of cases, mostly due to obesity or presence of ascites [50].

Magnetic resonance elastography (MRE) has become a safe, noninvasive, and reliable tool in predicting advanced fibrosis or cirrhosis [51]. Its use in the assessment of portal hypertension has not been extensively explored; however recent studies have suggested a correlation of liver MRE with HVPG results [52].

Finally, the combination of different noninvasive tests, including liver stiffness, spleen diameter, and platelet count, has been proposed with promising results. The portal hypertension risk score was calculated with the formula: $5.953 + 0.188 \times$ liver stiffness $+ 1.583 \times$ sex (1: male; 0: female) $+ 26.705 \times$ spleen diameter/platelet count ratio. In patients with compensated cirrhosis, this model demonstrated an AUROC of 0.935 [44].

Spleen Stiffness

Splenomegaly is a specific feature of portal hypertension, and therefore spleen stiffness has recently been explored as a new noninvasive tool for estimating portal pressure. Measurement of spleen stiffness by transient elastography was superior to liver stiffness, liver stiffness-spleen diameter to platelet count ratio and platelet count to spleen diameter ratio, in both the assessment of clinically significant portal hypertension and the presence of gastroesophageal varices [53]. Finally, assessment of viscoelastic parameters of the spleen by MRE was superior to liver MRE in detection of severe portal hypertension (HVPG > 12 mmHg) with an AUROC of 0.81 [52].

Etiology

In addition to cirrhosis, portal hypertension can be caused by a myriad of conditions which can be classified according to their anatomical location: prehepatic, intrahepatic, or posthepatic (Table 27.2).

Prehepatic

The most common cause of prehepatic portal hypertension is portal vein thrombosis (PVT). In the absence of cirrhosis, portal vein thrombosis usually results from a combination of prothrombotic and local factors. Common thrombophilic disorders associated with PVT include primary myeloproliferative disorders, antithrombin, or

Table 27.2 Causes of portal hypertension

Prehepatic
Portal vein thrombosis
Splenic vein thrombosis
Intrahepatic
Presinusoidal
Schistosomiasis
Idiopathic noncirrhotic portal hypertension
Primary biliary cirrhosis
Sarcoidosis
Congenital hepatic fibrosis
Nodular Regenerative Hyperplasia
Adult polycystic liver disease
Sinusoidal
Cirrhosis
Amyloidosis
Zellweger syndrome
Gaucher's disease
Vinyl Chloride toxicity
Postsinusoidal
Sinusoidal obstruction syndrome (veno-occlusive disease)
Posthepatic
Budd-Chiari syndrome
Cardiac disease (constrictive pericarditis, right sided heart failure, restrictive cardiomyopathy)

protein S deficiency, antiphospholipid syndrome, hyperhomocysteinemia, factor V Leiden, and factor II G20210 mutations. Local factors precipitating or favoring PVT include local inflammatory processes (neonatal omphalitis, pancreatitis, appendicitis, diverticulitis, peptic ulcer disease, sepsis, etc.), or injury to the portal vein system (splenectomy, colectomy, gastrectomy, etc.) [54]. Management of acute or chronic portal vein thrombosis includes the use of anticoagulation, which should be long-term if permanent prothrombotic conditions are identified [55].

Intrahepatic

Intrahepatic causes of portal hypertension can be further divided according to the location of increased vascular resistance: presinusoidal, sinusoidal, or postsinusoidal. Presinusoidal portal hypertension is characterized by fairly normal WVHP and FHVP, and therefore with normal or slightly elevated HVPG. The main causes of presinusoidal portal hypertension include nodular regenerative hyperplasia, schistosomiasis, sarcoidosis, primary biliary cirrhosis, autoimmune cholangiopathy, congenital hepatic fibrosis, tuberculosis, adult polycystic disease, and lymphoma.

The most common cause of sinusoidal portal hypertension is cirrhosis, but it can also result from infiltrative conditions (amyloidosis, mastocytosis, Gaucher's disease, etc.). Finally, postsinusoidal portal hypertension is usually caused by veno-occlusive disease, also called hepatic sinusoidal obstruction syndrome. Both, sinusoidal and postsinusoidal portal hypertension are characterized by elevated WHVP with normal FHVP, therefore resulting in high HVPG [56].

Posthepatic

The most frequent causes of posthepatic portal hypertension are Budd-Chiari syndrome and cardiac conditions (such as constrictive pericarditis, restrictive cardiomyopathy, complex congenital heart disease, and Fontan physiology). Posthepatic portal hypertension is characterized by a normal HVPG, with elevated WHVP and FHVP values.

Acknowledgments We acknowledge the American Association for the Study of Liver Diseases Foundation for the funding support through the Advanced/Transplant Hepatology Fellowship Award.

References

1. Gadano A, Hadengue A, Vachiery F, Moreau R, Sogni P, Soupison T, et al. Relationship between hepatic blood flow, liver tests, haemodynamic values and clinical characteristics in patients with chronic liver disease. J Gastroenterol Hepatol. 1997;12:167–71.
2. Bhathal PS, Grossman HJ. Reduction of the increased portal vascular resistance of the isolated perfused cirrhotic rat liver by vasodilators. J Hepatol. 1985;1:325–37.

3. Kowalski HJ, Abelmann WH. The cardiac output at rest in Laennec's cirrhosis. J Clin Invest. 1953;32:1025–33.

4. Lebrec D, Sogni P, Vilgrain V. Evaluation of patients with portal hypertension. Baillieres Clin Gastroenterol. 1997;11:221–41.

5. Lunderquist A, Vang J. Transhepatic catheterization and obliteration of the coronary vein in patients with portal hypertension and esophageal varices. N Engl J Med. 1974;291:646–9.

6. Perello A, Escorsell A, Bru C, Gilabert R, Moitinho E, Garcia-Pagan JC, et al. Wedged hepatic venous pressure adequately reflects portal pressure in hepatitis C virus-related cirrhosis. Hepatology. 1999;30:1393–7.

7. Iwao T, Toyonaga A, Ikegami M, Sumino M, Oho K, Sakaki M, et al. Wedged hepatic venous pressure reflects portal venous pressure during vasoactive drug administration in nonalcoholic cirrhosis. Dig Dis Sci. 1994;39:2439–44.

8. Thalheimer U, Leandro G, Samonakis DN, Triantos CK, Patch D, Burroughs AK. Assessment of the agreement between wedge hepatic vein pressure and portal vein pressure in cirrhotic patients. Dig Liver Dis. 2005;37:601–8.

9. Groszmann RJ, Wongcharatrawee S. The hepatic venous pressure gradient: anything worth doing should be done right. Hepatology. 2004;39:280–2.

10. Bosch J, Abraldes JG, Berzigotti A, Garcia-Pagan JC. The clinical use of HVPG measurements in chronic liver disease. Nat Rev Gastroenterol Hepatol. 2009;6:573–82.

11. Groszmann RJ, Bosch J, Grace ND, Conn HO, Garcia-Tsao G, Navasa M, et al. Hemodynamic events in a prospective randomized trial of propranolol versus placebo in the prevention of a first variceal hemorrhage. Gastroenterology. 1990;99:1401–7.

12. Garcia-Tsao G, Groszmann RJ, Fisher RL, Conn HO, Atterbury CE, Glickman M. Portal pressure, presence of gastroesophageal varices and variceal bleeding. Hepatology. 1985;5:419–24.

13. Merkel C, Bolognesi M, Bellon S, Zuin R, Noventa F, Finucci G, et al. Prognostic usefulness of hepatic vein catheterization in patients with cirrhosis and esophageal varices. Gastroenterology. 1992;102:973–9.

14. Lebrec D, De Fleury P, Rueff B, Nahum H, Benhamou JP. Portal hypertension, size of esophageal varices, and risk of gastrointestinal bleeding in alcoholic cirrhosis. Gastroenterology. 1980;79:1139–44.

15. Stanley AJ, Robinson I, Forrest EH, Jones AL, Hayes PC. Haemodynamic parameters predicting variceal haemorrhage and survival in alcoholic cirrhosis. QJM. 1998;91:19–25.

16. Moitinho E, Escorsell A, Bandi JC, Salmeron JM, Garcia-Pagan JC, Rodes J, et al. Prognostic value of early measurements of portal pressure in acute variceal bleeding. Gastroenterology. 1999;117:626–31.

17. Ripoll C, Banares R, Rincon D, Catalina MV, Lo Iacono O, Salcedo M, et al. Influence of hepatic venous pressure gradient on the prediction of survival of patients with cirrhosis in the MELD Era. Hepatology. 2005;42:793–801.

18. Bruix J, Castells A, Bosch J, Feu F, Fuster J, Garcia-Pagan JC, et al. Surgical resection of hepatocellular carcinoma in cirrhotic patients: prognostic value of preoperative portal pressure. Gastroenterology. 1996;111:1018–22.

19. Poynard T, Degott C, Munoz C, Lebrec D. Relationship between degree of portal hypertension and liver histologic lesions in patients with alcoholic cirrhosis. Effect of acute alcoholic hepatitis on portal hypertension. Dig Dis Sci. 1987;32:337–43.

20. Sen S, Mookerjee RP, Cheshire LM, Davies NA, Williams R, Jalan R. Albumin dialysis reduces portal pressure acutely in patients with severe alcoholic hepatitis. J Hepatol. 2005;43:142–8.

21. Rincon D, Lo Iacono O, Ripoll C, Gomez-Camarero J, Salcedo M, Catalina MV, et al. Prognostic value of hepatic venous pressure gradient for in-hospital mortality of patients with severe acute alcoholic hepatitis. Aliment Pharmacol Ther. 2007;25:841–8.

22. Ripoll C, Groszmann RJ, Garcia-Tsao G, Bosch J, Grace N, Burroughs A, et al. Hepatic venous pressure gradient predicts development of hepatocellular carcinoma independently of severity of cirrhosis. J Hepatol. 2009;50:923–8.

23. Lebrec D, Poynard T, Bernuau J, Bercoff E, Nouel O, Capron JP, et al. A randomized controlled study of propranolol for prevention of recurrent gastrointestinal bleeding in patients with cirrhosis: a final report. Hepatology. 1984;4:355–8.
24. Lebrec D, Hillon P, Munoz C, Goldfarb G, Nouel O, Benhamou JP. The effect of propranolol on portal hypertension in patients with cirrhosis: a hemodynamic study. Hepatology. 1982;2:523–7.
25. Feu F, Garcia-Pagan JC, Bosch J, Luca A, Teres J, Escorsell A, et al. Relation between portal pressure response to pharmacotherapy and risk of recurrent variceal haemorrhage in patients with cirrhosis. Lancet. 1995;346:1056–9.
26. Vorobioff J, Groszmann RJ, Picabea E, Gamen M, Villavicencio R, Bordato J, et al. Prognostic value of hepatic venous pressure gradient measurements in alcoholic cirrhosis: a 10-year prospective study. Gastroenterology. 1996;111:701–9.
27. Abraldes JG, Tarantino I, Turnes J, Garcia-Pagan JC, Rodes J, Bosch J. Hemodynamic response to pharmacological treatment of portal hypertension and long-term prognosis of cirrhosis. Hepatology. 2003;37:902–8.
28. Villanueva C, Lopez-Balaguer JM, Aracil C, Kolle L, Gonzalez B, Minana J, et al. Maintenance of hemodynamic response to treatment for portal hypertension and influence on complications of cirrhosis. J Hepatol. 2004;40:757–65.
29. Merkel C, Bolognesi M, Sacerdoti D, Bombonato G, Bellini B, Bighin R, et al. The hemodynamic response to medical treatment of portal hypertension as a predictor of clinical effectiveness in the primary prophylaxis of variceal bleeding in cirrhosis. Hepatology. 2000;32:930–4.
30. Villanueva C, Minana J, Ortiz J, Gallego A, Soriano G, Torras X, et al. Endoscopic ligation compared with combined treatment with nadolol and isosorbide mononitrate to prevent recurrent variceal bleeding. N Engl J Med. 2001;345:647–55.
31. Hicken BL, Sharara AI, Abrams GA, Eloubeidi M, Fallon MB, Arguedas MR. Hepatic venous pressure gradient measurements to assess response to primary prophylaxis in patients with cirrhosis: a decision analytical study. Aliment Pharmacol Ther. 2003;17:145–53.
32. de Franchis R. Revising consensus in portal hypertension: report of the Baveno V consensus workshop on methodology of diagnosis and therapy in portal hypertension. J Hepatol. 2010;53:762–8.
33. de Bruyn G, Graviss EA. A systematic review of the diagnostic accuracy of physical examination for the detection of cirrhosis. BMC Med Inform Decis Mak. 2001;1:6.
34. Berzigotti A, Gilabert R, Abraldes JG, Nicolau C, Bru C, Bosch J, et al. Noninvasive prediction of clinically significant portal hypertension and esophageal varices in patients with compensated liver cirrhosis. Am J Gastroenterol. 2008;103:1159–67.
35. Abraldes JG, Villanueva C, Banares R, Aracil C, Catalina MV, Garci APJC, et al. Hepatic venous pressure gradient and prognosis in patients with acute variceal bleeding treated with pharmacologic and endoscopic therapy. J Hepatol. 2008;48:229–36.
36. Zaman A, Hapke R, Flora K, Rosen HR, Benner K. Factors predicting the presence of esophageal or gastric varices in patients with advanced liver disease. Am J Gastroenterol. 1999;94:3292–6.
37. Verma V, Sarin SK, Sharma P, Kumar A. Correlation of aspartate aminotransferase/platelet ratio index with hepatic venous pressure gradient in cirrhosis. United European Gastroenterol J. 2014;2:226–31.
38. Abdelmoneim SS, Talwalkar J, Sethi S, Kamath P, Fathalla MM, Kipp BR, et al. A prospective pilot study of circulating endothelial cells as a potential new biomarker in portal hypertension. Liver Int. 2010;30:191–7.
39. Sethi S, Simonetto DA, Abdelmoneim SS, Campion MB, Kaloiani I, Clayton AC, et al. Comparison of circulating endothelial cell/platelet count ratio to aspartate transaminase/platelet ratio index for identifying patients with cirrhosis. J Clin Exp Hepatol. 2012;2:19–26.
40. Kondo M, Miszputen SJ, Leite-mor MM, Parise ER. The predictive value of serum laminin for the risk of variceal bleeding related to portal pressure levels. Hepatogastroenterology. 1995;42:542–5.

41. Kropf J, Gressner AM, Tittor W. Logistic-regression model for assessing portal hypertension by measuring hyaluronic acid (hyaluronan) and laminin in serum. Clin Chem. 1991;37:30–5.
42. Thabut D, Imbert-Bismut F, Cazals-Hatem D, Messous D, Muntenau M, Valla DC, et al. Relationship between the Fibrotest and portal hypertension in patients with liver disease. Aliment Pharmacol Ther. 2007;26:359–68.
43. Vilgrain V, Lebrec D, Menu Y, Scherrer A, Nahum H. Comparison between ultrasonographic signs and the degree of portal hypertension in patients with cirrhosis. Gastrointest Radiol. 1990;15:218–22.
44. Berzigotti A, Seijo S, Arena U, Abraldes JG, Vizzutti F, Garcia-Pagan JC, et al. Elastography, spleen size, and platelet count identify portal hypertension in patients with compensated cirrhosis. Gastroenterology. 2013;144:102–111.e1.
45. Castera L, Pinzani M, Bosch J. Non invasive evaluation of portal hypertension using transient elastography. J Hepatol. 2012;56:696–703.
46. Simonetto DA, Yang HY, Yin M, de Assuncao TM, Kwon JH, Hilscher M, et al. Chronic passive venous congestion drives hepatic fibrogenesis via sinusoidal thrombosis and mechanical forces. Hepatology. 2015;61:648–59.
47. Carrion JA, Navasa M, Bosch J, Bruguera M, Gilabert R, Forns X. Transient elastography for diagnosis of advanced fibrosis and portal hypertension in patients with hepatitis C recurrence after liver transplantation. Liver Transpl. 2006;12:1791–8.
48. Vizzutti F, Arena U, Romanelli RG, Rega L, Foschi M, Colagrande S, et al. Liver stiffness measurement predicts severe portal hypertension in patients with HCV-related cirrhosis. Hepatology. 2007;45:1290–7.
49. Shi KQ, Fan YC, Pan ZZ, Lin XF, Liu WY, Chen YP, et al. Transient elastography: a meta-analysis of diagnostic accuracy in evaluation of portal hypertension in chronic liver disease. Liver Int. 2013;33:62–71.
50. Castera L, Foucher J, Bernard PH, Carvalho F, Allaix D, Merrouche W, et al. Pitfalls of liver stiffness measurement: a 5-year prospective study of 13,369 examinations. Hepatology. 2010;51:828–35.
51. Yin M, Talwalkar JA, Glaser KJ, Manduca A, Grimm RC, Rossman PJ, et al. Assessment of hepatic fibrosis with magnetic resonance elastography. Clin Gastroenterol Hepatol. 2007;5:1207–1213.e2.
52. Ronot M, Lambert S, Elkrief L, Doblas S, Rautou PE, Castera L, et al. Assessment of portal hypertension and high-risk oesophageal varices with liver and spleen three-dimensional multifrequency MR elastography in liver cirrhosis. Eur Radiol. 2014;24:1394–402.
53. Colecchia A, Montrone L, Scaioli E, Bacchi-Reggiani ML, Colli A, Casazza G, et al. Measurement of spleen stiffness to evaluate portal hypertension and the presence of esophageal varices in patients with HCV-related cirrhosis. Gastroenterology. 2012;143:646–54.
54. Valla DC, Condat B. Portal vein thrombosis in adults: pathophysiology, pathogenesis and management. J Hepatol. 2000;32:865–71.
55. DeLeve LD, Valla DC, Garcia-Tsao G. Vascular disorders of the liver. Hepatology. 2009;49:1729–64.
56. Schouten JN, Garcia-Pagan JC, Valla DC, Janssen HL. Idiopathic noncirrhotic portal hypertension. Hepatology. 2011;54:1071–81.

Chapter 28
Endoscopic Management of Portal Hypertension

Murad Aburajab

Question 1: What is portal hypertension?

Patient level answer: Portal hypertension is the elevation of portal vein pressure that typically exceeds 6 mmHg as a result of the increased resistance of portal blood flow. Clinically, the hepatic venous pressure gradient (HVPG), which is the difference between the wedged and the free hepatic venous pressure measurement, gives an estimate of the portal pressure gradient in cases of liver cirrhosis. This gradient usually becomes clinically important when it exceeds 10 mmHg at which point it places patients at risk of decompensation by forming esophageal varices and ascites [1, 2]. Over 90 % of cases of portal hypertension in the western world are attributed to liver cirrhosis and there is a marked decrease in median 1-year survival when compensated cirrhosis transitions to decompensated cirrhosis [3, 4].

Question 2: When do esophageal varices form and what is the risk of bleeding?

Patient level answer: The risk of bleeding correlates with the HVPG. Once HVPG is above 10 mmHg, patients are at risk of forming gastroesophageal varices and of the development of ascites. The risk of bleeding escalates when the gradient is above 12 mmHg and correlates with increasing HVPG. Varices can develop in compensated cirrhotic patients at a rate of 5–7 % per year [4]. It is estimated that 30 % of patients with compensated cirrhosis have varices at the time of diagnosis, with a bleeding risk of 5–15 % depending on the size of the varices. Small varices can progress into larger ones at a rate of 8 % per year; several factors involved in this progression include higher Child–Pugh class, ongoing alcohol intake and the presence of red wale marks at the initial endoscopic evaluation [5]. The mortality rate after first variceal bleeding episodes is not negligible. Almost 20 % of patients die within 6 weeks of their first bleeding episode [4, 6].

M. Aburajab, M.D. (⊠)
Division of Gastroenterology and Hepatology, Medical College of Wisconsin,
Milwaukee, WI, USA
e-mail: maburajab@mcw.edu

© Springer International Publishing Switzerland 2017
K. Saeian, R. Shaker (eds.), *Liver Disorders*,
DOI 10.1007/978-3-319-30103-7_28

Question 3: What are the repercussions of bleeding from esophageal varices? What is meant by primary and secondary prophylaxis?

Patient level answer: The role of prevention is important in managing cirrhotic patients with esophageal varices. Every episode of variceal bleeding can increase the complications of liver cirrhosis, such as spontaneous bacterial peritonitis, hepatorenal syndrome, and hepatic encephalopathy, which can lead to increased patient morbidity and mortality. Prophylaxis is classified into two major strategies: primary prophylaxis indicates that the patient has esophageal varices, but has never bled from them previously, and secondary prophylaxis in which the patient has had a previous variceal bleeding episode and the aim is to prevent further bleeding episodes.

What Are the Options for Primary Prophylaxis?

Based on the American Association for the Study of Liver Diseases guidelines (AASLD), all patients diagnosed with liver cirrhosis should have a screening endoscopy for esophageal and gastric varices [4]. During an endoscopic evaluation, esophageal varices are graded according to their size. It is recommended to classify esophageal varices as small or large, with the latter described as being larger than 5 mm. Some physicians classify esophageal varices as small, medium, or large, depending on how much of the esophageal lumen they occupy. That classification is not helpful from a management standpoint, as medium and large varices are treated the same; the same applies to the previous grading system of 0–4. It is also necessary to identify high-risk stigmata such as red wale marks during an endoscopic evaluation, because such features are not only risk factors for bleeding, but also a predictor of variceal progression [7].

Primary prophylaxis is crucial to prevent the first bleeding episodes. This can be carried out either by using a nonselective beta-adrenergic blocker (NSBB) or endoscopic variceal banding (EVB). The management strategy for primary prevention is summarized in Table 28.1.

What Are the Medical Options for Primary Prophylaxis?

Nonselective beta-adrenergic blockers are the drugs of choice for primary prophylaxis. They lower the portal pressure by causing splanchnic arteriolar vasoconstriction through their β-2 effect and lower cardiac output by blocking β-1 receptors, which reduce portal venous inflow [8]. Propranolol and nadolol are the two most commonly used medications. Their role in preventing the progression of the size of varices and bleeding in small varices is controversial. A multi-center study showed no benefit of using NSBBs compared with placebo in preventing the development of esophageal varices in cirrhotic patients who did not have esophageal varices; on the

Table 28.1 Management strategy after the results of the first endoscopic evaluation in patients with liver cirrhosis (primary prophylaxis)

	Management		
No varices	Repeat endoscopy in 3 years (sooner if decompensation occurs)		
Small varices	In a CTP B/C patient or varices with red signs	Nonselective β-blockers (propranolol or nadolol)	Start propranolol (20 mg bid) or nadolol (20 mg qd)
			Titrate to maximal tolerable dose or a heart rate of 55–60 bpm
			No need to repeat EGD
	In a CTP A patient, without red signs	Nonselective β-blockers optional	Same as above
		If no β-blockers are given, repeat endoscopy in 2 years (sooner if decompensation occurs)	
Medium/large varices	All patients independent of CTP class	Nonselective β-blockers (propranolol, nadolol) or endoscopic variceal ligation	Same as above
			Ligate every 1–2 weeks until variceal obliteration. First surveillance endoscopy 1–3 months after obliteration, then every 6–12 months indefinitely

Choice depends on patient characteristics and preferences, and local resources
bid twice a day, *bpm* beats per minute, *CTP* Child–Turcotte–Pugh, *EGD* esophagogastroduodenoscopy, *qd* once daily

other hand, there were significant adverse outcomes in that group [9–11]. A recent meta-analysis performed by Qi et al. [12], which included a total of six randomized controlled studies, showed the NSBBs did not show any significant benefit on progression, bleeding events or mortality compared with the placebo group. Yet, some experts advocate using NSBBs in patients with small varices, who are a high risk, as in a Child–Pugh score of B or C, alcoholic liver disease, and in patients who had red wale marks at their initial endoscopic evaluation [13]. Merkel et al. [14] showed in a placebo-controlled trial that using nadolol was effective in reducing the progression and bleeding of small varices, but did not add significant survival benefit.

Nonselective beta-adrenergic blockers play a pivotal role in preventing bleeding in patients with medium and large varices. For esophageal varices to rupture and bleed, HVPG is generally ≥12 mmHg. There is a marked reduction in the risk of bleeding when HVPG was lowered either below 12 mmHg or >20 % from the baseline [15]. It has been shown that either nadolol or propranolol reduces the risk of the first variceal bleed compared with the placebo group (30 % in controls vs 14 % in patients receiving beta-blockers) by lowering the HVPG [8]. Additionally, there was a significant survival benefit in patients who received NSBBs [16]. The starting dose of propranolol is 20 mg twice a day and 40 mg once day for nadolol. The strategy is to reduce the heart rate by at least 20 % from the baseline and to adjust the medication to its maximal tolerated dose. Some 15–20 % of patients cannot tolerate the medication owing to side effects such as lightheadedness and asthma-related symptoms, which lead to complete withdrawal of the medication [17].

Besides nadolol and propranolol, carvedilol is an NSBB with intrinsic alpha-1 adrenergic blocking activity, the use of which for primary prophylaxis against variceal bleeding is becoming more widespread. In a recent study, in patients receiving carvedilol who had not initially responded to propranolol there was a greater reduction in HVPG compared with patients who had responded to propranolol treatment. Not only did patients who had received carvedilol achieved a better hemodynamic response, they also had a lower mortality rate compared with patients treated only with endoscopic variceal banding [18, 19]. More recent data suggest that NSBBs should be avoided in patients with refractory ascites as they result in poor outcomes [20].

To conclude, the use of NSBBs in patients with medium and large varices, in those with high-risk stigmata for bleeding, and in patients with small varices who have not had variceal bleeding results in decreased bleeding episodes and improved survival. Their use is limited to patients who tolerate the medications, requires a hemodynamic response to therapy, and is not advocated in cirrhotic patients with no esophageal varices and those with refractory ascites.

What Are the Endoscopic Options for Primary Prophylaxis?

As noted above, all patients with the diagnosis of cirrhosis should undergo screening for esophageal varices [3], but the role of EVB in primary prophylaxis is still controversial. It is clear that EVB is very effective in eradicating esophageal varices and reducing first bleeding events. However, most comparative studies have not shown superiority in reducing bleeding-related mortality compared with NSBBs for primary prophylaxis. A recent Cochrane review by Gluud and Krag [21] included 19 randomized trials comparing EVB with NSBBs for primary prevention. There was a greater reduction in bleeding events in the EVB group (RR=0.68, 95 % CI: 0.52–0.90); however, EVB was not superior to NSBBs with regard to bleeding-related mortality. Despite this evidence, there is clear agreement that EVB is the option of choice for primary prophylaxis in patients who either cannot tolerate or have a contraindication to NSBBs, those with refractory ascites, and those with high-risk esophageal varices. Of note, trials of endoscopic variceal sclerotherapy for primary prophylaxis do not support its use for primary prophylaxis.

What About Combining NSBBs and EVB?

Combination therapy using EVB in addition to NSBBs in primary prevention has been studied with conflicting results [22–24]. A recent retrospective study by Je et al. [25] investigated the long-term efficacy of the combination of EVB and propranolol compared with propranolol alone. A total of 504 patients were enrolled in the study. There was a marked difference in preventing the first variceal bleed in favor of a combination strategy, with no difference in overall mortality between the two groups. On the other hand, Lo et al. conducted a randomized study comparing combination therapy of EVB and nadolol with nadolol alone. There was no difference in bleeding events and bleeding-related mortality in the groups; however, in contrast to the report by Je et al [25]. there were more adverse events in the combined group related to EVB, including esophageal ulcerations [23]. Given the current evidence, there is no clear added benefit of combination EVB and NSBB therapy and it cannot be routinely recommended as the first-line modality for primary prevention.

What Are the Options for Secondary Prophylaxis?

Patients who survive the first episode of variceal bleeding are at a high risk of recurrent bleeding. This risk is greater than 60 % within the first 2 years, with a higher risk of bleeding within the first 6 weeks after the index bleed and 33 % mortality [15]. In this particular scenario, combination therapy using NSBBs and EVB is the standard treatment and has proved its superiority when compared with either treatment alone. This was shown in a meta-analysis of 9 trials where combination therapy reduced the risk of variceal rebleeding, but not overall mortality, when compared with the use of NSBBs or EVL alone [26]. The added benefit of NSBBs to that of EVB lies in reducing portal pressure, which reduces the risk of bleeding. Additionally, studies demonstrate that NSBBs reduce the risk of spontaneous bacterial peritonitis by 12 %, independent of their hemodynamic effect on HVPG [27].

Once patients recover from the first variceal bleed, treatment should be targeted at eradicating those varices. An endoscopic banding session should be scheduled at 2- to 4-week intervals after the index bleeding episode until the esophageal varices are completely eradicated. This process typically takes 2–4 sessions. Once they are eradicated, the patient should be back in 3 months for a first surveillance, and, if negative, this should be repeated every 6 months. Endoscopic variceal sclerotherapy is also an option that has been shown to decrease rebleeding, but is now infrequently employed (typically in cases in which EVB is not technically feasible) in light of the more favorable complication profile of EVB. The management strategy for secondary prevention is summarized in Table 28.2.

What Are the Complications of EVB?

Adverse events of esophageal variceal banding are observed in 14 % of patients. The two most common complications are chest pain and dysphagia, but both are short-lived complications [28]. Post-banding ulcers occur at the banding site in

Table 28.2 Management strategy in preventing rebleeding in patients with liver cirrhosis (secondary prophylaxis)

Treatment	Management	
First-line therapy	Nonselective β-blockers (propranolol, nadolol) and Endoscopic variceal ligation	Start propranolol (20 mg bid) or nadolol (20 mg qd)
		Titrate to the maximum tolerable dosage or a heart rate of 55–60 bpm
		No need to repeat endoscopy
		Ligate every 1–2 weeks until variceal obliteration
		First surveillance endoscopy 1–3 months after obliteration, then every 6–12 months
Second-line therapy (if combined pharmacological + endoscopic treatment has failed)	TIPS or shunt surgery (CTP class A patients, where available)	

TIPS transjugular intrahepatic portosystemic shunt

0.5–3.0 % of cases; these ulcers are shallow in nature and have the tendency to bleed in 5–6.6 % of treated patients. Studies showed that using pantoprazole daily for 9 days following the procedure can significantly reduce the size of post-banding ulcers and their bleeding risk [29]. Life-threatening bleeding associated with post-banding ulceration has been reported and requires urgent attention. Post-banding strictures have also been reported, but are typically easily managed. Endoscopic variceal sclerotherapy is associated with a higher rate of esophageal ulcers and with fever and chest and abdominal pain. It is also associated with risks of perforation, mediastinitis, and portal vein thrombosis.

What to Do If Those Varices Bleed

Patients with liver cirrhosis who present with suspected variceal bleeding should be admitted to the intensive care unit. After rapid stabilization and resuscitation of the patient, including assessing the need for airway protection with a low threshold for intubation and securing adequate intravenous access, urgent endoscopy with therapeutic intent should be undertaken. Blood transfusion should not be undertaken until the hemoglobin falls below 7 mg/dl and caution should be exercised not to over-resuscitate using crystalloids or other blood products so that the portal pressures are not elevated further, hence predisposing to more rebleeding, associated with increased mortality [30]. Once endoscopy is undertaken, EVB is now typically the standard of care if esophageal variceal bleeding is identified. Esophageal variceal sclerotherapy is also effective in this setting.

There is a major established role of using vasoactive pharmacological agents in the acute portal hypertensive bleeding event. Vasopressin and terlipressin have a vasoconstrictive effect on splanchnic circulation and octreotide prevents postprandial elevation and portal pressures. Thus, these agents either lower the portal pressure or prevent a rebound elevation in portal pressure in response to bleeding and subsequently enhance the efficacy of endoscopic therapy. Vasopressin is associated with significant side effects, including potential coronary vasoconstriction, and is thus now rarely used. Terlipressin is very effective, but is not available in the USA, leaving octreotide as the most common agent used in variceal bleeding there. The dose of octreotide is a 50-µg intravenous bolus followed by an infusion of 50 µg/h. Although the optimal duration of infusion has not been well established, given the risk of early rebleeding, which is approximately 50 % in the first 5 days after endoscopic intervention, it is reasonable to continue the octreotide infusion for 5 days, although some studies showed no difference in outcome if octreotide infusion was continued for 2 days or 3 days versus a 5-day strategy [31, 32] In our practice, we commonly continue the octreotide for at least 3 days. It is well-established that the short-term use of prophylactic antibiotics in cirrhotic patients and portal hypertensive bleeding with or without ascites not only decreases the risk of infectious complications, but also improves survival [33]. Antibiotics must be given to patients with liver cirrhosis who suffer from gastrointestinal bleeding irrespective of their ascites status. The use of oral norfloxacin at a dose of 400 mg BID for 7 days or intravenous ceftriaxone in a dose of 1 g/day for 7 days also diminish the incidence of bacterial peritonitis [34].

What Is the Classification Scheme of Gastric Varices?

Gastric varices are present in approximately 17 % of patients with cirrhosis [35]. Although they bleed less frequently than esophageal varices, the episodes of bleeding tend to be more severe, with higher mortality of almost 45 %. The most accepted and well-known classification for gastric varices is the Sarin system (Fig. 28.1). They are classified into: GOV1, esophageal varices that extend below the gastroesophageal junction into the lesser curvature of the stomach; GOV2 extends beyond the gastroesophageal junction into the fundus of the stomach; IGV1 are isolated gastric varices that are limited to the fundus of the stomach and have no contiguity with esophageal varices (Fig. 28.2); and isolated gastric varices in other areas of the stomach are called IGV2. The most prevalent type of gastric varix is GOV1 (75 %), followed by GOV2 (21 %), IGV2 (4 %), and IGV1 (<1 %).

How Do I Manage the Patient with Gastric Variceal Bleeding?

Initial management of suspected gastric variceal bleeding is similar to that for esophageal varices. Patients should be admitted to the intensive care unit and resuscitative measures taken in addition to using vasoactive agents and antibiotics.

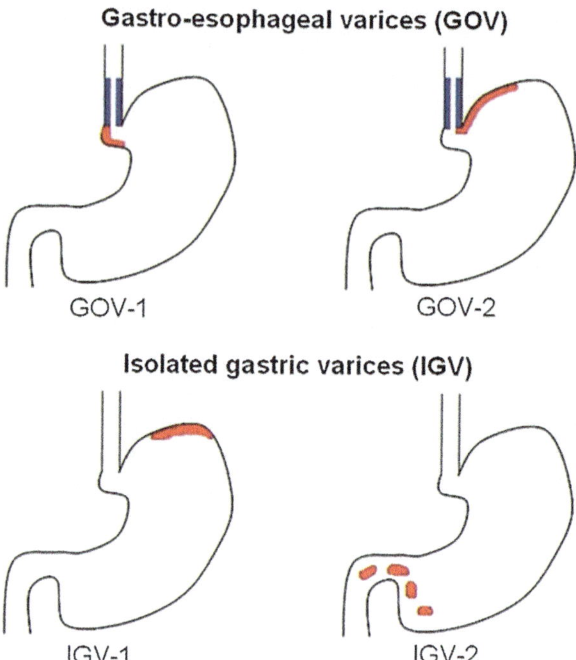

Fig. 28.1 Sarin classification for gastroesophageal varices

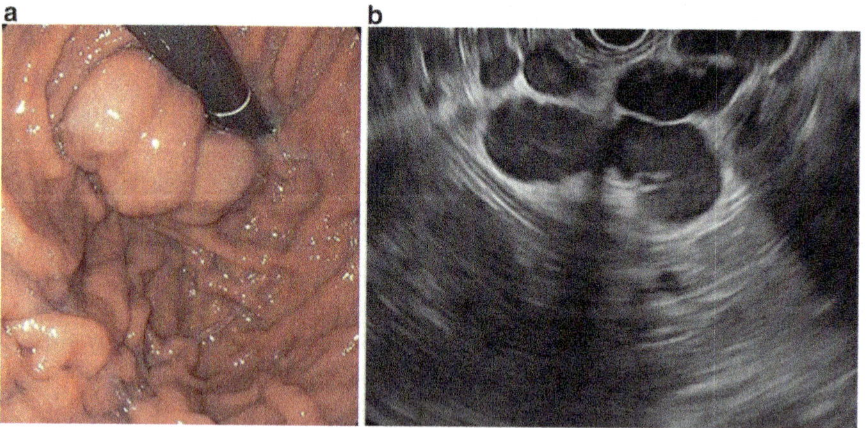

Fig. 28.2 Isolated gastric varices on (**a**) endoscopic view, (**b**) endoscopic ultrasound view

The typical endoscopic options to stop esophageal variceal bleeding including band ligation and sclerotherapy apply to GOV1, but are suboptimal in the management of gastric variceal bleeding due to GOV2, IGV2, and IGV1. It bears repeating that in the setting of GOV1, given the short segment of the gastric varices in continuity with esophageal varices, EVB and endoscopic variceal sclerotherapy are viable options for treatment. The reported success rate of endoscopic banding for GOV1 and achieving hemostasis was near 85 % [36]. Despite its effectiveness in controlling esophageal variceal bleeding, EVB should typically be avoided for the other forms of gastric varices, unless there are no other options. Several factors may play a role in its lack of efficacy in this setting, including the greater mucosal thickness overlying the varix in the stomach, along with the typically larger size of the varix, making it difficult and challenging to engulf the entire varix into the suction hood during the process of ligation.

Although endoscopic sclerotherapy has its place in the treatment of esophageal varices, its use has been less successful in the management of isolated and fundic gastric varices (non-GOV1). Studies have shown that the overall success rate for achieving initial hemostasis is between 60 and 100 %; however, the rebleeding rate was unacceptably high, approaching 90 % [37, 38]. Almost 50 % of the rebleeding is due to ulcers induced by sclerotherapy itself, exacerbating a situation that is already difficult to manage.

Can We Use Endoscopic Glue to Treat Gastric Varices?

The endoscopic injection of tissue adhesives such as cyanoacrylate (CA) has been successfully used for the cessation of bleeding from gastric varices, including GOV2, IGV2 and IGV1 obliteration. CA is a monomer that undergoes rapid polymerization when it comes into contact with hydroxyl ions, as in water or blood. Histoacryl (*N*-butyl-cyanoacrylate) and 2-octyl-cyanoacrylate have been used as tissue adhesives to be injected directly into a gastric varix. Studies have shown the efficacy of using CA in treating gastric varices with a success rate ranging between 91 and 100 % and a rebleeding rate of 8–23 % [39–42]. Tissue adhesives have been used both in the acute setting to control bleeding and to eradicate after a previous bleeding episode. Reported complications are infrequent and include ulceration, thromboembolic episodes in less than 1 % including cerebrovascular accidents, splenic infarction, pulmonary embolism, and adrenal abscesses [43]. Extrusion of the glue from the injection site can occur a few weeks following treatment, causing ulcerations that may bleed in 4.4 %; however, those events are controllable [43]. Other technical complications can occur if the injector needle becomes trapped in the varix during the process of injection, which can occur as a result of the polymerization and premature solidification of CA. Care must be taken not only to promptly removed the needle, but also to use irrigation with either normal saline or D5W, because entrapment of the needle may result in worsening the bleeding upon forceful removal. Currently, the use of CA for this indication has not been approved by the FDA, but a number of centers throughout the country offer the service for patients who have no other options.

Endoscopic ultrasound (EUS) has the ability to detect blood flow in gastric varices through its Doppler capability and allows the precise localization of gastric varices and their perforating veins (Fig. 28.2). Using this technology, not only does EUS allow for the accurate delivery of CA into the gastric varix, but it also detects residual blood flow following CA injection, which carries prognostic implications [44, 45]. There are different approaches to the EUS-guided therapy of gastric varices by injecting CA, placing fibered coils that are used in interventional radiology, or a combination of the two. Binmoeller et al. [46] shared their outstanding experience in 30 patients who underwent EUS-guided treatment for gastric fundic varices using a combined glue and coil approach. Initial hemostasis was achieved in 100 % of patients and gastric varices were obliterated in 96 % of patients in a single session.

Are There Non-endoscopic Approaches to Treating Gastric Varices?

Non-endoscopic treatments of gastric varices are grouped under rescue therapy. These include placement of a transjugular intrahepatic portosystemic shunt (TIPS) and balloon-occluded retrograde transverse obliteration (BRTO), in addition to temporizing measures such as balloon tamponade (e.g., the use of the Minnesota tube or the Sengstaken–Blakemore tube). Both TIPS and BRTO are very effective rescue measures when other treatments fail Chap. 34, particularly in the hands of experienced interventional radiologists, and are addressed elsewhere in this text.

Conclusion

Portal hypertension carries ominous complications as in esophageal and gastric variceal bleeding. It can lead to major morbidity and mortality. Using NSBBs remain the most appropriate approach in primary prevention with added benefit in secondary prevention.

References

1. Bosch J, et al. Portal hypertension and gastrointestinal bleeding. Semin Liver Dis. 2008;28(1):3–25.
2. Garcia-Pagan JC, De Gottardi A, Bosch J. Review article: the modern management of portal hypertension – primary and secondary prophylaxis of variceal bleeding in cirrhotic patients. Aliment Pharmacol Ther. 2008;28(2):178–86.
3. Garcia-Tsao G, Bosch J, Groszmann RJ. Portal hypertension and variceal bleeding – unresolved issues. Summary of an American Association for the study of liver diseases and European Association for the study of the liver single-topic conference. Hepatology. 2008;47(5):1764–72.

4. Garcia-Tsao G, et al. Prevention and management of gastroesophageal varices and variceal hemorrhage in cirrhosis. Hepatology. 2007;46(3):922–38.
5. North Italian Endoscopic Club for the Study and Treatment of Esophageal Varices. Prediction of the first variceal hemorrhage in patients with cirrhosis of the liver and esophageal varices. A prospective multicenter study. N Engl J Med. 1988;319(15):983–9.
6. Luigiano C, et al. Role of endoscopy in management of gastrointestinal complications of portal hypertension. World J Gastrointest Endosc. 2015;7(1):1–12.
7. D'Amico G, Garcia-Tsao G, Pagliaro L. Natural history and prognostic indicators of survival in cirrhosis: a systematic review of 118 studies. J Hepatol. 2006;44(1):217–31.
8. D'Amico G, Pagliaro L, Bosch J. Pharmacological treatment of portal hypertension: an evidence-based approach. Semin Liver Dis. 1999;19(4):475–505.
9. Triantos C, Kalafateli M. Primary prevention of bleeding from esophageal varices in patients with liver cirrhosis. World J Hepatol. 2014;6(6):363–9.
10. Cales P, et al. Lack of effect of propranolol in the prevention of large oesophageal varices in patients with cirrhosis: a randomized trial. French-Speaking Club for the Study of Portal Hypertension. Eur J Gastroenterol Hepatol. 1999;11(7):741–5.
11. Groszmann RJ, et al. Beta-blockers to prevent gastroesophageal varices in patients with cirrhosis. N Engl J Med. 2005;353(21):2254–61.
12. Qi XS, et al. Nonselective beta-blockers in cirrhotic patients with no or small varices: a meta-analysis. World J Gastroenterol. 2015;21(10):3100–8.
13. de Franchis R, Baveno VF. Revising consensus in portal hypertension: report of the Baveno V consensus workshop on methodology of diagnosis and therapy in portal hypertension. J Hepatol. 2010;53(4):762–8.
14. Merkel C, et al. A placebo-controlled clinical trial of nadolol in the prophylaxis of growth of small esophageal varices in cirrhosis. Gastroenterology. 2004;127(2):476–84.
15. Albillos A, et al. Value of the hepatic venous pressure gradient to monitor drug therapy for portal hypertension: a meta-analysis. Am J Gastroenterol. 2007;102(5):1116–26.
16. Chen W, et al. Beta-blockers reduce mortality in cirrhotic patients with oesophageal varices who have never bled (Cochrane review). J Hepatol. 2004;40 Suppl 1:67.
17. Garcia-Tsao G, Bosch J. Management of varices and variceal hemorrhage in cirrhosis. N Engl J Med. 2010;362(9):823–32.
18. Reiberger T, et al. Carvedilol for primary prophylaxis of variceal bleeding in cirrhotic patients with haemodynamic non-response to propranolol. Gut. 2013;62(11):1634–41.
19. Sinagra E, et al. Systematic review with meta-analysis: the haemodynamic effects of carvedilol compared with propranolol for portal hypertension in cirrhosis. Aliment Pharmacol Ther. 2014;39(6):557–68.
20. Serste T, et al. Deleterious effects of beta-blockers on survival in patients with cirrhosis and refractory ascites. Hepatology. 2010;52(3):1017–22.
21. Gluud LL, Krag A. Banding ligation versus beta-blockers for primary prevention in oesophageal varices in adults. Cochrane Database Syst Rev 2012;(8):CD004544.
22. Gheorghe C, et al. Primary prophylaxis of variceal bleeding in cirrhotics awaiting liver transplantation. Hepatogastroenterology. 2006;53(70):552–7.
23. Lo GH, et al. Controlled trial of ligation plus nadolol versus nadolol alone for the prevention of first variceal bleeding. Hepatology. 2010;52(1):230–7.
24. Sarin SK, et al. Endoscopic variceal ligation plus propranolol versus endoscopic variceal ligation alone in primary prophylaxis of variceal bleeding. Am J Gastroenterol. 2005;100(4):797–804.
25. Je D, et al. The comparison of esophageal variceal ligation plus propranolol versus propranolol alone for the primary prophylaxis of esophageal variceal bleeding. Clin Mol Hepatol. 2014;20(3):283–90.
26. Thiele M, et al. Meta-analysis: banding ligation and medical interventions for the prevention of rebleeding from oesophageal varices. Aliment Pharmacol Ther. 2012;35(10):1155–65.
27. Senzolo M, et al. beta-Blockers protect against spontaneous bacterial peritonitis in cirrhotic patients: a meta-analysis. Liver Int. 2009;29(8):1189–93.

28. Albillos A, Tejedor M. Secondary prophylaxis for esophageal variceal bleeding. Clin Liver Dis. 2014;18(2):359–70.
29. Shaheen NJ, et al. Pantoprazole reduces the size of postbanding ulcers after variceal band ligation: a randomized, controlled trial. Hepatology. 2005;41(3):588–94.
30. Villanueva C, et al. Transfusion strategies for acute upper gastrointestinal bleeding. N Engl J Med. 2013;368(1):11–21.
31. Rengasamy S, et al. Comparison of 2 days versus 5 days of octreotide infusion along with endoscopic therapy in preventing early rebleed from esophageal varices: a randomized clinical study. Eur J Gastroenterol Hepatol. 2015;27(4):386–92.
32. Chitapanarux T, et al. Three-day versus five-day somatostatin infusion combination with endoscopic variceal ligation in the prevention of early rebleeding following acute variceal hemorrhage: a randomized controlled trial. Hepatol Res. 2015;45:1276.
33. Bernard B, et al. Antibiotic prophylaxis for the prevention of bacterial infections in cirrhotic patients with gastrointestinal bleeding: a meta-analysis. Hepatology. 1999;29(6):1655–61.
34. Fernandez J, et al. Norfloxacin vs ceftriaxone in the prophylaxis of infections in patients with advanced cirrhosis and hemorrhage. Gastroenterology. 2006;131(4):1049–56. quiz 1285.
35. Sarin SK, et al. Prevalence, classification and natural history of gastric varices: a long-term follow-up study in 568 portal hypertension patients. Hepatology. 1992;16(6):1343–9.
36. Lo GH, et al. A retrospective comparative study of histoacryl injection and banding ligation in the treatment of acute type 1 gastric variceal hemorrhage. Scand J Gastroenterol. 2013;48(10):1198–204.
37. Sarin SK, Mishra SR. Endoscopic therapy for gastric varices. Clin Liver Dis. 2010;14(2):263–79.
38. Trudeau W, Prindiville T. Endoscopic injection sclerosis in bleeding gastric varices. Gastrointest Endosc. 1986;32(4):264–8.
39. Cheng LF, et al. Treatment of gastric varices by endoscopic sclerotherapy using butyl cyanoacrylate: 10 years' experience of 635 cases. Chin Med J (Engl). 2007;120(23):2081–5.
40. Kang EJ, et al. Long-term result of endoscopic Histoacryl (N-butyl-2-cyanoacrylate) injection for treatment of gastric varices. World J Gastroenterol. 2011;17(11):1494–500.
41. Kind R, et al. Bucrylate treatment of bleeding gastric varices: 12 years' experience. Endoscopy. 2000;32(7):512–9.
42. Paik CN, et al. The therapeutic effect of cyanoacrylate on gastric variceal bleeding and factors related to clinical outcome. J Clin Gastroenterol. 2008;42(8):916–22.
43. Cheng LF, et al. Low incidence of complications from endoscopic gastric variceal obturation with butyl cyanoacrylate. Clin Gastroenterol Hepatol. 2010;8(9):760–6.
44. Weilert F, Binmoeller F. Endoscopic management of gastric variceal bleeding. Gastroenterol Clin North Am. 2014;43(4):807–18.
45. Lee YT, et al. EUS-guided injection of cyanoacrylate for bleeding gastric varices. Gastrointest Endosc. 2000;52(2):168–74.
46. Binmoeller KF, et al. EUS-guided transesophageal treatment of gastric fundal varices with combined coiling and cyanoacrylate glue injection (with videos). Gastrointest Endosc. 2011;74(5):1019–25.

Chapter 29
Portosystemic Encephalopathy

Jawaid Shaw and Jasmohan S. Bajaj

What Is Portosystemic or Hepatic Encephalopathy?

Patient-Level Answer

In patients with liver disease, hepatic encephalopathy (HE) is a well-known condition in which changes in mental activity occur leading to confusion and other thinking problems. Alterations in sleep patterns, mood, and bodily movements may also occur.

Provider-Level Answer

In the United States (US) chronic hepatitis C and alcohol are the most common causes of chronic liver disease (CLD) and its resultant end stage of cirrhosis. The expanded diagnostic codes for cirrhosis indicate that it is the eighth leading cause of death in the US [1]. HE is a serious complication of cirrhosis and its relative contribution to the utilization of resources is rapidly growing [2, 3]. The updated definition for HE as per the 2014 American Association for the Study of Liver Diseases (AASLD) practice guidelines is "a brain dysfunction caused by

J. Shaw, M.D.
Department of Medicine, McGuire VA Medical Center, Richmond, VA, USA

J.S. Bajaj, M.D., M.S., F.A.C.G., A.G.A.F. (✉)
Division of Gastroenterology, Hepatology and Nutrition, Virginia Commonwealth University, Richmond, VA, USA

McGuire VA Medical Center, 1201 Broad Rock Boulevard, Richmond, VA 23249, USA
e-mail: jsbajaj@vcu.edu

© Springer International Publishing Switzerland 2017
K. Saeian, R. Shaker (eds.), *Liver Disorders*,
DOI 10.1007/978-3-319-30103-7_29

Table 29.1 Hepatic encephalopathy description

Type	Grade		Time course	Spontaneous or precipitated
A	MHE	Covert	Episodic	Spontaneous
	1			
B	2	Overt	Recurrent	Precipitated
C	3			
	4		Persistent	

liver insufficiency and/or portosystemic shunting (PSS); it manifests as a wide spectrum of neurological or psychiatric abnormalities ranging from subclinical alterations to coma" [4]. As per these guidelines, all cases of HE should be classified according to one component from each of the following underlying disease-based three axes [4]: type A (acute liver failure), type B (portosystemic bypass without intrinsic liver disease), and type C (cirrhosis). The latter two types (B and C) present similarly and can be classified according to the West Haven Criteria (WHC) clinical grading according to the severity ranging from mild confusion to comatose state (Grade 1–IV), with further subdivision into episodic, recurrent, and persistent forms depends on as to how HE appears spaced in time and further on qualifying the HE episode/s as precipitated or nonprecipitated (Table 29.1). HE may not always be simple to diagnose. Cases that are mild with no obvious clinical profile may be diagnosed by using neuropsychometric testing and are classified as covert hepatic encephalopathy (CHE). The previous terminology for CHE included minimal hepatic encephalopathy (MHE) or subclinical HE. On the other hand, overt HE (OHE) is readily identifiable to the clinician and does not need specific neuropsychometric testing. At times, HE may be difficult to diagnose given subtle signs and symptoms. Hence, under the new terminology called SONIC (Spectrum of Neuro-cognitive Impairment in Cirrhosis), CHE includes minimal and Grade I HE, and OHE encompass Grades II–IV HE [5, 6]. For the remainder of this chapter, we will use the terms MHE and CHE interchangeably. The term OHE refers to the decompensated phase of cirrhotic liver disease [7] which carries a poor prognosis compared to cirrhotics without HE even when adjusted for disease severity based on MELD score [8]. The prevalence of OHE is approximately 30–40 % during the clinical course of cirrhotic liver disease [9]. In a study from India, the 1-year risk of a recurrent episode of HE after a previous event was found to be 40 %[10]. The rate of CHE in the United States has been reported to be as high as 60–80 %[11, 12]. There is now an understanding that patients with CHE have a higher likelihood of eventually developing OHE [11, 13, 14]. After undergoing a transjugular intrahepatic portosystemic shunt (TIPS) procedure, the incidence of HE has been reported as 20–31 % [15]. Looking at the United States inpatient national admission data with HE from 2005 to 2009 (approx. 110, 000 patients), investigators found that despite the lack of increased inpatient mortality, resource utilization has risen during the same cycle putting an increased financial burden on the health care system [3].

What Are the Symptoms of Hepatic Encephalopathy?

Patient-Level Answer

The common symptoms of HE are related to mental activities (feeling slow, confusion, lethargy, slurred speech, difficulty drawing objects, changes in handwriting), changes in sleep patterns, slip-ups with memory, and mood issues such as feeling depressed and not wanting to eat. Difficulties in driving may also be noticed by the patient or family/friends. Problems with balance and coordination are frequent and may result in falls.

Provider-Level Answer

The presence of nonspecific neuropsychiatric signs and symptoms is the hallmark of HE [5, 16]. MHE is regarded as a preclinical stage of OHE in SONIC and is comprised of deficits in multiple domains including attention, vigilance, response inhibition, and executive function [11, 17, 18]. Over recent years, CHE has received more attention given its propensity to degenerate into OHE. The difficulty with CHE is that it is difficult to diagnose clinically even for an astute physician, given its characteristic cognitive profile [16, 19, 20]. Driving skills are known to be impaired in CHE patients hence, exposing the driver as well as others to danger [21–23]. Studies have demonstrated that patients with CHE have impaired quality of life as well as working capability [24–27]. Furthermore, not only does CHE predict the subsequent onset of OHE [14, 28, 29] but it is also associated with poor prognosis and is an independent predictor of survival [30]. The appearance of asterixis or disorientation as per consensus heralds the onset of OHE [5]. However, asterixis (flapping tremor) which reflects negative myoclonus is not seen in HE alone as it can be elicited in other metabolic conditions such as uremia and carbon dioxide narcosis [31]. Sleep–wake cycle disturbances (insomnia, hypersomnia, and excessive day time sleepiness) due to disturbance in the circadian rhythm are common even in early stages of HE and may precede other neuropsychiatric disturbances [32, 33]. With the progression of HE from covert to overt stages, more advanced neuro-psychiatric signs and symptoms emerge. These may include progressive disorientation, behavioral issues including confusion, irritability, apathy, disinhibition, depression, agitation, increased sleepiness, and finally stupor leading to coma [34, 35].

An initial thorough history and physical examination should be performed with specific questions directed to both the patient as well as the caregiver to assess for the presence of any cognitive or mental status changes. In the case of CHE, the caregiver may be better able to answer some of the questions about changes in sleep patterns, behavior, mood, and driving errors. The provider should pose direct questions about disturbances in cognition such as impairment in working memory, decrease in attention span, difficulty in driving leading to accidents, and/or problems working with machines potentially leading to work impairment. On examination, initially assess the general level of alertness and orientation. A detailed neurological examination may reveal upper motor neuron signs (hypertonia, brisk reflexes, positive Babinski sign) in many HE patients but maybe absent in coma. Extrapyramidal dysfunction manifested as expression-less masked facies, slowness of movements/speech, parkinsonian-like tremors, and dyskinesic movements can be observed [31]. In addition to examination findings due to other manifestations of cirrhosis, distinct and focal transient neurological deficits including hemiplegia have been reported with no evidence of abnormalities seen on brain imaging or cerebrospinal fluid analysis [36]. Seizures including those leading to status epilepticus are rare but are reported in patients with HE [37, 38] as are rapidly progressive Parkinsonian-like symptoms which have been shown in a study done using SPECT imaging to be related to disturbances at the pre- and postsynaptic level in the striatal region involved in dopaminergic neurotransmission. These symptoms are not responsive to ammonia lowering strategies and have been reported in around 4.2 % of patients [39]. A dramatic but rare pattern of spinal cord involvement in some patients with HE (wherein the mental status changes may be minimal) related to liver disease and PSS is characterized by progressive spastic lower limb weakness and termed as hepatic myelopathy (HM). MRI of spine is often normal in HM with no reported motor involvement of upper limbs. Hepatic myelopathy can predate OHE in some case. There are approximately 90 cases reported in literature since the first description in 1949 [40]. These motor manifestations of HM do not respond to usual ammonia lowering strategies but early liver transplantation (LT) does lead to better neurological outcomes hence, making a case for MELD exception for patients with HM [41].

What Are the Causes of Hepatic Encephalopathy?

Patient-Level Answer

Patients with underlying portal hypertension can have HE triggered by infections, bleeding in the GI tract (upper or lower GI), effects from medications (excessive use of pain medications and sleeping pills or lack of adherence to ammonia lowering regimens), dehydration, electrolyte disturbances (particularly low sodium and potassium levels), being constipated, and/or changes in diet.

Provider-Level Answer

The precipitation of HE may be secondary to multiple causes including infection, electrolyte abnormalities, medication nonadherence, gastrointestinal bleeding, excessive diuretic use, and constipation. In a US-based study lactulose nonadherence was the most common precipitating event after the first OHE episode [42] but infections are typically thought to be the most common cause of episodic OHE implicated in 56 % of cases [43] with electrolyte disorders more commonly implicated in recurrent cases [44–47]. The most common infectious triggers of OHE are SBP and urinary tract infections.

When approaching the patient with OHE, the clinician should ask focused questions to assess for other precipitants such as prescription/nonprescription drug usage (sedative medications like benzodiazepines, narcotics, recreational drugs), alcohol usage, reasons for being dehydrated (over-diuresis, GI losses), and history of procedures (iatrogenic/spontaneous shunts, recent large-volume paracentesis). However, it is not always possible to find a clear precipitant as reported in one study in which for 12 % patients no precipitant was found [46].

Overt hepatic encephalopathy has nonspecific neuropsychiatric manifestations but in the right clinical setting, the diagnosis remains straight forward. A number of other entities which can result in acute confusional states or delirium include metabolic causes (diabetes related: hypoglycemia or hyperglycemia, diabetic ketoacidosis, nonketotic hyperosmolar state), electrolyte abnormalities (hyponatremia or hypernatremia, hypokalemia, hypercalcemia), pulmonary issues (hypoxic or hypercarbic states), renal-mediated (uremia), toxin-related (acute alcohol intoxication, Wernicke's or Korsakoff syndromes, and delirium tremens), medications and illicit drugs (inappropriate use or over dosage of either prescription or over-the-counter medications, drugs of abuse like sedative-hypnotics, opiates, antihistamines, hallucinogens, heroine, cannabis, atypical alcohols) infectious (sepsis and meningo-encephalitic syndromes, severe systemic infections) CNS-related (cerebrovascular accidents including subdural hematomas, brain tumors, traumatic brain injuries, convulsive or nonconvulsive seizures, and dementing or psychiatric illnesses). In the end, any severe medical and physical stress (leading to organ failure or inflammation) can lead to altered mentation. Hyponatremia (serum sodium levels <130 mEq/l) is an independent risk factor for development of OHE and may be a target for preventive intervention [48]. Diabetes mellitus in patients with hepatitis C-related cirrhosis has been shown to be a risk factor for development of HE at earlier stages of liver decompensation. Patients with liver cirrhosis and renal dysfunction are also at an elevated risk of developing HE irrespective of the severity of the underlying liver disease [49].

Individual cases can follow different patterns of disease progression within the category of type C HE. And it appears that the pathogenesis of OHE and CHE is likely to be similar and the differences occur among levels of severity and stages of liver disease. Studies into the pathophysiology of HE and CHE have focused on the accumulation of toxins in the bloodstream and brains of patients with chronic liver disease. Ammonia is only a single component of this multifactorial disease and synergistic action of ammonia with other toxins may play a role in changing the metabolism of amino acid neurotransmitters and increasing the permeability of blood–brain barrier to these neurotransmitters. Ultimately, this leads to shifting of the balance towards the inhibitory gamma-aminobutyric acid (GABA) neurotransmission with suppression of the excitatory neurotransmitters like glutamate and catecholamine. The presence of the chronic neuro-inflammation, sepsis, oxidative stress, hyponatremia, and perturbations of gut flora could have a larger role in development of HE as well [50–53]. Although the mechanism by which ammonia cause brain dysfunction are not fully elucidated but there is some evidence of the association of ammonia with MHE [54]. The main source of ammonia in the body seems to be the gut microbiota, although animal model studies suggest alternative sources [55]. Glutamate is found mainly in the enterocytes of the small bowel and to a lesser extent in the colon and glutaminase from these multiple sources produces ammonia by metabolizing glutamine into glutamate and ammonia [56]. Ammonia is typically metabolized in the liver to urea, a water-soluble molecule that can be excreted by the kidneys. The diseased liver is not able to process the ammonia at normal capacity. It has been demonstrated that in patients with acute liver failure (ALF) brain and muscle cells get more involved in ammonia metabolism [57]. Studies have shown that after insertion of a portacaval shunt in rats there is increased expression of an intestinal glutaminase in rat enterocytes leading to increased ammonia levels, which may explain the increased risk of HE among patients who have undergone this procedure [58]. In the endoplasmic reticulum of brain astrocytes (only cells to metabolize ammonia in brain) glutamine synthetase produces equimolar ratios of ammonia and glutamine [57, 59]. Hence, with the advancing liver failure the intracellular levels of glutamine increase. As glutamine is an osmotic agent this increase is believed to be one of the putative reasons in the development of low-grade cerebral edema in patients with MHE or OHE [60].

The role of inflammation with or without hyperammonemia in the pathogenesis of HE is being recognized clearly more [61]. In patients with cirrhosis, inflammatory processes result mainly from infections but also from other causes like GI bleeding, obesity, and alterations in the intestinal flora. In a recent study by Merli et al., addressing the association between bacterial infections and cognitive dysfunction in cirrhotic ($n = 150$) vs. noncirrhotic patients ($n = 81$) found that neurocognitive changes were significantly increased in the cirrhotic group as compared to the noncirrhotics (90 % vs. 39 %) after the diagnoses of sepsis [62]. There were lowered scores on cognitive testing in patients with cirrhosis with systemic inflammatory response syndrome (SIRS) and induced hyperammonemia only when they also had increased levels of the inflammatory cytokines (tumor necrosis factor (TNF), interleukins (IL)-1 and IL-6) implying that hyperammonia only causes alterations in cognition in presence of neuro-inflammation and not alone [51]. This has been demonstrated in animal model studies as well where in administration of lipopolysaccharide in the liver damaged rats resulted in brain edema leading to altered consciousness but not in healthy rats [63]. Again, various other studies have demonstrated that the serum levels of various inflammatory cytokines (TNF-alfa, IL-6, and IL-18) in cirrhotic patients are associated with presence and severity of both OHE and CHE [64, 65]. In the end, it appears that infections promote the development of HE and cerebral edema in patients with ALF with inflammatory cytokines synergizing with hyper-ammonemia to produce cerebral edema [66, 67].

Are There Any Tests for Establishing the Diagnosis of Hepatic Encephalopathy?

Patient-Level Answer

While there are multiple tests available which help in establishing the diagnosis of HE including simple blood tests, electroencephalography (EEG) which measures brain electrical activity, brain CT or MRI scans, the diagnosis of OHE is ultimately made by physician based on examination and historical findings and no single test by itself establishes the diagnosis of OHE. The diagnosis of MHE, which cannot be detected simply on examination or questioning requires specialized paper and pencil or computerized tests for testing the thinking ability of the patient. The physician depending upon the circumstances may do none, one, some, or all of these tests.

Provider-Level Answer

The diagnosis of OHE requires clinical evaluation and exclusion of other etiologies as noted above with judicious use of additional testing depending on circumstances and the severity of mental status changes [68]. Laboratory testing should include basic metabolic panel (for renal function, hypokalemia, or hyponatremia), liver function tests, coagulation panel, CBC (for leukocytosis and platelet counts), urine analysis, ascitic fluid analysis to rule out SBP, culturing of blood, urine, ascitic fluid, and serum alphafetoprotein levels in the appropriate setting. The measurement of serum ammonia routinely in CLD patients suspected to have HE is not helpful as a high blood level of ammonia by itself does not provide any extra diagnostic or prognostic value [69]. However, in a case of OHE if the serum ammonia level is normal then the diagnosis of OHE should be reconsidered. Adding complexly to the utility of ammonia levels is that not only can other nonhepatic causes result in elevations of ammonia (such as medications) but problems with preservation and processing samples may also lead to difficulty with accurately determining ammonia levels. A study done in an emergency department (ED) setting to see whether elevated blood ammonia levels coincide with HE (additionally established by the WHC and the critical flicker frequency) found that ammonia blood levels do not reliably detect HE. The use of ammonia as sole indicator for HE in the ED may result in frequent errors in diagnosis [70]. Brain imaging (CT or MRI scans) do not contribute significantly to diagnosis or prognosis but should be considered in the appropriate clinical setting keeping in view the fact this subgroup of patients are at increased risk of intracranial bleeding [71].

Grading of OHE

The West Haven criteria (WHC) is the "gold standard" classification of hepatic encephalopathy classifying HE into five grades (0–IV) based upon impairment in consciousness, intellectual function, and behavior [16]. Grade 0 represents patients without detectable changes (unimpaired), grade I includes patients with trivial lack of awareness, shortened attention span, and altered sleep and mood, with grades II–IV representing progressive stages of overt HE and coma. This scale has been recommended by the Working Party on HE for assessment of OHE in clinical trials as well [16].

Other Classification Systems

The Hepatic Encephalopathy Scoring Algorithm (HESA): It may be particularly useful for assessing patients with low grades of HE and minimal variability was detected between the scores given at the different study sites [72]. The HESA combines clinical indicators with simple neuropsychological tests often used to detect milder grades of HE (grade I/II). The performance of each indicator was robust when compared across grades and sites [73]. HESA is simple, time efficient, and sensitive to subtle brain changes like the WHC but more objective, which should yield greater reliability across the spectrum of HE. However, the length of HESA makes it difficult to apply in clinical practice and thus it is predominantly used in research settings.

The Clinical Hepatic Encephalopathy Staging Scale (CHESS): This scale was designed to monitor the severity of HE on a linear scale from 0 (unimpaired) to 9 (deep coma) with each of the nine questions registering a value of 0 or 1. The test is considered to have good reproducibility and internal consistency with low inter observer variability [74].

The Modified-orientation log (MO-Log): This is an eight-question adaptation of the original orientation log devised for predicting outcomes in traumatic brain injury [75, 76]. The questions in MO-Log are heavily weighted towards disorientation to time (the earliest form of disorientation in OHE). The test is scored from 24 (highest) and 0 (lowest). A recent study found that MO-Log is a valid tool for assessing severity and is better than WHC in predicting outcomes in hospitalized HE patient [75].

Glasgow Coma Scale (GCS): For deeper grades of coma with nonverbal/minimally responsive patients wherein a questionnaire cannot be used, a validated GCS can be utilized. GCS adds to the assessment of severe HE by providing a wider separation for cases in grades III and IV.

CHE Testing Strategies

These tests are three types

1. Paper-pencil
2. Computerized
3. Neuro-physiological

Paper-And-Pencil Tests

Psychometric Hepatic Encephalopathy Score (PHES): This battery comprises of seven tests and measures psychomotor speed and precision, visual perception, visuo-spatial orientation, visual construction, concentration, attention, and memory. As there were concerns about the poor sensitivity of some of the subtests this led to the introduction of a revised battery called the Portosystemic Encephalopathy (PSE) Syndrome Test consisting of five tests. These tests are easy to administer and have been validated [18]. The test was originally developed in Germany and it has been shown that figure connection test can be used with similar results as number connection test in illiterate patients [77].

Repeatable Battery for the Assessment of Neuropsychological Status (RBANS): This test is used to diagnose neurocognitive disorders and evaluates global cognitive functioning based on language, visual perception, attention, immediate, and delayed memory. Some studies have confirmed its usefulness in characterizing cognitive impairment in liver transplant candidates [12, 78]. This, however, is not widely used given that two domains, delayed memory and language are not usually impaired in CHE.

Computerized Tests

Inhibitory Control Test (ICT): Tests attention, response inhibition, and working memory. On a computer screen every 500 ms, a continuous stream of letters are presented with targets (alternating X and Y) and lures (nontarget X and Y). Note is made of the percentage of target and lure response including the reaction time. With lower lure response along with higher target response and shorter reaction times indicating a good performance on the test [79]. ICT is a sensitive, inexpensive, with good validity but requires highly functional patients [80]. This test is available for free download at www.hecme.tv.

The EncephalApp Stroop Test: It measures psychomotor speed and cognitive flexibility evaluating the functioning of the anterior attention system [81]. Recently, the Stroop mobile application for smart phone or tablet computer (EncephalApp Stroop) has been used as a valid tool to screen for CHE compared to conventional paper-pencil tests [82]. A more recent study by the same group demonstrated that EncephalApp has good face validity, test-retest reliability, and external validity for the diagnosis of CHE [83]. This "app" is available for free download on iTunes and is not only easy to administer but also simple to score and interpret. The details of this test can be viewed as webcasts at www.chronicliverdisease.org.

The Scan Test: This test is a three-level-difficulty reaction time test that measures speed and accuracy to perform a digit recognition memory task of increasing complexity to diagnose varying degrees of HE [84]. In one study, this test was most closely related to central brain atrophy as compared to other psychometric tests (Trail-making Tests and Symbol Digit Modality Tests) [85]. This test has some prognostic value as well with patients who already had history of OHE performing significantly worse than those who never had a bout of OHE [30, 86].

Neurophysiological Tests

Critical flicker frequency (CFF) test: In this test, patients are presented with light pulses at a frequency of 60 Hz downward (being gradually reduced by 0.1 Hz decrements per second). Patients are asked to identify the time at which the fused light begins to flicker. A critical flicker frequency of below 39 Hz diagnoses CHE with high sensitivity and specificity [87]. In recent studies, CFF has been evaluated as an objective measure for grading for assessing recovery from MHE and from propofol sedation for cirrhotics undergoing endoscopy [88, 89]. Yet some other studies assessed the use of CFF as a marker for objective HE evaluation in patients undergoing TIPS with an aim to select the patients pre-TIPS to decrease the rate of post-TIPS HE and for early liver transplantation [87, 90]. A recent meta-analysis has shown that CFF is a diagnostically accurate test, which could be used as an adjunct to conventional psychometric test batteries such as PHES at this point in time till more research percolates [91]. CFF has the advantage of being simple and easy to use, not being dependent on language, verbal fluency, numeracy, and being independent of literacy, gender, and age.

The electroencephalogram (EEG): Is able to capture changes in the electric activity of cerebral cortex and classifies HE in five grades of severity from normal to coma without necessary need of patient cooperation [92]. The initial tracings of posterior dominant alpha rhythm slowing in mild HE degenerate into appearance of theta and high-amplitude irregular delta waves with the progression of HE into advanced stages and coma. However, this neurophysiological method may lack objectivity as not only metabolic issues and drugs influence the test but is also subject to both inter and intra-observer variability [93]. Hence, more objective quantitative methods of EEG analysis like spectral analysis (computerized analysis of the frequency distribution in the EEG) and digital analysis are being advocated [94, 95]. Another limiting factor of EEG is that it requires a proper set up and expertise to conduct and to interpret the tracing.

Strategies to Manage Test Results

By consensus, at least two validated tests (PHES and one of the computerized or neurophysiological tests) should be used for multicenter studies while for single center studies or clinical evaluation a validated test depending on the local familiarity with the test may be used [6]. Only properly trained persons should administer the tests and repeat testing for CHE or MHE should be done within 6 months if testing for these was negative initially [23].

What Are My Treatment Options?

Patient-Level Answer

It is important to address the potential trigger of the HE. Hence, actively seeking and treating the infections, correcting the electrolyte disturbances, avoiding medications causing excessive sleepiness, avoiding constipation by taking medications, and making appropriate dietary changes are the foundations of treatment.

Provider-Level Answer

While a majority of patients with episodic OHE may need to be hospitalized, the grade and severity of HE often determines the level of care, with patients who are not able to safely protect their airways preferably being managed in the intensive care unit. Since the majority (up to 90 %) of OHE episodes do have a precipitating trigger as outlined above [96], actively seeking and treating these precipitants is of paramount importance and may in itself result in resolution of the OHE episode. The main objectives of drug treatment in OHE are to reduce ammonia production and absorption. Thus a two-pronged approach is used.

Nonabsorbable Disaccharides

Despite lack of definitive randomized controlled trials, the use of lactulose is still prevalent as the first line treatment of acute episodes of OHE [4]. Both lactulose and lactitol (not available in US) have multifactorial mechanisms of action with the net result of reducing plasma ammonia levels. These mechanisms include acidification of the colonic lumen with resultant conversion of ammonia to nonabsorbable ammonium, modifying the colonic flora from urease to non-urease producing bacterial species, increasing the stool volume, and a cathartic effect diminishing transit time and subsequently ammonia absorption [97]. Clinical familiarity with the medication, long-standing clinical effectiveness based on years of experience, and a cost-friendly profile favor usage of lactulose [98]. The dose should be properly titrated to 2–3 soft bowel movements per day being cognizant of the fact that overuse may not only lead to serious side effects such as diarrhea, dehydration, perianal rash, but may also per se precipitate HE [42]. Alternative routes of administration like via nasogastric tube or by rectum may have to be resorted to if patient is not able to take the medications by mouth safely. Lactose in place of lactulose can be used in lactose intolerant patients [99]. Two recent, single center open label trials provide some evidence for lactulose usage as a secondary prevention agent for OHE in cirrhosis [10, 100].

Antibiotics

More research into the pathogenesis of HE is pointing towards the role of infections, alterations in the microbiome of cirrhotic patients, inflammation, and hyperammonemia [61, 101]. Hence, controlling inflammation, diminishing bacterial production of ammonia and altering the microbiota in cirrhotic patients underlies the rationale for antibiotic use in HE [102, 103].

Rifaximin is a gut-specific antimicrobial agent with broad spectrum activity, including against anaerobic enteric bacteria with less than 1 % of the drug being absorbed systemically after oral administration resulting in higher concentration in GI tract [104]. It has been demonstrated to be either superior or equivalent as compared to lactulose, other antimicrobials and placebo in numerous trials in patients with mild to moderate severe HE with the added advantage of having low side effect profile [105]. In a well designed trail, studying usage of rifaximin at a dose of 550 mg twice daily over 6 months duration in patients with two prior OHE episodes demonstrated superiority over placebo in preventing recurrent episodes and decreasing hospitalization [106]. Along with this, rifaximin usage has been show to improve the health-related quality of life (HRQOL) in patients versus placebo [107]. Rifaximin added to lactulose is the best documented agent to maintain remission in those who have already experienced one or more bouts of OHE while on lactulose treatment after their initial episode of overt hepatic encephalopathy [106].

Neomycin is an aminoglycoside with intestinal glutaminase inhibitor activity and has a spectrum against most gram-negative aerobes, except pseudomonas [108]. Although, this drug was used previously to treat HE and remains FDA approved, its use has fallen out of favor predominantly because of its toxicity profile (intestinal malabsorption, nephrotoxicity, and neurotoxicity) particularly with long-term use in the setting of cirrhosis. A randomized controlled study comparing neomycin to lactulose found no significant difference between the two agents [109]. Another agent, metronidazole was used in 11 patients with mild to severe HE who were treated for 1 week and had similar efficacy as compared to neomycin [110]. However, given its toxicity profile (ototoxicity, nephrotoxicity, and irreversible neurotoxicity) which gets exacerbated due to prolonged rate of elimination in cirrhotic patients metronidazole is not recommend for the management of HE [111]. Vancomycin use in acute episodes of HE may be less unsafe however, limited data along with cost and resistance issues preclude its routine clinical use and hence this is not FDA approved for this indication [112]. A well-done study addressed cost effectiveness of six different strategies in the management of HE (no HE treatment; lactulose monotherapy; lactitol monotherapy; neomycin monotherapy; rifaximin monotherapy; and or up front lactulose with crossover to rifaximin if there was a poor response or intolerance to lactulose). The study concluded that the no HE treatment arm was the least efficacious while as the rifaximin salvage being the most efficacious and that rifaximin monotherapy alone was not cost effective [98]. However, studies have shown that since rifaximin may be associated with a lower rate of hospitalizations, this could result in overall cost-savings [113]. If patients have recurrent episode of OHE being precipitated by well-recognized precipitants like variceal GI bleeds and good control of these precipitants is achieved prophylactic agents may be stopped. Another scenario is if patients liver function and nutritional status (muscle mass) improves prophylactic agents may be stopped. One may consider performing neuropsychometric testing prior to stopping HE medication as testing positive on these tests will predict recurrence of HE episodes, however this approach is not data driven [4].

Branched Chain Amino Acids (BCAAs)

These are essential amino acids (valine, leucine, and isoleucine) which are metabolized by the skeletal muscles and not by liver itself. In patients with cirrhosis, there occurs a flip in the plasma amino acids concentrations: aromatic amino acid (AAA), phenylalaninie, and tyrosine along with methionine are increased while as the BCAA are reduced [114]. This altered ratio ultimately contributes to alteration in the neuronal excitability. In a recent, updated cochrane systematic analysis comprising of 16 randomized clinical trials (827 participants) with both OHE and MHE showed that BCAA had a beneficial effect on hepatic encephalopathy. However, no effect was found on mortality, quality of life, or nutritional parameters with the note that additional trails need to be done to further explore the use of these medications [115]. An older study however, showed no clear value of using IV BCCA to treat episodes of OHE [116]. It is not considered as standard of care to use IV BCCA in treatment of HE. These are not available pharmacologically in the US.

L-ornithine L-aspartate (LOLA)

By enhancing the metabolism of ammonia to glutamine, LOLA helps to lower the plasma ammonia concentrations and is used in some countries other than US [117]. In a RCT, 126 patients with chronic OHE were assigned to get IV LOLA or a placebo found that patients in the treatment arm with mild OHE had improvements in the ammonia levels and clinical parameters [118]. However, authors concluded more studies were required in MHE and severe grades of OHE. A recent, RCT studied the utility of prophylactic LOLA infusion after TIPS placement and found that it significantly reduced the venous ammonia concentration hence benefiting patients mental status [119]. Another RCT, trying to address the reversal of MHE by rifaximin, probiotics, and L-ornithine L-aspartate (LOLA) individually by comparing it with placebo group found that these agents are better than placebo in MHE [120]. However, as of now oral supplementation with LOLA has not been found to be effective. These are not available pharmacologically in the US.

Prebiotics and Probiotics

While prebiotics are selectively fermented ingredients, probiotics are live microorganisms both of which modulate the gut microflora in a way, which is beneficial for the host. The combinations of both agents are called synbiotics. Lactulose which has know efficacy for HE treatment as per some, has probiotic properties as well [121]. A cochrane meta-analysis, reviewing use of probiotics in HE did not find convincing evidence for use as there were no beneficial and or harmful effects in HE [122]. A later study, focusing more on the usage of probiotics and synbiotics on MHE found that these might be effective treatments but need more vigorous randomized studies [123]. Yet another study has shown that Lactulose and probiotics are equally effective in secondary prophylaxis of HE as compared to a placebo [100]. Clearly, the use of prebiotics and probiotics seems to be an interesting field and may hold some promise for future. Hence, groups are working to find safer strains of probiotics for use in future studies [124].

Polyethylene Glycol (PEG)

PEG solution is a cathartic agent and in a recent single center trial, PEG was compared with Lactulose in patients hospitalized for OHE. Twenty-five patients were randomized to either arm to receive PEG (4 l over 4 h) versus Lactulose (20–30 g three to four doses over 24 h period). It was concluded that, PEG led to more rapid HE resolution as compared to Lactulose therapy (1 day vs. 2 days) suggestive of some superiority [125]. However, more trials are needed to validate these results in a larger population.

Molecular Adsorbent Recirculating System (MARS)

This is based on the concept of albumin dialysis which was designed to remove protein and albumin bound toxins such as bilirubin, bile acids, nitrous oxide, and endogenous benzodiazepines and also removes nonprotein bound ammonia that accumulates in liver failure. In a multicenter RCT, of extracorporeal albumin dialysis (ECAD) for hepatic encephalopathy in advanced cirrhosis using MARS; A total of 70 patients were randomized, 39 to ECAD and standard medical therapy (SMT) vs. 31 to SMT alone. The difference in improvement proportion of HE between the groups, the primary end was ascertained. The primary endpoint was met whereby a higher proportion of patients had a 2 grade improvement in HE in the ECAD+SMT arm (mean 34%) vs. SMT arm (19%) with a p value=0.044 and more rapid improvement (p=0.045) with good tolerability of MARS in this trail [126]. In the most recent, RELIEF Trail; evaluating effect of MARS in 189 patients with acute on chronic liver failure (ACLF) by randomizing into two groups MARS+SMT vs. SMT alone. The primary endpoints were LT free survival at 28 and 90 days. The survival endpoints were not met, but safety was demonstrated. However, looking at the proportion of patients with HE Grade III–IV HE improvement to HE Grade 0–I was higher in MARS treated patients (62.5 %) compared SMT (38.2 %) with trend towards statistical significance ($p=0.07$) [127]. Although, MARS system has FDA approval for usage in HE but its usage is precluded by high operating cost, availability, and the need for careful selection of patients who may tolerate this modality amongst others. Hence, this may be considered a reserve therapy for patients not responding to standard of care.

What Should I Eat?

Patient-Level Answer

You should keep on eating several small meals at regular intervals in a day and a late snack before going to bed at nighttime. This late snack should consist of complex carbohydrates such as whole-grain breads, starchy vegetables, and proteins.

Provider-Level Answer

Malnutrition is an under recognized problem in patients with HE and the presence of severe protein calorie malnutrition can exacerbate the manifestations of HE in turn. It is know that muscles have a role in clearing ammonia, hence loss of muscle mass may further exacerbate the manifestations of HE [59, 128]. Per se malnutrition may be an independent risk factor for survival in cirrhotic patients [129]. All patients with HE should get a formal evaluation of nutritional status with the involvement of dieticians, nutrition experts, or special teams. While as hand-grip dynamometer has a good sensitivity and specificity for providing information on depletion of body cell mass with its associated effect on survival in males but it cannot be held true for females [130, 131]. The best method of providing nutrition is orally however, alternative routes like nasogastric tubes and parenteral may be used in patients with higher levels of HE who are either not able to cooperate or able to maintain adequate oral intake. Avoidance of fasting state, along with small frequent meals and a late night snack has been shown to be beneficial in a recent systematic analysis [132]. The energy intake should be maintained at 35–40 kcal/kg/day of ideal body weight with a protein intake of 1.2–1.5 g/kg/day and these recommendation have been incorporated in the recent evidence-based guidelines by ISHEN [133]. The source of the dietary protein should be richer in vegetable and dairy proteins rather than meat based proteins. In patients not able to tolerate proteins, use of oral BCAA supplementation should be considered [134]. There is some overlap of signs and symptoms in both HE and Wernicke's encephalopathy (WE), also patients with cirrhosis (alcohol and nonalcohol related) may be deficient in water-soluble vitamins including thiamine. Hence, oral vitamin supplements may be considered in HE patients as vitamins are safe and cheap. In case of WE, parenteral thiamine supplementation prior to giving a glucose load is important. Correcting of electrolyte abnormalities in particularly, low sodium and potassium levels that are risk factors for development of HE is pertinent [48, 135]. However, extreme caution needs to be exercised while correcting low sodium levels, which should be done slowly as rapid corrections can lead to central pontine myelinolysis, which is a devastating condition.

Do Patients with MHE Need Treatment?

Patient-Level Answer

While as patients with MHE are not routinely offered treatment, in special cases treatment might be offered. If such is the case, the treating liver specialist will determine as to who such patients would be.

Provider-Level Answer

A recent prospective study found that despite controlling for MELD score, patients with CHE are at increased risk for development of OHE, worsened survival and increased risk of hospitalization and hence, strategies to detect and treat CHE early may improve these outcomes [136]. Falls are frequent among patients with MHE with debilitating consequences. A small prospective study, found that 40 % of patients vs. 13 % without MHE suffered falls requiring increasing utilization of health care resources [137]. Another recent study, examining the effects of underlying cognitive reserve on the HRQOL in patients with progression of CHE concluded that patients with lower cognitive reserve might benefit from early interventions to measures and improves HRQOL [138]. In the RIME trial, MHE patients were randomized into rifaximin vs. placebo arms and found that rifaximin therapy was associated with a significant improvement in both HRQOL and cognitive performance as compared to placebo [139]. Another study also demonstrated that use of lactulose associated with both improvement in cognition and HRQOL [140]. MHE is known to alter the driving capabilities and hence making them prone to traffic accidents. Rifaximin was found to improve the driving performance in a simulated setting along with cognition and psychosocial aspects of quality of life [141]. However, from a societal point of view as in CHE the need to hospitalizations is less and the therapy may be needed for longer time, rifaximin as compared to lactulose was not found to be a cost effective strategy for prevention of driving accidents [142]. The results of a small open-label study showing that lactulose used as a primary prophylactic agent may prevent the development of OHE need to be replicated in larger and well-controlled studies [143]. However, at this point in time as per the guidelines routine treatment of MHE patients is not offered but individual patients may be offered lactulose or lactitol therapy if their quality of life is impaired after undergoing psychometric testing [4].

Do I Need a Liver Transplant?

Patient-Level Answer

If despite optimal treatment strategies for HE there is no resolution of symptoms, liver transplantation (LT) may be considered by the liver doctors.

Provider-Level Answer

HE alone is not an indication for LT without underlying severely compromised liver function. However, exceptions to this rule are patients with severely impaired quality of life despite maximal therapy for HE who may still have good underlying liver function. Large spontaneous portosystemic shunts (like splenorenal shunts) can cause such a scenario and hence, these shunts should be actively sought and abolished by embolization in the pre-LT period, otherwise even after successful LT, HE may return [144]. LT is a complex exercise involving coordinated planning and is not without its associated risks and complications. Separate guidelines have been published by the AASLD for the evaluation of LT patients [145]. Meticulous assessment of patients in the pre-LT period should be embarked upon to differentiate HE from alternative causes like neurodegenerative or dementing illnesses using appropriate imaging studies and expertise. Another, observation is that HE induces structural and functional brain impairment and hence even after LT all the neurologic manifestations may not reverse [146]. This possibility should be discussed with the patient and care-givers ahead of time. In the end, a multifactorial confusional syndrome developing in the postoperative period has been defined which entails thoroughly search for the various causes so as to reverse them [147].

Can I Drive Safely?

Patient-Level Answer

There is association of driving errors and traffic accidents in people with MHE. Your liver doctor may be in a position to advise you further on continuation of driving safely or not.

Provider-Level Answer

In patients with subclinical HE earlier studies, done around a decade apart using neuropsychological testing reported that 44–60 % of the patients were unfit to drive [148, 149]. A study performed on road test using a blinded professional driving instructor (48 cirrhotic patients out of whom 14 had MHE) found that patients with MHE had impaired fitness to drive [150]. Similar results (50–60 % of patients with MHE and stage 1 HE, unfit to drive) were found in another study [22]. Patients with cirrhosis are significantly more prone to traffic accidents and violations as compared to controls with MHE patients being at the highest risk as also corroborated by the state driving agencies [21, 151]. The neurocognitive manifestation of HE results in impairment in attention, response inhibition, working memory, and visuomotor coordination [18]. All these impairments set up the stage for difficulty in driving, as there occurs impaired reaction time leading to navigational difficulties and psychomotor speed [148, 149, 152]. Even after successful therapy for an episode of OHE, not only is there persistence of residual cognitive issues but also treated OHE patients can easily be tipped over by precipitants to get recurrent episodes of OHE [16, 153, 154]. To add insult to the injury, not only do patients with both OHE and MHE report of higher fatigue while driving but also exhibit lack of insight about their driving capabilities [22, 155, 156]. All of these factors can potentially lead to deleterious consequences if these patients keep on driving. However, given the above discussion as per the current consensus the presence of MHE or CHE does not in itself mean that the affected person cannot drive [157]. The providers while following the state laws (only six states require physicians to report drivers with medical impairments at this time) should try to act in the best interests of their patients at both the individual and the societal levels [157, 158]. This is pertinent in view of the fact that physicians are not trained to evaluate for driving fitness. But this does not absolve them of counseling their HE patients about the dangers of driving to self and the others. If the provider is concerned, the best course of action is to ask stop driving with involvement of the caregiver in the discussion and to refer the difficult cases to the proper driving authorities for resolution [4].

Early readmissions to hospitals are considered a quality measure associated with penalties of reduced insurance reimbursements for some disease states, which could be extended to all the hospital readmissions soon. The 30-day readmission, for decompensated cirrhosis has been reported between 20 and 37 %: some of these readmissions may be avoidable, are costly and associated with increased mortality. The most common cause of re-admissions in this study was HE [159]. Hence, improving transitions of care and focusing on as to how to prevent readmissions is a huge challenge calling for urgent research. Newer technology tools like smart phones and tablets may play a role in future to achieve these goals. Recently, a validated model has been developed to identify patients at risk for OHE development using albumin levels, PHES, and history of previous episode of HE, which may help in some advance planning [160].

References

1. Asrani SK, Larson JJ, Yawn B, Therneau TM, Kim WR. Underestimation of liver-related mortality in the United States. Gastroenterology. 2013;145:375–382.e1-2.
2. Gines P, Quintero E, Arroyo V, Teres J, Bruguera M, Rimola A, et al. Compensated cirrhosis: natural history and prognostic factors. Hepatology. 1987;7:122–8.
3. Stepanova M, Mishra A, Venkatesan C, Younossi ZM. In-hospital mortality and economic burden associated with hepatic encephalopathy in the United States from 2005 to 2009. Clin Gastroenterol Hepatol. 2012;10:1034–1041.e1031.
4. Vilstrup H, Amodio P, Bajaj J, Cordoba J, Ferenci P, Mullen KD, et al. Hepatic encephalopathy in chronic liver disease: 2014 Practice Guideline by the American Association for the Study of Liver Diseases and the European Association for the Study of the Liver. Hepatology. 2014;60:715–35.
5. Bajaj JS, Wade JB, Sanyal AJ. Spectrum of neurocognitive impairment in cirrhosis: implications for the assessment of hepatic encephalopathy. Hepatology. 2009;50:2014–21.
6. Bajaj JS, Cordoba J, Mullen KD, Amodio P, Shawcross DL, Butterworth RF, et al. Review article: the design of clinical trials in hepatic encephalopathy--an International Society for Hepatic Encephalopathy and Nitrogen Metabolism (ISHEN) consensus statement. Aliment Pharmacol Ther. 2011;33:739–47.
7. D'Amico G, Morabito A, Pagliaro L, Marubini E. Survival and prognostic indicators in compensated and decompensated cirrhosis. Dig Dis Sci. 1986;31:468–75.
8. Stewart CA, Malinchoc M, Kim WR, Kamath PS. Hepatic encephalopathy as a predictor of survival in patients with end-stage liver disease. Liver Transpl. 2007;13:1366–71.
9. Amodio P, Del Piccolo F, Petteno E, Mapelli D, Angeli P, Iemmolo R, et al. Prevalence and prognostic value of quantified electroencephalogram (EEG) alterations in cirrhotic patients. J Hepatol. 2001;35:37–45.
10. Sharma BC, Sharma P, Agrawal A, Sarin SK. Secondary prophylaxis of hepatic encephalopathy: an open-label randomized controlled trial of lactulose versus placebo. Gastroenterology. 2009;137:885–91. 891.e881.
11. Bajaj JS, Saeian K, Verber MD, Hischke D, Hoffmann RG, Franco J, et al. Inhibitory control test is a simple method to diagnose minimal hepatic encephalopathy and predict development of overt hepatic encephalopathy. Am J Gastroenterol. 2007;102:754–60.
12. Meyer T, Eshelman A, Abouljoud M. Neuropsychological changes in a large sample of liver transplant candidates. Transplant Proc. 2006;38:3559–60.
13. Romero-Gomez M, Boza F, Garcia-Valdecasas MS, Garcia E, Aguilar-Reina J. Subclinical hepatic encephalopathy predicts the development of overt hepatic encephalopathy. Am J Gastroenterol. 2001;96:2718–23.
14. Saxena N, Bhatia M, Joshi YK, Garg PK, Dwivedi SN, Tandon RK. Electrophysiological and neuropsychological tests for the diagnosis of subclinical hepatic encephalopathy and prediction of overt encephalopathy. Liver. 2002;22:190–7.
15. Boyer TD, Haskal ZJ, American Association for the Study of Liver Diseases. The role of Transjugular Intrahepatic Portosystemic Shunt (TIPS) in the management of portal hypertension: update 2009. Hepatology. 2010;51:306.
16. Ferenci P, Lockwood A, Mullen K, Tarter R, Weissenborn K, Blei AT. Hepatic encephalopathy--definition, nomenclature, diagnosis, and quantification: final report of the working party at the 11th World Congresses of Gastroenterology, Vienna, 1998. Hepatology. 2002;35:716–21.
17. Schiff S, Vallesi A, Mapelli D, Orsato R, Pellegrini A, Umilta C, et al. Impairment of response inhibition precedes motor alteration in the early stage of liver cirrhosis: a behavioral and electrophysiological study. Metab Brain Dis. 2005;20:381–92.
18. Weissenborn K, Ennen JC, Schomerus H, Ruckert N, Hecker H. Neuropsychological characterization of hepatic encephalopathy. J Hepatol. 2001;34:768–73.

19. Ortiz M, Jacas C, Cordoba J. Minimal hepatic encephalopathy: diagnosis, clinical significance and recommendations. J Hepatol. 2005;42(Suppl):S45–53.
20. Bajaj JS. Management options for minimal hepatic encephalopathy. Expert Rev Gastroenterol Hepatol. 2008;2:785–90.
21. Bajaj JS, Hafeezullah M, Hoffmann RG, Saeian K. Minimal hepatic encephalopathy: a vehicle for accidents and traffic violations. Am J Gastroenterol. 2007;102:1903–9.
22. Kircheis G, Knoche A, Hilger N, Manhart F, Schnitzler A, Schulze H, et al. Hepatic encephalopathy and fitness to drive. Gastroenterology. 2009;137:1706–1715.e1-9.
23. Prakash RK, Brown TA, Mullen KD. Minimal hepatic encephalopathy and driving: is the genie out of the bottle? Am J Gastroenterol. 2011;106:1415–6.
24. Prakash RK, Mullen KD. Is poor quality of life always present with minimal hepatic encephalopathy? Liver Int. 2011;31:908–10.
25. Groeneweg M, Quero JC, De Bruijn I, Hartmann IJ, Essink-bot ML, Hop WC, et al. Subclinical hepatic encephalopathy impairs daily functioning. Hepatology. 1998;28:45–9.
26. Bajaj JS. Minimal hepatic encephalopathy matters in daily life. World J Gastroenterol. 2008;14:3609–15.
27. Schomerus H, Hamster W. Quality of life in cirrhotics with minimal hepatic encephalopathy. Metab Brain Dis. 2001;16:37–41.
28. Das A, Dhiman RK, Saraswat VA, Verma M, Naik SR. Prevalence and natural history of subclinical hepatic encephalopathy in cirrhosis. J Gastroenterol Hepatol. 2001;16:531–5.
29. Romero-Gomez M, Cordoba J, Jover R, del Olmo JA, Ramirez M, Rey R, et al. Value of the critical flicker frequency in patients with minimal hepatic encephalopathy. Hepatology. 2007;45:879–85.
30. Amodio P, Del Piccolo F, Marchetti P, Angeli P, Iemmolo R, Caregaro L, et al. Clinical features and survivial of cirrhotic patients with subclinical cognitive alterations detected by the number connection test and computerized psychometric tests. Hepatology. 1999;29:1662–7.
31. Weissenborn K, Bokemeyer M, Krause J, Ennen J, Ahl B. Neurological and neuropsychiatric syndromes associated with liver disease. AIDS. 2005;19 Suppl 3:S93–8.
32. Cordoba J, Cabrera J, Lataif L, Penev P, Zee P, Blei AT. High prevalence of sleep disturbance in cirrhosis. Hepatology. 1998;27:339–45.
33. Montagnese S, De Pitta C, De Rui M, Corrias M, Turco M, Merkel C, et al. Sleep-wake abnormalities in patients with cirrhosis. Hepatology. 2014;59:705–12.
34. Wiltfang J, Nolte W, Weissenborn K, Kornhuber J, Ruther E. Psychiatric aspects of portal-systemic encephalopathy. Metab Brain Dis. 1998;13:379–89.
35. Weissenborn K. Diagnosis of encephalopathy. Digestion. 1998;59 Suppl 2:22–4.
36. Cadranel JF, Lebiez E, Di Martino V, Bernard B, El Koury S, Tourbah A, et al. Focal neurological signs in hepatic encephalopathy in cirrhotic patients: an underestimated entity? Am J Gastroenterol. 2001;96:515–8.
37. Delanty N, French JA, Labar DR, Pedley TA, Rowan AJ. Status epilepticus arising de novo in hospitalized patients: an analysis of 41 patients. Seizure. 2001;10:116–9.
38. Eleftheriadis N, Fourla E, Eleftheriadis D, Karlovasitou A. Status epilepticus as a manifestation of hepatic encephalopathy. Acta Neurol Scand. 2003;107:142–4.
39. Tryc AB, Goldbecker A, Berding G, Rumke S, Afshar K, Shahrezaei GH, et al. Cirrhosis-related Parkinsonism: prevalence, mechanisms and response to treatments. J Hepatol. 2013;58:698–705.
40. Nardone R, Holler Y, Storti M, Lochner P, Tezzon F, Golaszewski S, et al. Spinal cord involvement in patients with cirrhosis. World J Gastroenterol. 2014;20:2578–85.
41. Caldwell C, Werdiger N, Jakab S, Schilsky M, Arvelakis A, Kulkarni S, et al. Use of model for end-stage liver disease exception points for early liver transplantation and successful reversal of hepatic myelopathy with a review of the literature. Liver Transpl. 2010;16:818–26.
42. Bajaj JS, Sanyal AJ, Bell D, Gilles H, Heuman DM. Predictors of the recurrence of hepatic encephalopathy in lactulose-treated patients. Aliment Pharmacol Ther. 2010;31:1012–7.

43. Merli M, Lucidi C, Giannelli V, Giusto M, Riggio O, Falcone M, et al. Cirrhotic patients are at risk for health care-associated bacterial infections. Clin Gastroenterol Hepatol. 2010;8:979–85.
44. Strauss E, da Costa MF. The importance of bacterial infections as precipating factors of chronic hepatic encephalopathy in cirrhosis. Hepatogastroenterology. 1998;45:900–4.
45. Maqsood S, Saleem A, Iqbal A, Butt JA. Precipitating factors of hepatic encephalopathy: experience at Pakistan Institute of Medical Sciences Islamabad. J Ayub Med Coll Abbottabad. 2006;18:58–62.
46. Mumtaz K, Ahmed US, Abid S, Baig N, Hamid S, Jafri W. Precipitating factors and the outcome of hepatic encephalopathy in liver cirrhosis. J Coll Physicians Surg Pak. 2010;20:514–8.
47. Onyekwere CA, Ogbera AO, Hameed L. Chronic liver disease and hepatic encephalopathy: clinical profile and outcomes. Niger J Clin Pract. 2011;14:181–5.
48. Guevara M, Baccaro ME, Torre A, Gomez-Anson B, Rios J, Torres F, et al. Hyponatremia is a risk factor of hepatic encephalopathy in patients with cirrhosis: a prospective study with time-dependent analysis. Am J Gastroenterol. 2009;104:1382–9.
49. Kalaitzakis E, Bjornsson E. Renal function and cognitive impairment in patients with liver cirrhosis. Scand J Gastroenterol. 2007;42:1238–44.
50. Norenberg MD, Jayakumar AR, Rama Rao KV, Panickar KS. New concepts in the mechanism of ammonia-induced astrocyte swelling. Metab Brain Dis. 2007;22:219–34.
51. Shawcross DL, Davies NA, Williams R, Jalan R. Systemic inflammatory response exacerbates the neuropsychological effects of induced hyperammonemia in cirrhosis. J Hepatol. 2004;40:247–54.
52. Ahboucha S, Butterworth RF. The neurosteroid system: implication in the pathophysiology of hepatic encephalopathy. Neurochem Int. 2008;52:575–87.
53. Shawcross DL, Shabbir SS, Taylor NJ, Hughes RD. Ammonia and the neutrophil in the pathogenesis of hepatic encephalopathy in cirrhosis. Hepatology. 2010;51:1062–9.
54. Lockwood AH, Yap EW, Wong WH. Cerebral ammonia metabolism in patients with severe liver disease and minimal hepatic encephalopathy. J Cereb Blood Flow Metab. 1991;11:337–41.
55. Weber Jr FL, Veach GL. The importance of the small intestine in gut ammonium production in the fasting dog. Gastroenterology. 1979;77:235–40.
56. Plauth M, Roske AE, Romaniuk P, Roth E, Ziebig R, Lochs H. Post-feeding hyperammonaemia in patients with transjugular intrahepatic portosystemic shunt and liver cirrhosis: role of small intestinal ammonia release and route of nutrient administration. Gut. 2000;46:849–55.
57. Cooper AJ, Plum F. Biochemistry and physiology of brain ammonia. Physiol Rev. 1987;67:440–519.
58. Romero-Gomez M, Jover M, Diaz-Gomez D, de Teran LC, Rodrigo R, Camacho I, et al. Phosphate-activated glutaminase activity is enhanced in brain, intestine and kidneys of rats following portacaval anastomosis. World J Gastroenterol. 2006;12:2406–11.
59. Olde Damink SW, Jalan R, Redhead DN, Hayes PC, Deutz NE, Soeters PB. Interorgan ammonia and amino acid metabolism in metabolically stable patients with cirrhosis and a TIPSS. Hepatology. 2002;36:1163–71.
60. Haussinger D, Kircheis G, Fischer R, Schliess F, von Dahl S. Hepatic encephalopathy in chronic liver disease: a clinical manifestation of astrocyte swelling and low-grade cerebral edema? J Hepatol. 2000;32:1035–8.
61. Shawcross DL, Sharifi Y, Canavan JB, Yeoman AD, Abeles RD, Taylor NJ, et al. Infection and systemic inflammation, not ammonia, are associated with Grade 3/4 hepatic encephalopathy, but not mortality in cirrhosis. J Hepatol. 2011;54:640–9.
62. Merli M, Lucidi C, Pentassuglio I, Giannelli V, Giusto M, Di Gregorio V, et al. Increased risk of cognitive impairment in cirrhotic patients with bacterial infections. J Hepatol. 2013;59:243–50.
63. Wright G, Davies NA, Shawcross DL, Hodges SJ, Zwingmann C, Brooks HF, et al. Endotoxemia produces coma and brain swelling in bile duct ligated rats. Hepatology. 2007;45:1517–26.

64. Odeh M, Sabo E, Srugo I, Oliven A. Serum levels of tumor necrosis factor-alpha correlate with severity of hepatic encephalopathy due to chronic liver failure. Liver Int. 2004;24:110–6.
65. Montoliu C, Piedrafita B, Serra MA, del Olmo JA, Urios A, Rodrigo JM, et al. IL-6 and IL-18 in blood may discriminate cirrhotic patients with and without minimal hepatic encephalopathy. J Clin Gastroenterol. 2009;43:272–9.
66. Blei AT. Infection, inflammation and hepatic encephalopathy, synergism redefined. J Hepatol. 2004;40:327–30.
67. Pedersen HR, Ring-Larsen H, Olsen NV, Larsen FS. Hyperammonemia acts synergistically with lipopolysaccharide in inducing changes in cerebral hemodynamics in rats anaesthetised with pentobarbital. J Hepatol. 2007;47:245–52.
68. Montagnese S, Amodio P, Morgan MY. Methods for diagnosing hepatic encephalopathy in patients with cirrhosis: a multidimensional approach. Metab Brain Dis. 2004;19:281–312.
69. Lockwood AH. Blood ammonia levels and hepatic encephalopathy. Metab Brain Dis. 2004;19:345–9.
70. Gundling F, Zelihic E, Seidl H, Haller B, Umgelter A, Schepp W, et al. How to diagnose hepatic encephalopathy in the emergency department. Ann Hepatol. 2013;12:108–14.
71. Gronbaek H, Johnsen SP, Jepsen P, Gislum M, Vilstrup H, Tage-Jensen U, et al. Liver cirrhosis, other liver diseases, and risk of hospitalisation for intracerebral haemorrhage: a Danish population-based case-control study. BMC Gastroenterol. 2008;8:16.
72. Hassanein TI, Hilsabeck RC, Perry W. Introduction to the hepatic encephalopathy scoring algorithm (HESA). Dig Dis Sci. 2008;53:529–38.
73. Hassanein T, Blei AT, Perry W, Hilsabeck R, Stange J, Larsen FS, et al. Performance of the hepatic encephalopathy scoring algorithm in a clinical trial of patients with cirrhosis and severe hepatic encephalopathy. Am J Gastroenterol. 2009;104:1392–400.
74. Ortiz M, Cordoba J, Doval E, Jacas C, Pujadas F, Esteban R, et al. Development of a clinical hepatic encephalopathy staging scale. Aliment Pharmacol Ther. 2007;26:859–67.
75. Salam M, Matherly S, Farooq IS, Stravitz RT, Sterling RK, Sanyal AJ, et al. Modified-orientation log to assess hepatic encephalopathy. Aliment Pharmacol Ther. 2012;35:913–20.
76. Novack TA, Dowler RN, Bush BA, Glen T, Schneider JJ. Validity of the orientation log, relative to the Galveston orientation and amnesia test. J Head Trauma Rehabil. 2000;15:957–61.
77. Dhiman RK, Saraswat VA, Verma M, Naik SR. Figure connection test: a universal test for assessment of mental state. J Gastroenterol Hepatol. 1995;10:14–23.
78. Mooney S, Hasssanein TI, Hilsabeck RC, Ziegler EA, Carlson M, Maron LM, et al. Utility of the Repeatable Battery for the Assessment of Neuropsychological Status (RBANS) in patients with end-stage liver disease awaiting liver transplant. Arch Clin Neuropsychol. 2007;22:175–86.
79. Bajaj JS, Hafeezullah M, Franco J, Varma RR, Hoffmann RG, Knox JF, et al. Inhibitory control test for the diagnosis of minimal hepatic encephalopathy. Gastroenterology. 2008;135:1591–1600.e1.
80. Montgomery JY, Bajaj JS. Advances in the evaluation and management of minimal hepatic encephalopathy. Curr Gastroenterol Rep. 2011;13:26–33.
81. Amodio P, Schiff S, Del Piccolo F, Mapelli D, Gatta A, Umilta C. Attention dysfunction in cirrhotic patients: an inquiry on the role of executive control, attention orienting and focusing. Metab Brain Dis. 2005;20:115–27.
82. Bajaj JS, Thacker LR, Heuman DM, Fuchs M, Sterling RK, Sanyal AJ, et al. The Stroop smartphone application is a short and valid method to screen for minimal hepatic encephalopathy. Hepatology. 2013;58:1122–32.
83. Bajaj JS, Heuman DM, Sterling RK, Sanyal AJ, Siddiqui M, Matherly S, et al. Validation of EncephalApp, Smartphone-based stroop test, for the diagnosis of covert hepatic encephalopathy. Clin Gastroenterol Hepatol. 2015;13:1828.

84. Montagnese S, Schiff S, Turco M, Bonato CA, Ridola L, Gatta A, et al. Simple tools for complex syndromes: a three-level difficulty test for hepatic encephalopathy. Dig Liver Dis. 2012;44:957–60.
85. Amodio P, Pellegrini A, Amista P, Luise S, Del Piccolo F, Mapelli D, et al. Neuropsychological-neurophysiological alterations and brain atrophy in cirrhotic patients. Metab Brain Dis. 2003;18:63–78.
86. Sakamoto M, Perry W, Hilsabeck RC, Barakat F, Hassanein T. Assessment and usefulness of clinical scales for semiquantification of overt hepatic encephalopathy. Clin Liver Dis. 2012;16:27–42.
87. Kircheis G, Bode JG, Hilger N, Kramer T, Schnitzler A, Haussinger D. Diagnostic and prognostic values of critical flicker frequency determination as new diagnostic tool for objective HE evaluation in patients undergoing TIPS implantation. Eur J Gastroenterol Hepatol. 2009;21:1383–94.
88. Sharma P, Sharma BC, Sarin SK. Critical flicker frequency for diagnosis and assessment of recovery from minimal hepatic encephalopathy in patients with cirrhosis. Hepatobiliary Pancreat Dis Int. 2010;9:27–32.
89. Sharma P, Singh S, Sharma BC, Kumar M, Garg H, Kumar A, et al. Propofol sedation during endoscopy in patients with cirrhosis, and utility of psychometric tests and critical flicker frequency in assessment of recovery from sedation. Endoscopy. 2011;43:400–5.
90. Berlioux P, Robic MA, Poirson H, Metivier S, Otal P, Barret C, et al. Pre-transjugular intrahepatic portosystemic shunts (TIPS) prediction of post-TIPS overt hepatic encephalopathy: the critical flicker frequency is more accurate than psychometric tests. Hepatology. 2014;59:622–9.
91. Torlot FJ, McPhail MJ, Taylor-Robinson SD. Meta-analysis: the diagnostic accuracy of critical flicker frequency in minimal hepatic encephalopathy. Aliment Pharmacol Ther. 2013;37:527–36.
92. Guerit JM, Amantini A, Fischer C, Kaplan PW, Mecarelli O, Schnitzler A, et al. Neurophysiological investigations of hepatic encephalopathy: ISHEN practice guidelines. Liver Int. 2009;29:789–96.
93. Amodio P, Pellegrini A, Ubiali E, Mathy I, Piccolo FD, Orsato R, et al. The EEG assessment of low-grade hepatic encephalopathy: comparison of an artificial neural network-expert system (ANNES) based evaluation with visual EEG readings and EEG spectral analysis. Clin Neurophysiol. 2006;117:2243–51.
94. Amodio P, Marchetti P, Del Piccolo F, de Tourtchaninoff M, Varghese P, Zuliani C, et al. Spectral versus visual EEG analysis in mild hepatic encephalopathy. Clin Neurophysiol. 1999;110:1334–44.
95. Kullmann F, Hollerbach S, Lock G, Holstege A, Dierks T, Scholmerich J. Brain electrical activity mapping of EEG for the diagnosis of (sub)clinical hepatic encephalopathy in chronic liver disease. Eur J Gastroenterol Hepatol. 2001;13:513–22.
96. Strauss E, Tramote R, Silva EP, Caly WR, Honain NZ, Maffei RA, et al. Double-blind randomized clinical trial comparing neomycin and placebo in the treatment of exogenous hepatic encephalopathy. Hepatogastroenterology. 1992;39:542–5.
97. Ferenci P, Herneth A, Steindl P. Newer approaches to therapy of hepatic encephalopathy. Semin Liver Dis. 1996;16:329–38.
98. Huang E, Esrailian E, Spiegel BM. The cost-effectiveness and budget impact of competing therapies in hepatic encephalopathy - a decision analysis. Aliment Pharmacol Ther. 2007;26:1147–61.
99. Uribe M, Campollo O, Vargas F, Ravelli GP, Mundo F, Zapata L, et al. Acidifying enemas (lactitol and lactose) vs. nonacidifying enemas (tap water) to treat acute portal-systemic encephalopathy: a double-blind, randomized clinical trial. Hepatology. 1987;7:639–43.
100. Agrawal A, Sharma BC, Sharma P, Sarin SK. Secondary prophylaxis of hepatic encephalopathy in cirrhosis: an open-label, randomized controlled trial of lactulose, probiotics, and no therapy. Am J Gastroenterol. 2012;107:1043–50.

101. Bajaj JS, Hylemon PB, Ridlon JM, Heuman DM, Daita K, White MB, et al. Colonic mucosal microbiome differs from stool microbiome in cirrhosis and hepatic encephalopathy and is linked to cognition and inflammation. Am J Physiol Gastrointest Liver Physiol. 2012;303:G675–85.
102. Jalan R. Rifaximin in hepatic encephalopathy: more than just a non-absorbable antibiotic? J Hepatol. 2010;53:580–2.
103. Kalambokis GN, Mouzaki A, Rodi M, Pappas K, Fotopoulos A, Xourgia X, et al. Rifaximin improves systemic hemodynamics and renal function in patients with alcohol-related cirrhosis and ascites. Clin Gastroenterol Hepatol. 2012;10:815–8.
104. Jiang ZD, DuPont HL. Rifaximin: in vitro and in vivo antibacterial activity--a review. Chemotherapy. 2005;51 Suppl 1:67–72.
105. Patidar KR, Bajaj JS. Antibiotics for the treatment of hepatic encephalopathy. Metab Brain Dis. 2013;28:307–12.
106. Bass NM, Mullen KD, Sanyal A, Poordad F, Neff G, Leevy CB, et al. Rifaximin treatment in hepatic encephalopathy. N Engl J Med. 2010;362:1071–81.
107. Sanyal A, Younossi ZM, Bass NM, Mullen KD, Poordad F, Brown RS, et al. Randomised clinical trial: rifaximin improves health-related quality of life in cirrhotic patients with hepatic encephalopathy - a double-blind placebo-controlled study. Aliment Pharmacol Ther. 2011;34:853–61.
108. Hawkins RA, Jessy J, Mans AM, Chedid A, DeJoseph MR. Neomycin reduces the intestinal production of ammonia from glutamine. Adv Exp Med Biol. 1994;368:125–34.
109. Orlandi F, Freddara U, Candelaresi MT, Morettini A, Corazza GR, Di Simone A, et al. Comparison between neomycin and lactulose in 173 patients with hepatic encephalopathy: a randomized clinical study. Dig Dis Sci. 1981;26:498–506.
110. Morgan MH, Read AE, Speller DC. Treatment of hepatic encephalopathy with metronidazole. Gut. 1982;23:1–7.
111. Loft S, Sonne J, Dossing M, Andreasen PB. Metronidazole pharmacokinetics in patients with hepatic encephalopathy. Scand J Gastroenterol. 1987;22:117–23.
112. Tarao K, Ikeda T, Hayashi K, Sakurai A, Okada T, Ito T, et al. Successful use of vancomycin hydrochloride in the treatment of lactulose resistant chronic hepatic encephalopathy. Gut. 1990;31:702–6.
113. Mantry PS, Munsaf S. Rifaximin for the treatment of hepatic encephalopathy. Transplant Proc. 2010;42:4543–7.
114. Morgan MY, Milsom JP, Sherlock S. Plasma ratio of valine, leucine and isoleucine to phenylalanine and tyrosine in liver disease. Gut. 1978;19:1068–73.
115. Gluud LL, Dam G, Les I, Cordoba J, Marchesini G, Borre M, Aagaard NK, Vilstrup H. Branched-chain amino acids for people with hepatic encephalopathy. Cochrane Database Syst Rev 2015; (2): CD001939.
116. Naylor CD, O'Rourke K, Detsky AS, Baker JP. Parenteral nutrition with branched-chain amino acids in hepatic encephalopathy. A meta-analysis. Gastroenterology. 1989;97:1033–42.
117. Khungar V, Poordad F. Hepatic encephalopathy. Clin Liver Dis. 2012;16:301–20.
118. Kircheis G, Nilius R, Held C, Berndt H, Buchner M, Gortelmeyer R, et al. Therapeutic efficacy of L-ornithine-L-aspartate infusions in patients with cirrhosis and hepatic encephalopathy: results of a placebo-controlled, double-blind study. Hepatology. 1997;25:1351–60.
119. Bai M, He C, Yin Z, Niu J, Wang Z, Qi X, et al. Randomised clinical trial: L-ornithine-L-aspartate reduces significantly the increase of venous ammonia concentration after TIPSS. Aliment Pharmacol Ther. 2014;40:63–71.
120. Sharma K, Pant S, Misra S, Dwivedi M, Misra A, Narang S, et al. Effect of rifaximin, probiotics, and l-ornithine l-aspartate on minimal hepatic encephalopathy: a randomized controlled trial. Saudi J Gastroenterol. 2014;20:225–32.
121. Shukla S, Shukla A, Mehboob S, Guha S. Meta-analysis: the effects of gut flora modulation using prebiotics, probiotics and synbiotics on minimal hepatic encephalopathy. Aliment Pharmacol Ther. 2011;33:662–71.

122. McGee RG, Bakens A, Wiley K, Riordan SM, Webster AC. Probiotics for patients with hepatic encephalopathy. Cochrane Database Syst Rev 2011; (11): CD008716.
123. Holte K, Krag A, Gluud LL. Systematic review and meta-analysis of randomized trials on probiotics for hepatic encephalopathy. Hepatol Res. 2012;42:1008–15.
124. Bajaj JS, Heuman DM, Hylemon PB, Sanyal AJ, Puri P, Sterling RK, et al. Randomised clinical trial: lactobacillus GG modulates gut microbiome, metabolome and endotoxemia in patients with cirrhosis. Aliment Pharmacol Ther. 2014;39:1113–25.
125. Rahimi RS, Singal AG, Cuthbert JA, Rockey DC. Lactulose vs polyethylene glycol 3350--electrolyte solution for treatment of overt hepatic encephalopathy: the HELP randomized clinical trial. JAMA Intern Med. 2014;174:1727–33.
126. Hassanein TI, Tofteng F, Brown Jr RS, McGuire B, Lynch P, Mehta R, et al. Randomized controlled study of extracorporeal albumin dialysis for hepatic encephalopathy in advanced cirrhosis. Hepatology. 2007;46:1853–62.
127. Banares R, Nevens F, Larsen FS, Jalan R, Albillos A, Dollinger M, et al. Extracorporeal albumin dialysis with the molecular adsorbent recirculating system in acute-on-chronic liver failure: the RELIEF trial. Hepatology. 2013;57:1153–62.
128. Merli M, Giusto M, Lucidi C, Giannelli V, Pentassuglio I, Di Gregorio V, et al. Muscle depletion increases the risk of overt and minimal hepatic encephalopathy: results of a prospective study. Metab Brain Dis. 2013;28:281–4.
129. Alberino F, Gatta A, Amodio P, Merkel C, Di Pascoli L, Boffo G, et al. Nutrition and survival in patients with liver cirrhosis. Nutrition. 2001;17:445–50.
130. Madden AMM, Morgan MY. Hand-grip strength in cirrhosis - its relationship to nutritional status and severity of liver disease. Hepatology. 1998;28(Suppl):609A.
131. Figueiredo FA, Dickson ER, Pasha TM, Porayko MK, Therneau TM, Malinchoc M, et al. Utility of standard nutritional parameters in detecting body cell mass depletion in patients with end-stage liver disease. Liver Transpl. 2000;6:575–81.
132. Tsien CD, McCullough AJ, Dasarathy S. Late evening snack: exploiting a period of anabolic opportunity in cirrhosis. J Gastroenterol Hepatol. 2012;27:430–41.
133. Amodio P, Bemeur C, Butterworth R, Cordoba J, Kato A, Montagnese S, et al. The nutritional management of hepatic encephalopathy in patients with cirrhosis: International Society for Hepatic Encephalopathy and Nitrogen Metabolism Consensus. Hepatology. 2013;58:325–36.
134. Dam G, Ott P, Aagaard NK, Vilstrup H. Branched-chain amino acids and muscle ammonia detoxification in cirrhosis. Metab Brain Dis. 2013;28:217–20.
135. Gabduzda GJ, Hall 3rd PW. Relation of potassium depletion to renal ammonium metabolism and hepatic coma. Medicine. 1966;45:481–90.
136. Patidar KR, Thacker LR, Wade JB, Sterling RK, Sanyal AJ, Siddiqui MS, et al. Covert hepatic encephalopathy is independently associated with poor survival and increased risk of hospitalization. Am J Gastroenterol. 2014;109:1757–63.
137. Roman E, Cordoba J, Torrens M, Torras X, Villanueva C, Vargas V, et al. Minimal hepatic encephalopathy is associated with falls. Am J Gastroenterol. 2011;106:476–82.
138. Patel AV, Wade JB, Thacker LR, Sterling RK, Siddiqui MS, Stravitz RT, et al. Cognitive reserve is a determinant of health-related quality of life in patients with cirrhosis, independent of covert hepatic encephalopathy and model for end-stage liver disease score. Clin Gastroenterol Hepatol. 2015;13:987.
139. Sidhu SS, Goyal O, Mishra BP, Sood A, Chhina RS, Soni RK. Rifaximin improves psychometric performance and health-related quality of life in patients with minimal hepatic encephalopathy (the RIME Trial). Am J Gastroenterol. 2011;106:307–16.
140. Prasad S, Dhiman RK, Duseja A, Chawla YK, Sharma A, Agarwal R. Lactulose improves cognitive functions and health-related quality of life in patients with cirrhosis who have minimal hepatic encephalopathy. Hepatology. 2007;45:549–59.
141. Bajaj JS, Heuman DM, Wade JB, Gibson DP, Saeian K, Wegelin JA, et al. Rifaximin improves driving simulator performance in a randomized trial of patients with minimal hepatic encephalopathy. Gastroenterology. 2011;140:478–487.e1.

142. Bajaj JS, Pinkerton SD, Sanyal AJ, Heuman DM. Diagnosis and treatment of minimal hepatic encephalopathy to prevent motor vehicle accidents: a cost-effectiveness analysis. Hepatology. 2012;55:1164–71.
143. Sharma P, Sharma BC, Agrawal A, Sarin SK. Primary prophylaxis of overt hepatic encephalopathy in patients with cirrhosis: an open labeled randomized controlled trial of lactulose versus no lactulose. J Gastroenterol Hepatol. 2012;27:1329–35.
144. Herrero JI, Bilbao JI, Diaz ML, Alegre F, Inarrairaegui M, Pardo F, et al. Hepatic encephalopathy after liver transplantation in a patient with a normally functioning graft: treatment with embolization of portosystemic collaterals. Liver Transpl. 2009;15:111–4.
145. Martin P, DiMartini A, Feng S, Brown Jr R, Fallon M. Evaluation for liver transplantation in adults: 2013 practice guideline by the American Association for the Study of Liver Diseases and the American Society of Transplantation. Hepatology. 2014;59:1144–65.
146. Garcia-Martinez R, Rovira A, Alonso J, Jacas C, Simon-Talero M, Chavarria L, et al. Hepatic encephalopathy is associated with posttransplant cognitive function and brain volume. Liver Transpl. 2011;17:38–46.
147. Amodio P, Biancardi A, Montagnese S, Angeli P, Iannizzi P, Cillo U, et al. Neurological complications after orthotopic liver transplantation. Dig Liver Dis. 2007;39:740–7.
148. Watanabe A, Tuchida T, Yata Y, Kuwabara Y. Evaluation of neuropsychological function in patients with liver cirrhosis with special reference to their driving ability. Metab Brain Dis. 1995;10:239–48.
149. Schomerus H, Hamster W, Blunck H, Reinhard U, Mayer K, Dolle W. Latent portasystemic encephalopathy. I. Nature of cerebral functional defects and their effect on fitness to drive. Dig Dis Sci. 1981;26:622–30.
150. Wein C, Koch H, Popp B, Oehler G, Schauder P. Minimal hepatic encephalopathy impairs fitness to drive. Hepatology. 2004;39:739–45.
151. Bajaj JS, Saeian K, Schubert CM, Hafeezullah M, Franco J, Varma RR, et al. Minimal hepatic encephalopathy is associated with motor vehicle crashes: the reality beyond the driving test. Hepatology. 2009;50:1175–83.
152. Bajaj JS, Hafeezullah M, Hoffmann RG, Varma RR, Franco J, Binion DG, et al. Navigation skill impairment: another dimension of the driving difficulties in minimal hepatic encephalopathy. Hepatology. 2008;47:596–604.
153. Bajaj JS, Schubert CM, Heuman DM, Wade JB, Gibson DP, Topaz A, et al. Persistence of cognitive impairment after resolution of overt hepatic encephalopathy. Gastroenterology. 2010;138:2332–40.
154. Bajaj JS. Review article: the modern management of hepatic encephalopathy. Aliment Pharmacol Ther. 2010;31:537–47.
155. Bajaj JS, Hafeezullah M, Zadvornova Y, Martin E, Schubert CM, Gibson DP, et al. The effect of fatigue on driving skills in patients with hepatic encephalopathy. Am J Gastroenterol. 2009;104:898–905.
156. Bajaj JS, Saeian K, Hafeezullah M, Hoffmann RG, Hammeke TA. Patients with minimal hepatic encephalopathy have poor insight into their driving skills. Clin Gastroenterol Hepatol. 2008;6:1135–9. quiz 1065.
157. Bajaj JS, Stein AC, Dubinsky RM. What is driving the legal interest in hepatic encephalopathy? Clin Gastroenterol Hepatol. 2011;9:97–8.
158. Cohen SM, Kim A, Metropulos M, Ahn J. Legal ramifications for physicians of patients who drive with hepatic encephalopathy. Clin Gastroenterol Hepatol. 2011;9:156–60. quiz e117.
159. Volk ML, Tocco RS, Bazick J, Rakoski MO, Lok AS. Hospital readmissions among patients with decompensated cirrhosis. Am J Gastroenterol. 2012;107:247–52.
160. Riggio O, Amodio P, Farcomeni A, Merli M, Nardelli S, Pasquale C, et al. A model for predicting development of overt hepatic encephalopathy in patients with cirrhosis. Clin Gastroenterol Hepatol. 2015;13:1346.

Chapter 30
Ascites

Adam J. Schiro

1. What causes ascites to develop?

    Patient-Level Answer: Fluid within the abdominal cavity, or ascites, can develop for many reasons including heart or kidney disease but is seen most commonly in patients with liver cirrhosis. Fluid accumulation happens because of increased pressures in the blood vessels that supply the liver causing leaking of fluid into the abdomen.

2. How is it treated?

    Patient-Level Answer: The first step is to follow a low-salt diet because excess salt leads to excess fluid within the abdomen. If this is not effective, the next step is to use diuretic medications to remove salt and fluid from the bloodstream. In certain patients who continue to have problems with ascites we may recommend a special procedure called a shunt or TIPS to relieve the high pressures which lead to ascites

3. Why does it keep coming back?

    Patient-Level Answer: The most common explanation is too much salt in the diet. If diuretic pills are being used to treat ascites, the dose may need to be increased to achieve better effect. Sometimes an ultrasound is needed to make sure there isn't another explanation for worsening ascites such as a blood clot in the vessels supplying the liver or a liver cancer.

A.J. Schiro, M.D. (✉)
Division of Gastroenterology & Hepatology, Department of Medicine,
Medical College of Wisconsin, 9200 W. Wisconsin Ave, Milwaukee, WI 53226, USA
e-mail: aschiro@mcw.edu

© Springer International Publishing Switzerland 2017
K. Saeian, R. Shaker (eds.), *Liver Disorders*,
DOI 10.1007/978-3-319-30103-7_30

Introduction

Ascites is defined as an excess of fluid within the peritoneal cavity. According to the International Club of Ascites grading is performed according to severity [1]. Grade 1 is defined as mild and is not clinically evident, diagnosed by imaging such as ultrasound or computerized tomography. Grade 2, moderate ascites, is defined as proportionate sensible abdominal distention. Grade 3, severe ascites, is defined as noticeable tense distension of the abdomen.

Pathogenesis

The development of ascites in patients with cirrhosis occurs via a complex mechanism and molecular pathway known as the "peripheral arterial vasodilation hypothesis." The initial event appears to be the development of portal hypertension. This occurs in the setting of advanced fibrosis which leads to architectural distortion and increased hepatic vascular tone via the release of various vasoconstrictive agents such as angiotensin, endothelin, and thromboxane, as well as reduced levels of hepatic nitric oxide. This elevation of portal pressures leads to a reflexive systemic vasodilatation. This process is primarily driven by peripheral release of nitric oxide leading to a diffuse vasodilatory state, especially dilatation of the splanchnic circulation. This vasodilation leads to perceived underfilling and a drop in mean systemic arterial pressure. This triggers a baroreceptor-mediated response involving activation of the renin-angiotensin-aldosterone system, release of anti-diuretic hormone, and activation of the sympathetic nervous system. Sodium and water retention is promoted, and in the setting of splanchnic vasodilatation, permeability and leakage of fluid into the peritoneal space occurs. This cycle leads to more vasodilation, more underfilling, and more retention of sodium and water, forming essentially a vicious cycle. The mechanism and pathogenesis for development of ascites in the noncirrhotic patient is quite distinct from that which occurs in the setting of cirrhosis and will not be discussed in further detail.

Diagnosis

In the United States ascites occurs due to underlying cirrhosis and portal hypertension in roughly 85 % of cases. The remaining cases of ascites include additional noncirrhotic causes of portal hypertension, cardiac disease, peritoneal carcinomatosis, and miscellaneous nonportal hypertension related disorders [2].

A thorough history including inquiry into specific risk factors for the development of cirrhosis including amount of alcohol consumption, history of intravenous drug use, tattoos, high-risk sexual behavior, blood transfusions received prior to

1992 when universal screening was implemented, presence of coexisting autoimmune disease, family history of iron or copper storage disorders, and country of origin. Assessment for underlying risk factors for nonalcoholic steatohepatitis (NASH) such as the presence of obesity, diabetes mellitus, and hyperlipidemia should also be made.

Presence of coexisting risk factors or medical comorbidities should guide the clinical evaluation in a patient with new onset ascites. A patient with known malignancy, especially of the colon, breast, pancreas, or lung, who suddenly develops ascites, should be suspected of having malignancy related ascites. Abdominal pain can be a useful distinguishing feature as patients with ascites due to malignancy are more likely than patients with ascites from cirrhosis to complain of abdominal pain. A patient with known cardiac disease or cardiac risk factors should be evaluated for heart failure or cardiomyopathy leading to ascites. Additional clinical clues suggesting pancreatitis, thyroid dysfunction, renal impairment, or risk factors for tuberculosis should prompt further investigation as to an underlying disorder leading to the development of noncirrhotic ascites.

Physical exam findings are typically readily apparent. Abdominal distention, bulging flanks, especially in the setting of known liver disease should prompt further investigation and work-up. Typically flank dullness to percussion is noted, often appreciated higher up the abdominal wall than normally expected and accompanied by shifting when the patient is repositioned. Generally 1500 mL of ascitic fluid is required to manifest as shifting dullness [3]. The presence of intraluminal gastrointestinal gas, increased central adiposity, and intra-abdominal masses can mimic ascites and make clinical investigation difficult. If exam findings are equivocal and there remains a high degree of suspicion to suspect underlying ascites, abdominal ultrasonography can be useful and is able to detect as little as 100 mL of free fluid within the abdominal cavity.

Once the presence of ascites is confirmed based on exam or imaging, abdominal paracentesis is recommended for further evaluation with appropriate diagnostic fluid testing. Per American Association for the Study of Liver Disease (AASLD) guidelines this should be performed in every case of newly diagnosed ascites whether inpatient or outpatient, and also during each hospitalization for patients with cirrhosis and ascites who are admitted to the hospital to exclude the presence of spontaneous bacterial peritonitis (SBP) [4]. This, in addition to patients who display clinically features suggestive of SBP (altered mental status, confusion, abdominal pain, fevers, peripheral leukocytosis, etc.).

The abdominal paracentesis procedure itself is quite safe and relatively few true contraindications exist. Coagulopathy is frequently cited as a precluding factor for safe performance of the procedure, as elevated international normalized ratio (INR) values are common in patients with cirrhosis and evidence of hepatic synthetic dysfunction. In reality, due to balanced deficiencies of both procoagulant and anticoagulant factors, the elevations of INR seen in cirrhotic patients likely overestimate a truly elevated bleeding risk, and paracentesis has been shown to be quite safe in this patient population [5]. Valid exclusionary criteria would, however, include the presence of clear evidence of fibrinolysis or disseminated intravascular coagulation

(DIC). In general the routine use of plasma transfusion prior to performing paracentesis is not recommended and has never been shown to prevent bleeding or improve outcomes. Serious complications including bowel perforation, hemoperitoneum, or death are exceedingly rare. The most common complication is abdominal wall hematoma occurring in 2 % of cases, and significant enough to require a blood transfusion in only 1 % of procedures [5]. Complications are typically less common when more experienced providers perform the procedure, and the use of ultrasonography guidance is strongly encouraged especially in obese patients or patients with abdominal surgical scars.

Routine laboratory analysis should include cell count, gram stain, total protein and albumin from ascitic fluid and serum (in order to calculate a serum-ascites albumin gradient), bacterial cultures, glucose, and lactate dehydrogenase (LDH). Depending on gross appearance of the ascitic fluid, or on other clinical factors which may be present, such as concern for malignancy or thoracic duct injury, additional values may be run as appropriate such as cytology, lipase and amylase levels, triglycerides, and/or bilirubin levels. The cutoff value for total PMN count in order to make a diagnosis of SBP is generally accepted to be 250 PMN's per mm^3. The total leukocyte count can be elevated in other conditions besides SBP, including in peritoneal carcinomatosis and in tuberculous peritonitis, though these entities typically display a lymphocyte predominance on differential [6]. If the specimen is grossly bloody, which typically occurs following a traumatic "tap," the total PMN count may be elevated due to the increased number of neutrophils within blood itself. A correction factor is employed to calculate the total number of polymorphonuclear cells (PMN's) by subtracting 1 PMN for every 250 red blood cells (RBC's) identified on the cell count.

Historically, characterization of ascites fluid was regarded similarly to pleural effusions, as either exudative or transudative using mainly total protein levels, as well as LDH, however, this was shown to be notoriously inaccurate [2]. A more effective classification scheme is based on calculation of the serum-ascites albumin gradient, or SAAG, which provides a representative estimation of hydrostatic-oncotic balance. The preferred classification terms now for ascites are high-albumin gradient and low-albumin gradient in place of transudative and exudative respectively. Calculation is accomplished by subtracting the level of albumin from the ascitic fluid from the serum albumin level at the time the paracentesis was performed (keeping in mind exogenous administration of intravenous albumin products could lead to inaccuracies). Serum and ascitic fluid samples should be obtained at least on the same day; preferably within the same hour. In patients with portal hypertension, an elevated hydrostatic pressure gradient is present between the portal system and the ascitic fluid. This requires balance in terms of colloid oncotic pressure, of which albumin serves as a representative marker for, therefore leading to a direct correlation of the SAAG value and portal pressures. A generally accepted cutoff SAAG value of ≥ 1.1 g/dL has been shown to be consistent with portal hypertension with an accuracy of 97 % [2]. Conditions which lead to falsely low SAAG value include systemic hypotension by reduction of the portal pressure gradient, as well as with hyperglobulinemia where oncotic pressures are elevated thus narrowing the gradient. Falsely elevated SAAG values can be seen in conditions such as chylous ascites where lipids interfere with the laboratory analysis of albumin.

Ascitic fluid culture is used most commonly to detect the presence of a specific organism in cirrhotic patients with SBP in order to tailor antibiotic therapy and track resistance patterns for various organisms. TSBP infections are typically monomicrobial and characterized by overall low bacterial concentration as compared to infections of the urine or stool. As a result, typical culture methods tend to yield lower diagnostic results. It has been shown that, as with blood cultures for the detection of bacteremia, the practice of bedside inoculation of ascitic fluid samples into culture tubes dramatically improves diagnostic capabilities and this practice is recommended as standard of care when performing diagnostic paracentesis [7].

Total protein levels from ascitic fluid are useful in several circumstances. In patients with ascites of unclear etiology, and an elevated SAAG ≥1.1 g/dL, a low total protein level is mores suggestive of underlying cirrhosis whereas an elevated total protein level >2.5 g/dL is more suggestive of ascites from underlying heart failure [8]. This cutoff is less absolute and there are a significant number of patients with ascites due to cirrhosis who also have an ascitic fluid total protein of >2.5 g/dL. SAAG values tend to narrow with diuresis in patients with ascites from right-sided heart failure, whereas SAAG is generally unaffected by diuresis in cirrhotic patients. In patients with ascites and a SAAG value <1.1 g/dL, a low total protein level <2.5 g/dL is most consistent with nephrotic syndrome. Total protein levels are also inversely related to risk of development of SBP, through deficiency in opsonins, among other factors. Conversely, infections resulting from secondary bacterial peritonitis, which are often polymicrobial, tend to correlate with higher levels of ascitic fluid total protein. Highly sensitive diagnostic criteria exist to aid in identification of patients with intra-abdominal infection resulting from secondary bacterial peritonitis from perforated viscous [9]. The criteria include total protein >1 g/dL, glucose <50 mg/dL, and LDH >upper limit of normal for serum, and are associated with sensitivity of nearly 100 % and specificity of 45 % in identifying secondary bacterial peritonitis.

Glucose levels from ascitic fluid can be helpful for confirming a suspected diagnosis of SBP. Generally sterile ascitic fluid should have similar concentrations of glucose to serum; however, in the case of bacterial infection, levels of glucose typically fall to very low or undetectable levels. This can happen with either SBP or with secondary bacterial peritonitis from intestinal perforation, and is not generally helpful at distinguishing the two. LDH levels are typically reduced in sterile ascites, as the molecule is not easily released from the bloodstream. Levels of LDH in SBP are generally increased due to release of LDH from neutrophils. These levels are even more significantly elevated in cases of secondary bacterial peritonitis.

In cases where pancreatic ascites is suspected, amylase levels are generally found to be significantly elevated above serum levels as compared to uncomplicated ascites, where amylase values are generally around half of serum values.

Gram stain of ascitic fluid is routinely performed, but its sensitivity for detection of a causative organism in the setting of SBP is limited. The gram stain is positive in roughly 10 % of cases of SBP owing to the low inoculum requirements for this type of infection [10]. Gram stain is more useful for the diagnoses of cases of secondary peritonitis or intestinal perforation were multiple types of organisms (polymicrobial) are noted.

For cases of suspected *Mycobacterium tuberculosis* infection of the peritoneal cavity, ascitic fluid culture or smear for acid-fast bacilli are largely insensitive for solidifying the diagnosis. For adequate diagnostic yield the gold standard is obtained via laparoscopic biopsies of the peritoneum. Tuberculous peritonitis can be easily confused for SBP, which is compounded by the fact that it occurs 50 % of the time in a setting of underlying cirrhosis. Additional diagnostic clues suggesting tuberculous peritonitis include a mononuclear predominance on cell count and a negative bacterial culture [11]. Unlike tuberculous pleural effusions, testing of ascitic fluid for adenosine deaminase (ADA) levels has not been shown to be helpful as it is far less sensitive than peritoneal biopsy.

Malignant ascites develops in the setting of direct malignant infiltration of the lining of the peritoneal cavity with the prototypical example being peritoneal carcinomatosis. This is distinguished from the scenario of massive hepatic tumor infiltration leading to portal hypertension and the development of ascites, as no malignant cells would be expected to be isolated from the ascitic fluid in this situation. Malignancy-related ascites may also present with an elevated white cell count, though this is often predominately lymphocytic.

If there is concern for injury to the thoracic duct or lymphatic system, or if the ascites fluid has a milky appearance to it, a fluid triglyceride level should be obtained. Chylous ascites is characterized by fluid triglyceride levels of $\geq$200 mg/dL, though observed values often exceed 1000 mg/dL. Similarly, if bile injury is suspected or if the ascites fluid has a dark brown hue, a bilirubin level should be obtained. Levels $\geq$6 mg/dL or levels greater than serum concentration are suggestive of a bile leak.

Complications

The development of infection in previously sterile ascitic fluid is the most important complication resulting from the presence of ascites. The pathogenesis, diagnosis, management, and prophylaxis of SBP are discussed separately. Additional complications include cellulitis, abdominal wall hernias, hepatic hydrothorax, and the development of tense ascites.

Patients with ascites and peripheral edema are especially prone to developing superficial skin infections of the lower extremities and abdominal wall. This risk is compounded in obese patients and patients with a greater degree of edema. One retrospective analysis of cirrhotic patients who developed cellulitis found a significantly higher risk of development of renal failure (21.7 % versus 5.4 %, $p=0.001$) as well as death or transplant at 3 months (23 % versus 4 %, $p<0.001$) [12].

Increased intra-abdominal pressure as a result of ascites leads to abdominal wall defects in approximately 20 % of patients [13]. The most common site of herniation is at the umbilicus, but incisional hernias and less commonly inguinal hernias are also seen. Incarceration and necrosis is of concern especially in the setting of ascites, and typically elective hernia repair is recommended to prevent these complications but of course patients may be at high operative risk. Paracentesis with complete removal of existing ascites is recommended given high rates of hernia recurrence if fluid is present at the time of surgery. Transjugular intrahepatic portosystemic shunt (TIPS) can also be a consideration for management of problematic umbilical hernias if surgery is felt to be prohibitively high risk.

Ascites in the setting of portal hypertension and hypoalbuminemia with decreased colloid oncotic pressures can lead to the development of pleural effusions as well. Classically hepatic hydrothorax manifests as an isolated right-sided pleural effusion (70–85 %) although isolated left-sided (10–15 %) and bilateral effusions are also encountered and are believed to result from defects in the diaphragm. They tend to occur in patients with refractory or diuretic resistant ascites, and can lead to dyspnea, hypoxia, respiratory failure, and infection. Management of hepatic hydrothorax can be problematic as it almost uniformly recurs following therapeutic thoracentesis and carries a poor prognosis. Tube thoracostomy has not been shown to be helpful in this setting and should be avoided especially as it may result in copious fluid loss and electrolyte abnormalities. For patients who are unable to be managed with dietary sodium restriction, diuretics, and intermittent thoracentesis, placement of TIPS should be considered as should consideration of liver transplantation.

Tense ascites refers to development of critical amount of intra-abdominal fluid leading to symptoms of abdominal pain, respiratory compromise, and potentially abdominal compartment syndrome. The treatment is urgent therapeutic paracentesis.

Treatment

The goals of therapy for management of ascites include improving quality of life, reducing abdominal discomfort, preventing umbilical hernia development, reducing the risk of infections such as SBP, and ultimately improving survival. Management strategies center on control of the offending etiology. In alcoholic cirrhosis, abstinence from alcohol is imperative. Similarly, patients with cirrhosis from underlying treatable conditions such as Wilson's disease, autoimmune hepatitis, or hepatitis B virus, need these disorders addressed and may see resolution or a significant improvement in ascites with a focus on underlying disease management.

Reversible or iatrogenic causes of ascites development in a setting of cirrhosis should be sought out and addressed. These would include dietary indiscretion and lack of adherence to a sodium restricted diet, noncompliance with diuretic therapy, intravenous fluid infusion with normal saline, infection, gastrointestinal hemorrhage, or hepatocellular carcinoma.

Dietary sodium restriction is a cornerstone of therapy, and is crucial to combating the renal retention of sodium seen in portal hypertension. Patient's need strict adherence to a low-sodium diet, typically limited to 2000 mg daily, and formal dietician-led education on this topic is strongly recommended. The major limitation with this strategy is compliance. Patients following a 2000 mg daily sodium diet ingest 88 mmol of sodium per day. Roughly 10 mmol are lost through nonrenal mechanisms such as via the stool or perspiration. If a patient with a serum sodium level of 130 mEq/L undergoes a 5 L paracentesis, this entails the removal of 650 mmol of sodium. Assuming a patient is completely anuric, these 650 mmol should take over 8 days to re-accumulate on an 88 mmol per day diet. Patients requiring paracentesis more frequently than this are therefore not compliant with the 2000 mg sodium diet. Urinary sodium excretion can also be assessed. Patients who excrete more than 78 mmol of sodium per day and who are adherent to a 2000 mg sodium diet should expect their weight to remain stable or decline. If this is not the case despite excretion of 78 mmol of sodium per day, then this suggests dietary indiscretion. While 24-h urine excretion is the gold-standard, random urine sodium to potassium ratio has been shown to correlate well. A ratio of >1 in the setting of dietary sodium compliance should lead to weight and fluid losses. For this minority of patients, ascites can be managed with diet alone, and without diuretics.

In general fluid restriction is not routinely recommended, except in cases of severe hyponatremia with serum sodium levels <120 mEq/L. Hyponatremia results from water retention (as a result of ADH release) out of proportion to sodium retention (as a result of renin-angiotensin-aldosterone activation), and in these cases fluid restriction is warranted. Cirrhotic patients typically tolerate low levels of serum sodium as a result of chronic hyponatremia and rarely develop symptoms or consequences unless there is a rapid fluctuation in serum levels.

For ascites which persists despite strict dietary adherence to a low-sodium diet, the mainstay of therapy is diuretic agents. Typically a combination of the aldosterone antagonist spironolactone and the loop diuretic furosemide are used in combination. Given the opposing effects on serum potassium levels of the two agents, a ratio of 5:2 in terms of spironolactone to furosemide dose is generally preferred. Goals of therapy should include both total body weight reduction, as well as an increase in urinary sodium concentration. It is postulated that diuretics may play a role in preventing SBP via concentration of ascitic fluid opsonin activity which plays a critical role in preventing the development of SBP [14]. Intravenous administration of diuretics is employed commonly in the inpatient setting, and while generally effective for patients with congestive heart failure, this should be employed with caution in cirrhotic patients. The alternations in renal physiology and hemodynamics among cirrhotic patients readily predispose them to the development of azotemia. The concomitant use of intravenous administration of colloidal substance such as albumin, to which furosemide is highly bound to in serum, has not been shown to be of benefit in the cirrhotic population [15]. In addition to electrolyte abnormalities, other potential adverse effects from diuretics used in the management of ascites center around intravascular volume depletion in the setting of over-diuresis. This scenario is a common precipitant of hepatic encephalopathy, azotemic renal failure, and severe hyponatremia. It is generally recommended that the presence of a serum creatinine of greater than 2.0 mg/dL, a serum sodium less than 120 mmol/L, or new hepatic encephalopathy should prompt discontinuation of diuretics, and in many cases should be followed by an attempt at intravascular volume expansion.

Refractory ascites is defined by the persistence of abdominal ascites despite adherence to a low-sodium diet and high-dose diuretic regimen, and occurs in less than 10 % of patients [16]. This diagnosis should prompt a thorough evaluation of a patient's medications, with particular attention to anti-hypertensive agents. In patients with baseline hypotension as defined by systolic blood pressure less than 100 mmHg, these agents should be discontinued, which allows for improved renal hemodynamics and an improved or effective response to diuretics. The alpha-adrenergic agonist midodrine has been suggested to be of potential benefit in patients who continue to have refractory ascites in the setting of hypotension after discontinuation of antihypertensive medications [17].

Therapeutic abdominal paracentesis can be safely performed to allow for large volume removal of abdominal ascites fluid. There is generally no limit on the amount of fluid volume which can safely be removed in a single procedure, though concerns tend to arise regarding electrolyte abnormalities resulting from fluid shifts after removal of more than 5 L of fluid. Cases of removal of up to 41 L in a single session have previously been reported [18]. In an effort to combat electrolyte abnormalities and large fluid shifts, co-administration of colloidal substances has been proposed for large volume paracentesis. Absolute guidelines for this practice remain controversial as the clinical benefit is somewhat unclear, though this practice aims to prevent post-paracentesis circulatory dysfunction syndrome. A randomized trial comparing administration of albumin to placebo found fewer changes in electrolytes and serum creatinine, though ultimately mortality and morbidity did not differ between the two groups [19]. A subsequent meta-analysis of the use of albumin during paracentesis specifically in tense ascites, as compared to alternative volume expansion agents and vasoconstrictors found that use of albumin resulted in decreased mortality (OR 0.64; 95 % CI 0.41–0.98) [20]. As a result it is generally advisable to administer albumin (6–8 g/L of fluid removed) in large-volume paracentesis. Removal of volumes of 5 L or less are generally felt to be safe to perform without administering albumin, as this small volume has not been shown to alter post-procedure hemodynamics, namely plasma renin levels [21].

In patients with refractory ascites who require intermittent therapeutic abdominal paracentesis, attention should be brought to patients requiring increasingly frequent paracentesis as this may suggest underlying dietary indiscretion in terms of adherence to low-sodium diet. The following example will explain the molecular reasoning to support this inference. A removal of 5 L of abdominal ascites in a patient with a serum sodium concentration of 130 mmol/L will removed 650 mmol of sodium. A 2000 mg sodium diet will afford 88 mmol of sodium intake daily, of which typically 10 mmol are lost through nonrenal mechanisms. Assuming a patient were completely anuric, the time required to re-accumulate the 5 L of fluid removed during paracentesis would be approximately 8.3 days. It can be assumed that with preserved renal function this time interval would be significantly longer. For patients requiring paracentesis more frequently than this, it is therefore physiologically impossible that the patient is adhering to a low-salt diet.

For difficult to manage ascites that is refractory to diuretics, requiring frequent paracentesis, or with which other complications such as hepatic hydrothorax have arisen, consideration should be given to portal-caval shunt formation in the form of transjugular intrahepatic portosystemic shunt (TIPS). TIPS was initially developed as a method to relieve portal pressure gradients in an effort to abate variceal hemorrhage, but was subsequently adopted for patients with refractory ascites requiring frequent paracentesis. Outcomes from this intervention have overall been mixed in terms of survival advantage. A 2006 meta-analysis from the Cochrane Review found that in cirrhotic patients with ascites, compared to repeated paracentesis, TIPS was more effective a fluid removal without an improvement in overall mortality, rate of GI hemorrhage, renal failure, or infection. There was a significant increase in incidence of hepatic encephalopathy among patients undergoing TIPS, however [22]. Another meta-analysis of trials comparing TIPS to repeated paracentesis again found superiority with TIPS in terms of treatment of ascites, and also showed a trend toward improved overall survival, though this did not reach statistical significance (OR 0.74, 95 % CI 0.40–1.37) [23]. Some of the controversy among survival from early trials involving TIPS placement may be attributed to the use of uncovered stents early on, which have since been replaced by polytetrafluoroethylene (PTFE)-coated stents with subsequent improvement in patency and reintervention rates. A retrospective analysis assessing PTFE-coated compared to uncovered stents found improved survival at 3 months, 1 year, and 2 years (93 %, 88 %, 76 % respectively) for the PTFE group compared to the uncovered group (83 %, 73 %, 62 % respectively) [24]. A subsequent randomized trial of 80 patients comparing covered versus uncovered stents again found improved clinical outcomes, and a trend toward improved survival in the covered stent group which did not reach statistical significance [25]. Only 32 of the 80 patients underwent TIPS placement for refractory ascites in this trial, however, as GI bleeding was the most common indication for TIPS among patients enrolled. Overall TIPS is a useful tool for patients with refractory ascites and should be considered for appropriate patients who do not otherwise have contraindications such as heart failure, severe tricuspid regurgitation, severe coagulopathy, hepatic encephalopathy. It should be performed with caution in patients with very elevated MELD score as well as outcomes in this group tend to be poorer [26]. TIPS can also be considered for conditions resulting for complications of ascites including hepatic hydrothorax and symptomatic umbilical hernia. Patients with refractory ascites who are not transplant candidates, and who are either not candidates for TIPS or have had previously failed attempt at TIPS placement may be candidates for a peritoneovenous shunt, though these procedures are fraught with complications and high rate of shunt failure as well as a lack of survival advantage [16].

Future Trends

New strategies for the management of ascites are an attractive area of research interest due to the significant morbidity, mortality, and health care utilization associated with ascites. One strategy which has previously been suggested has been albumin infusion therapy concomitantly with diuretics. A trial of 100 consecutive patients with new onset ascites found that weekly albumin infusion combined with oral diuretics compared to diuretics alone portended a significant survival advantage of 16 months at mean follow-up of 7 years [27]. Another area of research interest has been with splanchnic vasoconstrictor Terlipressin. This agent has been used overseas to improve renal function in patients with hepatorenal syndrome (HRS). A small trial aimed to investigate its use in patients with ascites without HRS, and found that Terlipressin effectively induced natriuresis as indicated by sodium clearance and change in urine sodium concentration [28]. It has been hypothesized that this agent may provide a novel method of managing ascites, though further randomized clinical trials are needed, and this agent is currently not available in the United States.

References

1. Moore KP et al. The management of ascites in cirrhosis: report on the consensus conference of the International Ascites Club. Hepatology. 2003;38(1):258–66.
2. Runyon BA, Montano AA, Akriviadis EA, et al. The serum-ascites albumin gradient is superior to the exudate-transudate concept in the differential diagnosis of ascites. Ann Intern Med. 1992;117:215–20.
3. Cattau E, Benjamin S, Knuff T, et al. The accuracy of the physical exam in the diagnosis of suspected ascites. JAMA. 1982;247:1164–6.
4. Runyon BA. Introduction to the revised American Association for the Study of Liver Diseases Practice Guideline management of adult patients with ascites due to cirrhosis 2012. Hepatology. 2013;57(4):1651–3.
5. Runyon BA. Paracentesis of ascitic fluid: a safe procedure. Arch Intern Med. 1986;146:2259–61.
6. Runyon BA, Hoefs JC, Morgan TR. Ascitic fluid analysis in malignancy-related ascites. Hepatology. 1988;8:1104–9.
7. Runyon BA, Antillon MR, Akriviadis EA, et al. Bedside inoculation of blood culture bottles with ascitic fluid is superior to delayed inoculation in the detection of spontaneous bacterial peritonitis. J Clin Microbiol. 1990;8:2811–2.
8. Runyon BA. Cardiac ascites: a characterization. J Clin Gastroenterol. 1988;10:410–2.
9. Akriviadis EA, Runyon BA. The value of an algorithm in differentiating spontaneous from secondary bacterial peritonitis. Gastroenterology. 1990;98:127–33.
10. Runyon BA, Canawati HN, Akriviadis EA. Optimization of ascitic fluid culture technique. Gastroenterology. 1988;95:1351–5.
11. Hillebrand DJ, Runyon BA, Yasmineh WG, et al. Ascitic fluid adenosine deaminase insensitivity in detecting tuberculous peritonitis in the United States. Hepatology. 1996;24:1408–12.
12. Pereira G, Guevara M, Fagundes C, Solá E, Rodríguez E, Fernández J, et al. Renal failure and hyponatremia in patients with cirrhosis and skin and soft tissue infection. A retrospective study. J Hepatol. 2012;56:1040–6.

13. Belghiti J, Rueff B, Fekete F. Umbilical hernia in cirrhotic-patients with ascites-prevalence, course, and management. *Gastroenterology*. 1983;84:1363A.
14. Runyon BA, Antillon MR, Montano AA. Effect of diuresis versus therapeutic paracentesis on ascitic fluid opsonic activity and serum complement. Gastroenterology. 1989;97(1):158–62.
15. Chalasani N et al. Effects of albumin/furosemide mixtures on responses to furosemide in hypoalbuminemic patients. J Am Soc Nephrol. 2001;12(5):1010–6.
16. Stanley MM et al. Peritoneovenous shunting as compared with medical treatment in patients with alcoholic cirrhosis and massive ascites. N Engl J Med. 1989;321(24):1632–8.
17. Singh V et al. Midodrine in patients with cirrhosis and refractory or recurrent ascites: a randomized pilot study. J Hepatol. 2012;56(2):348–54.
18. Smith GS, Barnard GF. Massive volume paracentesis (up to 41 liters) for the outpatient management of ascites. J Clin Gastroenterol. 1997;25(1):402–3.
19. Ginès P et al. Randomized comparative study of therapeutic paracentesis with and without intravenous albumin in cirrhosis. Gastroenterology. 1988;94:1493–502.
20. Bernardi M et al. Albumin infusion in patients undergoing large-volume paracentesis: a meta-analysis of randomized trials. Hepatology. 2012;55(4):1172–81.
21. Peltekian KM et al. Cardiovascular, renal, and neurohumoral responses to single large-volume paracentesis in patients with cirrhosis and diuretic-resistant ascites. Am J Gastroenterol. 1997;92(3):394–9.
22. Saab S, et al. TIPS versus paracentesis for cirrhotic patients with refractory ascites. Cochrane Database Syst Rev 2006;(4):CD004889.
23. D'Amico G et al. Uncovered transjugular intrahepatic portosystemic shunt for refractory ascites: a meta-analysis. Gastroenterology. 2005;129(4):1282–93.
24. Angermayr B et al. Survival in patients undergoing transjugular intrahepatic portosystemic shunt: ePTFE-covered stentgrafts versus bare stents. Hepatology. 2003;38(4):1043–50.
25. Bureau C et al. Improved clinical outcome using polytetrafluoroethylene-coated stents for TIPS: results of a randomized study. Gastroenterology. 2004;126(2):469–75.
26. Montgomery A et al. MELD score as a predictor of early death in patients undergoing elective transjugular intrahepatic portosystemic shunt (TIPS) procedures. Cardiovasc Intervent Radiol. 2005;28(3):307–12.
27. Romanelli RG et al. Long-term albumin infusion improves survival in patients with cirrhosis and ascites: an unblinded randomized trial. World J Gastroenterol. 2006;12(9):1403–7.
28. Krag A et al. Terlipressin improves renal function in patients with cirrhosis and ascites without hepatorenal syndrome. Hepatology. 2007;46(6):1863–71.

Chapter 31
Spontaneous Bacterial Peritonitis (SBP)

Adam J. Schiro

1. How do I know I have SBP?

    Patient-Level Answer: In order to get SBP, you have to have ascites or fluid in the abdomen as a result of your liver disease. Once this fluid is present it runs the risk of becoming infected. The most common signs of infection include abdominal pain, fevers, or confusion. The only way to diagnose SBP is with a paracentesis where a sample of fluid is removed from the abdomen and analyzed to see if an infection is present.

2. How is it treated?

    Patient-Level Answer: SBP is a serious infection and can lead to death if not treated promptly and aggressively. Typically once the diagnosis is suggested based on preliminary findings from a paracentesis, antibiotics should be started. The length of treatment depends on how well a patient is responding to the treatment but is typically between 5 and 10 days.

3. What can be done to prevent me from getting SBP again?

    Patient-Level Answer: The most effective way to prevent SBP is to prevent the development of ascites or fluid in the abdomen from accumulating in the first place. Once fluid is present, there are certain patients who may benefit from taking antibiotics regularly to prevent an infection from developing including those who have had prior episodes of SBP.

A.J. Schiro, M.D. (✉)
Division of Gastroenterology & Hepatology, Department of Medicine,
Medical College of Wisconsin, 9200 W. Wisconsin Ave, Milwaukee, WI 53226, USA
e-mail: aschiro@mcw.edu

© Springer International Publishing Switzerland 2017
K. Saeian, R. Shaker (eds.), *Liver Disorders*,
DOI 10.1007/978-3-319-30103-7_31

Pathogenesis and Risk Factors

Spontaneous bacterial peritonitis (SBP) is defined as an intraperitoneal infection of ascitic fluid without underlying anatomic or pathologic cause. The term was initially described by Conn in 1964 who postulated that translocation of enteric pathogens in decompensated cirrhotic patients could lead to peritonitis and bacteremia, a vastly underreported syndrome at the time [1]. Initial reports suggested an exceedingly high mortality rate of greater than 90 % associated with SBP. Despite advances in management and more widespread use of antimicrobial prophylaxis, mortality continues to range from 10 to 30 % making it a significant cause of death in patients with end-stage liver disease [2].

At least 90 % of cases of SBP are monomicrobial with the most common causative organisms including gram negative enteric flora such as *Escherichia coli* and *Klebsiella pneumoniae*, as well as various Streptococcal species [3]. Studies seem to suggest a role for bacterial overgrowth and delayed intestinal motility as predisposing factors for the development of SBP. A study by Chang, et al. from 2003 compared cirrhotic patients with and without a history of SBP and found significantly higher rates of bacterial overgrowth and small intestinal dysmotility as assessed by hydrogen breath testing and small bowel manometry respectively among patients with a history of SBP [4]. The study was limited by significantly higher Child-Pugh score in the group with a history of SBP. A subsequent analysis using jejunal aspirates from cirrhotic patients found an association between bacterial overgrowth and acid-suppressive therapy, but no association with the development of SBP [5]. Independent of bacterial overgrowth concerns, the phenomena of bacterial translocation of enteric pathogens in patients with cirrhosis has been well documented. For example, analysis of mesenteric lymph node sampling has revealed increased levels of bacteria in cirrhotic compared to noncirrhotic patients [6].

SBP typically develops in patients with advanced liver disease, and risk is directly proportional to Child-Pugh score which has been shown to be an independent risk factor for bacterial infections in general including SBP [7]. An elevated Model for End-Stage Liver Disease (MELD) score has also been implicated. A retrospective case–control analysis found that for every 1-point increase in MELD score there is an associated 11 % increased risk of developing SBP [8].

There has also been considerable interest in the role of acid-suppressive therapy in the development of SBP. A retrospective case–control analysis of cirrhotic patients admitted with SBP compared to matched control cirrhotic patients admitted for other reasons found on multivariate analysis that PPI use was associated with an increased risk of SBP (odds ratio 4.31, 95 % CI 1.34–11.7) [9]. A more recent large, multicenter prospective analysis found no increase in risk of SBP among patients taking proton-pump inhibitors [10].

Additional known risk factors predisposing to the development of SBP include: low ascitic fluid total protein concentrationcoagulopathy, hyperbilirubinemia, gastrointestinal hemorrhage, and prior episode of SBP [11–14]. Several randomized trials were analyzed and based on results showing mortality benefit and reduced rate of infection, primary prophylaxis with antibiotics to prevent SBP is recommended in patients with cirrhosis and ascites whose ascitic total protein level is less than 1.0 g/dL, in addition to evidence of either impaired renal function (serum creatinine $\geq$1.2 mg/dL, blood urea nitrogen $\geq$25 mg/dL, or serum sodium $\leq$130 mEq/L) or hepatic failure (Child-Pugh score $\geq$9 or total bilirubin $\geq$3 mg/dL) [14, 15]. Genetic variability in terms of inflammatory signaling may play a role in terms of SBP risk as well. A recent genotypic analysis showed that specific variants of a Toll-Like Receptor 4 gene were associated with lower serum levels of tumor necrosis factor-alpha (TNF-α) and a significantly decreased risk of severe bacterial infections among patients awaiting liver transplant. Zero deaths as a result of severe bacterial infections were observed while awaiting transplant in this group [16].

Immune dysfunction is thought to play a significant role in cirrhotic patients by predisposing them to the development of infections including SBP. For example, complement deficiency has been well documented in the cirrhotic population and has been demonstrated to correlate with elevated rates of SBP [17]. A variety of other host factors play a role as well including malnutrition, decreased phagocyte activity, neutrophil dysfunction, and altered inflammatory cytokine levels [18].

True SBP in patients with ascites due to noncirrhotic causes, or elevated ascitic protein levels >2.5 g/dL is very uncommon and limited in the literature to case reports and small series [19]. Typically when there is an infection in this setting, an underlying predisposing anatomic defect leading to secondary bacterial peritonitis should be sought.

Clinical Manifestations

SBP tends to develop only in cases of clinically apparent and preexisting ascites. Its most common presenting features include abdominal pain, fevers, encephalopathy, diarrhea or ileus, and hemodynamic instability or sepsis, and it should be strongly considered in any patient with cirrhosis and clinically apparent ascites who presents with these complaints. Common laboratory findings include peripheral leukocytosis with or without left shift, acidosis, and renal failure. A significant number of patients present without symptoms, and more routine use of paracentesis for hospitalized cirrhotic patients with ascites has led to increased recognition of this clinical entity. Despite this, mortality rates related to SBP have remained high [20].

Diagnosis

SBP is associated with high mortality and early identification and initiation of appropriate antibiotics is critical to mitigating this risk. Based on AASLD guidelines it is recommended that all hospitalized patients with cirrhosis and ascites receive a diagnostic paracentesis during their admission, and paracentesis should also be obtained any time a patient shows clinical signs or laboratory evidence suggestive of possible SBP. Despite these recommendations a recent large retrospective database analysis found that paracentesis remains underutilized, being performed in 61 % of the 17,711 cirrhosis-related hospitalizations included in the study. Patients who received a paracentesis had a 24 % reduction of in-hospital mortality, though their length of stay and cost of hospitalization were slightly higher [21]. Paracentesis should ideally be performed prior to the administration of antibiotics if clinically feasible to prevent false negative results from partially treated sample specimens. Procedural delay should be avoided, and in general, an elevated prothrombin time or international normalized ratio is not a contraindication to diagnostic paracentesis as it has been shown to be safe despite presence of abnormal coagulation factors [22]. Patients with SBP who had paracentesis performed >12 h after admission had a 2.7-fold higher mortality compared to those who received early paracentesis [23].

It is important to utilize sterile technique to prevent contamination from skin flora. Direct bedside inoculation of the sample into culture media has been shown to be superior to conventional inoculation of sample sent to a clinical laboratory with increased sensitivity for diagnosing SBP [24]. Fluid sample should be sent for aerobic and anaerobic culture, cell count with differential, gram stain, and if the initial sampling albumin and total protein levels, in addition to other values relevant on a case by case basis (i.e. cytology for cases of suspected metastatic malignancy, etc.).

The diagnosis of SBP is made by the finding of $\geq$250 polymorphonuclear (PMN) cells per mm^3 with positive culture results and potential causes of secondary peritonitis excluded. Patients meeting criteria based on cell count alone should be presumed to have SBP and treatment with antibiotics should be initiated empirically while awaiting culture results. Correction for grossly blood specimens as occurs during a traumatic paracentesis can be performed by subtracting one PMN from the total count for every 250 red blood cells per mm^3 present in the specimen. Additional ascitic fluid chemistries can also be helpful in confirming or excluding the presence of SBP. For example, the serum-ascites albumin gradient (SAAG) is calculated by subtracting the ascitic fluid albumin level from the serum level. A value of >1.1 g/dL indicates the presence of portal hypertension with 97 % certainty. As SBP rarely develops in patients without portal hypertension, a SAAG of <1.1 g/dL makes the diagnosis of SBP unlikely [25]. Additionally, the total protein concentration of ascitic fluid has been shown to inversely correlate with the risk of development of SBP [11].

Management

It is imperative that intravenous antibiotics be initiated promptly following diagnostic paracentesis in cases of suspected SBP due to the high mortality associated with this disease, especially in patients with fevers, abdominal pain, or altered mental status. Patients who are asymptomatic but are found to have bacterascites (defined as the presence of bacteria on culture or gram stain in the setting of PMN count less than 250 cells per mm^3) should have a repeat paracentesis performed within 48 h and antibiotics should be initiated if symptoms develop or the PMN count rises above 250 cells per mm^3. Initial therapy regimen should consist of broad antimicrobial coverage such as a third generation cephalosporin or floroquinolone, though local resistance patterns should be taken into account when selecting an agent. Choice of antibiotic should be rapidly narrowed when culture results and sensitivities become available to prevent the development of bacterial resistance.

There is a relative dearth of large, prospective, randomized controlled trials available to guide initial antibiotic selection, and a 2009 Cochrane review was unable to provide clear evidence in favor of any specific regimen [26]. One small prospective trial found improved efficacy with IV cefotaxime as compared to ampicillin-tobramycin (clinical cure in 85 % as compared to 56 %, $p < 0.02$) as well as fewer superinfections and lower rates of renal failure [27]. In general, aminoglycosides are avoided due to their accumulation in the ascitic fluid and thus difficulty in measuring true levels with the potential development of renal failure.

Duration of Treatment

SBP typically responds rapidly to appropriate antibiotic administration, and clinical resolution is typically readily apparent. Typical treatment regimens consist of 5 days of therapy based on findings from a prospective, randomized trial which found equivalent outcomes among patients with SBP who were treated with either 5 or 10 days of antibiotics. Clinical cure was obtained in 93.1 % with 5 days of therapy versus 91.2 % with 10 days of therapy. The groups had similar rates of recurrence (11.6 % and 12.8 % respectively) as well as hospital mortality (32.6 % and 42.5 % respectively), neither of which were statistically significant [28]. Short treatment duration has the added benefit of reduced costs as well as minimizing the development of antimicrobial resistance. After completion of therapy, repeat clinical assessment should be performed and if persistent symptoms or signs of ongoing infection are present (abdominal pain, fevers, leukocytosis, altered mental status) then repeat paracentesis should be performed. Antibiotics should be continued if the polymorphonuclear cell count remains elevated above 250 cells per mm^3. For the majority of patients who respond promptly to treatment and have clinical resolution of symptoms, a repeat paracentesis is not typically needed despite previous recommendations of follow-up paracentesis to guide therapy.

Renal failure is common among patient with SBP, occurring in approximately one-third of patients [29]. A recent meta-analysis found that the development of renal failure was the highest independent predictor of mortality among patients with SBP, followed by MELD score. Mortality among those with renal dysfunction in the analysis was 67 % compared to 11 % in patients without renal impairment [30]. Altered renal hemodynamics that occur during infection are thought to play a role, including activation of the renin-angiotensin system as well as release of norepinephrine, effectively reducing renal perfusion [31]. Volume expansion using

IV albumin has been shows to improve outcomes among sub-groups of patients with SBP who develop renal failure. A randomized controlled analysis assessed administration of intra-venous albumin concomitantly with antibiotics in patients with SBP who also have evidence of elevated serum creatinine >1.0 mg/dL, blood urea nitrogen >30 mg/dL, or serum bilirubin >4 mg/dL. The treatment arm who received albumin had lower risk of progression to renal failure as well as lower overall mortality [32]. These findings have been corroborated in other randomized trials including a meta-analysis as well [33]. Thus, albumin at a dose of 1.5 g/kg IV within 6 h of diagnosis followed by 1 g/kg IV on day 3 should be administered.

Nonselective beta-blockers are commonly used for prophylaxis of esophageal varices in certain scenarios. This class of medications has myriad influences on systemic hemodynamics and on circulatory reserve. The role of nonselective beta-blocker usage in outcomes among patients with SBP has been investigated. A retrospective analysis of 607 consecutive patients with cirrhosis undergoing paracentesis found that nonselective beta-blocker usage in patients without SBP was associated with increased survival (HR 0.75, 95 % CI 0.581–0.968). Conversely, among patients who were diagnosed with SBP, beta-blocker use reduced survival (HR 1.58, 95 % CI 1.098–2.274), led to more prolonged length of hospitalization (mean 29.6 days per person year versus 23.7 days per person year) and increased incidence of hepatorenal syndrome (24 % versus 11 %) [34]. Therefore, patients who are taking nonselective beta-blockers for prophylaxis of esophageal varices should have this medication discontinued at the time that SBP is first suspected.

Prophylaxis

Patients who are considered to be at high risk for the development of SBP have been shown to benefit from antimicrobial prophylaxis to prevent infections and reduce mortality. High risk groups include patients with a history of prior episode of SBP, patients with GI bleeding, and patients with a low ascitic fluid total protein concentration.

Patients with a history of prior episode of SBP are at particularly high risk of developing recurrent infection. One study of consecutive cirrhotic patients who survived and recovered from an initial episode of SBP found a 43 % incidence of recurrent SBP at 6 months and 69 % incidence at 1 year with overall 1 year survival of only 38 % [12]. Similar risk of SBP recurrence at 1 year was found in a randomized, controlled trial assessing prophylactic norfloxacin versus placebo in patients with a history of prior episode of SBP. Risk of development of SBP at 1 year in the placebo arm was 68 % compared to 20 % in the arm receiving prophylactic norfloxacin 400 mg daily [35].

Patients with low ascitic fluid total protein concentration have a significantly increased risk of development of SBP and have been demonstrated to benefit from prophylactic antibiotic administration as well. A prospective trial assessing use of norfloxacin versus placebo in patients with low protein ascites found rates of SBP in the placebo group to be 22.7 % as compared to 0.0 % in the group receiving antimicrobial prophylaxis. There was a trend toward improved mortality as well in the treatment group; however, this did not reach statistical significance [36].

Advanced cirrhosis and renal dysfunction are additional patient subsets that have been suggested to benefit from prophylaxis against SBP. A randomized controlled trial including patients with advanced cirrhosis (Child-Pugh score ≥ 9, with serum bilirubin ≥ 3 mg/dL) or impaired renal function (serum creatinine ≥ 1.2 mg/dL, blood urea nitrogen ≥ 25 mg/dL, or serum sodium level of ≤ 130 mEq/L) compared prophylactic treatment with norfloxacin to placebo in the prevention of SBP [15]. Primary endpoints were 3-month and 1-year survival, and secondary endpoints included the probability of development of SBP or hepatorenal syndrome at 1-year. The risk of developing SBP at 1-year was 7 % in the treatment group compared to 61 % with placebo ($p<0.001$), and overall survival was significantly improved at 3-months (94 % versus 62 %, $p=0.003$) and at 1-year (60 % and 48 %, $p=0.05$). The trial served for the basis of the AASLD guideline statement suggesting antimicrobial prophylaxis for patients meeting the clinical criteria required for inclusion into the study.

In general, regimens with coverage against gram negative organisms have been preferred for use as prophylactic agents including quinolones and trimethoprim-sulfamethoxazole. A randomized trial assessing the use of trimethoprim-sulfamethoxazole five times per week (Monday–Friday) for prophylaxis in patients at high risk for SBP (low ascitic protein level, renal dysfunction, hyperbilirubinemia, etc.) found that treatment reduced the risk of development of SBP from 27 % in the placebo group to 3 % in the treatment group. There was a trend toward improved mortality as well, though this was not statistically significant [37]. Another trial looking at once-weekly ciprofloxacin among cirrhotic patients with low protein ascites found similar reduction in risk of development of SBP from 22 % in the placebo group to 3.6 % in the treatment group [38].

Gastrointestinal bleeding and variceal hemorrhage predispose patients to the development of SBP and prophylactic antibiotics have been shown to improve outcomes in these patients. A meta-analysis consisting of a total of five trials and 534 patients with cirrhosis and gastrointestinal bleeding found that short course antibiotic prophylaxis administration reduces rates of infections including SBP and improves overall survival [14]. A Cochrane systematic review from 2010 confirmed these findings. A total of 12 trials and 1241 patients were included in this analysis. Overall mortality was improved with use of antibiotics among patients with cirrhosis and gastrointestinal bleeding (RR 0.79, 95 % CI 0.63–0.98), as well as improvements in infection-related morality (RR 0.43, 95 % CI 0.19–0.97) and risk of SBP (RR 0.29, 95 % CI 0.15–0.57). Length of hospitalization and rebleeding risks were also improved among patients receiving prophylactic antibiotics [39]. As practice habits have changed and antimicrobial prophylaxis in the setting of gastrointestinal bleeding in cirrhotic patients has become more routine, improved outcomes over the years have been observed among these patients. In-hospital mortality from variceal hemorrhage in 1980 at a single center in Europe was 42.6 %, and had improved by year 2000 to 14.5 % [40]. Although direct causality has not been proven, prophylactic antibiotics are postulated to play a role in this observed improvement.

Current updated practice guidelines from the AASLD in 2012 recommend prophylactic antibiotics be given to all patients with cirrhosis who present with gastrointestinal bleeding, whether or not they have ascites, with a recommended duration of therapy of 7 days. These recommendations are also endorsed by the ASGE as reflected in the recent guideline statement regarding use of antibiotics for GI endoscopy [41].

Current guidelines do not comment on the routine use of antibiotic prophylaxis to prevent SBP in the setting of patients awaiting liver transplant who do not already have an indication. A small trial that assessed the effect of daily administration of ciprofloxacin in patients with advanced liver disease awaiting transplant found that, compared to placebo, treatment with ciprofloxacin was not associated with improvements in hepatic function, though rates of hospitalization were improved (5 % in Ciprofloxacin group versus 32 % in placebo group, $p=0.02$) [42]. The trial did not look at perioperative or posttransplant outcomes, and at this time there is a lack of data to support routine use of antibiotics in this setting. Another area where routine antibiotic prophylaxis is not routinely recommended is among patient receiving treatment with sclerotherapy. A trial comparing use of antibiotics to prevent post-sclerotherapy bacteremia found no significant difference among patients receiving prophylactic imipenem/cilastatin. A higher risk of infection was observed in patients who underwent emergent as compared to elective sclerotherapy, which was likely reflective of increased risk of infection among cirrhotic patients with active gastrointestinal bleeding [43].

Future Trends

Evolving research and active investigation is underway involving several areas of SBP. One particular area of interest involves the use of enhanced diagnostic tools for the detection and diagnosis of patients with SBP, as early identification and implementation of appropriate therapy has consistently been shown to improve outcomes as previously discussed. Serum procalcitonin concentration has been identified as an important tool in the early identification of patients with sepsis from a bacterial infection, and has been increasingly integrated into sepsis protocols among emergency rooms and intensive care units [44]. Research has suggested a role for this biomarker in the diagnosis of patients with SBP as well. The identification of a diagnostic marker easily obtained from the serum would potentially be of benefit given the challenges sometimes associated with obtaining a prompt diagnostic paracentesis specimen. A recent meta-analysis identified three relevant trials and found pooled sensitivity and specificity values for use of this marker in the diagnosis of SBP of 86 % and 80 % respectively [45]. This finding suggests a high diagnostic accuracy and the authors note that further larger trials are warranted.

Additional investigation has suggested a role for ascitic fluid markers as well, citing the possibility of false negatives obtained from a manual cell count if lysis of PMN's has occurred during prolonged transport or specimen processing. One trial assessed the use of ascitic lactoferrin concentration among consecutive ascitic fluid samples [46]. Among the 22 samples meeting diagnostic criteria for SBP, an ascitic lactoferrin level of $\geq$242 ng/mL had a sensitivity and specificity of 95 % and 97 % respectively with an area under the receiver operating characteristic curve of 0.98.

For even more rapid identification of SBP, investigation into the use of dipsticks for ascitic fluid analysis is also underway. One such product is designed to detect leukocyte esterase from ascitic fluid, and calibrated to a PMN count of 250 cells per mL. An analysis of 1089 ascitic fluid samples found a sensitivity and specificity of 100 % and 59 % respectively for the detection of samples positive for SBP [47]. At this point the product remains investigational and further investigation is underway.

Identification of additional antimicrobial agents given ongoing concerns for resistance, side-effect profiles, and cost, is an area of interest as well. A commonly used agent among patients with cirrhosis and hepatic encephalopathy is rifaximin. Recent literature has suggested that this agent may reduce incidence of SBP and may impact the bacterial flora as well. In one retrospective study, consecutive patients with cirrhosis and large-volume ascites were analyzed, excluding patients with a history of SBP or patients already receiving prophylactic antibiotics. The authors identified 49 patients who received rifaximin and after mean follow-up of 4.2 months, 89 % remained SBP-free compared to 68 % of those not on rifaximin ($p=0.002$) [48]. Another study prospectively assessed patients undergoing diagnostic paracentesis and found that treatment with rifaximin did not reduce incidence of SBP compared to no antibiotics [49]. The predominate species isolated among patients not receiving antibiotics were *Escherichia coli* and enterococci whereas those on rifaximin tended to grow Klebsiella species, suggesting that rifaximin plays a role in modulating the bacterial flora and impacting pathogenesis. Further studies are needed to better delineate the role of rifaximin in patients with or at risk for SBP.

References

1. Conn HO. Spontaneous peritonitis and bacteremia in Laennec's cirrhosis caused by enteric organisms: a relatively common but rarely recognized syndrome. Ann Intern Med. 1964;60(4):568–80.
2. Garcia-Tsao G. Current management of the complications of cirrhosis and portal hypertension: variceal hemorrhage, ascites, and spontaneous bacterial peritonitis. Gastroenterology. 2001;120(3):726–48.
3. McHutchison JG, Runyon BA. Spontaneous bacterial peritonitis. In: Surawicz CM, Owen RL, editors. Gastrointestinal and hepatic infections. Philadelphia, PA: WB Saunders Company; 1994.
4. Chang C-S et al. Small intestine dysmotility and bacterial overgrowth in cirrhotic patients with spontaneous bacterial peritonitis. Hepatology. 1998;28(5):1187–90.
5. Bauer TM et al. Small intestinal bacterial overgrowth in patients with cirrhosis: prevalence and relation with spontaneous bacterial peritonitis. Am J Gastroenterol. 2001;96(10):2962–7.
6. Cirera I et al. Bacterial translocation of enteric organisms in patients with cirrhosis. J Hepatol. 2001;34(1):32–7.
7. Caly WR, Strauss E. A prospective study of bacterial infections in patients with cirrhosis. J Hepatol. 1993;18(3):353–8.

8. Obstein KL et al. Association between model for end-stage liver disease and spontaneous bacterial peritonitis. Am J Gastroenterol. 2007;102(12):2732–6.
9. Bajaj JS et al. Association of proton pump inhibitor therapy with spontaneous bacterial peritonitis in cirrhotic patients with ascites. Am J Gastroenterol. 2009;104(5):1130–4.
10. Terg R et al. Proton pump inhibitor therapy does not increase the incidence of spontaneous bacterial peritonitis in cirrhosis: a multicenter prospective study. J Hepatol. 2015;62:1056.
11. Runyon BA. Low-protein-concentration ascitic fluid is predisposed to spontaneous bacterial peritonitis. Gastroenterology. 1986;91(6):1343–6.
12. Tító L et al. Recurrence of spontaneous bacterial peritonitis in cirrhosis: frequency and predictive factors. Hepatology. 1988;8(1):27–31.
13. Rimola A et al. Oral, nonabsorbable antibiotics prevent infection in cirrhotics with gastrointestinal hemorrhage. Hepatology. 1985;5(3):463–7.
14. Bernard B et al. Antibiotic prophylaxis for the prevention of bacterial infections in cirrhotic patients with gastrointestinal bleeding: a meta-analysis. Hepatology. 1999;29(6):1655–61.
15. Fernández J et al. Primary prophylaxis of spontaneous bacterial peritonitis delays hepatorenal syndrome and improves survival in cirrhosis. Gastroenterology. 2007;133(3):818–24.
16. Senkerikova R et al. Genetic variation in TNFA predicts protection from severe bacterial infections in patients with end-stage liver disease awaiting liver transplantation. J Hepatol. 2014;60(4):773–81.
17. Such J et al. Low C 3 in cirrhotic ascites predisposes to spontaneous bacterial peritonitis. J Hepatol. 1988;6(1):80–4.
18. Bonnel AR, Bunchorntavakul C, Rajender Reddy K. Immune dysfunction and infections in patients with cirrhosis. Clin Gastroenterol Hepatol. 2011;9(9):727–38.
19. Woolf GM, Runyon BA. Spontaneous Salmonella infection of high-protein noncirrhotic ascites. J Clin Gastroenterol. 1990;12(4):430–2.
20. Thuluvath PJ, Morss S, Thompson R. Spontaneous bacterial peritonitis—in-hospital mortality, predictors of survival, and health care costs from 1988 to 1998. Am J Gastroenterol. 2001;96(4):1232–6.
21. Orman ES et al. Paracentesis is associated with reduced mortality in patients hospitalized with cirrhosis and ascites. Clin Gastroenterol Hepatol. 2014;12(3):496–503.
22. Grabau CM et al. Performance standards for therapeutic abdominal paracentesis. Hepatology. 2004;40(2):484–8.
23. Kim JJ et al. Delayed paracentesis is associated with increased in-hospital mortality in patients with spontaneous bacterial peritonitis. Am J Gastroenterol. 2014;109(9):1436–42.
24. De A, Bankar S, Baveja S. Comparison of three culture methods for diagnosis of Spontaneous Bacterial Peritonitis (SBP) in adult patients with cirrhosis. Int J Curr Microbiol Appl Sci. 2014;3(7):156–60.
25. Runyon BA et al. The serum-ascites albumin gradient is superior to the exudate-transudate concept in the differential diagnosis of ascites. Ann Intern Med. 1992;117(3):215–20.
26. Chavez-Tapia NC, et al. Antibiotics for spontaneous bacterial peritonitis in cirrhotic patients. Cochrane Database Syst Rev 2009; (1): CD002232.
27. Felisart J et al. Cefotaxime is more effective than is ampicillin-tobramycin in cirrhotics with severe infections. Hepatology. 1985;5(3):457–62.
28. Runyon BA et al. Short-course versus long-course antibiotic treatment of spontaneous bacterial peritonitis. A randomized controlled study of 100 patients. Gastroenterology. 1991;100(6):1737–42.
29. Follo A et al. Renal impairment after spontaneous bacterial peritonitis in cirrhosis: incidence, clinical course, predictive factors and prognosis. Hepatology. 1994;20(6):1495–501.
30. Tandon P, Garcia-Tsao G. Renal dysfunction is the most important independent predictor of mortality in cirrhotic patients with spontaneous bacterial peritonitis. Clin Gastroenterol Hepatol. 2011;9(3):260–5.
31. Ruiz-del-Arbol L et al. Systemic, renal, and hepatic hemodynamic derangement in cirrhotic patients with spontaneous bacterial peritonitis. Hepatology. 2003;38(5):1210–8.

32. Sort P et al. Effect of intravenous albumin on renal impairment and mortality in patients with cirrhosis and spontaneous bacterial peritonitis. N Engl J Med. 1999;341(6):403–9.
33. Salerno F, Navickis RJ, Wilkes MM. Albumin infusion improves outcomes of patients with spontaneous bacterial peritonitis: a meta-analysis of randomized trials. Clin Gastroenterol Hepatol. 2013;11(2):123–30.
34. Mandorfer M et al. Nonselective β blockers increase risk for hepatorenal syndrome and death in patients with cirrhosis and spontaneous bacterial peritonitis. Gastroenterology. 2014;146(7):1680–90.
35. Ginés P et al. Norfloxacin prevents spontaneous bacterial peritonitis recurrence in cirrhosis: results of a double-blind, placebo-controlled trial. Hepatology. 1990;12(4):716–24.
36. Soriano G et al. Selective intestinal decontamination prevents spontaneous bacterial peritonitis. Gastroenterology. 1991;100(2):477–81.
37. Singh N et al. Trimethoprim-sulfamethoxazole for the prevention of spontaneous bacterial peritonitis in cirrhosis: a randomized trial. Ann Intern Med. 1995;122(8):595–8.
38. Rolachon A et al. Ciprofloxacin and long-term prevention of spontaneous bacterial peritonitis: results of a prospective controlled trial. Hepatology. 1995;22(4):1171–4.
39. Chavez-Tapia NC, et al. Antibiotic prophylaxis for cirrhotic patients with upper gastrointestinal bleeding. Cochrane Database Syst Rev 2010; (9): CD002907.
40. Carbonell N et al. Improved survival after variceal bleeding in patients with cirrhosis over the past two decades. Hepatology. 2004;40(3):652–9.
41. Khashab MA et al. Antibiotic prophylaxis for GI endoscopy. Gastrointest Endosc. 2015;81(1):81.
42. Minuk GY et al. Daily ciprofloxacin treatment for patients with advanced liver disease awaiting liver transplantation reduces hospitalizations. Dig Dis Sci. 2011;56(4):1235–41.
43. Rolando N et al. Infectious sequelae after endoscopic sclerotherapy of oesophageal varices: role of antibiotic prophylaxis. J Hepatol. 1993;18(3):290–4.
44. Dellinger RP et al. Surviving Sepsis Campaign: international guidelines for management of severe sepsis and septic shock, 2012. Intensive Care Med. 2013;39(2):165–228.
45. Su D-H et al. Value of serum procalcitonin levels in predicting spontaneous bacterial peritonitis. Hepatogastroenterology. 2013;60(124):641–6.
46. Parsi MA et al. Ascitic fluid lactoferrin for diagnosis of spontaneous bacterial peritonitis. Gastroenterology. 2008;135(3):803–7.
47. Mendler MH et al. A new highly sensitive point of care screen for spontaneous bacterial peritonitis using the leukocyte esterase method. J Hepatol. 2010;53(3):477–83.
48. Hanouneh MA et al. The role of rifaximin in the primary prophylaxis of spontaneous bacterial peritonitis in patients with liver cirrhosis. J Clin Gastroenterol. 2012;46(8):709–15.
49. Lutz P et al. Impact of rifaximin on the frequency and characteristics of spontaneous bacterial peritonitis in patients with liver cirrhosis and ascites. PLoS One. 2014;9(4):e93909.

Chapter 32
Hepatorenal Syndrome

Michael M. Yeboah

Patient Questions and Answers

1. What is hepatorenal syndrome?

    The hepatorenal syndrome is a potentially life-threatening but reversible kidney disease which usually develops in patients with advanced liver disease. It occurs when the worsening liver disease leads to constriction of the blood vessels in the kidney and causes diversion of blood supply away from the kidneys. Generally, correction of the liver problem leads to resolution of the kidney problem. The condition therefore emphasizes the close relationship between the liver and the kidney in the body.

2. What are the symptoms of hepatorenal syndrome?

    There are 2 types of hepatorenal syndrome. The first one is called type 1 hepatorenal syndrome. Type 1 hepatorenal syndrome tends to progress very rapidly and may lead to death within 2–3 weeks if no treatment is given. Patients with this type of hepatorenal syndrome have nonspecific symptoms including general malaise and will usually notice reduction in their urine volume. These patients are often very sick overall and will need to be admitted to the hospital if they are not already hospitalized. The diagnosis is then made by the doctor after full assessment, including the results of urine and blood tests. The second type, called type 2 hepatorenal syndrome is relatively less aggressive and progresses rather slowly over weeks to several months. Type 2 hepatorenal syndrome usually does not cause specific symptoms apart from some reduction in urine volume and increasing swelling of the belly. Patients with type 2 hepatorenal syndrome are usually well enough to stay at home and are followed-up in the clinic from time to time.

M.M. Yeboah, M.B.Ch.B., Ph.D. (✉)
Division of Nephrology, Medical College of Wisconsin, Milwaukee, WI, USA
e-mail: mmyeboah@mcw.edu

© Springer International Publishing Switzerland 2017
K. Saeian, R. Shaker (eds.), *Liver Disorders*,
DOI 10.1007/978-3-319-30103-7_32

3. How is hepatorenal syndrome treated?

   Patients with type 1 hepatorenal syndrome are usually very sick and need to be admitted to hospital immediately for treatment. The most effective and ideal treatment option is liver transplantation. This helps to reverse the liver failure and leads to resolution of the hepatorenal syndrome, and more importantly prevents death in most people with hepatorenal syndrome.

   In situations where the person cannot have liver transplantation for whatever reason, maximum medical management will be given that includes medicines that help the body to redirect more blood flow to the kidneys. Also some of these patients will undergo some form of dialysis where a machine helps in doing the work of the kidney by removing toxins from the blood, at least temporarily. This is especially the case when the patient is awaiting liver transplantation. The dialysis on its own will neither cure the liver nor the kidney problem.

   Patients with type 2 hepatorenal syndrome may remain overall well for several months. In some of them, however, the kidney condition worsens over time and may switch to become type 1 hepatorenal syndrome and will need to be treated as above. Treatment options for type 2 hepatorenal syndrome include attempts at improving the liver function by treating underlying viral hepatitis, stopping alcohol use, or addressing any other reversible cause of the liver problem. If improvement in liver function cannot be achieved through such means, liver transplantation will be necessary in suitable patients. Some patients who have had hepatorenal syndrome for several weeks will ultimately develop chronic kidney failure and will need long-term dialysis treatment or combined liver and kidney transplantation.

4. Does one need to take specific medications daily?

   Patients with the type 1 hepatorenal syndrome are usually very sick and are admitted to the hospital for treatment. For those who have resolution of the hepatorenal syndrome (either through medical treatment or after liver transplantation), no specific ongoing medications will be necessary; however, the patient may be on medications for other reasons. For instance those who undergo liver transplantation will need to take regular medications to prevent rejection of the liver. Patients with type 2 hepatorenal syndrome are usually at home and are followed in the outpatient clinic periodically. Those with very low blood pressure may be given a particular medicine to help improve their blood pressure but most of them will not need any specific medications.

5. What is the prognosis for hepatorenal syndrome?

   Unfortunately, the prognosis for persons with the hepatorenal syndrome is generally poor. Most of those who develop the type 1 hepatorenal syndrome die within a couple weeks unless they respond to medical treatment their liver condition resolves in a timely manner or if they receive a liver transplantation urgently. Patients with the type 2 hepatorenal syndrome tend to be relatively well for several weeks to months but will ultimately need liver transplantation to stay alive unless the liver failure resolves one way or the other. Some of these patients will also need kidney transplantation or will require long-term dialysis because the hepatorenal syndrome would have progressed to chronic kidney failure over time. Persons with the hepatorenal syndrome have to abstain from alcohol ingestion and avoid any medications that could affect the function of the liver or kidney.

Summary

Approximately 5.5 million people in the United States have cirrhosis, a condition that is associated with very high morbidity, healthcare costs, and death. Kidney dysfunction is a major complication of cirrhosis, with the incidence increasing as the severity of cirrhosis progresses. The prevalence is highest in cirrhotic patients with ascites. The onset of kidney dysfunction in liver failure portends a poor prognosis. Patients with advanced liver disease and kidney failure are at increased risk for death while awaiting liver transplantation and are at a higher risk for complications and reduced survival after transplantation when compared with patients without kidney failure. Kidney dysfunction in the setting of liver failure is due mostly to conditions that lead to reduced kidney blood flow (pre-renal causes) or from problems within the kidney (intrinsic renal causes).

The pathophysiologic hallmark of cirrhosis complicated by renal dysfunction is portal hypertension. The development of portal hypertension is associated with splanchnic vasodilatation and reduction in effective blood volume, a hyperdynamic systemic circulation which is characterized by increased heart rate and cardiac output and also intense renal vasoconstriction due the activation of neurohumoral vasoconstrictor systems like the sympathetic nervous system (SNS), renin-angiotension-aldo sterone-system (RAAS), and vasopressin, which is aimed at counteracting the hemodynamic effects of splanchnic vasodilatation. The foregoing establishes a tenuous background renal blood flow and makes the kidneys overly sensitive to further hemodynamic compromise occurring either spontaneously from progression of the underlying portal hypertension or as precipitated by sepsis or hypovolemia among others. These patients also have increased sensitivity to both endogenous and exogenous nephrotoxins, including intravenous contrast and nonsteroidal anti-inflammatory drugs.

The hepatorenal syndrome is one of the many potential causes of renal dysfunction in patients with chronic liver disease. It is relatively less common but is a potentially life-threatening complication. Identifying the specific cause of acute renal dysfunction is difficult in the clinical setting as the initial clinical findings and test results are usually nonspecific. The patients may also have intrinsic renal diseases that are commonly associated with chronic renal dysfunction, including diabetic nephropathy, IgA nephropathy, and glomerulonephritis from hepatitis B or hepatitis C infection.

Introduction: Hepatorenal Syndrome

The occurrence of kidney failure in the setting of advanced liver failure has been known for over 150 years [1]. The modern description of the hepatorenal syndrome which laid down the foundation for our present understanding of its pathophysiology is attributed to Sherlock and Hecker [2]. Over the years, most of their original findings have been confirmed, including the underlying hemodynamic disturbances. Considerable effort has also gone into clearly defining the hepatorenal syndrome in order to distinguish patients with the hepatorenal syndrome from other patients who have renal dysfunction from causes other than the hepatorenal syndrome. This is important as the treatment and clinical course is very different. To this end the diagnostic criteria for the hepatorenal syndrome has undergone some modifications over this period [3]. Current medical treatment of the hepatorenal syndrome is based on an attempt to correct the systemic and splanchnic vasodilatation and to improve the circulating blood volume. However, despite the advances made over the last 2–3 decades, only about 40 % of patients respond to the available treatments which generally speaking are only seen as bridge therapy pending liver transplantation [4, 5].

Definition

The hepatorenal syndrome (HRS) is a severe and potentially life-threatening complication of advanced cirrhosis, alcoholic hepatitis, and fulminant acute liver failure. It is one of the many possible causes of renal dysfunction in subjects with chronic liver disease and occurs in approximately 11 % of cirrhotics with refractory ascites. HRS is characterized by significant reduction in renal blood flow due to an intense renal vasoconstriction on the background of marked systemic and splanchnic vasodilation. HRS is associated with very poor prognosis. Two subtypes (types 1 and 2) of HRS are described based on the clinical presentation and overall clinical course. There are no specific diagnostic tests and treatment options are limited. Although HRS presents clinically with a pre-renal hemodynamic picture, it is unresponsive to volume expansion. The diagnosis needs to be made as early as possible in order to initiate treatment.

Pathophysiology

The HRS represents the culmination of significant hemodynamic derangement that is initiated by portal hypertension. It is characterized by intense intrarenal vasoconstriction in association with overt splanchnic vasodilatation and a relatively insufficient cardiac output [6–10]. Increased pressure in the portal system due to worsening cirrhosis causes increased shear stress in the splanchnic vasculature.

This, in addition to bacterial translocation from the bowel and the associated inflammatory response lead to the elaboration of endogenous vasodilators including nitric oxide, prostacyclins, glucagon, and carbon monoxide that contribute to splanchnic vasodilatation, pooling of blood, and reduced effective circulating blood volume [9–14]. The body compensates for the effective hypovolemia by the establishment of a hyperdynamic circulation, including increased heart rate and cardiac output. As portal hypertension progresses, the splanchnic vasodilatation and associated reduction in systemic vascular resistance worsen, and with time, the heart is unable to generate adequate output to maintain the arterial pressure. The cause of this so-called cirrhotic cardiomyopathy is unclear [13–18]. Relative adrenal insufficiency is common in patients with cirrhosis and worsens as the cirrhosis progresses. This subclinical adrenal insufficiency state could affect cardiac function and may play a role in the development of the cardiomyopathy and the circulatory dysfunction [19]. Also, with advancing cirrhosis, neurohumoral vasoconstrictor systems like the sympathetic nervous system (SNS), renin-angiotension-aldosterone-system (RAAS), and vasopressin are activated. These vasoconstrictor mechanisms while helping to achieve and maintain an adequate circulating blood volume, are associated with detrimental vasoconstriction in various organs including the kidney, brain, and liver. In the kidney, the consequences include intense vasoconstriction, reduction in blood flow, reduced GFR, and salt and water retention that causes ascites and the oligoanuric state typical of the hepatorenal syndrome [19–24].

Epidemiology

The typical patient at risk of HRS is one with advanced, decompensated chronic liver disease. These patients usually have resistant ascites and other complications of cirrhosis, including spontaneous bacteria peritonitis (SBP), esophageal varices, and hepatic encephalopathy. HRS may also complicate fulminant liver failure and severe alcoholic hepatitis. The incidence of hepatorenal syndrome increases with advancing cirrhosis and is estimated to occur in approximately 20 % and 40 % of cirrhotics at 1 year and 5 years respectively. HRS occurs in 11 % of hospitalized patients with cirrhosis and ascites [6, 7]. Risk factors for development of HRS include orthostatic hypotension and hyponatremia. Common precipitating clinical events include SBP, gastrointestinal bleeding, and large-volume paracentesis.

Current Diagnostic Criteria and Clinical Subtypes

For some time now, the definition of HRS has been based on the International Club of Ascites (ICA) 2007 guidelines [3]. HRS is a diagnosis of exclusion with no specific diagnostic test. In patients with advanced liver cirrhosis or fulminant acute liver failure, the diagnosis of HRS may be made if the following criteria are met:

- Serum creatinine >1.5 mg/dl
- No improvement of serum creatinine (decrease to a level of ≤1.5 mg/dl) after at least 2 days with diuretic withdrawal and volume expansion with albumin
- No signs of shock
- No recent use of nephrotoxic drugs
- Absence of parenchymal kidney disease as indicated by proteinuria >500 mg/day, microhematuria (>50 red blood cells per high power field)

Very recently, the ICA published new guidelines for the definition of AKI in patients with cirrhosis and also the diagnosis of HRS [45]. In the new guidelines, the definition of AKI is based on the ICA-AKI criteria which is a modification of the Kidney Disease Improving Global Outcomes (KDIGO) criteria. The major change in the diagnostic criteria of HRS noted in the 2015 guidelines compared to the 2007 criteria is that the threshold of serum creatinine ≥1.5 mg/dl has been abandoned.

The 2015 ICA definition of AKI and diagnostic criteria for HRS are as follows:

ICA-AKI criteria: Increase in serum creatinine ≥0.3 mg/dl (≥26.5 μmol/l) within 48 h; or a ≥50 % increase in serum creatinine from baseline which is known, or presumed to have occurred within the prior 7 days.

The new HRS diagnostic criteria are:

- Diagnosis of cirrhosis and ascites
- Diagnosis of AKI according to ICA-AKI criteria
- No response after 2 consecutive days of diuretic withdrawal and plasma volume expansion with albumin 1 g/kg body weight
- Absence of shock
- No current or recent use of nephrotoxic drugs (NSAIDs, aminoglycosides, iodinated contrast media etc.)
- No macroscopic signs of structural kidney injury*, defined as:

  - absence of proteinuria (>500 mg/day)
  - absence of microhaematuria (>50 RBCs per high power field)
  - normal findings on renal ultrasonography

*Patients who fulfill these criteria may still have structural damage such as tubular damage. Urine biomarkers will become an important element in making a more accurate differential diagnosis between HRS and acute tubular necrosis.

Renal biopsy is not required to make the diagnosis and is usually avoided because of the significant risk of bleeding in this group of patients. HRS has long been designated as a "functional" condition because no major histological abnormalities were evident on biopsy. Also the return of renal function after liver transplantation and the ability of the affected kidney to function in a recipient without liver failure are consistent with this [25, 26]. Of note, most of the information used to identify HRS as a functional condition was based on data from several decades ago; at a time when HRS was not particularly well-defined as is true currently. It may therefore not be entirely true that HRS uniformly has normal histological findings as the biopsies might have been done in patients with renal dysfunction but who did not have

HRS as per current diagnostic criteria. Also, per current knowledge, the rate of recovery of renal function following liver transplantation is rather variable in patients with a presumed diagnosis of HRS [27, 28]. Possible explanations for this are (1) inability to routinely identify when HRS progresses to ATN. (2) HRS is not as "functional" as we think [28, 29]. In a review of autopsy series, Kanel et al. noted reflux of proximal convoluted tubular epithelium into Bowman's space in 71.4 % of cases with the hepatorenal syndrome, while this lesion was only present in 0–27.3 % of other autopsy categories [30]. They suggested that since this lesion had been previously described with experimental renal ischemic change and terminal hypotension, it is possible that it is caused in part by the decreased or altered renal blood flow known to be associated with the hepatorenal syndrome.

Clinically, two distinct subtypes of HRS are encountered based on the rate of decline in renal function and the overall prognosis. Type 1 HRS is associated with rapidly progressing renal failure with a natural course that lead to death at a median of 2 weeks. It usually develops in the presence of a precipitating event such as SBP, gastrointestinal bleeding, and large-volume paracentesis and is defined as at least a twofold increase in serum creatinine to a level greater than 2.5 mg/dl (221 μmol/l) in less than 2 weeks. In many subjects, the occurrence of the HRS is associated with deterioration of function in other organs, including the liver, heart, and brain.

Type 2 HRS is a more chronic form of HRS and is associated with a slower progression of renal failure and without treatment, the median survival is about 6 months [31, 32]. It is common in patients with refractory ascites.

Clinical Presentation

At presentation, there are no obvious clinical features that may differentiate patients with HRS from those with other causes of acute kidney dysfunction. Diligent assessment of the patient together with tests to exclude other causes of kidney dysfunction will help to make the diagnosis using the criteria noted above. Urine output decreases over time and most patients with type 1 HRS become oligo-anuric within a relatively short time. Patients with type 2 HRS may not have any significant decrease in urine output at the time of the initial presentation with the main finding being the elevation is serum creatinine. The urine sodium is usually very low, consistent with pre-renal hemodynamic state. The urine sediment is bland.

Treatment

HRS was previously a terminal condition but improvements in our understanding of the pathophysiology over the last 2–3 decades has led to improvement in management which has helped to change the prognosis of this condition. Despite the advances made, however, only about 40–50 % of patients with HRS respond to treatment, and at best, current pharmacologic agents have only modest effects on survival, and for most patients their use is only aimed as a bridge to liver transplantation [33, 34]. Unfortunately most of these patients will die before a suitable liver becomes available. Therefore, novel treatment options are needed to improve the long-term survival of these patients.

Following the diagnosis of HRS (see above for diagnostic criteria), initial medical management should focus on identifying and managing any precipitating factors. Fluid management is essential and strict charting of fluid input and output is required. In patients with hyponatremia free water restriction will be necessary. Development of tense ascites can contribute to poor renal perfusion (consistent with abdominal compartment syndrome) and needs to be treated appropriately. Concomitant infusion of intravenous albumin will help to reduce the degree of intravascular hypovolemia in those who undergo large-volume paracentesis (>4 l of ascitic fluid) or who undergo anything more than a diagnostic paracentesis in the setting of already established renal insufficiency. Underlying infections should be treated aggressively. Spontaneous bacterial peritonitis is a common precipitant of type 1 HRS and should be actively looked for and treated including administration of intravenous albumin (1.5 mg/kg within 6 h of diagnosis and 1 mg/kg on day 3) in addition to appropriate antibiotics. In patients with type 1 HRS, the urine output may decline rapidly and the need for RRT will permeate the discussions. Initiation of aggressive medical treatment in this situation should be made after discussions at the multidisciplinary level. Median survival in such patients is very limited and apart from specific clinical situations where there is a very high possibility of liver recovery in the short-term as in acute fulminant liver failure or acute alcoholic hepatitis, initiation of a treatment like RRT may be futile, unless the patient is a candidate for liver transplantation. Currently available medical and other treatment options are discussed below.

Medical Therapy

Based on its underlying pathophysiology, both renal vasodilators and systemic vasoconstrictors have been tried in patients with HRS. The renal vasodilators (including dopamine, endothelin-A receptor antagonists, and prostaglandin analogues) had minimal benefits together with significant adverse effects and have been abandoned. The mainstay of pharmacologic treatment for HRS is therefore based on systemic vasoconstrictors. These agents are used with the aim of reversing splanchnic vasodilatation to improve the circulating blood volume and the target is to raise the mean arterial pressure by approximately 10–15 mmHg. All the vasoconstrictors are given in combination with intravenous albumin. Of the available systemic vasoconstrictors, the vasopressin analogue, terlipressin is the most widely used worldwide. In situations where terlipressin cannot be used or in countries like the United States where terlipressin is not available, other options include vasopressin, norepinerphrine, octreotide, and midorine. Norepinerphrine is specifically a good option to consider in patients admitted to the intensive care unit. Octreotide is a nonspecific inhibitor of endogenous vasodilators. It is usually given subcutaneously in combination with the alpha-adrenergic agonist, midodrine. Most of the data related to the use of these agents have come from single center studies with very few patients and there were no control groups in most of the studies. A recent head-to-head randomized trial found that terlipressin plus albumin was significantly more effective than octreotide and midodrine plus albumin in improving renal function in patients with HRS [35–37]. A meta-analysis involving a total of 154 patients with type 1 HRS did not find any statistically significant difference between terlipressin and norepinerphrine in terms of resolution of HRS and 30-day mortality [36].

The optimal duration of medical therapy is unknown but in most instances, treatment is continued for 2–4 weeks, depending on the clinical response. Patients who do not have any response after 2 weeks of therapy are unlikely to benefit from this treatment and the therapy should be discontinued. Of those who respond to treatment, approximately half of them will relapse and most of these patients will respond to a repeat course of treatment. In patients who relapse and for those with rather low baseline mean arterial blood pressure, consideration should be given to ongoing treatment with midodrine.

Transjugular Intrahepatic Portosystemic Shunt (TIPS)

TIPS is a potential treatment for refractory ascites. Insertion of TIPS has been associated with reduction of portal pressure and improvement in hemodynamic and neurohumoral parameters in cirrhotic patients. TIPS has also been shown to improve urine output, sodium excretion, and GFR in patients with HRS. Although the data remains limited, there is evidence that TIPS may improve short-term outcomes in patients with the HRS. Indeed in some cases long-term improvement in survival has been noted. In one report, placement of TIPS after initial response to medical treatment with octreotide and midodrine in combination with albumin in patients with type 1 HRS resulted in improved long-term survival and sustained improvement in renal function compared with patients who did not undergo TIPS [38]. Despite the reassuring results, TIPS has many complications, including encephalopathy, heart failure, and worsening of renal function from contrast exposure and many of these patients have contraindications to this procedure. Selected patients who have failed pharmacologic treatment and who are deemed not candidates for liver transplantation may be considered for TIPS if there are no major contraindications including absence of overt hepatic encephalopathy and any evidence of right-sided heart failure or pulmonary hypertension on echocardiography.

Renal Replacement Therapy (RRT)

RRT does not change the clinical course of HRS and may be associated with significant morbidity and increased hospital length of stay. In patients with type 1 HRS, it should only be offered as a bridge therapy in those awaiting liver transplantation and in selected patients where the liver failure is expected to resolve as in those with acute alcoholic hepatitis. Patient survival on RRT is dependent on the severity of the liver failure. The choice of RRT modality in patients with type 1 HRS is controversial but continuous renal replacement therapy (CRRT) tends to be tolerated better than hemodialysis on account of the underlying hemodynamic instability. Patients with type 2 HRS who progress to ESRD generally tolerate hemodialysis. When no contraindications are present, such patients should be listed for combined liver and kidney transplantation.

Molecular Adsorbent Recirculation System (MARS)

MARS is a specialized dialysis technique which enables the removal of water-soluble and albumin-bound substances of molecular weight <50 kDa. It is hoped that removal of such vasodilators would help to reverse the hemodynamic situation in HRS. So far, in patients with type 1 HRS, MARS has failed to show any significant benefit in randomized controlled trials.

Liver Transplantation

Despite the improved short-term outcomes associated with the use of current available medical treatment, to date, liver transplantation remains the best treatment option for suitable patients with HRS as it affords the chance for cure of the liver failure and also leads to resolution of the HRS if performed in a timely manner. Unfortunately this superior treatment modality is limited by availability of organs and in practice, most patients with type 1 HRS will die before a suitable organ becomes available. Liver transplantation seem to offer a clear survival benefit to patients with type 1 HRS regardless of which medical therapy they had received and this is also independent of whether HRS had been reversed or not prior to the liver transplantation [39, 40]. The rate of recovery of renal function after liver transplantation is variable and is likely dependent on the time that had elapsed prior to liver transplantation [41]. The variability in the reports may also be due to the underlying difficulties in making a definitive diagnosis of HRS. In established cases of HRS complicated by anuria, it is not routinely possible to identify those who subsequently develop superimposed to acute tubular necrosis (ATN). Clearly the outcome in such patients will be different from those without ATN. The relatively prolonged clinical course in patients with type 2 HRS means they are more likely to survive to liver transplantation. Patients with HRS and who are dialysis-dependent for a prolonged period (>8 weeks) should be considered for combined liver and kidney transplantation as their chance of developing end-stage kidney disease in the future is higher. New guidelines for combined liver and kidney transplantation in such patients are being considered by the united network for organ sharing (UNOS). Since the introduction of the Model of end-stage liver disease (MELD) scores (which incorporates serum creatinine) into the liver allocation system in the United States in 2002 with the aim of giving priority to the sickest patients, more patients with renal dysfunction, including those with HRS have been transplanted. Similarly, the number of combined liver and kidney transplantations has increased.

Prevention

Once it is established, the hepatorenal syndrome is generally associated with poor outcomes and thus it behooves providers place emphasis on its prevention in the first place. To achieve this, it is important to identify the presence of known precipitating factors (e.g. SBP, gastrointestinal bleeding, large-volume paracentesis, and alcoholic hepatitis) and manage them appropriately. Indeed, a precipitating event can be identified in most cases of type 1 HRS. SBP is common in cirrhotic patients and is a common precipitant of type 1 HRS. Approximately a third of patients with who have SBP will go on to develop HRS. A high level of suspicion is always necessary to make the diagnosis as a number of patients will present nonspecifically and without overt abdominal pain. Empiric antibiotics should be initiated as soon as possible until the sensitivity test result is available. Concomitant administration of intravenous albumin with the antibiotic (1.5 g/kg) within 6 h of diagnosis of infection and another dose of albumin (1 g/kg) on day 3 of antibiotic treatment has been shown to reduce the incidence of both renal dysfunction and mortality in such patients [42]. Also primary prophylaxis with norfloxacin (400 mg daily) reduced the incidence of SBP, delayed the development of HRS, and improved survival in selected patients with advanced cirrhosis and low ascitic fluid protein levels [43]. Although significant gastrointestinal bleeding tends to cause acute tubular necrosis in patients with advanced cirrhosis, it may also precipitate HRS especially in the setting of superimposed bacterial infection. Large-volume paracentesis (>5 l) is commonly complicated by HRS in predisposed patients due to its effect on the existing tenuous hemodynamic state. Administration of intravenous albumin (e.g. 8 g/l of ascitic fluid removed) at the time of the procedure can reduce this risk. Severe alcoholic hepatitis (SAH) is a life-threatening condition and may be complicated by hepatorenal syndrome. Treatment with a corticosteroid has short-term survival benefit and is the recommended treatment for SAH. Pentoxifylline is an alternative treatment where corticosteroids are contraindicated. Despite a suggestion of benefit, a recent, relatively large study failed to detect a significant difference in incidence of hepatorenal syndrome in patients with severe alcoholic hepatitis who were treated with pentoxifylline [44].

Conclusion

The hepatorenal syndrome is a severe complication that occurs in patients with advanced cirrhosis, severe alcoholic hepatitis, and fulminant liver failure. It is one of many possible causes of renal dysfunction in patients with cirrhosis.

Improvements in our understanding of the underlying pathophysiology over the last 2–3 decades has led to development of current treatment that has changed the natural history of HRS from what was a uniformly terminal condition to one that is potentially reversible. Despite the advances made, however, at best, the current treatment options have only modest effects on survival, and for most patients, their use is only aimed as a bridge to liver transplantation. Further research is required in order to develop novel treatment for this condition. For example, a better understanding of the causes of cirrhotic cardiomyopathy with the view to preventing or treating it may help to reduce the incidence of HRS. The role of subclinical adrenal insufficiency in enhancing the hemodynamic derangement is not entirely clear and will need to receive attention. The reasons for the varied renal outcome after liver transplantation will also need further studies.

References

1. Flint A. Clinical report on hydro-peritoneum, based on analysis of forty-six cases. Am J Med Sci. 1863;45:306–39.
2. Hecker R, Sherlock S. Electrolyte and circulatory changes in terminal liver failure. Lancet. 1956;271:1121–5.
3. Salerno F, Gerbes A, Ginès P, Wong F, Arroyo V. Diagnosis, prevention and treatment of hepatorenal syndrome in cirrhosis. Gut. 2007;56(9):1310–8.
4. Colle I, Durand F, Pessione F, Rassiat E, Bernuau J, Barriere E, et al. Clinical course, predictive factors and prognosis in patients with cirrhosis and type 1 hepatorenal syndrome treated with Terlipressin: a retrospective analysis. J Gastroenterol Hepatol. 2002;17:882–8.
5. Solanki P, Chawla A, Garg R, Gupta R, Jain M, Sarin SK. Beneficial effects of terlipressin in hepatorenal syndrome: a prospective, randomized placebo-controlled clinical trial. J Gastroenterol Hepatol. 2003;18:152–6.
6. Ginès P, Schrier RW. Renal failure in cirrhosis. N Engl J Med. 2009;361(13):1279–90.
7. Moreau R, Lebrec D. Acute renal failure in patients with cirrhosis: perspectives in the age of MELD. Hepatology. 2003;37(2):233–43.
8. Arroyo V, Ginès P, Gerbes AL, Dudley FJ, Gentilini P, Laffi G, et al. Definition and diagnostic criteria of refractory ascites and hepatorenal syndrome in cirrhosis. International Ascites Club. Hepatology. 1996;23:164–76.
9. Nair S, Verma S, Thuluvath PJ. Pretransplant renal function predicts survival in patients undergoing orthotopic liver transplantation. Hepatology. 2002;35(5):1179–85.
10. Martin PY, Ginès P, Schrier RW. Nitric oxide as a mediator of hemodynamic abnormalities and sodium and water retention in cirrhosis. N Engl J Med. 1998;339(8):533–41.
11. Ros J, Clària J, To-Figueras J, Planagumà A, Cejudo-Martín P, Fernández-Varo G, et al. Endogenous cannabinoids: a new system involved in the homeostasis of arterial pressure in experimental cirrhosis in the rat. Gastroenterology. 2002;122(1):85–93.
12. Guarner C, Soriano G, Tomas A, Bulbena O, Novella MT, Balanzo J, et al. Increased serum nitrite and nitrate levels in patients with cirrhosis: relationship to endotoxemia. Hepatology. 1993;18(5):1139–43.

13. Ruiz-del-Arbol L, Urman J, Fernández J, González M, Navasa M, Monescillo A, et al. Systemic, renal, and hepatic hemodynamic derangement in cirrhotic patients with spontaneous bacterial peritonitis. Hepatology. 2003;38(5):1210–8.
14. Wiest R, Das S, Cadelina G, Garcia-Tsao G, Milstien S, Groszmann RJ. Bacterial translocation in cirrhotic rats stimulates eNOS-derived NO production and impairs mesenteric vascular contractility. J Clin Invest. 1999;104(9):1223–33.
15. Ruiz-del-Arbol L, Monescillo A, Arocena C, Valer P, Ginès P, Moreira V, et al. Circulatory function and hepatorenal syndrome in cirrhosis. Hepatology. 2005;42(2):439–47.
16. Krag A, Bendtsen F, Henriksen JH, Møller S. Low cardiac output predicts development of hepatorenal syndrome and survival in patients with cirrhosis and ascites. Gut. 2010;59(1):105–10.
17. Møller S, Henriksen JH. Cirrhotic cardiomyopathy: a pathophysiological review of circulatory dysfunction in liver disease. Heart. 2002;87(1):9–15.
18. Alqahtani SA, Fouad TR, Lee SS. Cirrhotic cardiomyopathy. Semin Liver Dis. 2008;28(1):59–69.
19. Lang F, Tschernko E, Schulze E, Ottl I, Ritter M, Völkl H, et al. Hepatorenal reflex regulating kidney function. Hepatology. 1991;14(4 Pt 1):590–4.
20. Schneider AW, Kalk JF, Klein CP. Effect of losartan, an angiotensin II receptor antagonist, on portal pressure in cirrhosis. Hepatology. 1999;29(2):334–9.
21. Epstein M, Weitzman RE, Preston S, DeNunzio AG. Relationship between plasma arginine vasopressin and renal water handling in decompensated cirrhosis. Miner Electrolyte Metab. 1984;10(3):155–65.
22. Bichet D, Szatalowicz V, Chaimovitz C, Schrier RW. Role of vasopressin in abnormal water excretion in cirrhotic patients. Ann Intern Med. 1982;96(4):413–7.
23. Henriksen JH, Ring-Larsen H. Hepatorenal disorders: role of the sympathetic nervous system. Semin Liver Dis. 1994;14(1):35–43.
24. Bichet DG, Van Putten VJ, Schrier RW. Potential role of increased sympathetic activity in impaired sodium and water excretion in cirrhosis. N Engl J Med. 1982;307(25):1552–7.
25. Koppel MH, Coburn JW, Mims MM, Goldstein H, Boyle JD, Rubini ME. Transplantation of cadaveric kidneys from patients with hepatorenal syndrome. Evidence for the functional nature of renal failure in advanced liver disease. N Engl J Med. 1969;280:1367–71.
26. Iwatsuki S, Popovtzer MM, Corman JL, Ishikawa M, Putnam CW, Katz FH, et al. Recovery from "hepatorenal syndrome" after orthotopic liver transplantation. N Engl J Med. 1973;289:1155–9.
27. Marik PE, Wood K, Starzl TE. The course of type 1 hepato-renal syndrome post liver transplantation. Nephrol Dial Transplant. 2005;25:25–365.
28. Adebayo D, Morabito V, Davenport A, Jalan R. Renal dysfunction in cirrhosis is not just a vasomotor nephropathy. Kidney Int. 2015;87(3):509–15.
29. Mandal AK, Lansing M, Fahmy A. Acute tubular necrosis in hepatorenal syndrome: an electron microscopy study. Am J Kidney Dis. 1982;2:363–74.
30. Kanel GC, Peters RL. Glomerular tubular reflux--a morphologic renal lesion associated with the hepatorenal syndrome. Hepatology. 1984;4:242.
31. Gines P, Guevara M, Arroyo V, Rodes J. Hepatorenal syndrome. Lancet. 2003;362:1819–27.
32. Gines A, Escorsell A, Gines P, Salo J, Jimenez W, Inglada L, et al. Incidence, predictive factors, and prognosis of the hepatorenal syndrome in cirrhosis with ascites. Gastroenterology. 1993;105:229–36.
33. Wadei HM. Hepatorenal syndrome: a critical update. Semin Respir Crit Care Med. 2012;33(1):55–69.
34. Nazar A, Pereira GH, Guevara M, Martín-Llahi M, Pepin MN, Marinelli M, et al. Predictors of response to therapy with terlipressin and albumin in patients with cirrhosis and type 1 hepatorenal syndrome. Hepatology. 2010;51(1):219–26.
35. Duvoux C, Zanditenas D, Hézode C, et al. Effects of noradrenalin and albumin in patients with type I hepatorenal syndrome: a pilot study. Hepatology. 2002;36:374.

36. Nassar Junior AP, Farias AQ, D'Albuquerque L, Carrilho FJ, Malbouisson LM. Terlipressin versus norepinephrine in the treatment of hepatorenal syndrome: a systematic review and meta-analysis. PLoS One. 2014;9(9):e107466.
37. Cavallin M, Kamath PS, Merli M, Fasolato S, Toniutto P, Salerno F, Bernardi M, Romanelli RG et al; for the Italian Association for the Study of the Liver Study Group on Hepatorenal Syndrome. Terlipressin plus albumin versus midodrine and octreotide plus albumin in the treatment of hepatorenal syndrome: a randomized trial. Hepatology 2015; 62: 567.
38. Wong F, Pantea L, Sniderman K. Midodrine, octreotide, albumin, and TIPS in selected patients with cirrhosis and type 1 hepatorenal syndrome. Hepatology. 2004;40(1):55–64.
39. Gonwa TA, Morris CA, Goldstein RM, Husberg BS, Klintmalm GB. Long-term survival and renal function following liver transplantation in patients with and without hepatorenal syndrome--experience in 300 patients. Transplantation. 1991;51(2):428–30.
40. Gonwa TA, Klintmalm GB, Levy M, Jennings LS, Goldstein RM, Husberg BS. Impact of pretransplant renal function on survival after liver transplantation. Transplantation. 1995;59(3):361–5.
41. Wong F, Leung W, Al Beshir M, et al. Outcomes of patients with cirrhosis and hepatorenal syndrome type 1 treated with liver transplantation. Liver Transpl. 2015;21:300.
42. Sort P, Navasa M, Arroyo V, Aldeguer X, Planas R, Ruiz-del-Arbol L, et al. Effect of intravenous albumin on renal impairment and mortality in patients with cirrhosis and spontaneous bacterial peritonitis. N Engl J Med. 1999;341(6):403–9.
43. Fernández J, Navasa M, Planas R, et al. Primary prophylaxis of spontaneous bacterial peritonitis delays hepatorenal syndrome and improves survival in cirrhosis. Gastroenterology. 2007;133:818.
44. Mathurin P, Louvet A, Duhamel A, Nahon P, Carbonell N, Boursier J, et al. Prednisolone with vs without pentoxifylline and survival of patients with severe alcoholic hepatitis: a randomized clinical trial. JAMA. 2013;310(10):1033–41.
45. Angela P, Genes P, Wong F, Bernarda M, Boyer TD, Grebes A, et al. Diagnosis and management of acute kidney injury in patients with cirrhosis: revised consensus recommendations of the International Club of Ascites. Gut. 2015;64(4):531–7.

Chapter 33
Hepatopulmonary Syndrome

Rahul Sudhir Nanchal and Tessa Damm

Patient-Level Questions

1. What is hepatopulmonary syndrome and what causes it?
   Hepatopulmonary syndrome is a condition that may be present in patients with liver disease. It is characterized by low levels of oxygen in the body. We think that the diseased liver is responsible for changes in the lungs that cause the low oxygen levels. Oxygen enters the body through transfer from the airspaces in the lung to small blood vessels that are a part of the lung circulation. These small blood vessels in the pulmonary circulation are affected by this condition and become enlarged or dilated and are not able to efficiently participate in receiving oxygen from the lung airspaces leading to low oxygen levels in the body

2. What are the consequences of hepatopulmonary syndrome?
   The most important consequence of hepatopulmonary syndrome is the low level of oxygen in the body. This may lead to shortness of breath at rest or with exercise. The shortness of breath may become worse on standing up from a supine or sitting position. Frequently patients may have to wear supplemental oxygen to raise the levels of oxygen in their body and alleviate their shortness of breath. The definitive cure for heptaopulmonary syndrome is liver transplantation; however, complete resolution may take several months after liver transplant.

3. How do I know if I have hepatopulmonary syndrome?
   The most commonly used method of diagnosing hepatopulmonary syndrome is contrast-enhanced echocardiography. In this test, tiny air bubbles are injected into a peripheral vein while visualizing the heart via echocardiography at the

R.S. Nanchal, M.D. (✉)
Division of Pulmonary & Critical Care, Medical College of Wisconsin, Milwaukee, WI, USA
e-mail: rnanchal@mcw.edu

T. Damm, M.D.
Department of Critical Care Medicine, Aurora St. Luke's Medical Center,
Milwaukee, WI, USA

© Springer International Publishing Switzerland 2017
K. Saeian, R. Shaker (eds.), *Liver Disorders*,
DOI 10.1007/978-3-319-30103-7_33

same time. Normally the tiny injected bubbles pass through the right side of the heart and into pulmonary circulation where they are trapped by the small vessels of the lungs. This is because the bubbles are usually larger than the small lung vessels. However, in hepatopulmonary syndrome, the lung vessels are dilated and allow passage of the air bubbles into the left side of the heart. This is seen on echocardiography.

Historical Perspectives

Observations linking chronic liver disease to pulmonary abnormalities first appeared in the medical literature in 1884 when Fluckiger reported cyanosis and finger clubbing in patients with cirrhosis [1]. This was followed by confirmation of arterial hypoxemia and elegant autopsy studies describing widespread vasodilation of the pre-capillary pulmonary arterioles in 13 patients with cirrhosis [2]. Seminal observations from these histopathological studies included normal lung structures (alveoli and connective tissue) and increase in number of vessels along the alveolar wall caused by pre-capillary arteriolar vasodilation. Hepatopulmonary (HPS) syndrome was recognized as a clinical entity when the intellectual leap of intrapulmonary vasodilation causing arterial hypoxemia was made [3].

Epidemiology and Natural History

There remains a lack of large prospective series defining the epidemiology of HPS. Retrospective series mostly from single centers report prevalence ranges between 5 and 32 % [4]. The wide variance in prevalence is likely secondary to variability in cutoffs used to define gas exchange abnormalities. Although most commonly associated with cirrhosis and portal hypertension, HPS has been described in hepatitis without cirrhosis and portal hypertension as well as in noncirrhotic portal hypertension without underlying chronic liver disease [5–8]. Further neither the presence nor the degree of hypoxemia in HPS correlate well with the severity of liver disease as adjudicated by the Child-Pugh's or Model for End-Stage Liver Disease (MELD) classification [9]. However, the presence of HPS confers an increased risk of mortality when compared to similar patients who do not have HPS [9, 10]. Moreover, survival is markedly worse if the room air partial pressure of oxygen is less than 50 mmHg at the time of diagnosis. Reasons for demise in patients with HPS are usually related to complications of liver disease and are rarely secondary to arterial hypoxemia. Although, the exact biological pathways that lead to the development of HPS need to be elucidated, a recent study found that polymorphisms in candidate genes involved in the regulation of angiogenesis was associated with a higher risk of HPS [11].

Pathophysiology

The main pathological features of HPS are gross dilatation of the pulmonary precapillary and capillary vessels as well as an increase in the absolute number of dilated vessels [2]. Additionally, some pleural and pulmonary arteriovenous communications (true shunts) may also be observed. Reduced tone of the pulmonary vasculature and inhibition of hypoxic pulmonary vasoconstriction are some other findings that characterize HPS [12]. The arterial hypoxemia seen in HPS is secondary to intrapulmonary vascular dilatations (IPVD) resulting in ventilation-perfusion inequality [13, 14]. Blood flow or lung perfusion is increased while ventilation remains preserved. The ventilation perfusion mismatch may be exacerbated by true shunting of deoxygenated blood through pulmonary arteriovenous communications [13, 14]. The severity of arterial hypoxemia is related to the extent of the intrapulmonary mechanisms in play.

Animal Models

A rat common bile duct ligation (CBDL) model has features akin to human HPS [15]. In this model, proliferating cholangiocytes secrete endothelin-1 (ET-1), which binds to upregulated endothelin B receptors [16]. This enhances nitric oxide (NO) production through endothelial nitric oxide synthetase (NOS) [17]. Further an increase in pulmonary monocytes is observed which enhance nitric oxide and carbon monoxide production through inducible NOS and heme-oxygenase-1 respectively [18]. Moreover, an increase in blood levels of vascular endothelial growth factor is observed (VEGF) [19]. These mechanisms in concert are responsible for the development of IPVD and de novo pulmonary angiogenesis resulting in hypoxemia [20]. The anti-angiogenesis factor sorafenib has shown to be associated with improvements in oxygenation in CBDL rats with HPS [21].

Human Disease

Besides autopsy studies demonstrating the presence of vascular dilatations and shunts, the understanding of molecular mechanisms leading to HPS in humans is limited. Several lines of indirect evidence implicate NO and angiogenesis as likely contributors. Exhaled nitric oxide levels in patients with HPS are higher compared to those without HPS and these levels normalize after liver transplantation [22, 23]. Polymorphisms in genes associated with angiogenesis have now been linked to the presence of HPS [11]. Often, hypoxemia post liver transplantation takes several months to resolve suggesting that there is perhaps remodeling of the pulmonary vasculature, lending credence to the theory of angiogenesis. In one study, ET-1 levels in the hepatic vein were higher in patients with HPS and IPVD compared to patients without IPVD and blood ET-1 levels corresponded with the degree of bile duct proliferation in liver biopsy specimens [24]. It is, however, important to understand that a causal relationship between the aforementioned mechanisms and hypoxemia in HPS has yet to be established.

Diagnostic Criteria

Formal accepted diagnostic criteria for HPS comprise of three components—(1) documentation of impaired oxygenation, (2) presence of intrapulmonary vasodilation (IPVD), and (3) evidence of cirrhosis or portal hypertension [25].

Because patients with liver disease hyperventilate and this phenomenon may increase the arterial tension of oxygen, milder forms of HPS may be missed if hypoxemia is used as the sole criterion. It is therefore important to use the sensitive alveolar-arterial (A-a) oxygen gradient to document defects in oxygenation for milder forms. A cut-off value of 15 mmHg for younger patients and 20 mmHg for patients aged 64 or older while breathing ambient air (21 % oxygen) is agreed upon as being diagnostic of impaired oxygenation in the right clinical setting [25].

The severity of the oxygenation defect is associated with survival and is a guide to the timing and risks of liver transplantation. Therefore the technique of alveolar-arterial gradient for the diagnosis of impaired oxygenation in HPS is used to classify patients into the following 4 categories of severity [25]

(a) Mild disease—$PaO_2 > 80$ mmHg
(b) Moderate disease—$PaO_2 > 60$ to <80 mmHg
(c) Severe disease—$PaO_2 > 50$ to <60 mmHg
(d) Very severe disease—$PaO_2 < 50$ mmHg (or <300 mmHg while breathing 100 % oxygen)

Demonstration of IPVD

There are two commonly used tests to demonstrate the presence of IPVD—contrast-enhanced echocardiography (CEE) [26] and nuclear medicine lung perfusion scan using technetium-labeled macro-aggregates of albumin [27].

CEE is the most sensitive test and is more commonly used. Agitated saline which creates microbubbles is infused into a peripheral vein causing opacification of the right atrium and ventricles. Normally as the microbubbles move through the pulmonary circulation they are trapped by the pulmonary capillaries and should not appear on the left side of the heart. Appearance of microbubbles in the left atrium within 3–6 cardiac cycles is indicative of passage through an abnormally dilated pulmonary vascular bed. Earlier appearance of microbubbles on the left side (<3 cardiac cycles) indicates a right to left intra-cardiac shunt. Almost 60 % of patients referred for liver transplantation have a positive CEE, but only half meet the diagnostic criteria for HPS (IPVD with normal A-a gradient). The clinical significance of these subclinical IPVD is currently not known [4, 28].

Using the lung perfusion approach involves injecting macro-aggregates of albumin into the peripheral venous circulation. These macro-aggregates should not pass into systemic circulation as they are trapped by the pulmonary vasculature. Appearance in the systemic circulation as measured by scintigraphy is indicative of either IPVD or a right to left shunt at the cardiac or pulmonary level. A shunt fraction (brain/total body macro-aggregates) of greater than 6 % denotes a positive result. This test is less sensitive than CEE and maybe useful in the determining the degree of contribution of IPVD to hypoxemia in patients with coexisting lung disease and other causes of hypoxemia.

Pulmonary angiography is another modality that may be used but is not generally recommended. It is reserved for patients whose hypoxemia is poorly responsive to 100 % oxygen and may demonstrate true arteriovenous (AV) communications that may be amenable to coil embolization. The appearance of the pulmonary vasculature in HPS with pulmonary angiography has two patterns—Type I HPS characterized by pre-capillary dilatations without AV communications and Type 2 HPS characterized by true localized pulmonary AV communications. Type 2 HPS is poorly responsive to oxygen therapy and consideration should be given to coil embolization in these cases [29, 30].

Clinical Manifestations and Laboratory Testing

In addition to the general manifestations of chronic liver disease such as spider nevi, dyspnea is the most common complaint of patients with HPS, occurring in nearly 70 % patients [31]. However, this complaint is nonspecific and may result from a variety of coexisting conditions. These conditions may be complications of chronic liver disease and portal hypertension such as ascites and hepatic hydrothorax or independent associated entities such as volume overload, muscle wasting, anemia, and intrinsic lung disease. HPS may be concurrent with these pleural and pulmonary complications of advanced liver disease and therefore clinical judgment may be necessary in several cases in the attribution of the degree of hypoxemia to HPS versus one of the concomitant conditions.

Physical examination findings are nonspecific as well and include the presence of digital clubbing, cyanosis, and spider nevi. Two phenomena associated with HPS are orthodeoxia (hypoxemia that worsens in the upright position) and platypnea (increased shortness of breath in the seated versus supine position). These occur because change in position from supine to upright result in redistribution of pulmonary blood flow to lung bases, preferentially perfusing dilated vasculature and worsening ventilation perfusion defects [32]. Although classically described in HPS, both platypnea and orthodeoxia are not sensitive indicators of disease [28].

The single most consistent laboratory abnormality is a decrease in the diffusing capacity for carbon monoxide [28]. However, this is not specific and unlike other gas exchange indexes may not normalize after liver transplantation [33, 34]. The chest radiograph may demonstrate an interstitial reticular pattern in the lower lung zones reflecting the presence of IPVD. Often chest imaging and pulmonary function tests may be representative of other conditions that coexist with HPS and contribute to hypoxemia. In these cases demonstration of IVPD via CEE and judgment is essential to attribute clinical manifestations to HPS [35].

Treatment

Pharmacological Therapies

Patients with significant degrees of hypoxemia at rest or with exercise are universally treated with supplemental oxygen therapy. However, oxygen therapy has never been demonstrated to reliably improve dyspnea or improve quality of life in patients with HPS. Although a variety of pharmacological agents targeting putative biological pathways have been tested in uncontrolled studies, effects have been variable and none have shown to dependably improve oxygenation. These interventions include pentoxifylline [36], mycophenolate mofetil [37], somatostatin [29], methylene blue [38], almitrine [39], cyclo-oxygenase inhibitors [40], antibiotics [41], propranolol [42] and garlic [43, 44].

Transjugular Intrahepatic Portosystemic Shunt (TIPS)

Since HPS can occur in noncirrhotic portal hypertension, portal decompression has been evaluated as a therapy to reduce portal pressures and alleviate hypoxemia in patients with HPS. However, like pharmacological interventions, studies are limited to case reports and have had variable results [45, 46]. A recent meta-analysis concluded that although TIPS may have promise as a treatment strategy, future prospective studies were warranted [47]. Coupled with the fact that TIPS could potentially increase venous return and exacerbate the hyperdynamic circulatory state thereby exacerbating the severity of HPS, it is not currently recommended as a treatment alternative for HPS. It may, however, still be used for other indications such as refractory ascites and variceal bleeding in patients with concomitant HPS.

Liver Transplantation (LT)

Liver transplantation remains the only viable option that improves both oxygenation and survival in HPS [48]. In the past severe hypoxemia (room air $PaO_2 < 50$ mmHg) was considered a contraindication to LT. However, several reports have documented complete resolution of hypoxemia after LT [49]. Moreover poor 5 year survival of nontransplanted patients with HPS compared to those receiving LT [9], combined with the absence of correlation between the severity of HPS and degree of hepatic dysfunction resulted in HPS becoming a standard indication for LT. Since the severity of liver disease does not correlate well with the degree of hypoxemia and HPS detrimentally affects overall survival, patients with HPS and significant hypoxemia (room air $PaO_2 < 60$ mmHg) are eligible for MELD exception points [50], which gives them priority on the liver transplantation list. Currently, a standard MELD score increase amounting to a 10% wait list mortality equivalent is granted every 3 months if the repeat PaO_2 remains less than 60. To be eligible for the MELD exception, patients need to be free of underlying primary lung disease that may account for the hypoxemia [51]. Controversy currently exists around whether the severity of pre-transplant hypoxemia is predictive of post-transplant mortality [9, 51]. Most studies reporting outcomes post-transplant are single center, have small numbers of patients and have significant heterogeneity in definitions of HPS, thus comparisons are difficult [52–54]. A recent large retrospective study reported that the severity of pre-transplant hypoxemia did not predict post-transplant mortality and that the MELD exception policy may have resulted in improved outcomes [55]. Investigators have also demonstrated that patients with HPS eligible for LT have minimal wait list mortality, resolve their hypoxemia post-transplant, and do well long term [48]. Although the degree of hypoxemia does not appear to affect post LT mortality, there is expert agreement that the severity of pre-transplant hypoxemia is directly related to the time it takes for the hypoxemia to resolve post-transplant.

It is important to note that resolution of hypoxemia post LT is slow, often taking up to 12 months [51, 52], or longer in some case reports [53]. During the immediate postoperative period, hypoxemia can be severe requiring high concentrations of inspired oxygen. Paradoxically, there are now several case reports of inhaled pulmonary vasodilators especially inhaled nitric oxide leading to hypoxemia reversal and reduction in the amount of supplemental oxygen required [56, 57]. Post LT, patients with HPS may require extubation at higher than traditional oxygen concentrations and use of high flow oxygen delivery systems as a bridge to hypoxemia resolution. Use of trans-tracheal oxygen therapy has been recently reported as an efficient way of providing oxygen post LT [58].

Future Directions

Currently MELD exception is available only to patients with diagnosed HPS and no concurrent additional pulmonary disease. This may exclude many patients with HPS and mild lung disease such as COPD who have the potential to do well long term after LT. A more precise measurement of the contribution of HPS to hypoxemia could be accomplished through macro-aggregate albumin nuclear perfusion scanning; thus reconsideration of how MELD exception is granted in HPS is warranted. Finally better insights into the biological pathways that underpin HPS are needed so that intelligent therapies may be developed.

References

1. Fluckiger M. Vorkommen von trommelschagel formigen fingerendphalangen ohne chronische veranderungen an der lungen oder am herzen. Wien Med Wochenschr. 1884;34:1457.
2. Berthelot P, Walker JG, Sherlock S, et al. Arterial changes in the lungs in cirrhosis of the liver–lung spider nevi. N Engl J Med. 1966;274:291–8.
3. Kennedy TC, Knudson RJ. Exercise-aggravated hypoxemia and orthodeoxia in cirrhosis. Chest. 1977;72:305–9.
4. Schenk P, Fuhrmann V, Madl C, et al. Hepatopulmonary syndrome: prevalence and predictive value of various cut offs for arterial oxygenation and their clinical consequences. Gut. 2002;51:853–9.
5. Fuhrmann V, Madl C, Mueller C, et al. Hepatopulmonary syndrome in patients with hypoxic hepatitis. Gastroenterology. 2006;131:69–75.
6. Regev A, Yeshurun M, Rodriguez M, et al. Transient hepatopulmonary syndrome in a patient with acute hepatitis A. J Viral Hepat. 2001;8:83–6.
7. Gupta D, Vijaya DR, Gupta R, et al. Prevalence of hepatopulmonary syndrome in cirrhosis and extrahepatic portal venous obstruction. Am J Gastroenterol. 2001;96:3395–9.
8. Krowka MJ. Hepatopulmonary syndrome and extrahepatic vascular abnormalities. Liver Transpl. 2001;7:656–7.
9. Swanson KL, Wiesner RH, Krowka MJ. Natural history of hepatopulmonary syndrome: impact of liver transplantation. Hepatology. 2005;41:1122–9.
10. Schiffer E, Majno P, Mentha G, et al. Hepatopulmonary syndrome increases the postoperative mortality rate following liver transplantation: a prospective study in 90 patients. Am J Transplant. 2006;6:1430–7.
11. Roberts KE, Kawut SM, Krowka MJ, et al. Genetic risk factors for hepatopulmonary syndrome in patients with advanced liver disease. Gastroenterology. 2010;139(1):130–9.
12. Rodriguez-Roisin R, Roca J, Agusti AG, Mastai R, Wagner PD, Bosch J. Gas exchange and pulmonary vascular reactivity in patients with liver cirrhosis. Am Rev Respir Dis. 1987;135:1085–92.
13. Edell ES, Cortese DA, Krowka MJ, Rehder K. Severe hypoxemia and liver disease. Am Rev Respir Dis. 1989;140:1631–5.
14. Whyte MK, Hughes JM, Peters AM, Ussov W, Patel S, Burroughs AK. Analysis of intrapulmonary right to left shunt in the hepatopulmonary syndrome. J Hepatol. 1998;29:85–93.
15. Fallon MB, Abrams GA, McGrath JW, et al. Common bile duct ligation in the rat: a model of intrapulmonary vasodilatation and hepatopulmonary syndrome. Am J Physiol. 1997;272:G779–84.
16. Zhang M, Luo B, Chen SJ, et al. Endothelin-1 stimulation of endothelial nitric oxide synthase in the pathogenesis of hepatopulmonary syndrome. Am J Physiol. 1999;277:G944–52.
17. Fallon MB, Abrams GA, Luo B, et al. The role of endothelial nitric oxide synthase in the pathogenesis of a rat model of hepatopulmonary syndrome. Gastroenterology. 1997;113:606–14.
18. Zhang J, Ling Y, Luo B, et al. Analysis of pulmonary hemeoxygenase-1 and nitric oxide synthase alterations in experimental hepatopulmonary syndrome. Gastroenterology. 2003;125:1441–51.
19. Zhang J, Yang W, Luo B, et al. The role of CX(3)CL1/CX(3)CR1 in pulmonary angiogenesis and intravascular monocyte accumulation in rat experimental hepatopulmonary syndrome. J Hepatol. 2012;57:752–8.
20. Zhang J, Luo B, Tang L, et al. Pulmonary angiogenesis in a rat model of hepatopulmonary syndrome. Gastroenterology. 2009;136:1070–80.
21. Chang CC, Chuang CL, Lee FY, et al. Sorafenib treatment improves hepatopulmonary syndrome in rats with biliary cirrhosis. Clin Sci (Lond). 2013;124:457–66.
22. Rolla G, Brussino L, Colagrande P, et al. Exhaled nitric oxide and oxygenation abnormalities in hepatic cirrhosis. Hepatology. 1997;26:842–7.

23. Rolla G, Brussino L, Colagrande P, et al. Exhaled nitric oxide and impaired oxygenation in cirrhotic patients before and after liver transplantation. Ann Intern Med. 1998;129:375–8.
24. Koch DG, Bogatkevich G, Ramshesh V, et al. Elevated levels of endothelin-1 in hepatic venous blood are associated with intrapulmonary vasodilatation in humans. Dig Dis Sci. 2012;57(2):516–23.
25. Rodriguez-Roisin R, Krowka MJ, Herve P, et al. Pulmonary-hepatic vascular disorders (PHD). Eur Respir J. 2004;24:861–80.
26. Abrams GA, Jaffe CC, Hoffer PB, et al. Diagnostic utility of contrast echocardiography and lung perfusion scan in patients with hepatopulmonary syndrome. Gastroenterology. 1995;109:1283–8.
27. Abrams GA, Nanda NC, Dubovsky EV, et al. Use of macroaggregated albumin lung perfusion scan to diagnose hepatopulmonary syndrome: a new approach. Gastroenterology. 1998;114: 305–10.
28. Martinez GP, Barbera JA, Visa J, et al. Hepatopulmonary syndrome in candidates for liver transplantation. J Hepatol. 2001;34:651–7.
29. Krowka MJ, Dickson ER, Cortese DA. Hepatopulmonary syndrome. Clinical observations and lack of therapeutic response to somatostatin analogue. Chest. 1993;104:515–21.
30. Ryu JK, Oh JH. Hepatopulmonary syndrome: angiography and therapeutic embolization. Clin Imaging. 2003;27:97–100.
31. Sood G, Fallon MB, Niwas S, et al. Utility of dyspnea-fatigue index for screening liver transplant candidates for hepatopulmonary syndrome. Hepatology. 1998;28:2319 [abstract].
32. Gomez FP, Martinez-Palli G, Barbera JA, et al. Gas exchange mechanism of orthodeoxia in hepatopulmonary syndrome. Hepatology. 2004;40:660–6.
33. Hourani JM, Bellamy PE, Tashkin DP, Batra P, Simmons MS. Pulmonary dysfunction in advanced liver disease: frequent occurrence of an abnormal diffusing capacity. Am J Med. 1991;90:693–700.
34. Martinez-Palli G, Gomez FP, Barberà JA, et al. Sustained low diffusing capacity in hepatopulmonary syndrome after liver transplantation. World J Gastroenterol. 2006;12:5878–83.
35. Martinez G, Barberà JA, Navasa M, Roca J, Visa J, Rodriguez-Roisin R. Hepatopulmonary syndrome associated with cardiorespiratory disease. J Hepatol. 1999;30:882–9.
36. Tanikella R, Philips GM, Faulk DK, et al. Pilot study of pentoxifylline in hepatopulmonary syndrome. Liver Transpl. 2008;14:1199–203.
37. Moreira Silva H, Reis G, Guedes M, et al. A case of hepatopulmonary syndrome solved by mycophenolate mofetil (an inhibitor of angiogenesis and nitric oxide production). J Hepatol. 2013;58:630–3.
38. Jounieaux V, Leleu O, Mayeux I. Cardiopulmonary effects of nitric oxide inhalation and methylene blue injection in hepatopulmonary syndrome. Intensive Care Med. 2001;27:1103–4.
39. Nakos G, Evrenoglou D, Vassilakis N, et al. Haemodynamics and gas exchange in liver cirrhosis: the effect of orally administered almitrine bismesylate. Respir Med. 1993;87:93–8.
40. Shijo H, Sasaki H, Yuh K, et al. Effects of indomethacin on hepatogenic pulmonary angiodysplasia. Chest. 1991;99:1027–9.
41. Anel RM, Sheagren JN. Novel presentation and approach to management of hepatopulmonary syndrome with use of antimicrobial agents. Clin Infect Dis. 2001;32:E131–6.
42. Lambrecht GL, Malbrain ML, Coremans P, et al. Orthodeoxia and platypnea in liver cirrhosis: effects of propranolol. Acta Clin Belg. 1994;49:26–30.
43. Abrams GA, Fallon MB. Treatment of hepatopulmonary syndrome with Allium sativum L. (garlic): a pilot trial. J Clin Gastroenterol. 1998;27:232–5.
44. De BK, Dutta D, Pal SK, et al. The role of garlic in hepatopulmonary syndrome: a randomized controlled trial. Can J Gastroenterol. 2010;24(3):183–8.
45. Allgaier HP, Haag K, Ochs A, et al. Hepatopulmonary syndrome: successful treatment by transjugular intrahepatic portosystemic stentshunt (TIPS). J Hepatol. 1995;23:102.
46. Corley DA, Scharschmidt B, Bass N, et al. Lack of efficacy of TIPS for hepatopulmonary syndrome. Gastroenterology. 1997;113:728–30.

47. Tsauo J, Weng N, Ma H, Jiang M, Zhao H, Li X. Role of transjugular intrahepatic portosystemic shunts in the management of hepatopulmonary syndrome: a systemic literature review. J Vasc Interv Radiol. 2015;26(9):1266–71.
48. Gupta S, Castel H, Rao RV, et al. Improved survival after liver transplantation in patients with hepatopulmonary syndrome. Am J Transplant. 2010;10:354–63.
49. Laberge JM, Brandt ML, Lebecque P, Moulin D, Veykemans F, Paradis K, et al. Reversal of cirrhosis-related pulmonary shunting in two children by orthotopic liver transplantation. Transplantation. 1992;53:1135–8.
50. Fallon MB, Mulligan DC, Gish RG, et al. Model for end-stage liver disease (MELD) exception for hepatopulmonary syndrome. Liver Transpl. 2006;12 Suppl 3:S105–7.
51. Arguedas MR, Abrams GA, Krowka MJ, et al. Prospective evaluation of out-comes and predictors of mortality in patients with hepatopulmonary syndrome undergoing liver transplantation. Hepatology. 2003;37:192–7.
52. Collisson EA, Nourmand H, Fraiman MH, et al. Retrospective analysis of the results of liver transplantation for adults with severe hepatopulmonary syndrome. Liver Transpl. 2002;8:925–31.
53. Taille C, Cadranel J, Bellocq A, et al. Liver transplantation for hepatopulmonary syndrome: a ten-year experience in Paris, France. Transplantation. 2003;75:1482–9 [discussion: 46–7].
54. Krowka MJ, Mandell MS, Ramsay MA, et al. Hepatopulmonary syndrome and portopulmonary hypertension: a report of the multicenter liver transplant data-base. Liver Transpl. 2004;10:174–82.
55. Iyer VN, Swanson KL, Cartin-Ceba R, et al. Hepatopulmonary syndrome: favorable outcomes in the MELD exception era. Hepatology. 2013;57:2427–35.
56. Nayyar D, Man HS, Granton J, Lilly LB, Gupta S. Proposed management algorithm for severe hypoxemia after liver transplantation in the hepatopulmonary syndrome. Am J Transplant. 2015;15(4):903–13.
57. Karnatovskaia LV, Matharu J, Burger C, Keller CA. Inhaled nitric oxide as a potential rescue therapy for persistent hepatopulmonary syndrome after liver transplantation. Transplantation. 2014;27:98(6).
58. Udoji TN, Berkowitz DM, Bechara RI, Hanish S, Subramanian RM. The use of transtracheal oxygen therapy in the management of severe hepatopulmonary syndrome after liver transplantation. Transplant Proc. 2013;45(9):3316–9.

Chapter 34
Endoscopy and the Liver Patient

Abdul H. Khan

Patient Questions

1. Is endoscopic therapy for varices painful and can I eat afterwards?

   Patient-Level Answer: Generally banding of varices is painless and patients do not feel the bands at all. The bands are also not large enough to cause blockage of food passing through. In a small percentage of patients, a small ulcer can be left behind when the band falls off and this may be painful or bleed. An acid suppressing medication can help heal an ulcer if present. There is no specific diet restriction after banding but a reasonable approach is to allow clear liquids on the day of banding and then soft foods for a day or two afterwards before resuming a general diet.

2. Can varices get big enough to block my food pipe?

   Patient-Level Answer: No, varices do not cause blockage of the esophagus even when becoming large. Varices are large veins but they are soft and easily compressible so the pressure associated with food passage is large enough to overcome the varices and allow food to pass. Varices do not cause any symptoms unless they rupture.

3. My doctor says I have varices. What can I do to prevent variceal bleeding?

   Patient-Level Answer: To prevent varices from bleeding, you can treat the underlying liver disease to whatever extent possible. If you have varices that are at high risk of bleeding based on their endoscopic appearance or the severity of your liver disease, you may benefit from starting a class of medications called nonselective beta-blockers that reduce the pressure in the varices. Alternatively, your doctor may recommend you undergo serial endoscopy for placement of rubber bands on the varices until they shrink and disappear. The best choice for

A.H. Khan, M.D. (✉)
Division of Gastroenterology, Gastroenterology and Hepatology – Froedtert, Medical College of Wisconsin, 9200 West Wisconsin Avenue, Milwaukee, WI 53226, USA
e-mail: ahkhan@mcw.edu

you depends on a number of factors that your doctor will discuss with you such as the presence of ascites (fluid in the belly), your tolerance of beta-blockers, your other medical conditions, and your risk of undergoing endoscopy.

Introduction

Portal hypertension is abnormally elevated pressure in the portal venous system as a result of several conditions but most often due to cirrhosis in the United States. In the case of cirrhosis, there is increased resistance to blood flow through the hepatic sinusoids due to fibrosis causing a pressure gradient from the inflowing portal vein to the outflowing hepatic vein. This gradient is considered abnormal above 5 mmHg and generally becomes clinically significant portal hypertension at 10 mmHg [1]. Due to this increased resistance to blood flow through the liver, blood is shunted through collateral routes back to the heart, which can result in a number of endoscopic findings: esophageal varices, gastric varices, portal hypertensive gastropathy, and less common findings of ectopic varices, portal hypertensive colopathy, and hemorrhoids. The clinical relevance of all these findings is that they can result in GI hemorrhage of variable severity, which in some instances can be life-threatening. GAVE (gastric antral vascular ectasia), commonly known as "watermelon stomach," is also seen in cirrhotic patients, but is not due to portal hypertension and thus does not improve with reduction of portal pressure.

Esophageal varices are the most important consequence of portal hypertension in the GI tract as they are responsible for the most morbidity and mortality. The prevalence of gastric varices is less clear but significantly less than esophageal varices. Portal hypertensive gastropathy, while quite common in cirrhosis, is much less life-threatening. Portal hypertensive colopathy, and varices in other parts of the GI tract are uncommon. Clinicians have sought to determine the natural history, severity, and efficacy of endoscopic and non-endoscopic intervention on these gastrointestinal sequelae of portal hypertension to reduce morbidity and mortality of cirrhotic patients.

Esophageal Varices

Esophageal varices are veins in the submucosa of the esophageal wall that become enlarged due to increased collateral return of blood to the heart as a result of portal hypertension. Varices can suddenly rupture resulting in bleeding that is most often overt, manifested by hematemesis and/or melena, along with anemia. In some cases, the bleeding may be so severe that it results in loss of consciousness, hemodynamic shock, and death. It so happens that variceal bleeding is common enough among cirrhotics to result in significant mortality making it a natural target for intervention. Ideally, clinicians would be able to identify those cirrhotics that have varices, stratify those patients according to their risk of bleeding, and treat cirrhotics where appropriate, to reduce the risk of developing varices, progression of varices, and both bleeding and re-bleeding from varices. However, clinicians cannot rely on patients to inform them of symptoms that would suggest the presence of varices since varices are completely asymptomatic until they bleed. Furthermore, when bleeding does occur from varices, it tends to occur without warning and be quite significant, even life-threatening. Therefore, management of varices involves screening tests to detect varices and monitor their change over time, and to apply interventions where appropriate, to reduce the risk of variceal hemorrhage.

Epidemiology

The problem of variceal bleeding among cirrhotics is not rare. Approximately 40 % of asymptomatic cirrhotics have varices and the prevalence is even higher in those with ascites [2]. Among cirrhotics with varices, 25–40 % will bleed at some point [3]. It has been shown that varices can change over time. Those cirrhotics who do not already have varices, develop varices at a rate of 5–8 % per year and those with small varices may progress to large varices at a rate of 10–15 % per year [2]. A prospective study evaluating the natural history of esophageal varices in 206 patients with cirrhosis found that over the course of 3 years, almost a third of patients without varices developed varices, and almost a third of patients with small varices progressed to large varices [4].

The mortality rate from bleeding esophageal varices in cirrhotics was historically 30–60 % but has significantly dropped in the past three decades to a 6 week mortality after the first variceal bleeding episode of roughly 15–20 % [5, 6]. A retrospective French study of all cirrhotics admitted to a single hospital ICU with variceal bleeding comparing the years 1985 and 2000, found a significant in-hospital mortality reduction from 42.6 % in 1985 to 14.5 % in 2000 ($p < 0.05$), reduced re-bleeding rate from 47 to 13 %, and reduced bacterial infection rate from 38 to 14 % [7]. Even in the past decade, a significant improvement in outcome has been demonstrated. A retrospective cohort study comparing cirrhotics admitted with variceal bleeding admitted in 2000 ($N = 57$) vs. 2010 ($N = 64$) showed that the 2010 group had significantly more use of octreotide, antibiotics, band ligation in place of sclerotherapy, and less blood transfusions. The re-bleeding rate at 6 months improved from 31.4 % in 2000 to 18.0 % in 2010 ($p = 0.01$) and the 6 week mortality also improved significantly from 24.6 to 10.9 % ($p = 0.05$) [8]. These improvements can be attributed to improvements in endoscopic therapy specifically band ligation, pharmacological therapy, and supportive care, as will be discussed.

Diagnosis

The ideal screening test for esophageal varices in cirrhotics would be painless, inexpensive, and accurate. Currently, the most reliable test is upper endoscopy where a camera is used to directly view the esophagus for varices which appear as bulging submucosal veins in the distal esophagus. It is a controlled dynamic test in that the esophagus is observed over a period of minutes to allow passage of esophageal contractions, suction of fluid, and air insufflation of the lumen to ensure relative certainty in detecting the presence or absence of varices and thus is considered the gold standard. It does require sedation and passage of an endoscope which carries some cardiopulmonary risk and low risks of bleeding, infection, and gastrointestinal perforation. Other less-invasive tests have been studied as a possible alternative to standard endoscopy since half of cirrhotics do not have varices and only some fraction will need intervention. A French prospective multicenter study of 120 patients with portal hypertension of which 74 (61.6 %) had esophageal varices on endoscopy, underwent capsule endoscopy to detect esophageal varices resulting in a sensitivity of 77 % with a false positive rate of 14 % [9]. A prospective study for variceal screening comparing EGD as a gold standard to multidetector CT on 102 cirrhotics found that CT was 90 % sensitive in detecting large esophageal varices but with only 50 % specificity [10]. An even less-invasive screening test that has been evaluated is the ratio of platelet count to spleen length on the basis that it takes into account two modalities, a biochemical marker and ultrasound imaging, that are abnormal in portal hypertension so this should cause a low platelet count and large spleen length resulting in a much lower ratio than in a normal person. A retrospective study of 145 patients with compensated cirrhotics found that using a ratio <909 was associated with a sensitivity of 100 % and a specificity of 71 % for predicting esophageal varices so it was deemed to be especially helpful in ruling out varices in cirrhotics due to its strong negative predictive value [11]. Endoscopy remains the diagnostic test of choice as it is the most reliable in detecting varices and in addition can stage the varices for bleeding risk, and allow intervention where appropriate.

Risk Factors/Natural History

A test that predicts not only the presence of varices in cirrhotics but also the risk of bleeding is the HVPG (hepatic venous pressure gradient) which estimates portal pressure via a catheter passed into the hepatic vein. The free hepatic vein pressure, or posthepatic pressure, is measured and subtracted from the wedge pressure, or prehepatic pressure, which is measured after inflating an occlusive balloon. This difference is the portal pressure gradient. Portal hypertension occurs at a gradient greater than 5 mmHg but it has been found that esophageal varices tend to form at pressures greater than 10 mmHg, and they are unlikely to bleed unless the pressure gradient is at least 12 mmHg [1]. Furthermore, several studies including a meta-analysis have

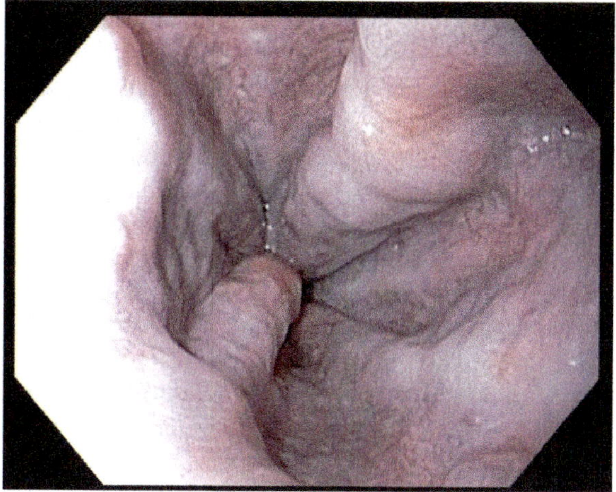

Fig. 34.1 Endoscopic view of grade 2 varices in distal esophagus

shown that in patients with elevated HVPG > 12 mmHg, reducing the HVPG to less than 12 mmHg or a reduction by more than 20 % of baseline results in a significant reduction in bleeding risk and mortality [12].

Cirrhotics with esophageal varices are not all at the same risk for bleeding and this has implications on management. There are endoscopic and clinical factors that independently affect bleeding risk. As the severity of cirrhosis increases, the risk of variceal bleeding increases at least 50 % for each successive step in Child's class from A to B to C [13]. Not surprisingly, a history of variceal bleeding is also a strong risk factor for variceal bleeding [14].

Endoscopically, varices are graded based on size and mucosal appearance when the esophageal lumen is insufflated and without contraction waves. Several classification systems evaluate varices and the Japanese classification is the most detailed as it incorporates variceal size, shape, color, and additional features; grade 1 are small straight varices that flatten with insufflation, grade 2 are medium size that occupy less than one-third of the lumen (Fig. 34.1), and grade 3 are large varices that occupy more than one-third of the lumen [15]. Larger variceal size and presence of a red spot or red wale, which are linear red marks on a varix, are associated with higher bleeding risk [14].

Prevention of Variceal Hemorrhage

Screening for Esophageal Varices in Cirrhotics

A great deal of research has been performed on cirrhotics to determine what interventions can be done to prevent the development of varices in those who have no varices (pre primary prophylaxis), prevent bleeding from varices in those who have varices that have never bled (primary prophylaxis), and to prevent re-bleeding in those who have a history of variceal bleeding (secondary prophylaxis).

Cirrhotics commonly develop portal hypertension as part of their disease and thus, are at risk for development of esophageal varices. If there was a safe and cost-effective intervention to significantly reduce the risk of esophageal variceal bleeding, it could be applied to all cirrhotics and endoscopy could be forgone, but such a treatment is not currently available. Endoscopy is a safe and effective method of screening cirrhotic patients for varices and can be done with moderate IV sedation unless the patient has significant cardiopulmonary disease, encephalopathy, or high tolerance to sedatives due to alcoholism or medications such as opioids and benzodiazpeines, in which case they should be sedated with monitored anesthesia. The patient is risk stratified based on the severity of cirrhosis and endoscopic exam to guide management of their varices.

In cirrhotics that do not have varices on endoscopy, the question arises as to how often they should be screened for development of varices, but there is no clear recommendation for screening interval. A prospective study 321 cirrhotics without history of bleeding were followed for a median of 2 years during which time 26.5 % had variceal bleeding. The three independent risk factors for bleeding were presence of red wales, large-sized varices, and advanced Child's class. Of the etiologies of cirrhosis, alcohol was most associated with bleeding. Thus consensus guidelines recommend screening cirrhotics who have no or small varices every 2–3 years, but yearly if they have Child's class C cirrhosis, alcoholic cirrhosis, or small varices with red wale sign [13, 16].

Nonselective Beta-Blockers

The class of medications most studied and found to be most useful in preventing variceal bleeding is nonselective beta-blockers (NNSB), such as propranolol, timolol, and nadolol. The effect of NNSB on varices has been studied due to their effect of blocking the increased cardiac output effect of beta-1 adrenergic receptors and the splanchnic venous dilation effect of beta-2 adrenergic receptors thus reducing blood flow through varices [17]. When researching the effect of any medication or treatment for variceal bleeding prophylaxis, a physiologic marker used has been HVPG which is the accepted surrogate of portal pressure, and as stated earlier, effective treatment should result in a drop in HVPG to less than 12 mmHg or a reduction from baseline HVPG by at least 20 %. Due to HVPG being relatively invasive, some studies use the simple physiologic marker of a change in baseline heart rate to signify an adequate dose of NSBB based on an early study showing cirrhotics that were given propranolol sufficient to reduce baseline heart rate by 25 % resulted in a persistent reduction in portal, venous pressure [18]. Unfortunately, it has also been shown that 15 % of patients have at least relative contraindications to NSBB such as insulin dependent diabetes or emphysema, and 15 % may develop side effects that prevent reaching efficacious doses. Furthermore, there are recent studies showing a deleterious effect of NSBB on cirrhotics with refractory ascites in terms of mortality, perhaps due to the already compromised cardiac output of these patients, but large randomized controlled trials are lacking [17].

Pre-primary Prophylaxis

There has been interest in therapies to prevent the development of varices in cirrhotics who have no varices on screening endoscopy. This is based on the logic that if the formation of varices can be prevented, then variceal bleeding is not possible.

A study of 213 patients with minimal portal hypertension based on HVPG of 6 mmHg and no varices at baseline endoscopy were randomized to timolol or placebo to assess for development of varices. Over a median time of 4.5 years, approximately 40 % of patients developed varices in both groups but serious adverse events were more common in the timolol group (18–6 %) and this was statistically significant [19]. Similarly, another randomized double blind trial found no reduction in the rate of variceal formation when comparing cirrhotics on propranolol vs. placebo, although a third of patients were lost to follow-up [20]. Thus attempting to prevent the formation of varices using beta-blockers for patients with portal hypertension is not recommended. In contrast, a 12 year study of 218 compensated HCV cirrhotics found that none of the 34 patients who achieved sustained virologic response (SVR) developed esophageal varices, compared with 22/69 (31.8 %) untreated cirrhotics and 45/115 (39.1 %) non-SVR cirrhotics [21]. Therefore, the only recommended intervention to prevent development of varices in cirrhotics that do not have varices is to treat the underlying liver disease to whatever extent possible.

Primary Prophylaxis

In contrast to pre-primary prophylaxis, medical intervention has had success in preventing bleeding in select patients with cirrhosis who have varices (primary prophylaxis). Many treatments have been studied, but the two most effective treatments have been found to be NNSB and endoscopic band ligation (Fig. 34.2).

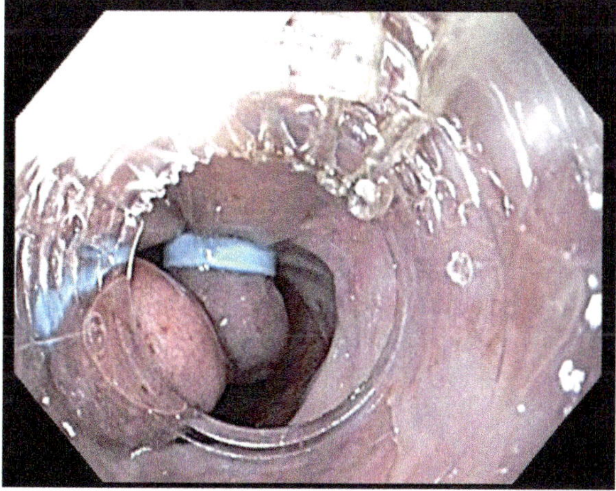

Fig. 34.2 Endoscopic view through cap of bands ligating two esophageal varices

A randomized controlled trial of 161 cirrhotics randomized to nadolol vs. placebo for a median period of 3 years, showed the rate of variceal growth from small to large was 37.2 % in the placebo group but only 10.8 % in the nadolol group, although there was no mortality difference and more adverse events in the nadolol group [22]. However, two more recent randomized controlled trials did not show positive results in cirrhotics with small varices [20, 23]. In one of the studies, 150 cirrhotics with small varices defined as <5 mm in diameter, were followed for 2 years and the growth to large varices was similar: 11 % in the propranolol group and 16 % in the placebo group ($p=0.79$). This study also evaluated the role of HVPG measurements in these patients and found that a baseline HVPG could not reliably predict which patients would respond to NSBB, nor did a significant drop in HVPG due to NSBB therapy correlate with prevention of variceal growth [23]. A recent meta-analysis of six randomized controlled trials of cirrhotics without history of GI bleeding with either no or small varices that were treated with NSBB vs. placebo found no significant difference in the development of large varices, prevention of first variceal bleeding, or mortality, and even a subgroup analysis showed no differences between patients with no varices or small varices. However, there was a significant increase in adverse events in the NSBB group (OR 3.47; 95 % CI 0.08–3.70) [24].

The results are much more favorable for NSBB used in primary prophylaxis in cirrhotics with large varices. In such patients, nadolol was shown to significantly reduce the rate of first bleeding when compared to controls in a prospective, randomized trial of 79 patients followed for 2 years [25]. A multicenter, randomized trial comparing propranolol to placebo in preventing first bleeding from large varices included 174 patients, and in 3.5 years, 26 % in the propranolol group had bled while 41 % in the placebo group bled, although this was not statistically significant [26]. A larger, similar multicenter, randomized study of 230 Child's C cirrhotics with large varices over 2 years showed that 26 % in the propranolol group bled, as in the previous study, but 61 % in the placebo group bled, and the survival difference was also statistically significant at 72 % in the propranolol group vs. 51 % in the placebo group [27]. A meta-analysis of 589 cirrhotics further supported the efficacy of both propranolol and nadolol in primary prophylaxis of variceal bleeding and improved mortality compared to placebo in high-risk patients [28]. Using a Markov model, propranolol for primary prophylaxis of variceal bleeding was found to be cost effective compared to placebo over a 5 year period [29].

There is emerging concern that although NSBB are effective in primary prophylaxis for variceal bleeding, they may induce a poor outcome in the subset of cirrhotics with refractory ascites. It is thought that these patients have low systemic blood pressure that is more sensitive to the drop in cardiac output induced by beta blockade. A prospective nonrandomized study of 151 cirrhotics with refractory ascites compared the outcomes of those on propranolol versus those not on beta-blockers with a median follow-up of 8 months and they found a significant difference in 1 year morality of 19 % vs. 29 % in favor of those who did not receive propranolol [30]. There was some criticism regarding lack of HVPG analysis of patients and

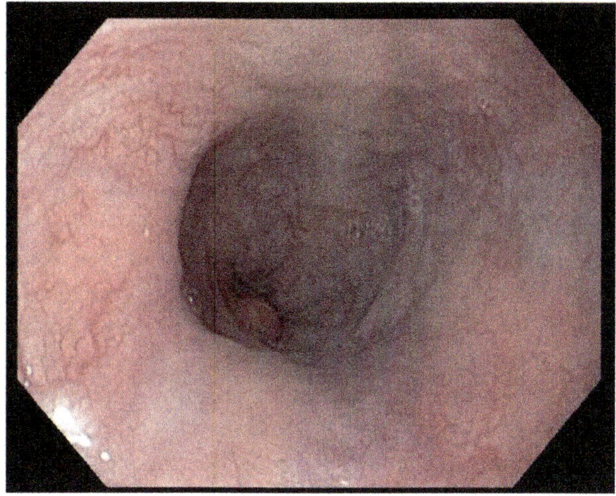

Fig. 34.3 Endoscopy showing resolved esophageal varices 1 month after band ligation

perhaps more severe liver disease in the propranolol group so more studies would be helpful [17].

Other treatments for primary prophylaxis have not been found to be effective, either on their own or in combination with NSBB. Based on the physiological finding of greater reduction in portal pressure with the combination of nitrates and beta-blockers compared to beta-blockers alone, it was theorized that this combination may also be effective in primary prophylaxis of variceal bleeding. However, a double blind randomized control trial of 349 cirrhotics that received a combination of propranolol and isosorbide mononitrate or propranolol with placebo showed nearly identical rates of variceal bleeding and mortality, while the nitrate group experienced significant more headaches [31].

Endoscopic sclerotherapy, where a sclerosant is directly injected into the varix to cause its obliteration by inducing fibrosis, has been found to be effective in controlling actively bleeding esophageal varices. However, in primary prophylaxis, sclerotherapy has not been effective in reducing the rate of variceal bleeding and its complication rate is as high as 50 % mainly due to chest pain [32]. Sclerotherapy is not recommended for prophylaxis of varices.

Endoscopic band ligation has been extensively studied for primary prophylaxis and is clearly effective in cirrhotics with high-risk varices (Fig. 34.3). An early randomized controlled trial of 68 cirrhotics with high-risk varices showed significant reduction in first bleed (8.6 % vs. 39.4 %) during the mean follow-up period of just over a year [33]. A meta-analysis of band ligation compared to placebo for primary prophylaxis consisting of 601 cirrhotics showed a relative risk reduction of first bleed of 64 % and risk reduction in mortality from upper GI bleeding of 80 %. The same study showed band ligation was more effective than propranolol for primary prophylaxis of variceal bleeding with a relative risk reduction of 52 % but there was no significant difference in bleeding related mortality or overall mortality between these two treatments [34].

A prospective randomized control study from India for primary prophylaxis of cirrhotics with medium or large (at least 3 mm diameter) esophageal varices was conducted comparing band ligation (41 patients) to propranolol (41 patients). They found the probability of variceal bleeding was 43 % in the propranolol group and 17 % in the ligation group over 18 months of follow-up, and this was statistically significant [35]. Another randomized control trial of 62 cirrhotics with high-risk varices were followed for a mean of 15 months and was terminated early due to an interim analysis showing a significant failure rate for propranolol with four deaths from variceal bleeding out of 31 patients compared to no deaths in the ligation group [36]. A meta-analysis of 16 randomized control trials of cirrhotics with high-risk varices, looked into this issue of primary prophylaxis, but focused on three trials with careful randomization to minimize selection bias, which the authors suspected were influencing the outcomes of many trials. In these three trials, they found no difference between band ligation and NSBB in mortality or rates of variceal bleeding. About half of the patients in the band ligation group developed superficial ulcers while 12 % of the NSBB group had to stop therapy and 20 % had to reduce dosage due to adverse effects [37].

The problem with the band ligation strategy is that it is costly, there is some risk of sedation and endoscopy, and the patient has to be compliant since it often requires multiple sessions to obliterate the varices. The banding itself results in sloughing of the mucosa leaving a shallow ulcer that tends to heal within 2 weeks; however the ulceration can potentially be deeper resulting in significant bleeding in 2–5 % of patients. A randomized, double blind, placebo-controlled trial of proton pump inhibitor therapy for 10 days after elective variceal banding followed by repeat endoscopy to assess for varices and ulcers showed that both groups had similar number of postbanding ulcers but the size of the ulcers in the placebo group was twice as large, and there were three patients with postband ligation bleeding in the placebo group but none in the pantoprazole group [38]. Therefore, PPI therapy after banding is recommended.

Since the two most effective treatments for primary prophylaxis of esophageal variceal bleeding have been found to be band ligation and NSBB, it was thought the combination of the two may be even more effective, and several trials have studied this possibility. A small single blind randomized controlled trial of 66 cirrhotics with medium to large varices were treated with band ligation alone or band ligation and propranolol until eradication of varices and then were followed up for a mean of 12 months to evaluate for variceal bleeding and recurrence of varices. All 66 patients achieved eradication of varices with no difference in time or number of endoscopic sessions needed to eradicate the varices. Only two patients experienced adverse effects from beta-blockers. There was no difference in bleeding with only a total of three patients who bled during the study of which only one was from variceal bleeding, and there was also no difference in mortality. Recurrence of varices, however, favored the combination group, 9–38 % with $p=0.003$ [39]. A similarly designed randomized control trial of 144 patients was conducted requiring a mean of 3.3 endoscopic sessions over 2 months to achieve variceal eradication. Bleeding occurred evenly in both groups and all were from esophageal varices: 5 in combination group and 6 in the band ligation group with two bleeding deaths in the band ligation group. This study also found recurrence of varices favored the combination group, 19–33 % ($p=0.03$). In the combination group, six patients discontinued propranolol due to side effects [40]. These studies show a modest benefit of combination therapy in select patients, but currently combination therapy of endoscopic band ligation and NSBB is not recommended for primary prophylaxis of esophageal varices.

More recently, an increased interest has developed in carvedilol, a NSBB that also has an alpha1-adrenergic receptor blocking effect that reduces vascular resistance causing both a reduction in both portal pressure and systemic pressure, and this effect seems to be stronger than propranolol [41]. A study of 104 patients was conducted to evaluate the efficacy of carvedilol in propranolol nonresponders. It included cirrhotics with esophageal varices without prior bleeding who were given propranolol as primary prophylaxis with a desired dose of 80–160 mg/day in order to achieve efficacy, which was evaluated after 4 weeks on the maximal tolerated dose by obtaining an HVPG measurement. If the HVPG was <12 mmHg or dropped by 20 %, the patient was deemed a propranolol responder and continued on that dose. If these parameters were not reached, the patient was switched to carvedilol, and the HVPG was again measured after 4 weeks on a stable dose, and continued if adequate drop in HVPG was reached. Of the 104 patients started on propranolol, only 37 (35.6 %) were propranolol responders with adequate HVPG response. Of the remaining 67 switched to carvedilol, 38 (56.7 %) showed adequate HVPG response, suggesting that carvedilol may be better tolerated and more efficacious than propranolol for primary prophylaxis [42]. Carvedilol has also been compared to band ligation for primary prophylaxis of esophageal variceal bleeding in cirrhotics. One such multicenter randomized control trial in Scotland of cirrhotics with medium or large varices followed for 2 years included 77 patients in the carvedilol group with a goal dose of 12.5 mg daily, and 75 patients in the band ligation group, who underwent band ligation every 2 weeks until eradication. Eleven patients (14.2 %) in the carvedilol group had to discontinue due to adverse reactions, while 23 patients (30.7 %) were unable to complete the endoscopy protocol in the band ligation group and 58 % reached variceal eradication. The study found no difference in mortality: 35 % in the carvedilol group and 37 % in the band ligation group. However, incidence of variceal bleeding during the follow-up period favored carvedilol 10–23 % ($p=0.04$) [41].

In summary, cirrhotics without varices or small varices without high-risk stigmata are considered low risk for bleeding do not require primary prophylaxis for variceal bleeding, just periodic screening endoscopy. Cirrhotics with large varices or with high-risk stigmata can be treated with band ligation or NSBB. If tolerated, NSBB are a reasonable first option. Band ligation is appropriate in the 15 % of patients with contraindications to NSBB and in the 15–20 % who are unable to reach therapeutic doses due to side effects. Band ligation may also be a better choice in patients with refractory ascites [43]. Carvedilol may be the most effective NSBB. Combination therapy may have some benefit in reducing recurrence of varices but currently there is insufficient data showing a reduction in variceal bleeding or mortality compared to band ligation or NSBB alone.

Surveillance

Over time, the severity of liver disease progresses at variable rates, and this can result in the development and progression of esophageal varices. Studies have shown that in cirrhotics without varices, varices develop at a rate of 5–8 % per year. Furthermore, patients with small varices progress to large varices at a rate of 5–20 % per year. Because varices are not stable over time and do not cause symptoms until they rupture, periodic endoscopy is necessary to monitor for change. There is no strong data to determine the optimal frequency of surveillance but guidelines have been developed to assist in management depending on endoscopic findings:

No varices: every 2–3 years
Small varices, no red wale: every 1–2 years
Small varices with red wale or alcoholic cirrhosis: every 1 year

If large varices are present, then primary prophylaxis should be initiated. If NSBB is chosen for primary prophylaxis, then endoscopic surveillance is not necessary. If band ligation is chosen, then yearly endoscopy after variceal obliteration is reasonable [44].

Acute Variceal Hemorrhage

Any cirrhotic who presents with signs of overt gastrointestinal bleeding such as hematemesis, melena, hematochezia, and/or hemodynamic instability should raise a strong suspicion for variceal hemorrhage. In fact, 60–65 % of upper GI bleeding in cirrhotics is due to varices [45]. Variceal hemorrhage is a potentially fatal and the cause of death is usually due to direct consequence of acute blood loss with hypovolemic shock, or the immediate complications of acute blood loss including renal failure, liver failure, hepatic encephalopathy, and sepsis [46].

As in any patient with upper GI bleeding, the patient initially has to be stabilized. Volume status has to be quickly assessed and good IV access obtained for volume resuscitation and possible blood transfusion. The patient's condition has to be optimized as quickly as possible to prepare for upper endoscopy which not only confirms the diagnosis but allows intervention in an effort to resolve the bleeding. There are a few special steps that have been shown to be important in cirrhotics with possible of variceal bleeding, compared to upper GI bleeding in other circumstances.

Intubation

Due to the proximal location of esophageal varices in the GI tract along with the potentially compromised mental state in cirrhotics from hepatic encephalopathy and/or volume loss, variceal bleeding poses a significant aspiration risk which has been shown to be 2.4–3.3 % during endoscopy [47]. A retrospective study was performed to analyze whether all cirrhotics with variceal bleeding should be intubated. This study of 69 hospital admissions with confirmed active variceal bleeding within 12 h of admission all had less than stage II hepatic encephalopathy, no signs of alcohol or drug intoxication, normal chest X-rays, and no signs of respiratory distress or aspiration prior to admission. Of these 69 hospital admissions, 47 underwent elective intubation for the endoscopy while 22 did not, and their characteristics were similar except that the non-intubation group had a significantly higher Child's Pugh score of 9.1–8.0. Nonetheless, it was the intubation group which had the worse outcome with aspiration pneumonia in 19–0 % and nine deaths compared to just one in the non-intubation group. The reason for this worse outcome with intubation is unclear but it was not a prospective trial so there may have been factors leading to physicians selecting intubation that did not reveal themselves in the study [48]. Intubation of patients with suspected variceal bleeding for airway protection is reasonable in any cirrhotic with altered mental status, but is not necessary for all cirrhotics.

Restricted Resuscitation

There is an understandable reaction on the part of clinicians to overt gastrointestinal hemorrhage, especially hematemesis, to aggressively resuscitate the patient with IV fluids and blood products to reduce the risk of circulatory shock and symptomatic anemia. This assumption has been studied objectively to determine the optimal resuscitation strategy. A randomized controlled trial of 889 patients admitted with gastrointestinal bleeding were randomized to liberal transfusion in which blood was transfused when the hemoglobin level dropped to 9 g/dl, or restrictive transfusion in which blood was transfused only when the hemoglobin level dropped to 7 g/dl. The study period was 45 days and included 277 cirrhotics of which 190 were found to have esophageal variceal bleeding. There was a significant mortality difference among cirrhotics favoring the restrictive strategy regardless of Child's class by more than a 2:1 margin, 12–22 % [49]. Similarly, aggressive volume replacement with IV fluids may cause rebound portal hypertension which can exacerbate variceal bleeding, so it has been suggested that a patient should be resuscitated such that the heart rate be kept less than 100 bpm with a systolic blood pressure of 90–100 mmHg [50].

Antibiotics

It has been found that cirrhotics admitted with GI bleeding are at significantly increased risk of infection during hospitalization, and this is associated with both variceal re-bleeding and increased mortality. Several studies have shown better outcomes in those treated empirically with antibiotics. A meta-analysis evaluated five randomized controlled trials comparing antibiotics to no treatment in 534 cirrhotics hospitalized with upper GI bleeding. Four of the studies used fluoroquinolones as the antibiotic which was given for a median of 7 days. The results favored the antibiotic group for several outcomes: remaining infection-free 86–55 %, free of spontaneous bacterial peritonitis (SBP) and bacteremia 92–73 %, and short-term survival up to 14 days 85–76 % [51]. Out of concern that there is emerging fluoroquinolone resistance, a randomized controlled trial of decompensated cirrhotics admitted with GI bleeding compared the outcome of 63 patients receiving oral norfloxacin to 61 patients receiving IV ceftriaxone. Over the course of 10 days, the norfloxacin group had a higher rate of infection, 33 % vs. 11 %, reaching statistical significance [52]. The available data strongly supports short-term antibiotic prophylaxis for all cirrhotics admitted with upper GI bleeding to reduce infection, re-bleeding, and improve survival. Fluoroquinolones are acceptable but if the patient is already on fluoroquinolones or there is concern for resistance, IV ceftriaxone is a reasonable choice.

Encephalopathy

Like SBP, variceal bleeding can precipitate hepatic encephalopathy in cirrhotics. Patients with hepatic encephalopathy should obviously continue therapy with lactulose if they develop upper GI bleeding. A study was conducted to determine if cirrhotics without known hepatic encephalopathy would also benefit from lactulose during hospitalization for acute variceal bleeding. It was a prospective, randomized trial of 35 patients each in the lactulose group and placebo group. Randomization was performed at time of endoscopy and the endoscopist and patient were not blinded but the clinician performing twice daily assessment of encephalopathy during hospitalization remained blinded. They found that 14 (40 %) patients in the control group but only 5 (14 %) patients in the treatment group developed clinical evidence of encephalopathy ($p=0.03$) with a median encephalopathy grade of two, and a median time to development of encephalopathy of 2 days. This study supports a low threshold for starting lactulose in any cirrhotic admitted with variceal bleeding, but more data is needed to make it the standard of care [53].

Vasoactive Drugs

Medications that acutely reduce portal pressure and hepatic blood flow in patients with portal hypertension have been given at the time of acute variceal bleeding in an attempt to reduce severity of bleeding in order to improve outcomes [54]. Vasoactive drugs include anti diuretic hormone analogues such as vasopressin and terlipressin, and somatostain analogues such as octreotide. Somatostatin tends to be well tolerated but vasopressin is known to cause many serious side effects due to intense systemic vasoconstriction including mesenteric and peripheral ischemia, myocardial infarction, and arrhythmias in over a third of patients, and this has limited its use [50]. An early randomized trial comparing vasopressin to octreotide as an adjunct to endoscopy for acute variceal bleeding was published in 1992. It included 48 cirrhotics with active variceal bleeding randomized to continuous infusion of octreotide or vasopressin after endoscopy. Complete bleeding control was achieved in 63 % of the octreotide group and 46 % in the vasopressin group, although there was no difference in mortality after 42 days. Serious side effects were more frequent in the vasopressin group, 40–12 % [55]. A meta-analysis comparing somatostatin analogues in addition to endoscopy compared to endoscopy alone for acute variceal bleeding evaluated eight randomized trials with a total of 939 patients and found that combination therapy was associated with a significant improvement in early hemostasis but no difference in mortality or adverse events [56]. Thus, a somatostatin analogue is the preferred vasoactive drug for any cirrhotic hospitalized with suspicion of variceal bleeding and should be given as an IV infusion for 3–5 days if variceal bleeding is confirmed on endoscopy [16]. Vasoactive drugs are not, however, adequate as a replacement to endoscopy.

Endoscopy for Acute Esophageal Variceal Hemorrhage

Optimal Time

As in any patient admitted with acute upper GI bleeding, endoscopy must be done in a timely manner to allow not only diagnosis of the cause of bleeding but to apply intervention to stop the bleeding. A retrospective cohort study evaluated 101 cirrhotics admitted with upper GI bleeding that were found to have active variceal bleeding at time of endoscopy, and found that "door-to-endoscopy" time <12 h was associated with lower re-bleeding rates and lower mortality in patients that presented with hematemesis and in patients with first time variceal bleeding [57]. Another retrospective study of 311 cirrhotics admitted with upper GI bleeding found that 25 patients died during hospitalization in a median time of 20 days after admission. The median time to endoscopy was significantly shorter for survivors (12.9 h vs. 17.7 h, $p = 0.001$) [58]. Current guidelines recommend that as soon as the patient is hemodynamically stable, endoscopy should be performed, ideally within 12 h of presentation [16, 59].

Endoscopic Therapy

Once the patient has been stabilized, resuscitated, and intubated if necessary, endoscopy is performed. The diagnosis of variceal bleeding is made if active bleeding is seen from the varices or if there are varices with large fresh blood in the stomach without other explanation. The traditional treatment in this setting was sclerotherapy where a sclerosing agent such as ethanolamine is injected directly into the varix just below the site of bleeding to induce fibrosis and obliterate the varix. Many studies have shown sclerotherapy to be effective in variceal bleeding cessation [60]. The main drawback with sclerotherapy are the considerable side effects including chest pain, ulceration, esophageal stricture, pleuritis, perforation, portal vein thrombosis, emboli, and bacteremia [61]. Band ligation has emerged as the preferred treatment.

Band ligation allows endoscopic placement of a rubber band directly on the varix resulting in its obliteration. This can be applied directly on to the site of bleeding for immediate bleeding control. The multiband device allows several bands to be deployed quickly in succession rather than endoscope removal and re-intubation, making this technique more efficient and effective. A randomized control trial of 179 cirrhotics with acute esophageal variceal bleeding was conducted in which patients were treated with vasoactive drugs and underwent endoscopy within 6 h. At endoscopy, they were randomized to receive sclerotherapy or band ligation. The outcomes favored band ligation in terms of initial failure to stop bleeding (4–15 %, $p=0.02$), serious side effects (4–13 %, $p=0.04$), and 6 week survival (83–67 %, $p=0.01$) [62]. There have been some studies that found no difference [63] or better outcomes for sclerotherapy [64] in the setting of acute variceal bleeding. Generally both are acceptable but band ligation is favored due to fewer complications [16, 59].

Severe Acute Bleeding with Endoscopic Failure to Stop Hemorrhage

When acute variceal bleeding is severe, initial endoscopic therapy with band ligation or sclerotherapy may fail to stop the active bleeding or the patient may show evidence of rebleeding (within 72 h). The mortality rate in these patients is very high. The most definitive way to reduce blood flow through the varices is to shunt the blood from the portal venous system into the systemic circulation and this was traditionally done by a surgical shunt between the splenic vein and the gastric vein. Later, the less-invasive technique of TIPS (transhepatic porto-systemic shunt) became available, allowing blood to bypass the high resistance to flow in the liver. If the bleeding is severe, a temporizing measure may be necessary prior to TIPS being available to the patient. Traditionally, this was achieved by balloon tamponade where a rubber tube with a dual esophageal and gastric balloon are passed and inflated to apply compressive pressure to the varices, and distal migration is prevented by application of traction on the tube by a string that emerges from the mouth and is attached to a helmet. It has been shown to be effective in the short term but must be removed within 48 h to prevent esophageal necrosis and rupture. It is generally considered a bridge to definitive therapy, mainly TIPS.

More recently, studies have been performed to evaluate the efficacy of covered metal esophageal stents for uncontrolled bleeding esophageal varices based on the same concept of applying compressive pressure to the esophageal varices to stop the bleeding until more definitive therapy can be offered. One of the earlier studies using covered esophageal metal stents involved 20 cirrhotics with history of variceal bleeding who had acute recurrence of variceal bleeding that could not be controlled endoscopically. The stents were successfully placed in all patients resulting in immediate cessation of esophageal variceal bleeding, and there was no stent related complication or recurrence of esophageal variceal bleeding. Partial stent migration distally occurred in five patients and was corrected endoscopically. One patient required surgery for gastric variceal bleeding. Two deaths within a week of stent placement were due to liver failure. All other patients had the stent removed uneventfully in 1 week and underwent further treatment such as TIPS [65]. A covered metal stent can also be useful in patients as definitive therapy in patients with recurrent esophageal variceal bleeding refractory to endoscopic therapy who are not candidates for TIPS, since it is relatively better tolerated with less risk of esophageal necrosis and rupture than balloon tamponade [66]. There are no studies to date comparing balloon tamponade to covered metal stents for esophageal variceal bleeding refractory to endoscopic therapy.

Patients with advanced cirrhosis and history of variceal bleeding are known to be at higher risk of failing to achieve a durable response to endoscopic therapy when presenting with esophageal variceal bleeding. The predictors of early re-bleeding (within 5 days) in a study of 256 patients were a high MELD score greater than 17 and transfusion requirement of 4 or more units of blood in first 24 h, along with active variceal bleeding at the time of initial endoscopy [67]. Thus, a study was conducted to evaluate optimal standard medical/endoscopic therapy for such patients compared to just directly proceeding to TIPS under the hypothesis that this subset may be better served by TIPS as upfront therapy. In this randomized multi-center trial, patients were included if they were admitted with upper GI bleeding and had a history of Child's C cirrhosis or had Child's B cirrhosis with active variceal bleeding at time of endoscopy. All patients were given vasoactive drugs and antibiotics upfront. The 31 patients in the endoscopy arm were treated with band ligation or sclerotherapy and continued on vasoactive drugs for at least 24 h after cessation of bleeding at which time they were transitioned to medical therapy of an NNSB plus a nitrate and serial band ligation sessions until varices were obliterated. The 32 patients in the TIPS arm underwent TIPS within 72 h of the diagnostic endoscopy with placement of a coated endoprosthesis with dilation of the stent to ensure HVPG < 12 mmHg. During the median 16 months of follow-up, re-bleeding occurred in 14 (50 %) of the endoscopy group and just one patient in the TIPS group ($p = 0.001$), and 1 year survival also favored the TIPS group 86 % vs. 61 % ($p < 0.001$). Delaying TIPS did seem to affect the outcome as 4 of the 7 endoscopic failures who received TIPS as a rescue therapy died. The rate of hepatic encephalopathy, which is a known risk in TIPS due to shunting of blood past the liver, was actually higher in the endoscopy group 40 % vs. 28 % at 1 year, though this did not reach statistical significance ($p = 0.13$) [68]. Another study was performed comparing upfront TIPS to endoscopic therapy in 126 cirrhotics (mostly Child's B and due to HBV) admitted with esophageal variceal bleeding. These patients differed from the previous study in that they did not have a history of variceal bleeding. This study, with average follow-up of about 1.5 years, also found better outcomes in the TIPS group in terms of rebleeding (11 vs. 31 patients) and survival (80.6 % vs. 64.9 %) which reached statistical significance [69]. If early re-bleeding occurs within 5 days of endoscopic therapy where esophageal variceal bleeding was initially controlled,

TIPS is likely the best long-term option with balloon tamponade or metal stent as a bridge to TIPS.

Secondary Prophylaxis

If endoscopic therapy does control variceal bleeding without early re-bleeding, the question arises as to the best strategy for secondary prophylaxis to prevent re-bleeding of varices. The risk of re-bleeding from esophageal varices is as high as 60 % in 2 years and highest in the first 6 weeks after each episode of variceal bleeding, with a mortality of 15–20 % with each bleeding episode [70]. As stated earlier, both NSBB and endoscopic band ligation are effective in primary prophylaxis although not in combination. This combined approach has also been tested for secondary prophylaxis but with greater success. A randomized prospective trial of cirrhotics with esophageal bleeding were treated successfully and then randomized at discharge to serial band ligation with the intent of variceal eradication (37 patients) or the combination of band ligation and nadolol (43 patients). After a mean of 16 months, the results favored the combination group for recurrent bleeding 38–14 % without a difference in mortality [71]. Another randomized trial comparing the combination drugs of isosoribide mononitrate and propranolol vs. endoscopic band ligation for secondary prophylaxis with about 60 patients in each arm found that band ligation was more effective for preventing rebleeding, 20 % vs. 42 %, over a mean of 2 years [72]. A meta-analysis of nine trials and 955 patients found that the combination of band ligation and NSBB does reduce the risk of overall bleeding and bleeding specifically from varices and just a slight reduction in bleeding related mortality, but still, no improvement in overall mortality [73]. The type of NSBB does not seem to matter nor does the addition of a nitrate seem necessary. A randomized study of 121 cirrhotics compared a similar drug combination of isosoribide mononitrate and nadolol to carvedilol for secondary prophylaxis but over a longer median of 2.5 years, and found equal bleeding rates of about 61 % and no difference in adverse events or mortality [74]. Guidelines recommend a combination of NSBB and band ligation for secondary prophylaxis of esophageal variceal bleeding [16, 59]. Another option is TIPS but due to the risk of hepatic encephalopathy, remains best suited for cirrhotics with other complications of portal hypertension or if they have already failed secondary prophylaxis with combination therapy of band ligation and NSBB [70].

Gastric Varices

The second most common site of varices after the esophagus, is in the stomach. Although the rate of bleeding is less than for esophageal varices, the severity and mortality rate may be higher [75]. Gastric varices can occur with or without esophageal varices. There are several types of gastric varices based on location. The most common are varices extending from the GE junction into the cardia along the lesser curvature accounting for three-fourths of gastric varices, but these are essentially treated like esophageal varices. Discussion of gastric varices, most often refers to varices involving the fundus (fundic and cardiofundic varices) as they are managed differently. Isolated gastric varices elsewhere in the stomach are rare.

Unlike the linear ascending orientation of esophageal varices, gastric varices have a web-like arrangement making it more difficult to target. Thus, endoscopic control of variceal bleeding has proven more difficult. Endoscopic treatments that have been used for gastric varices include sclerotherapy, band ligation, and injection of tissue adhesives. The most studied and used tissue adhesive is cyanoacrylate. The combination of cyanoacrylate with lipoidol is endoscopically injected with a needle directly into the varix and forms a space-occupying cast within the varix to seal off the site of bleeding. Radiologic therapies of balloon retrograde transvenous obliteration (BRTO) and TIPS are also options.

Primary Prophylaxis

If effective, primary prophylaxis against gastric variceal bleeding would be useful for the same reasons as for esophageal varices, namely, bleeding can be sudden and severe with the possibility of death. There are not many studies evaluating this issue but a randomized control trial for primary prophylaxis of gastric varices with about 30 patients in each arm was performed, comparing placebo, NSBB, and endoscopic injection of cyanoacrylate on patients with gastrofundal or isolated fundal varices. Over a median follow-up of about 2 years, the probability of bleeding was 13 % for cyanoacrylate, 28 % for NSBB, and 45 % for placebo which was a statistically significant difference. There was also a survival benefit in the cyanoacrylate group compared to placebo of 90–72 % [76]. This was a relatively small study however, and more data is needed. Cyanoacrylate is not without complications. In a study of 753 patients, rebleeding occurred in 4.4 %, sepsis in 1.3 %, and embolization of the glue cast to other sites in 0.7 % [77]. Prophylactic antibiotics should be given when using cyanoacrylate [16].

Acute Variceal Hemorrhage

For acute gastric variceal bleeding, pre-endoscopic management is the same as for esophageal varices in terms of resuscitation with restrictive fluid strategy, prophylactic antibiotics, and vasoactive drugs. These measures by themselves are generally not adequate to control gastric variceal bleeding [78]. Like for primary prophylaxis, the endoscopic therapy that has emerged as the best for acute bleeding despite generally small numbers in randomized controlled trials, is cyanoacrylate injection. A randomized prospective study of about 100 patients comparing band ligation to cyanoacrylate injection for cirrhotics with acutely bleeding gastric varices found no difference in immediate bleeding control for those with active bleeding at time of endoscopy (93 % for both groups), but the rate of rebleeding in 2 years was 63.1 % for band ligation but just 26.8 % for cyanoacrylate ($p=0.01$) [79]. A retrospective analysis of 105 patients admitted with gastric variceal hemorrhage compared endoscopic injection of cyanoacrylate ($N=61$) to TIPS ($N=44$) and found no difference in rebleeding rate or mortality [80]. It should be noted that cyanoacrylate treatment is limited to where there is available expertise and it is not yet approved for use in gastric varices by the FDA [16].

If endoscopic control of gastric variceal bleeding fails, interventional radiology is consulted for consideration of BRTO vs. TIPS. BRTO (bollon-occluded retrograde transvenous obliteration) is a procedure where a catheter is advanced in a retrograde fashion through the veins draining the gastric cardia to the site of hemorrhage and a balloon is inflated to stop flow from the vessel followed by injection of a sclerosant to obliterate the blood vessel. TIPS remains the most definitive therapy but is more invasive and carries the risk of hepatic encephalopathy [16].

Secondary Prophylaxis

Similar to esophageal varices, studies have evaluated secondary prophylaxis for gastric varices to determine best management of patients after recovering from gastric variceal hemorrhage. Due to emerging data supporting cyanoacrylate injection for gastric varices, a randomized comparative trial was conducted comparing cyanoacrylate injection to TIPS for secondary prophylaxis of gastric variceal bleeding. Patients admitted with gastric variceal bleeding from fundic or cardiofundic varices were treated somatostatin, antibiotics, lactulose, and underwent endoscopy with cyanoacrylate injection if acutely bleeding at the time. After the bleeding had been controlled for 3 days, patients were randomized to serial endoscopy with cyanoacrylate injection or TIPS with 37 patients in each arm. The results favored TIPS in terms of higher rate of gastric variceal obliteration, 51–20 % ($p<0.02$) and less rebleeding 43–59 % (p 0.12). The overall complication rate was the same at 40 % but far more in the TIPS group developed hepatic encephalopathy, and there was no significant mortality difference over 3 years [75]. Another randomized study of secondary prophylaxis compared propranolol to serial endoscopic cyanoacrylate injection with 32 patients in each group. They had an unusually high gastric variceal obliteration rate in the cyanoacrylate arm of 100 % and a beta-blocker compliance rate of 100 %. In a median follow-up of about 2 years, rebleeding results favored cyanoacrylate 9–44 % [81]. Where the expertise is available, cyanoacrylate injection for secondary prophylaxis in gastric varices is reasonable as it does not have the complication of hepatic encephalopathy that TIPS does.

A newer endoscopic technique is endoscopic ultrasound guided therapy which allows injection directly into the gastric varix under ultrasound guidance. A retrospective study evaluated EUS-guided injection of cyanoacrylate vs. stainless steel coils into patients with gastric varices to determine efficacy in preventing bleeding and adverse events. Coil injection was only possible in patients in whom a single feeding vein could be identified leading directly into the varix. There were 19 patients in the cyanoacrylate group and 11 in the coil group. All ten cases with active gastric variceal bleeding were in the cyanoacrylate group. Intervention was technically successful in nearly all patients and none had gastric variceal bleeding during the mean follow-up period of 17 months. There were nine asymptomatic glue emboli in the cyanoacrylate group and two others had fever or pain, whereas the only adverse event in the coil group was a patient with chest pain [82]. This is a technique that requires more study.

Portal HTN Gastropathy/Colopathy

In addition to varices, portal hypertension can cause changes to the mucosa of the GI tract as well, predominantly in the stomach but also in the small bowel and colon. Pathologically, there develops an engorgement of capillaries and venules within the mucosal and submucosal layers without inflammatory infiltrate. Portal hypertensive gastropathy (PHG) can be classified based on its endoscopic appearance. Mild PHG (Fig. 34.4a) is the usual diffusely edematous appearance of the mucosa sometimes described as a snakeskin or mosaic pattern. In severe PHG (Fig. 34.4b), there additionally is acid hematin, bulging red and black spots, or active oozing in the stomach. This occurs in the fundus and body and does not involve the antrum. Portal hypertensive gastropathy is commonly seen in cirrhotics to at least a mild degree; its exact prevalence is uncertain but is likely at least 20 %. Unlike true gastritis, it does not cause pain nor does it ulcerate. Its clinical relevance is that it can slowly bleed in which case it

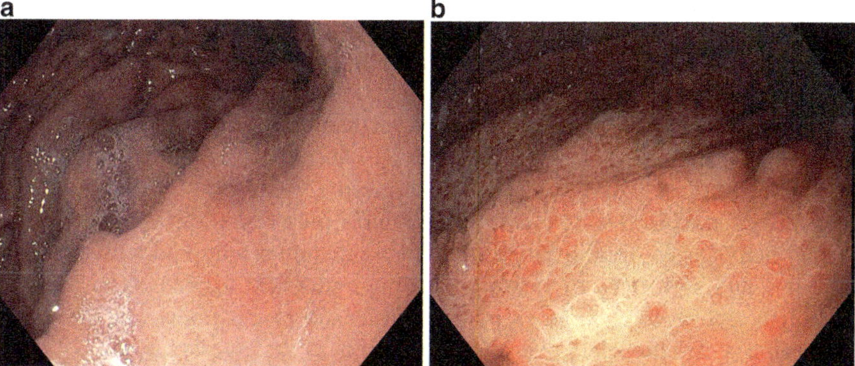

Fig. 34.4 (a) Mild portal hypertensive gastropathy; (b) Severe portal hypertensive gastropathy

can lead to chronic iron deficiency anemia and hemoccult positivity, but overt signs of bleeding would be highly uncommon. Virtually all symptomatic patients have the severe form of PHG [83].

When screening patients endoscopically for varices, PHG is often found. It is not recommended to start primary prophylaxis based on the finding of PHG. In patients with chronic iron deficiency in which PHG seems to be the cause, the best treatment is oral iron supplementation and NSBB based on a few studies. One of those studies was a trial of 54 cirrhotics with acute GI blood loss or chronic anemia secondary to PHG who were randomized to propranolol or placebo. The percentage of patients free of rebleeding favored propranolol 65–38 % at 1 year [84]. Due to the diffuse nature of PHG, endoscopic options are limited. There was a small study of just 11 patients admitted with GI bleeding attributed to PHG who were endoscopically treated with argon plasma coagulation in an effort to burn the gastropathic mucosa to stop bleeding. Over a median follow-up of 22 months, they reported a success rate of 86 % in preventing further bleeding and rebound of hematocrit to baseline levels [85]. In severe cases of bleeding from PHG in which other causes of anemia and GI blood loss have been ruled out and the patient is transfusion dependent despite iron therapy and NSBB, TIPS can be considered. Multiple studies have shown that in such situations, TIPS results in improvement in PHG and reduction in transfusions [83].

Portal hypertensive colopathy is a manifestation of the same pathological process in the colon. It is less common than PHG and seems to cause symptoms less often. Similar to PHG, acute overt bleeding is extremely rare, but it can cause chronic blood loss resulting in anemia. The endoscopic appearance is more variable than PHG and nonspecific, and therefore can often go unrecognized. It can appear as erythema, solitary red spots, irregular vascularity, and mucosal edema. There are no established guidelines for treatment so it is often treated similarly to PHG with iron supplementation and NSBB, with TIPS reserved for the most severe refractory cases [83].

Future Directions

Research will continue to find medications and interventions to treat cirrhosis and portal hypertension to prevent varices and mucosal congestion. A new endoscopic treatment for active gastrointestinal bleeding, including variceal bleeding, is hemospray. It is a granular, water-absorbent powder that is directly administered through the endoscope on to the site of bleeding. It increases clotting factors and platelets to create a mechanical plug and allow immediate temporary hemostasis. A prospective study of 14 cirrhotics admitted with upper GI bleeding and no history of variceal bleeding underwent upper endoscopy confirming active bleeding from esophageal varices in nine patients, and they were all treated with hemospray over the distal 15 cm of the esophagus and GE junction. Immediate hemostasis was achieved in all nine and there was no bleeding on follow-up EGD in 24 h at which time band ligation was able to be performed.

They also reported no deaths in 2 weeks follow-up [86]. This seems to be a promising technique in speed of application, technical ease of use, and efficacy of hemostasis. Larger, controlled studies using this technique are expected.

Summary

Portal hypertension due to liver disease can result in several endoscopic findings in the GI tract, all of which are similar in that they do not cause symptoms except for GI bleeding, which can sometimes be acute and severe. Endoscopic screening for esophageal varices is recommended and primary prophylaxis is indicated with either NSBB or endoscopic banding for select cirrhotics depending on the severity of underlying liver disease and endoscopic features of the varices. Acute esophageal variceal bleeding can be life-threatening and requires inpatient management with resuscitation with judicious use of IV fluids and blood transfusions, vasoactive drugs such as somatostatin, antibiotics, and endoscopic evaluation and/or therapy within 12 h of presentation. Secondary prophylaxis, after bleeding is controlled, includes both NSBB and endoscopic therapy. Refractory bleeding may require temporizing measures such as a covered esophageal stent or balloon tamponade as a bridge to definitive therapy, usually TIPS. Gastric variceal bleeding is more difficult to control endoscopically but tissue adhesives such as cyanoacrylate have an emerging role; TIPS is still often required. Portal hypertensive gastropathy/colopathy may cause chronic GI blood loss and rarely requires treatment but NSBB and endoscopic ablation along with iron supplementation are usually effective.

References

1. Garcia-Tsao G, Groszmann RJ, Fisher RL, Conn HO, Atterbury CE, Glickman M. Portal pressure, presence of gastroesophageal varices and variceal bleeding. Hepatology. 1985;5(3):419–24.
2. Ilyas JA, Kanwal F. Primary prophylaxis of variceal bleeding. Gastroenterol Clin North Am. 2014;43:783–94.
3. Graham DY, Smith JL. The course of patients after variceal hemorrhage. Gastroenterology. 1981;80(4):800–9.
4. Merli M, Nicolini G, Angeloni S, Rinaldi V, De Santis A, Merkel C, et al. Incidence and natural history of small esophageal varices in cirrhotic patients. J Hepatol. 2003;38(3):266–72.
5. Chalasani N, Kahi C, Francois F, Pinto A, Marathe A, Bini EJ, et al. Improved patient survival after acute variceal bleeding: a multicenter, cohort study. Am J Gastroenterol. 2003;98(3):653–9.
6. Thomopoulos K, Theocharis G, Mimidis K, Lampropoulou-Karatza C, Alexandridis E, Nikolopoulou V. Improved survival of patients presenting with acute variceal bleeding. Prognostic indicators of short- and long-term mortality. Dig Liver Dis. 2006;38(12):899–904.
7. Carbonell N, Pauwels A, Serfaty L, Fourdan O, Levy VG, Poupon R. Improved survival after variceal bleeding in patients with cirrhosis over the past two decades. Hepatology. 2004;40:652–9.

8. Vuachet D, Cervoni JP, Vuitton L, Weil D, Dritsas S, Dussaucy A, et al. Improved survival of cirrhotic patients with variceal bleeding over the decade 2000-2010. Clin Res Hepatol Gastroenterol. 2015;39(1):59–67.

9. Lapalus MG, Ben Soussan E, Gaudric M, Saurin JC, D'Halluin PN, Favre O, et al. Esophageal capsule endoscopy vs. EGD for the evaluation of portal hypertension - a French prospective multicenter comparative study. Am J Gastroenterol. 2009;104(5):1112–8.

10. Perri RE, Chiorean MV, Fidler JL, Fletcher JG, Talwalkar JA, Stadheim L, et al. A prospective evaluation of computerized tomographic (CT) scanning as a screening modality for esophageal varices. Hepatology. 2008;47(5):1587–94.

11. Giannini E, Botta F, Borro P, Risso D, Romagnoli P, Fasoli A, et al. Platelet count/spleen diameter ratio: proposal and validation of a non-invasive parameter to predict the presence of oesophageal varices in patients with liver cirrhosis. Gut. 2003;52(8):1200–5.

12. D'Amico G, Garcia-Pagan JC, Luca A, Bosch J. Hepatic vein pressure gradient reduction and prevention of variceal bleeding in cirrhosis: a systematic review. Gastroenterology. 2006;131(5):1611–24.

13. North Italian Endoscopic Club for the Study and Treatment of Esophageal Varices. Prediction of the first variceal hemorrhage in patients with cirrhosis of the liver and esophageal varices. A prospective multicenter study. N Engl J Med. 1988;319(15):983–9.

14. De Franchis R, Primignani M. Why do varices bleed? Gastroenterol Clin North Am. 1992;21(1):85–101.

15. Beppu K, Inokuchi K, Koyanagi N, Nakayama S, Sakata H, Kitano S, et al. Prediction of variceal hemorrhage by esophageal endoscopy. Gastrointest Endosc. 1981;27(4):213–8.

16. ASGE Standards of Practice Committee. The role of endoscopy in the management of variceal hemorrhage. Gastrointest Endosc. 2014;80(2):221–7.

17. Giannelli V, Lattanzi B, Thalheimer U, Merli M. Beta-blockers in liver cirrhosis. Ann Gastroenterol. 2014;27(1):20–6.

18. Lebrec D, Nouel O, Corbic M, Benhamou JP. Propranolol--a medical treatment for portal hypertension? Lancet. 1980;2(8187):180–2.

19. Groszmann RJ, Garcia-Tsao G, Bosch J, Grace ND, Burroughs AK, Planas R, et al. Beta-blockers to prevent gastroesophageal varices in patients with cirrhosis. N Engl J Med. 2005;353(21):2254–61.

20. Calés P, Oberti F, Payen JL, Naveau S, Guyader D, Blanc P, et al. Lack of effect of propranolol in the prevention of large oesophageal varices in patients with cirrhosis: a randomized trial. French-Speaking Club for the Study of Portal Hypertension. Eur J Gastroenterol Hepatol. 1999;11(7):741–5.

21. Bruno S, Crosignani A, Facciotto C, Rossi S, Roffi L, Redaelli A, et al. Sustained virologic response prevents the development of esophageal varices in compensated, Child-Pugh class A hepatitis C virus-induced cirrhosis. A 12-year prospective follow-up study. Hepatology. 2010;51(6):2069–76.

22. Merkel C, Marin R, Angeli P, Zanella P, Felder M, Bernardinello E, et al. A placebo-controlled clinical trial of nadolol in the prophylaxis of growth of small esophageal varices in cirrhosis. Gastroenterology. 2004;127(2):476–84.

23. Sarin SK, Mishra SR, Sharma P, Sharma BC, Kumar A. Early primary prophylaxis with beta-blockers does not prevent the growth of small esophageal varices in cirrhosis: a randomized controlled trial. Hepatol Int. 2013;7(1):248–56.

24. Bao YX, Bai M, Xu WD, Dai JN, Guo XZ. Nonselective beta-blockers in cirrhotic patients with no or small varices: a meta-analysis. World J Gastroenterol. 2015;21(10):3100–8.

25. Idéo G, Bellati G, Fesce E, Grimoldi D. Nadolol can prevent the first gastrointestinal bleeding in cirrhotics: a prospective, randomized study. Hepatology. 1988;8(1):6–9.

26. The Italian Multicenter Project for Propranolol in Prevention of Bleeding. Propranolol prevents first gastrointestinal bleeding in non-ascitic cirrhotic patients. Final report of a multicenter randomized trial. J Hepatol. 1989;9(1):75–83.

27. Pascal JP, Cales P. Propranolol in the prevention of first upper gastrointestinal tract hemorrhage in patients with cirrhosis of the liver and esophageal varices. N Engl J Med. 1987;317(14):856–61.

28. Poynard T, Calès P, Pasta L, Ideo G, Pascal JP, Pagliaro L, et al. Beta-adrenergic-antagonist drugs in the prevention of gastrointestinal bleeding in patients with cirrhosis and esophageal varices. An analysis of data and prognostic factors in 589 patients from four randomized clinical trials. Franco-Italian Multicenter Study Group. N Engl J Med. 1991;324(22):1532–8.
29. Teran JC, Imperiale TF, Mullen KD, Tavill AS, McCullough AJ. Primary prophylaxis of variceal bleeding in cirrhosis: a cost-effectiveness analysis. Gastroenterology. 1997;112(2):473–82.
30. Sersté T, Melot C, Francoz C, Durand F, Rautou PE, Valla D, et al. Deleterious effects of beta-blockers on survival in patients with cirrhosis and refractory ascites. Hepatology. 2010;52:1017–22.
31. García-Pagán JC, Morillas R, Bañares R, Albillos A, Villanueva C, Vila C, et al. Propranolol plus placebo versus propranolol plus isosorbide-5-mononitrate in the prevention of a first variceal bleed: a double-blind RCT. Hepatology. 2003;37(6):1260–6.
32. Avgerinos A, Armonis A, Manolakopoulos S, Rekoumis G, Argirakis G, Viazis N, et al. Endoscopic sclerotherapy plus propranolol versus propranolol alone in the primary prevention of bleeding in high risk cirrhotic patients with esophageal varices: a prospective multicenter randomized trial. Gastrointest Endosc. 2000;51(6):652–8.
33. Sarin SK, Guptan RK, Jain AK, Sundaram KR. A randomized controlled trial of endoscopic variceal band ligation for primary prophylaxis of variceal bleeding. Eur J Gastroenterol Hepatol. 1996;8(4):337–42.
34. Imperiale TF, Chalasani N. A meta-analysis of endoscopic variceal ligation for primary prophylaxis of esophageal variceal bleeding. Hepatology. 2001;33(4):802–7.
35. Sarin SK, Lamba GS, Kumar M, Misra A, Murthy NS. Comparison of endoscopic ligation and propranolol for the primary prevention of variceal bleeding. N Engl J Med. 1999;340(13):988–93.
36. Jutabha R, Jensen DM, Martin P, Savides T, Han SH, Gornbein J. Randomized study comparing banding and propranolol to prevent initial variceal hemorrhage in cirrhotics with high-risk esophageal varices. Gastroenterology. 2005;128(4):870–81.
37. Gluud LL, Klingenberg S, Nikolova D, Gluud C. Banding ligation versus beta-blockers as primary prophylaxis in esophageal varices: systematic review of randomized trials. Am J Gastroenterol. 2007;102:2842–8.
38. Shaheen NJ, Stuart E, Schmitz SM, Mitchell KL, Fried MW, Zacks S, et al. Pantoprazole reduces the size of postbanding ulcers after variceal band ligation: a randomized, controlled trial. Hepatology. 2005;41(3):588–94.
39. Bonilha DQ, Lenz L, Correia LM, Rodrigues RA, de Paulo GA, Ferrari AP, et al. Propranolol associated with endoscopic band ligation reduces recurrence of esophageal varices for primary prophylaxis of variceal bleeding: a randomized-controlled trial. Eur J Gastroenterol Hepatol. 2015;27(1):84–90.
40. Sarin SK, Wadhawan M, Agarwal SR, Tyagi P, Sharma BC. Endoscopic variceal ligation plus propranolol versus endoscopic variceal ligation alone in primary prophylaxis of variceal bleeding. Am J Gastroenterol. 2005;100:797–804.
41. Tripathi D, Ferguson JW, Kochar N, et al. Randomized controlled trial of carvedilol versus variceal band ligation for the prevention of the first variceal bleed. Hepatology. 2009;50:825–33.
42. Reiberger T, Ulbrich G, Ferlitsch A, Payer BA, Schwabl P, Pinter M, et al. Carvedilol for primary prophylaxis of variceal bleeding in cirrhotic patients with haemodynamic non-response to propranolol. Gut. 2013;62(11):1634–41.
43. Garcia-Tsao G, Grace ND, Groszmann RJ, Conn HO, Bermann MM, Patrick MJ, et al. Short-term effects of propranolol on portal venous pressure. Hepatology. 1986;6(1):101–6.
44. Poza Cordon J, Froilan Torres C, Burgos García A, Gea Rodriguez F, Suárez de Parga JM. Endoscopic management of esophageal varices. World J Gastrointest Endosc. 2012;4(7):312–22.
45. Garcia-Tsao G, Sanyal A, Grace N, Carey W, Practice Guidelines Committee of the American Association for the Study of Liver Diseases, the Practice Parameters Committee of the American College of Gastroenterology. Prevention and management of gastroesophageal varices and variceal hemorrhage in cirrhosis. Hepatology. 2007;46(3):922–38.

46. Kumar S, Asrani SK, Kamath PS. Epidemiology, diagnosis and early patient management of esophagogastric hemorrhage. Gastroenterol Clin North Am. 2014;43(4):765–82.
47. Sorbi D, Gostout CJ, Peura D, Johnson D, Lanza F, Foutch PG, et al. An assessment of the management of acute bleeding varices: a multicenter prospective member based study. Am J Gastroenterol. 2003;98(11):2424–34.
48. Koch DG, Arguedas MR, Fallon MB. Risk of aspiration pneumonia in suspected variceal hemorrhage: the value of prophylactic endotracheal intubation prior to endoscopy. Dig Dis Sci. 2007;52(9):2225–8.
49. Villanueva C, Colomo A, Bosch A, Concepción M, Hernandez-Gea V, Aracil C, et al. Transfusion strategies for acute upper gastrointestinal bleeding. N Engl J Med. 2013;368:11–21.
50. Satapathy SK, Sanyal AJ. Non endoscopic mgmt strategies for acute esophagogastric variceal bleeding. Gastroenterol Clin North Am. 2014;43(4):819–33.
51. Bernard B, Grange JD, Khac EN, Amiot X, Opolon P, Poynard T. Antibiotic prophylaxis for the prevention of bacterial infections in cirrhotic patients with gastrointestinal bleeding: a meta-analysis. Hepatology. 1999;29:1655–61.
52. Fernández J, Ruiz del Arbol L, Gómez C, Durandez R, Serradilla R, Guarner C, et al. Norfloxacin vs ceftriaxone in the prophylaxis of infections in patients with advanced cirrhosis and hemorrhage. Gastroenterology. 2006;131:1049–56.
53. Sharma P, Agrawal A, Sharma BC, Sarin SK. Prophylaxis of hepatic encephalopathy in acute variceal bleed: a randomized controlled trial of lactulose versus no lactulose. J Gastroenterol Hepatol. 2011;26(6):996–1003.
54. Bosch J, Kravetz D, Rodes J. Effects of somatostatin on hepatic and systemic hemodynamics in patients with cirrhosis of liver: comparison with vasopressin. Gastroenterology. 1981;80:518–25.
55. Hwang SJ, Lin HC, Chang CF, Lee FY, Lu CW, Hsia HC, et al. A randomized controlled trial comparing octreotide and vasopressin in the control of acute esophageal variceal bleeding. J Hepatol. 1992;16(3):320–5.
56. Bañares R, Albillos A, Rincón D, Alonso S, González M, Ruiz-del-Arbol L, et al. Endoscopic treatment versus endoscopic plus pharmacologic treatment for acute variceal bleeding: a meta-analysis. Hepatology. 2002;35:609–15.
57. Chen PH, Chen WC, Hou MC, Liu TT, Chang CJ, Liao WC, et al. Delayed endoscopy increases re-bleeding and mortality in patients with hematemesis and active esophageal variceal bleeding: a cohort study. J Hepatol. 2012;57(6):1207–13.
58. Hsu YC, Chung CS, Tseng CH, Lin TL, Liou JM, Wu MS, et al. Delayed endoscopy as a risk factor for in-hospital mortality in cirrhotic patients with acute variceal hemorrhage. J Gastroenterol Hepatol. 2009;24(7):1294–9.
59. de Franchis R. Baveno V Faculty. Revising consensus in portal hypertension: report of the Baveno V consensus workshop on methodology of diagnosis and therapy in portal hypertension. J Hepatol. 2010;53:762–8.
60. Helmy A, Hayes PC. Review article: current endoscopic therapeutic options in the management of variceal bleeding. Aliment Pharmacol Ther. 2001;15:575–94.
61. Baillie J, Yudelman P. Complications of endoscopic sclerotherapy of esophageal varices. Endoscopy. 1992;24(4):284–91.
62. Villanueva C, Piqueras M, Aracil C, Gómez C, López-Balaguer JM, Gonzalez B, et al. A randomized controlled trial comparing ligation and sclerotherapy as emergency endoscopic treatment added to somatostatin in acute variceal bleeding. J Hepatol. 2006;45:560–7.
63. Luz GO, Maluf-Filho F, Matuguma SE, Hondo FY, Ide E, Melo JM, et al. Comparison between endoscopic sclerotherapy and band ligation for hemostasis of acute variceal bleeding. World J Gastrointest Endosc. 2011;3(5):95–100.
64. Triantos CK, Goulis J, Patch D, Papatheodoridis GV, Leandro G, Samonakis D, et al. An evaluation of emergency sclerotherapy of varices in randomized trials: looking the needle in the eye. Endoscopy. 2006;38:797–807.
65. Hubmann R, Bodlaj G, Czompo M, Benkö L, Pichler P, Al-Kathib S, et al. The use of self-expanding metal stents to treat acute esophageal variceal bleeding. Endoscopy. 2006;38(9):896–901.
66. Holster IL, Kuipers EJ, van Buuren HR, Spaander MC, Tjwa ET. Self-expandable metal stents as definitive treatment for esophageal variceal bleeding. Endoscopy. 2013;45(6):485–8.

67. Bambha K, Kim WR, Pedersen R, Bida JP, Kremers WK, Kamath PS. Predictors of early re-bleeding and mortality after acute variceal hemorrhage in patients with cirrhosis. Gut. 2008;57:814–20.
68. García-Pagán JC, Caca K, Bureau C, Laleman W, Appenrodt B, Luca A, et al. Early use of TIPS in patients with cirrhosis and variceal bleeding. N Engl J Med. 2010;362(25):2370–9.
69. Xue H, Zhang M, Pang JX, Yan F, Li YC, Lv LS, et al. Transjugular intrahepatic portosystemic shunt vs endoscopic therapy in preventing variceal rebleeding. World J Gastroenterol. 2012;18(48):7341–7.
70. Albillos A, Tejedor M. Secondary prophylaxis for esophageal variceal bleeding. Clin Liver Dis. 2014;18(2):359–70.
71. de la Peña J, Brullet E, Sanchez-Hernández E, Rivero M, Vergara M, Martin-Lorente JL, et al. Variceal ligation plus nadolol compared with ligation for prophylaxis of variceal rebleeding: a multicenter trial. Hepatology. 2005;41:572–8.
72. Lo GH, Chen WC, Chen MH, Hsu PI, Lin CK, Tsai WL, et al. Banding ligation versus nadolol and isosorbide mononitrate for the prevention of esophageal variceal rebleeding. Gastroenterology. 2002;123(3):728–34.
73. Thiele M, Krag A, Rohde U, Gluud LL. Meta-analysis: banding ligation and medical interventions for the prevention of rebleeding from oesophageal varices. Aliment Pharmacol Ther. 2012;35(10):1155–65.
74. Lo GH, Chen WC, Wang HM, Yu HC. Randomized, controlled trial of carvedilol versus nadolol plus isosorbide mononitrate for the prevention of variceal rebleeding. J Gastroenterol Hepatol. 2012;27(11):1681–7.
75. Lo GH, Liang HL, Chen WC, et al. A prospective, randomized controlled trial of transjugular intrahepatic portosystemic shunt versus cyanoacrylate injection in the prevention of gastric variceal rebleeding. Endoscopy. 2007;39(8):679–85.
76. Mishra SR, Sharma BC, Kumar A, Sarin SK. Primary prophylaxis of gastric variceal bleeding comparing cyanoacrylate injection and beta-blockers: a randomized controlled trial. J Hepatol. 2011;54:1161–7.
77. Cheng L, Wang Z, Chang-Zheng L, Wu L, Yeo A, Jin B. Low incidence of complications from endoscopic gastric variceal obturation with butyl cyanoacrylate. Clin Gastroenterol Hepatol. 2010;8:760–6.
78. Garcia-Pagán JC, Barrufet M, Cardenas A, Escorsell A. Management of gastric varices. Clin Gastroenterol Hepatol. 2014;12:919–28.
79. Tan PC, Hou MC, Lin HC, Liu TT, Lee FY, Chang FY, et al. A randomized trial of endoscopic treatment of acute gastric variceal hemorrhage: N-butyl-2-cyanoacrylate injection versus band ligation. Hepatology. 2006;43(4):690–7.
80. Procaccini NJ, Al-Osaimi AM, Northup P, Argo C, Caldwell SH. Endoscopic cyanoacrylate versus transjugular intrahepatic portosystemic shunt for gastric variceal bleeding: a single-center U.S. analysis. Gastrointest Endosc. 2009;70(5):881–7.
81. Mishra SR, Chander Sharma B, Kumar A, Sarin SK. Endoscopic cyanoacrylate injection versus beta-blocker for secondary prophylaxis of gastric variceal bleed: a randomised controlled trial. Gut. 2010;59(6):729–35.
82. Romero-Castro R, Ellrichmann M, Ortiz-Moyano C, Subtil-Inigo JC, Junquera-Florez F, Gornals JB, et al. EUS-guided coil versus cyanoacrylate therapy for the treatment of gastric varices: a multicenter study. Gastrointest Endosc. 2013;78(5):711–21.
83. Pérez-Ayuso RM, Piqué JM, Bosch J, Panés J, González A, Pérez R, et al. Propranolol in prevention of recurrent bleeding from severe portal hypertensive gastropathy in cirrhosis. Lancet. 1991;337(8755):1431–4.
84. Urrunaga NH, Rockey DC. Portal hypertensive gastropathy and colopathy. Clin Liver Dis. 2014;18(2):389–406.
85. Herrera S, Bordas JM, Llach J, Ginès A, Pellisé M, Fernández-Esparrach G, et al. The beneficial effects of argon plasma coagulation in the management of different types of gastric vascular ectasia lesions in patients admitted for GI hemorrhage. Gastrointest Endosc. 2008;68(3):440–6.
86. Ibrahim M, El-Mikkawy A, Mostafa I, Devière J. Endoscopic treatment of acute variceal hemorrhage by using hemostatic powder TC-325: a prospective pilot study. Gastrointest Endosc. 2013;78(5):769–73.

Chapter 35
Liver Resection

Amir H. Fathi and T. Clark Gamblin

Liver resection has been transformed from a procedure with substantial mortality risk to one that is now performed frequently with less morbidity and mortality. This chapter aims to underscore important aspects of preoperative evaluation for patients undergoing liver surgery. Operative guidelines and essential techniques are also addressed in addition to alternative management approaches to patients who are not surgical candidates.

Patient Selection and Assessment

Preoperative Considerations

Preoperative care of patients with liver pathology requires a multidisciplinary approach to formulate the best individual treatment plan. Assessing patient candidacy for surgical intervention begins with a thorough evaluation of overall health, history and physical exam, medications, comorbid conditions, and patient's functional capacity. Comorbid health conditions are a major determinant of postoperative morbidity and mortality. Anesthesiology and perioperative medicine, in addition to the surgical team should evaluate each patient to stratify the risks and optimize outcomes. Serious or untreated medical conditions such as recent myocardial, cerebral infarction or advanced renal disease may exclude select patients from surgical resection [1, 2].

Comorbid illnesses are particularly prevalent in the elderly population. Advanced age alone should not be an exclusion criterion; however, age does carry a higher risk

A.H. Fathi, M.D. • T.C. Gamblin, M.D., M.S. (✉)
Division of Surgical Oncology, Medical College of Wisconsin,
9200 West Wisconsin Avenue, Milwaukee, WI 53226-3596, USA
e-mail: ahf59@yahoo.com; tcgamblin@mcw.edu

© Springer International Publishing Switzerland 2017
K. Saeian, R. Shaker (eds.), *Liver Disorders*,
DOI 10.1007/978-3-319-30103-7_35

Table 35.1 ECOG performance status scale

Grade	ECOG
0	Fully active, able to carry all pre-disease performance without restriction
1	Restricted in physically strenuous activity but ambulatory and able to carry out work of a light or sedentary nature such as light house work, office work
2	Ambulatory and capable of all self-care but unable to carry out any work activities. Up and about more that 50 % of walking hours
3	Capable of only limited self-care, confined to bed or chair more than 50 % of waking hours
4	Completely disabled. Cannot carry on any self-care. Totally confined to bed or chair
5	Dead

Oken M, Creech R, Tormey D, et al. Toxicity and response criteria of the Eastern Cooperative Oncology Group. Am J Clin Oncol. 1982;5:649–655

for postoperative complications [3, 4]. Patients' functional status and reserve is of much greater importance than the numeric age. Functional status refers to an individual's ability to perform normal daily activities required to meet basic needs, such as maintaining well-being and daily routines. Decline in functional status is measured by an individual's loss of independence in activities of daily living (ADL) over a certain period of time. Several tools have been developed to score the ability of patients to maintain their independence in the context of their daily life. They numerically rate physical, emotional, and cognitive status of patients. One of the most commonly used tools is the Eastern Cooperative Oncology Group (ECOG) performance status scale [5]. The ECOG scale is a simple way to quickly assess the patients' current status and when used longitudinally, it illustrates how the disease and/or treatment are affecting the daily living abilities of patients (Table 35.1).

After comprehensive assessment of patients' overall health and functional status, in-depth evaluation of patients' liver health is vital. Assessment starts by examining the risk factors for liver diseases such as congenital or familial syndromes, hepatitis, and alcohol intake. Please see Chap. 9 for liver diseases and syndromes. All patients should be specifically asked about alcohol intake history. These questions have a particularly important impact on treatments such as liver transplantation. Hepatitis testing can be selective, based on the presence of risk factors such as intravenous drug abuse, history of tattoos, high-risk sexual behavior, past episode of jaundice, or history of blood transfusions prior to 1990. All of the patients with hepatocellular carcinoma should be tested for hepatitis due to the known association.

The presence of cirrhosis and/or portal hypertension introduces unique challenges for liver surgery. In cirrhotic patients, a firm, nodular and enlarged liver poses technical difficulties in mobilization and parenchymal transection. Impairment of liver function after resection in cirrhotic patients is greater, may last longer and could result in liver failure. Additionally, potential liver regeneration is negatively impacted by cirrhosis. Therefore, the principles of parenchymal sparing should be strictly followed for cirrhotic patients. Portal hypertension imposes an increased risk for bleeding during surgery and in the postoperative period. A decreased platelet count is often used as a surrogate marker for portal hypertension rather than invasive measurement of hepatic vein pressure gradients.

Patients with biliary instrumentation have an increased risk of infections due to the colonized biliary tree associated with manipulation and/or stent placement. Postoperative alterations of immune system are thought to be a potential predisposing factor to infections. The risk of postoperative infection is particularly high in patients with cirrhosis and ascites or jaundice.

Assessment of Liver Function

There is no individual test to completely assess the liver's functional status. Assessment requires analysis and interpretation of multiple factors. Accurate estimation of liver resection extent and the predicted remnant volume assists in prediction of the potential postoperative complications. It also guides the therapeutic decisions which may include a staged resection or hybrid procedures with incorporation of ablation techniques.

Recent improvements in anesthesia support, surgical techniques, and ICU care have led to a surgical mortality of less than 3 % following liver resections at many high volume institutions. However, overall morbidity related to liver failure following resection remains between 16 and 50 % [6, 7].

Currently, measures to assess preoperative liver function are broadly divided to three major categories: (1) Classification systems, (2) Dynamic Liver tests, (3) Predicting postoperative liver volume.

Classification Systems

While many systems have been proposed for risk stratification and selection of patients undergoing liver surgery, the Child-Turcotte-Pugh (CTP) scoring system is most commonly utilized [8, 9]. The parameters measured in this classification include presence or absence of clinical ascites and encephalopathy, serum albumin, total bilirubin, and the international normalized ratio (INR). Based on clinical severity or measured laboratory value, each parameter will earn points. The final point total (which is a summation of all five categories) will classify the patient into three groups (A, B or C). These groups are used to stratify the patients' liver synthetic and detoxification function (Table 35.2). Numerous studies have demonstrated the predictive validity of the CTP score as a surrogate for liver function and prognostic of outcomes. For example, in patients with cirrhosis, the 1-year mortality related to liver failure is less than 5 % for Child-Pugh class A patients, compared with 20 % and 55 % for class B and C patients, respectively. Child-Pugh class B cirrhosis limits candidates for liver resection, and prohibits a major hepatectomy. Class C cirrhosis is a contraindication for surgical intervention.

Another classification system is the MELD (Model for End-Stage Liver Disease) [10]. This system is used to assess patients for liver transplantation and estimates the 3-month predicted mortality. It is a logarithmic equation comprised of serum creatinine, total bilirubin and INR values to predict the anticipated mortality. MELD

Table 35.2 Child-Turcotte-Pugh (CTP) scoring system

Points	1	2	3
Ascites	None	Mild to Moderate (diuretic controlled)	Severe
Encephalopathy	None	Mild	Severe
Bilirubin (mg/dL)	<2	2–3	>3
Albumin (g/L)	>3.5	2.8–3.5	<2.8
PT (sec >control) *or*	<4	4–6	>6
INR	<1.7	1.7–2.3	>2.3

INR international normalized ratio, *PT* prothrombin time

Class A: 5–6 points; Class B: 7–9 points; Class C: 10–15 points

score has been increasingly used to provide a complementary predictive value to Child-Pugh score. Patients with a MELD score above 14 may be excluded from major surgical interventions.

Dynamic Liver Tests

Although not routinely used in North America, dynamic tests can provide additional information on the future liver remnant by evaluating hepatic uptake, metabolism and excretion capacity. Indocyanine green (ICG) clearance and Galactose Elimination Capacity (GEC) are two most commonly utilized quantitative tests.

ICG clearance test is validated as a valuable adjunct in quantifying liver function. ICG is a dye that is selectively taken up and cleared from the circulation by the liver and its clearance is an indicator of hepatocyte function. Studies, suggest that an ICG retention values after intravenous injection above 10–15 % at 15 min are considered abnormal and are used as a cutoff to identify patients at high risk for liver failure following liver resection [11].

Predicting Postoperative Liver Volume

Future liver remnant (FLR) refers to the residual liver volume after hepatic resection. It is one of the most important determinants of postoperative liver function. Underlying liver disease and its inherent impaired liver functional capacity requires a larger remnant liver to achieve the necessary hepatic function. Studies have suggested that for patients with normal liver parenchyma, FLR >20–30 % is sufficient to avoid postoperative liver insufficiency. In cirrhotic patients with impaired baseline liver function, at least a 40 % FLR is recommended to compensate [12]. For patients who have received extensive systemic chemotherapy, FLR >30 % reduces the rate of postoperative hepatic insufficiency (PHI) and may provide enough functional reserve for clinical rescue [13].

Three-dimensional Computed Tomography (CT) scan or Magnetic Resonance Imaging (MRI) has been utilized to perform preoperative volumetric analyses.

Based on the predicted anatomical resection planes, software can calculate the corresponding remnant volumes. Image guided volumetry does not account for underlying parenchymal dysfunction and should not be used as the single decision variable. Inconsistencies can also occur when multiple, large or infiltrating tumors replace a large volume of the liver.

A number of techniques have been utilized to improve an insufficient FLR, in order to achieve a safe liver resection. These include portal vein embolization (PVE) and recently introduced ALPPS (Associated Liver Partition and Portal vein ligation for Staged hepatectomy). Portal vein embolization or ligation interrupts the flow and diverts the portal blood flow to the liver remnant, causing remnant growth. This effect is maximized in 4–6 weeks and is most effective for the patients with a normal liver [14]. ALPPS (Associated Liver Partition and Portal vein ligation for Staged hepatectomy) is a recent modification of staged liver resections that approaches resection in two steps. It relies on the regenerative capacity of the remnant liver after parenchymal transection and portal vein ligation in a short period of 1–2 weeks during a single hospitalization [15].

Imaging Modalities

The last critical component to the proper patient selection for liver surgery is to delineate the liver anatomy. It is crucial to outline the topography and characterize the liver pathology with its anatomical relationship to the critical structures. High quality preoperative cross-sectional imaging is imperative for this assessment.

Ultrasound (US) is an inexpensive, high resolution imaging technique that does not use ionizing radiation. Its versatility and real time imaging capability make it a useful screening tool. However, its sensitivity and specificity are lower than CT. Therefore it is not routinely used for preoperative planning. Intraoperative ultrasonography is an essential component of liver surgery. It is used for identifying the lesions, screen the remnant liver for occult disease, and ultimately determine resectability (Fig. 35.1a).

To date, CT scan and MRI are the most reliable preoperative imaging modalities to evaluate the liver. In addition to the information gained about the liver, they are also used to evaluate for extrahepatic disease. CT volumetry is one of the most common means of predicting the volume of functional liver remnant following a proposed resection [16]. It typically involves the ratio of remaining volume to total liver volume (Fig. 35.1b). MRI is a cross-sectional scanning technique that uses magnetic fields and radiofrequency pulses to generate images with tissue contrast (Fig. 35.1c). MRI cholangiography (MRCP) is a technique that is utilized to specifically evaluate the biliary and pancreatic systems. Diagnostic quality images are obtained via this technique with high sensitivity and specificity for assessment of biliary duct dilations, strictures and other abnormalities (Fig. 35.1d) [17]. The images obtained by MRCP are very similar to ones acquired by Endoscopic Retrograde CholangioPancreatography (ERCP) (Fig. 35.1e) or Percutaneous

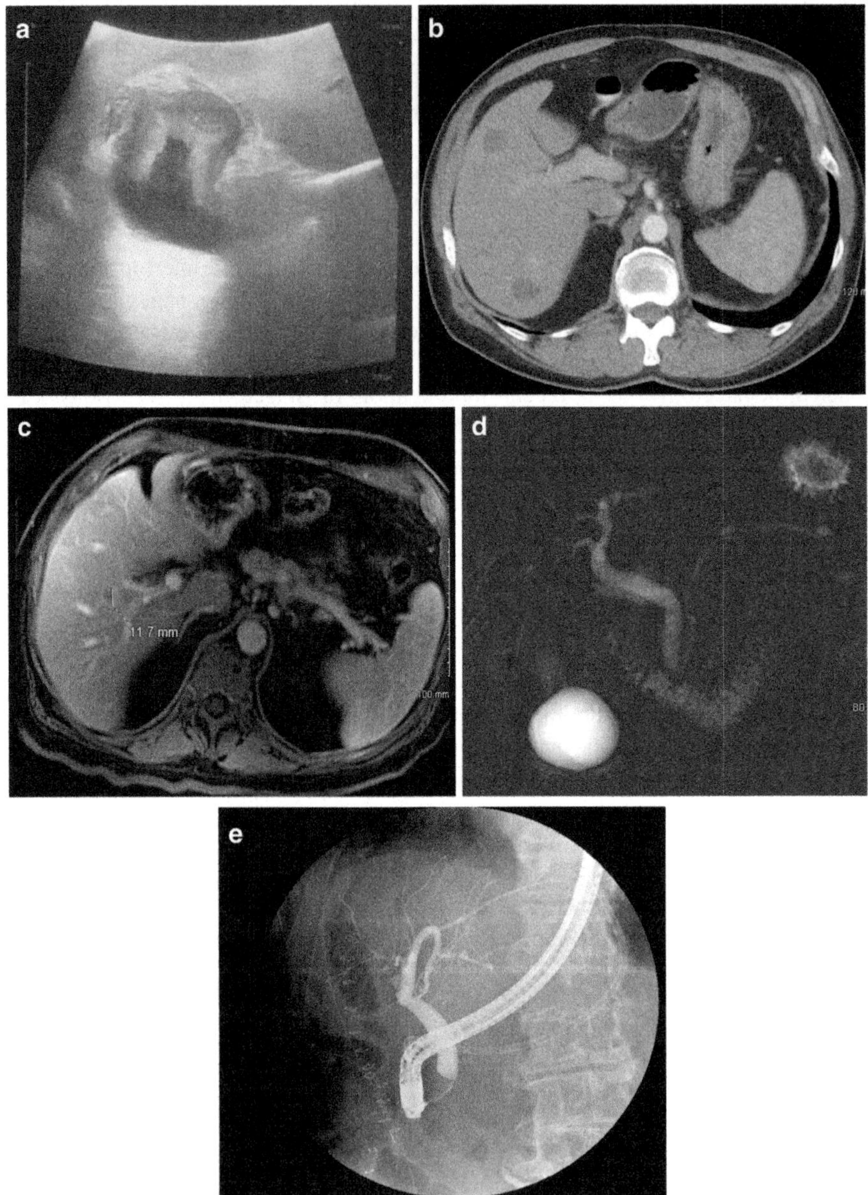

Fig. 35.1 Examples of different liver imaging modalities. (**a**) CT scan image of a liver lesion. (**b**) MRI imaging showing a solid liver tumor. (**c**) Ultrasonic image of a solid gallbladder lesion with posterior enhancement. (**d**) MRCP reconstruction of biliary tree. (**e**) ERCP imaging of biliary tree

Transhepatic Cholangiography (PTC). In contrast to those invasive procedures, MRCP is noninvasive and avoids morbidities such as post procedural pancreatitis. MRCP also provides the ability of visualization of the extrabiliary anatomy, allowing for exclusion or inclusion of alternative diagnoses. However, this modality does not provide the potential of a tissue diagnosis and the opportunity for therapeutic interventions such as stent placement.

General Principles

The liver is the largest solid organ in the human body. It lies protected under lower ribs, closely molded to the undersurface of the diaphragm. Most of liver bulk is located in the right side of the body, secured by multiple ligaments.

Liver is divided into right and left lobes by Cantlie's line which runs from gallbladder fossa anterior, to the IVC fossa posterior. These lobes are subdivided by the Couinaud classification into eight functionally independent segments. Each segment has its own vascular inflow, outflow, and biliary drainage. In the center of each segment, there is a branch of the portal vein, hepatic artery, and bile duct. In the periphery of each segment, there is vascular outflow through the hepatic veins.

Indications for liver resection vary widely from trauma to oncologic treatments (Table 35.3). Liver resections are divided into two major categories: Anatomic and non-anatomic. Anatomic resections follow the mentioned segmental divisions and could range from a single segment resection (Segmentectomy), to over six segment resections (Right Trisegmentectomy). Major hepatectomy is defined as resection of three or more Couinaud liver segments. Non-anatomic resection planes are not limited by these segmentations. For example, a wedge resection of liver parenchyma is considered non-anatomical resection. The International Hepato-Pancreato-Biliary Association (IHPBA) Brisbane 2000 terminology committee classifies the liver resections to five main categories [18]: (1) Right Hepatectomy: resection of segments V–VIII, (2) Left Hepatectomy: Resection of segments II–IV, (3) Extended Right Hepatectomy (Right Trisegmentectomy): Resection of segments IV–VIII, (4) Left Lateral Segmentectomy: Resection of segments II and III, (5) Extended Left Hepatectomy (Left Trisegmentectomy): Resection of segments II, V, and VIII.

Liver resection for treatment of benign tumors or cystic lesions is performed for symptomatic patients, when malignancy is suspected, or diagnostic dilemmas exist. Lesions with potential for malignant transformation, such as adenomas may also be an indication for resection. In such cases, parenchymal preservation should be stressed and removal of normal liver tissue should be minimized. Liver resection may be necessary in the management of some complex benign biliary strictures as well.

In malignant cases, oncologic appropriateness of liver resection and patient performance status are key determinants. Preoperative transcutaneous needle biopsy of liver tumor masses is not routinely necessary. Preoperative biopsy should be

Table 35.3 Most common indications for liver resection

1. Traumatic Injury
2. Living Donor Liver Resection for Transplanting
3. Malignant Liver Neoplasms
(a) Primary
• Hepatocellular carcinoma
• Intrahepatic cholangiocarcinoma
• Cyst adenocarcinoma
(b) Metastatic, from
• Colorectal cancer (CRS)
• Neuroendocrine neoplasms or non-colorectal cancers
• Tumors directly invading the liver
– Adrenal tumors
– Renal carcinoma
– Gastric cancer
– Colonic cancer
– Retroperitoneal and inferior vena cava sarcoma
4. Benign Liver Neoplasms
(a) Hemangioma
(b) Adenoma
(c) (FNH) Focal nodular hyperplasia
(d) Cystadenoma
5. Gallbladder Cancer
6. Extrahepatic Cholangiocarcinoma
7. Benign Conditions
(a) Intrahepatic biliary strictures/fistulae
(b) Hepatolithiasis
(c) Recurrent pyogenic cholangitis
(d) Liver cysts/polycystic liver disease
(e) Parasitic infections

pursued only if the information gained will alter the treatment plan. In the presence of a strong presumptive and clinical diagnosis of a potentially resectable liver tumor, it is preferred to avoid percutaneous methods, which could result in possible tumor dissemination, rupture, or hemorrhage.

Diagnostic laparoscopy has also emerged as a significant technique for revealing occult disease burden which has escaped preoperative imaging studies. Its benefits, when the occult disease is found, include decreased procedure-related morbidity and shorter time to initiation of adjuvant therapy [19].

Operative Guidelines

Perioperative Preparation and Anesthesia Considerations

Perioperative preparation includes intravenous antibiotic administration prior to skin incision and deep venous thrombosis prophylaxis. Coagulopathy is ruled out and blood products should be available for possible transfusion. Patients with a significant history of cardiopulmonary disease should undergo preoperative evaluation.

To minimize bleeding during parenchymal transection, central venous pressure less than five mmHg is desirable. Routine perioperative blood transfusion should be avoided, as allogeneic red blood cell transfusion has been associated with worse perioperative outcome and a possible impact on cancer-related survival [20].

Normothermia should be maintained with warmed fluids and external warming devices. Low body temperatures are associated with coagulopathy and postoperative complications such as surgical site infections [21].

Postoperative analgesia can be delivered by intravenous or epidural routes. The ability to metabolize narcotics after major liver resections may be reduced, thus the patient must be monitored carefully for oversedation and respiratory depression.

Operating Room Details

Patient Positioning

Patient is positioned supine on the operating room table. Both arms extended perpendicularly to the body and secured on arm boards. Care is taken to avoid overextension of the arms and to prevent any potential injury to the brachial plexus nerves in the axilla. Proper padding should be applied to all of the body pressure points, such as elbows and heals to prevent any iatrogenic pressure ulcers. For large posteriorly lying tumors, a shoulder roll or lateral decubitus position may be utilized. Central venous catheters and arterial lines are commonly used for major resections. The prepping and draping includes the lower chest from nipple line down to the both groins.

Surgical Technique

Incision

The incision length and type depends on the tumor location, type of planned resection and history of prior abdominal procedures. A xiphoid to umbilicus, upper midline incision should suffice for left sided or central resections. However, larger tumors of the right side of the liver will require a right subcostal incision with vertical midline extensions for an open resection. Incisions and port placements for minimally invasive liver surgery will be described later in the chapter.

Critical Steps of Operation

There are four defined steps for liver surgery.

Step One: *Exploration*

Upon entering the abdomen, the peritoneal cavity should be carefully explored to rule out distant disease.

Step Two: *Mobilization, exposure and reassessment*

In order to gain adequate exposure, it is essential to divide the suspensory hepatic ligaments. The extent of liver mobilization is determined by the tumor location and the planned anatomical resection. Visual and manual exploration of liver follows the mobilization. Intraoperative ultrasound (IOUS) is used in every case. It assists in evaluating the number and location of tumors along with their exact relation with the major vasculature and biliary structures.

Step Three: *Inflow, Outflow control and preservation of biliary tree integrity*

Prior to parenchymal transection, the vascular and biliary drainage division should be planned and arterial and venous blood supply should be controlled. Intraoperative cholangiogram as well as intraoperative ultrasound are valuable adjunct diagnostic methods to delineate the biliary and vascular anatomy before any transection. It is recommended to encircle the Porta Hepatis via foramen of Winslow for a Pringle maneuver, if necessary.

Control of the hepatic arterial and portal venous blood supply to the portion of liver to be removed could be obtained by extrahepatic dissection or alternatively by ligation within liver parenchyma. Special attentions should be exercised during dissection to preserve the adjacent vascular and biliary structures, associated with the future liver remnant. The remnant liver must maintain intact arterial and portal inflow, biliary drainage and at least one of three hepatic veins. Extrahepatic dissection and control of these veins is possible in the majority of cases. However, intrahepatic control of the veins, carried out during parenchymal transection, is also feasible and acceptable. Furthermore, there are multiple short hepatic veins draining directly from the posterior surface of the liver to the IVC. These veins should be individually identified and ligated, if right lobe mobilization is necessary.

Step Four: *Parenchymal transection*

A number of methods and tools are available to transect the liver parenchyma. Historically, the one that has been used most extensively is the crush-clamp technique. In this method, the Glisson capsule is scored with diathermy along the line of proposed transection and a Kelly clamp is used to crush the liver tissue and expose small vessels, biliary channels, and larger pedicles. Once exposed, these structures are divided using a variety of techniques, including clips and/or suture ligation. Recently, several devices have been developed to facilitate this process, such as: (1) bipolar cautery (LigaSure; Valleylab, Boulder, CO); (2) Saline-linked radiofrequency ablation monopolar device (TissueLink; TissueLink Medical, Dover, NH), or a bipolar variation (Aquamantys, TissueLink Medical); (3) Harmonic Scalpel (SonoSurg; Olympus Key Med, New York, NY). Ultrasonic or water-jet dissectors also have been used for parenchymal dissection. Ultrasonic dissector has some advantages in dissecting vessels, particularly in the performance of segmental and subsegmental resections, especially in the cirrhotic liver. The water-jet dissector (Helix Hydro-Jet ERBE; USA Inc., Marietta, GA) is another efficient device and is valuable in the exposure of major pedicles.

Use of vascular staplers for safely securing and dividing inflow and outflow vessels in major liver resections is well described in the literature. In addition to vascular division, application of surgical stapling devices for parenchymal transection in hepatic surgery has also been reported. This technique has multiple advantages including the speed in which the transection can be performed. This accelerated transection potentially eliminates the necessity for prolonged inflow occlusion (Pringle's maneuver). Furthermore, any secondary biliary radicals will also be sealed with the staple cartridges. One potential disadvantage of the stapled technique is the cost of multiple stapler cartridges. The cost issue should be weighed in light of impact on ICU admission, blood transfusion, and OR time, which if minimized, potentially offsets the cost of the stapler cartridges [22].

Minimally Invasive Approaches in Liver Resection

General Principles

Michel Gagner is credited for the first laparoscopic partial hepatectomy in 1992 [23]. Despite close to 20 years of development and over 3000 reported cases internationally, minimally invasive liver surgery remains an emerging field [24].

In 2008, a consensus statement divided minimally invasive liver procedures into three categories: (1) pure, (2) hand-assisted, and (3) hybrid laparoscopy [25]. Pure laparoscopy involves complete mobilization and resection via laparoscopic ports, with an incision for specimen extraction only. Hand-assisted laparoscopy involves the elective placement of a hand port for mobilization or resection, which is then used for specimen extraction. Hybrid laparoscopy refers to a procedure in which the mobilization of liver is done laparoscopically, but resection and extraction are performed through a mini-laparotomy. This classification was reiterated in the report of Second International Consensus Conference held in Morioka, Japan, 2014 [26].

The indications for laparoscopic resection do not vary from open hepatic surgery and the same oncologic principles are utilized. Appropriate oncologic resection must include negative margins and maintenance of maximal hepatic remnant (Table 35.4).

Table 35.4 Indications and contraindications for laparoscopic partial hepatectomy

Indications
Location
1. Segments I through VIII
Pathology
1. Benign and malignant neoplasms
2. Cystic lesions
3. Parasitic lesions
Size
1. Any size lesion, not in proximity to major vascular structures
2. Pedunculated lesions, not in proximity to major vascular structures
Relative contraindications
Location
1. Lesions near the inferior vena cava (IVC), hilum, or hepatic veins insertion site to IVC
2. Multiple bilateral lesions
Pathology
1. Coagulopathy or thrombocytopenia
2. Moderate to severe portal hypertension
Absolute contraindications
1. Gallbladder cancer and hilar cholangiocarcinoma
2. Inability to obtain a negative surgical margin that would otherwise be possible in an open approach
3. Patient unable to tolerate pneumoperitoneum

Laparoscopic liver resection provides the potential advantages including: shorter operative times, shorter lengths of hospitalization, less operative blood loss, reduced transfusion requirements, a reduced need for analgesia, improved maintenance of abdominal wall integrity, earlier access to adjuvant therapy because of quicker recovery, fewer postoperative adhesions, and improved cosmesis. Multiple large studies have compared the open technique to the laparoscopic approach and demonstrated similar outcomes [27].

Positioning

Patient positioning for minimal invasive liver procedures is similar to that described for open technique.

Port Placement and Conduct of Operation

A single laparoscopic port is placed in order to carefully inspect the peritoneal cavity and provided no occult disease is present, additional ports are placed accordingly. If the hand-assisted technique is required, the hand port will be placed in accordance with planned resection and the patient's body habits.

Following port placement, the four steps and principles for open liver surgery are pursued. This process will include: Laparoscopic exploration of abdominal cavity for any possible disease spread, mobilization and exposure of the liver by proper ligament division and retraction, reassessment of the disease process with the use of laparoscopic IOUS, inflow, outflow control and preservation of biliary tree integrity by laparoscopic dissection, parenchymal transection with the use of laparoscopic energy devises, dissectors, and staplers. When the resection is completed and hemostasis achieved, the umbilical access port is enlarged for specimen removal within a specimen bag, if necessary.

In conclusion, laparoscopic liver surgery is a safe procedure for thoughtfully selected patients, when performed by experienced surgeons. It offers considerable perioperative benefits compared to laparotomy. In addition, oncologic outcomes and survival for HCC and colorectal metastases have been demonstrated to be equivalent in nonrandomized trials.

Complications and Hazards of Liver Surgery

Three major complications of liver resection are bleeding, biliary complications, and liver failure. Hemorrhage may occur during the operation from open branches of hepatic artery, portal vein, or hepatic veins and requires immediate attention. There are multiple techniques to halt bleeding ranging from manual compression and suture repair of the bleeding vessel to vascular isolation. As mentioned before, Pringle maneuver can provide helpful inflow control to the liver. This technique will temporarily occlude arterial and portal venous flow to the liver, which in return will facilitate the identification and control of bleeding source.

Biliary fistula, strictures, or leakage can also occur postoperatively. This may require drainage, endoscopic stenting, percutaneous transhepatic biliary drainage, or rarely a second surgical procedure.

Postoperative liver failure and postoperative mortality are related to the extent of remnant liver preserved. Minimal risk of postoperative liver failure is present if the majority of the resection volume has been replaced by an extensive tumor mass. In such patients, compensatory hypertrophy of the unaffected residual liver already may have occurred prior to resection and the loss of functional parenchyma is limited. The incidence of other surgical complications such as intraabdominal infections may also trigger postoperative liver failure. Furthermore, cirrhosis predisposes patients to multiorgan failure after major hepatic resections.

Ascites accumulation after liver resection is one of the most frequent complications encountered after liver resection in cirrhotic patients, occurring in up to 80 % of patients. Gross abdominal distension can interfere with respiratory function and may result in leakage, infection and/or disruption of the surgical incision. Large volume ascites may also lead to major fluid, protein, and electrolyte imbalances.

Most common types of postoperative infections include: surgical site and soft tissue infections, bacteremia and blood stream infections, intraabdominal and/or

Table 35.5 Treatment options for unresectable liver tumors

– Transplantation
– Percutaneous cryosurgery, radiofrequency, or microwave ablative techniques
– Percutaneous ethanol injection
– Systemic chemotherapy
– Liver-directed chemotherapy including chemoembolization, regional chemotherapy, and isolated hepatic perfusion
– Radioembolization
– External Radiation Beam therapy

deep organ/space infections such as liver abscesses. Alteration of humoral and cellular immunity is common in cirrhotic patients. Therefore, infections should be treated aggressively with broad-spectrum antibiotics after liver surgery, to avoid subsequent complications.

Alternatives for Liver Resection

Transplantation and surgical resection are the gold-standard curative treatment options for any primary or metastatic liver lesion. Unfortunately, resection is only feasible in approximately 30 % of patients at diagnosis. Tumor size, location, and/or quantity may preclude a surgical resection. The patients' general condition and concurrent comorbidities also may prevent liver resection. Multiple treatment options exist for those patients deemed unresectable (Table 35.5).

Chemotherapy and radiation therapy are the mainstay of adjuvant treatment sequencing. In addition, these treatment options could be used as a palliative approach or in an effort to downstage the tumors. Regional therapies such as transarterial chemoembolization (TACE), radioembolization, or ablative techniques are also utilized as bridging treatments, while patients wait on the liver transplantation list.

In summary, liver resection is a curative approach for thoughtfully selected patients. It can be performed safely with low mortality and acceptable morbidity rates in specialized centers. Unfortunately, it is only feasible in approximately 30 % of patients at diagnosis. Therefore, other treatment options such as liver directed therapies and liver transplantation must also be present for comprehensive management.

References

1. Belghiti J et al. Seven hundred forty-seven hepatectomies in the 1990s: an update to evaluate the actual risk of liver resection. J Am Coll Surg. 2000;191(1):38–46.
2. Bruix J, Sherman M, Practice Guidelines Committee, American Association for the Study of Liver Diseases. Management of hepatocellular carcinoma. Hepatology. 2005;42(5):1208–36.
3. Srinevas K, Andrew S, Ryan S, Gamblin TC, et al. Major liver resection in elderly patients: a multi-institutional analysis. J Am Coll Surg. 2011;212(5):787–95.

4. Cho S, Steel J, Tsung A, et al. Safety of liver resection in the elderly: how important is age? Ann Surg Oncol. 2011;18(4):1088–95.
5. Oken MM, Creech RH, Tormey DC, et al. Toxicity and response criteria of the Eastern Cooperative Oncology Group. Am J Clin Oncol. 1982;5(6):649–55.
6. Nordlinger B et al. Surgical resection of colorectal carcinoma metastases to the liver: a prognostic scoring system to improve case selection based on 1,568 patients. Association Française de Chirurgie. Cancer. 1996;77(7):1254–62.
7. Nagao T et al. Hepatic resection for hepatocellular carcinoma: clinical features and long-term prognosis. Ann Surg. 1987;205(1):33–40.
8. Child CG et al. Surgery and portal hypertension. Major Probl Clin Surg. 1964;1:1–85.
9. Pugh RN et al. Transection of the oesophagus for bleeding oesophageal varices. Br J Surg. 1973;60(8):646–9.
10. Kamath PS et al. A model to predict survival in patients with end-stage liver disease. Hepatology. 2001;33(2):464–70.
11. Lam CM et al. Major hepatectomy for hepatocellular carcinoma in patients with an unsatisfactory indocyanine green clearance test. Br J Surg. 1999;86(8):1012–7.
12. Shoup M et al. Volumetric analysis predicts hepatic dysfunction in patients undergoing major liver resection. J Gastrointest Surg. 2003;7(3):325–30.
13. Shindoh J, Tzeng CW, Aloia T, et al. Optimal future liver remnant in patients treated with extensive preoperative chemotherapy for colorectal liver metastases. Ann Surg Oncol. 2013;20(8):2493.
14. Azoulay D et al. Percutaneous portal vein embolization increases the feasibility and safety of major liver resection for hepatocellular carcinoma in injured liver. Ann Surg. 2000;232(5):665–72.
15. Schnitzbauer AA, Lang SA, Goessmann H, Nadalin S, et al. Right portal vein ligation combined with in situ splitting induces rapid left lateral liver lobe hypertrophy enabling 2-staged extended right hepatic resection in small-for-size settings. Ann Surg. 2012;255(3):405–14.
16. Rubin GD. 3-D imaging with MDCT. Eur J Radiol. 2003;45 Suppl 1:S37–41.
17. Palmucci S et al. Magnetic resonance cholangiopancreatography and contrast-enhanced magnetic resonance cholangiopancreatography versus endoscopic ultrasonography in the diagnosis of extrahepatic biliary pathology. Radiol Med. 2010;115:732–46.
18. Strasberg S. Nomenclature of hepatic anatomy and resections: a review of the Brisbane 2000 system. J Hepatobiliary Pancreat Surg. 2005;12:351–5.
19. Jarnagin WR et al. A prospective analysis of staging laparoscopy in patients with hepatobiliary primary and secondary malignancies. J Gastrointest Surg. 2000;4:34–43.
20. Kooby DA et al. Influence of transfusions on perioperative and long-term outcome in patients following hepatic resection for colorectal metastases. Ann Surg. 2003;237(6):860–9.
21. Jarnagin W et al. Improvement in perioperative outcome after hepatic resection: analysis of 1,803 consecutive cases over the past decade. Ann Surg. 2002;236:397–407.
22. Balaa FK, Gamblin TC, Tsung A, et al. Right hepatic lobectomy using the staple technique in 101 patients. J Gastrointest Surg. 2008;12(2):338–43.
23. Gagner M, Rheault M, Dubuc J. Laparoscopic partial hepatectomy for liver tumor. Surg Endosc. 1992;6:97–8.
24. Nguyen KT, Gamblin TC, Geller DA. World review of laparoscopic liver resection: 2,804 patients. Ann Surg. 2009;250(5):831–41.
25. Buell JF et al. The international position on laparoscopic liver surgery: the Louisville Statement, 2008. Ann Surg. 2009;250(5):825–30.
26. Wakabayashi G, Cherqui D, Geller DA, et al. Recommendations for laparoscopic liver resection: a report from the second international consensus conference held in Morioka. Ann Surg. 2015;261(4):619–29.
27. Nguyen KT et al. Minimally invasive liver resection for metastatic colorectal cancer: a multi-institutional, international report of safety, feasibility, and early outcomes. Ann Surg. 2009;250(5):842–8.

Chapter 36
Liver Transplantation: An Overview

Joohyun Kim and Johnny C. Hong

Who Should Be Considered for Liver Transplantation?

For patients with irreversible liver disease, either secondary to acute or chronic causes, orthotopic liver transplantation (OLT) is a durable life-saving treatment modality with excellent long-term survival outcomes [1–3]. Furthermore, OLT provides/restores long-term physiologic and psychological well-being as well as superior quality of life compared to patients with liver disease or other chronic conditions [4, 5]. The general indications for OLT include: end-stage liver disease, hepatic encephalopathy, hyper-bilirubinemia, portal hypertension, hepatic synthetic dysfunction, poor quality of life due to liver disease, and specific liver and bile duct cancers.

Viral Hepatitis

Viral hepatitis is the most common primary liver disease in cirrhotic patients. In 2014, 20 % of all liver transplantation cases in the United States (US) were for hepatitis C-related cirrhosis and 13 % were for alcohol-related cirrhosis. Chronic hepatitis C

J. Kim, M.D., Ph.D.
Division of Transplant Surgery, Department of Surgery, Medical College of Wisconsin,
9200 W. Wisconsin Ave., Suite E5700, Milwaukee, WI 53226, USA
e-mail: jokim@mcw.edu

J.C. Hong, M.D., F.A.C.S. (✉)
Division of Transplant Surgery, Department of Surgery, Medical College of Wisconsin,
9200 W. Wisconsin Ave., Suite E5700, Milwaukee, WI 53226, USA

A Joint Program of Froedtert & Medical College of Wisconsin, Children's Hospital of
Wisconsin & Blood Center of Wisconsin, 9200 W. Wisconsin Ave., Suite E5700, Milwaukee,
WI 53226, USA
e-mail: jhong@mcw.edu

© Springer International Publishing Switzerland 2017
K. Saeian, R. Shaker (eds.), *Liver Disorders*,
DOI 10.1007/978-3-319-30103-7_36

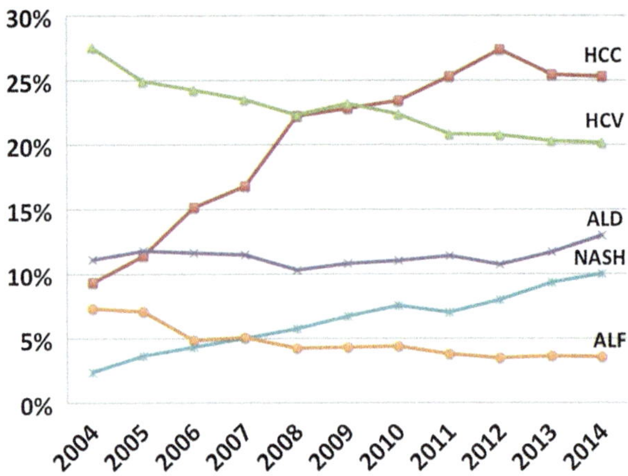

Fig. 36.1 Trends in the distribution of major indications for liver transplantation over the past decade in the United States. *HCC* hepatocellular carcinoma, *HCV* hepatitis C, *ALD* alcoholic liver disease, *NASH* nonalcoholic steatohepatitis, *ALF* acute liver failure

recurs universally after liver transplantation, between 80 and 100 % of cases recur within 4 years after OLT and 20–40 % of patients develop cirrhosis in the graft after 5 years [6, 7]. With the recent introduction of direct-acting antivirals in the treatment of hepatitis C, it is likely that the rates of recurrence as well as progression to cirrhosis will diminish [8]. In contrast, recurrence of hepatitis B infection after OLT (<5 %) has been effectively controlled with the use of a combination of long-term antivirals and intravenous anti-hepatitis B immunoglobulin after OLT [9].

Nonalcoholic Fatty Liver Disease

While hepatitis C-related cirrhosis remains the most common indication for OLT, there has been a downward trend over the past decade as shown in Fig. 36.1. Interestingly, the proportion of OLT for nonalcoholic steatohepatitis has markedly increased. Nonalcoholic steatohepatitis commonly recurs after OLT, but it rarely progresses to cirrhosis. This group of patients is frequently associated with metabolic syndrome, obesity, and chronic diabetic kidney disease.

Alcohol-Related Cirrhosis

Alcoholic liver disease is another common cause of cirrhosis. Patients with alcoholic liver disease commonly have comorbidities such as Wernicke's encephalopathy, malnutrition (including vitamin deficiency), and cardiomyopathy. It is important to maintain abstinence prior to transplantation, and some patients show stabilization and improvement of liver function such that transplantation is not required. Patients with substance abuse issues need an appropriate referral for a comprehensive evaluation and treatment. A multidisciplinary approach is required to address the multiple medical comorbidities related to cirrhosis and chronic illness as well as to ensure adequate psychosocial coping and a support structure to minimize the risk for recidivism. Any concern related to the patient's compliance should be addressed before the patient is placed on the recipient list.

Acute Liver Failure

Hepatic failure occurs in patients without any previous history of chronic liver disease, and this rare disease entity is called fulminant hepatic failure or acute liver failure (ALF). Traditionally, fulminant liver failure was defined as severe liver injury in which hepatic encephalopathy occurred less than 8 weeks after the onset of symptoms in an individual without preexisting liver disease, whereas subfulminant liver failure was defined as an onset of encephalopathy after 8 weeks but before 26 weeks after the onset of symptoms. The previous subcategories of ALF based on timing and severity of clinical presentation—hyperacute as the onset of encephalopathy within 7 days, acute as the onset between 7 and 28 days, and subacute as the onset between 28 days and 24 weeks—are no longer advocated by the National Institutes of Health (NIH) working group [10].

In 2008, the NIH working group on acute liver failure recommended that the term "acute liver failure" is preferable and that the most reliable signs of severe acute liver injury are the presence of coagulopathy (international normalized ratio [INR] >1.5) and any degree of encephalopathy occurring within 24 weeks of the first onset of symptoms in patients without underlying liver disease [10]. In 2014, acute liver failure accounted for 4% of all liver transplantation indications in the United States. Acetaminophen (APAP) toxicity is the leading cause (40%) of ALF. The other common etiologies are idiosyncratic drug-induced liver injury (13%), hepatitis B infection (6%), ischemic hepatitis (6%), autoimmune hepatitis (4%), Wilson's disease (3%), pregnancy (2%), Budd-Chiari syndrome (2%), malignancy (1%), and indeterminate (17%). Multiorgan failure is the most common cause of death from ALF, accounting for >50%, followed by intracranial hypertension and infection. The progress of the disease is rapid once the patient develops encephalopathy and is associated with an extremely high mortality without OLT. With timely OLT, the long-term patient survival ranges from 60 to 80%. As such, it is recommended to identify the etiology of ALF (i.e., APAP toxicity, mushroom poisoning, etc.), initiate an etiology-specific therapy for patients with ALF, and transfer the patients to a liver transplantation center as soon as ALF is suspected [10].

When Should Liver Transplantation Be Considered for Treatment of Liver and Bile Duct Cancers?

Curative treatment of hepatobiliary malignancy, complete extirpation of the tumor including all microscopically detectable disease, requires a multidisciplinary approach to provide the best chance for long-term tumor recurrence-free survival. It is prudent to have a comprehensive treatment plan in place prior to tumor manipulation. Incomplete resection (residual tumor) or invasive procedures (i.e. biopsy, locoregional therapy) increase the risk for tumor cell seeding that may negatively impact the overall patient survival. As such, all therapeutic modalities, including OLT, should be included in the initial treatment decision algorithm.

Hepatocellular carcinoma (HCC) is the most common type of liver cancer and a common indication for OLT. Hepatocellular carcinoma (HCC) accounts for 90 % of all primary liver cancers and it is projected to become the third leading cause of cancer-related death in the US by 2030. It is estimated that 80–90 % of all HCC cases result from cirrhosis. This explains the relatively high HCC morality rate, because management options are more limited in the setting of cirrhosis [11, 12]. Liver resection plays a limited role in HCC because of the higher rate of recurrence and post-hepatectomy liver failure in cirrhosis [12, 13].

OLT offers the best oncologic resection of HCC, treats cirrhosis, and restores normal hepatic function. The proportion of OLT for HCC has remarkably increased. In 2014, 25 % of OLTs in the US were for HCC (Fig. 36.1). HCC may recur even when OLT is performed without evidence of extrahepatic spread (e.g., major vascular invasion or distant metastasis). The Milan criteria were introduced to select patients with early HCC who would benefit from OLT. These criteria are based on the size and number of tumors: one lesion ≤5 cm or two or three lesions ≤3 cm. A systemic review reported a 5-year survival rate ranging from 65 to 78 % for patients who underwent OLT for HCC within the Milan criteria, which is comparable to the survival rate of patients with noncancer indications [14].

The current MELD system allows exception points to a patient with HCC meeting one of the following criteria: one lesion ≥2 cm and ≤5 cm or two or three lesions ≥1 cm and ≤3 cm. All eligible patients with HCC meeting specific criteria are immediately granted MELD exception points (independent of the patient's calculated laboratory MELD score). In patients with localized HCC, OLT provides an excellent curative treatment for eligible patients, 5-year tumor recurrence-free survival between 60 and 70 %.

Cholangiocarcinoma (CCA) is a malignant neoplasm arising from epithelial cells of the extrahepatic and intrahepatic bile ducts, excluding the papilla of Vater and the gallbladder [15]. CCA is the second most common primary hepatobiliary malignancy in the US. The incidence of CCA is increasing, and its prognosis remains grim without surgical treatment [16, 17]. Early diagnosis has been a constant challenge, because there is no effective screening test, and most patients with unresectable disease die within 6–12 months of diagnosis. Anatomically, CCA is classified into the proximal type, also known as hilar (HCCA), perihilar, or Klatskin tumors, that accounts for 60–70 % of cases; distal type for 20–30 %; and intrahepatic (ICCA) or peripheral for the remaining 5–10 %. The three different types of CCA have distinct pathophysiology, differ in their epidemiological features and clinical presentations, and vary in surgical treatments [18]. The primary modality of treatment for HCCA is radical bile duct resection with partial hepatectomy; for ICCA, partial hepatectomy; and for the distal type of CCA, pancreaticoduodenectomy. For patients with unresectable

Table 36.1 Criteria for MELD exception for liver transplant candidates with cholangiocarcinoma

- Centers must submit a written protocol for patient care to the UNOS Liver and Intestinal Committee before requesting a MELD score exception for a candidate with CCA. This protocol should include selection criteria, administration of neoadjuvant therapy before transplantation, and operative staging to exclude patients with regional hepatic lymph node metastases, intrahepatic metastases, and/or extrahepatic disease. The protocol should include data collection as deemed necessary by UNOS.
- Candidates must satisfy diagnostic criteria for hilar CCA: malignant-appearing stricture on cholangiography and biopsy or cytology results demonstrating malignancy, carbohydrate antigen 19-9 >100 U/mL, or aneuploidy. The tumor should be considered unresectable on the basis of technical considerations or underlying liver disease (e.g., PSC).
- If cross-sectional imaging studies (CT scan, ultrasound, MRI) demonstrate a mass, the mass should be ≤3 cm.
- Intra- and extrahepatic metastases should be excluded by cross-sectional imaging studies of the chest and abdomen at the time of initial exception and every 3 months before score increases.
- Regional hepatic lymph node involvement and peritoneal metastases should be assessed by operative staging after completion of neoadjuvant therapy and before LT. Endoscopic ultrasound-guided aspiration of regional hepatic lymph nodes may be advisable to exclude patients with obvious metastases before neoadjuvant therapy is initiated.
- Transperitoneal aspiration or biopsy of the primary tumor (either by endoscopic ultrasound, operative, or percutaneous approaches) should be avoided because of the high risk of tumor seeding associated with these procedures.

HCCA or ICCA, OLT presents a viable option and has been reported to provide survival benefits [19]. A predictive index for tumor recurrence after liver transplantation for locally advanced intrahepatic and hilar cholangiocarcinoma has been reported to facilitate patient selection. Based on this patient-tumor stratification system, a survival benefit of 5-year tumor recurrence-free of up to 78 % can be achieved with neoadjuvant therapy followed by OLT in the low risk category. There was no long-term survivor for patients in the high-risk group [20]. However, current MELD allocation only grants exception points for patients with HCCA meeting stringent Mayo Criteria (Table 36.1).

When Should Evaluation for Liver Transplantation Be Considered?

Regardless of the etiology of cirrhosis, patients may suffer from complications of portal hypertension and hepatic dysfunction, including hepatic encephalopathy, variceal bleeding, ascites, spontaneous bacterial peritonitis and/or hepatorenal syndrome. While the initial episodes of hepatic decompensation typically respond well to medical treatments, the underlying liver disease progresses, which leads to more frequent and severe occurrences of these complications. For patients with decompensated cirrhosis, the annual mortality and 5-year patient survival rates are approximately 20 % and 50 %, respectively.

The etiology of the patient's liver disease generally dictates the timing for referral to a transplant center or specialist. In patients with cirrhosis, the progression of the disease is initially slow and may take many years. However, once the patient shows the first signs of complications of cirrhosis, it is difficult to predict the clinical course of the patient, and the patient's health condition may rapidly deteriorate. Furthermore, chronic illness frequently leads to multiple patient comorbidities, i.e., malnutrition, debilitation, psychosocial issues, cardiopulmonary risk factors, that need to be addressed prior to orthotopic liver transplantation (OLT). As such, it is recommended to start the evaluation of the patient's candidacy for OLT after the first episode of hepatic decompensation, defined a major complication of cirrhosis, i.e., variceal hemorrhage, and hepatorenal syndrome.

In those with acute (fulminant) liver failure, the course of the disease is rapid and the risk of death without transplantation is extremely high. Whenever this diagnosis is suspected, early transfer to a transplant center is imperative in order to ensure timely evaluation and if deemed suitable for liver transplantation, medical optimization, and subsequent OLT. It is important to take into consideration the inherent waiting time for organ availability for transplantation due to an ongoing organ crisis.

How Long Is the Waiting Time for a Deceased-Donor Liver After Placement on the Waiting List?

For patients with end-stage liver disease, OLT is the only life-saving treatment modality. With the scarcity of organs for transplantation, the current Model for End-Stage Liver Disease/Pediatric End-Stage Liver Disease (MELD/PELD) liver allocation system prioritizes the organ based on medical urgency based on the patient's risk of death while awaiting liver transplantation. In short, the deceased donor liver graft is allocated for the sickest patient on the waiting list, based on the patient's MELD score, to reduce the number of patients dying while on the waiting list.

For patients 12 years of age and older, the MELD scoring system uses the patient's values for serum bilirubin, serum creatinine, and the international normalized ratio to predict the 90-day mortality risk while on the waiting list. It is calculated according to the following formula [21]:

$$\begin{aligned}
\text{MELD Score} \ &= 0.957 \times \log_e \left(\text{creatinine mg}/\text{dL} \right) \\
&+ 0.378 \times \log_e \left(\text{bilirubin mg}/\text{dL} \right) \\
&+ 1.120 \times \log_e \left(\text{INR} \right) \\
&+ 0.643
\end{aligned}$$

UNOS has made the following modifications to the score:

- For candidates with an initial MELD score greater than 11, the MELD score is then re-calculated as follows:

  $$\text{MELD Score} = \text{MELD(i)} + 1.32*(137-\text{Na}) - [0.033*\text{MELD(i)}*(137-\text{Na})]$$

- MELD(i) is initial MELD score without consideration of serum sodium values. Sodium values less than 125 mmol/L will be set to 125, and values greater than 137 mmol/L will be set to 137.

- If the patient has been dialyzed twice within the last 7 days, then the value for serum creatinine used should be 4.0
- Any value less than 1 is given a value of 1 (i.e., if bilirubin is 0.8, a value of 1.0 is used) to prevent the occurrence of scores below 0 (the natural logarithm of 1 is 0, and any positive value below 1 would yield a negative result)

MELD score ranges from 6 to ≥40. Patients having a MELD score <9 are associated with 1.9 % mortality whereas patients having a MELD score ≥40 are associated with a mortality rate of >70 %.

For patients less than 12 years of age, the PELD scoring system uses the values for serum bilirubin, serum albumin, INR, whether or not the patient is less than 1 year old, and whether or not the patient has growth failure (<−2 standard deviation) to predict survival.

$$
\begin{aligned}
\text{PELD Score} \quad =\ &0.480 \times \log_e (\text{creatinine mg}/\text{dL}) \\
&+1.857 \times \log_e (\text{INR}) \\
&-0.687 \times \log_e (\text{albumin g}/\text{dL})
\end{aligned}
$$

+0.436 if the patient is less than 1 year old (scores for patients listed for liver transplantation before the patient's first birthday continue to include the value assigned for age ($<1\,\text{Year}$) until the patient reaches

the age of 24 months)
+0.667 if the patient has growth failure (<-2 Standard deviation)

While the MELD score correlates well with a 3-month risk of mortality for the majority of the patients on the waiting list, there are some conditions associated with chronic liver disease that may diminish patient survival but that are not directly accounted for in the MELD scoring system. In short, the severity of illness in patients with certain liver disease types and comorbidities may not be reflected on the patient's calculated laboratory MELD score. For patients who meet these specific disease-related criteria, MELD exceptions points maybe granted. These standard MELD exceptions were developed to more accurately reflect the patient's mortality risk while awaiting OLT. Standard MELD exceptions include: HCC, hepatopulmonary syndrome, portopulmonary hypertension, familial amyloid polyneuropathy, primary hyperoxaluria, hilar cholangiocarcinoma, and hepatic artery thrombosis occurring within 14 days after OLT.

The implementation of the MELD/PELD system has decreased the mortality rate while on the waiting list. It is important to note that while the MELD scoring system is a powerful predictor of pre-transplant survival, it does not predict survival rate after OLT.

Allocation of Liver Grafts

It is estimated that approximately 3000 patients on the liver transplantation waiting list become too sick and die every year in the US. Therefore, it is imperative to have an effective and fair organ allocation system. The first national computer-based matching system was introduced in 1977 by the United Network for Organ Sharing (UNOS), an independent nonprofit organization. The organ allocation policy has been revised multiple times, and allocations are based on three major factors: geographic location, ABO blood type, and the severity of illness of the patients. UNOS divided the US into 11 regions and 59 service areas, and organs are primarily allocated by this geographic system. Blood type is another important consideration. In general, ABO-incompatible deceased liver transplantation is not performed due to the high incidence of posttransplant liver failure and severe ischemic cholangiopathy. The third and the most important factor is the severity of illness of a patient, and to improve the allocation efficiency, UNOS has been using the model for end-stage liver disease (MELD) score to prioritize candidates for liver transplantation since 2002. The MELD score was originally introduced to predict mortality in cirrhotic patients undergoing a transjugular intrahepatic postosystemic shunt procedure. Multiple follow-up studies have validated that the MELD score correlates to the 3-month mortality rate of cirrhotic patients in a variety of settings. For example, a prospective observational study of 3437 adult liver transplant candidates reported that the 3-month mortality rate in patients with a MELD score of less than 9 was 2 %; in contrast, the mortality rate of patients with a MELD score of 40 or higher was 71 % [22]. The MELD score is based on the results of three blood tests: the prothrombin time international normalized ratio (PT-INR) and the serum levels of total bilirubin and creatinine. Because this score is based on objective laboratory findings, the process has become more transparent and efficient. An Internet-based calculation tool is also available at the Organ Procurement and Transplantation Network (OPTN) website, and it notes that a candidate for liver transplantation has a MELD score ranging from 6 to 40 [21]. The MELD score has also been utilized to stratify the risk of patients. Waitlist and posttransplant mortality analyses have demonstrated that patients with a MELD score that is less than 15 do not gain survival benefit from liver transplantation [23]. On the other hand, if a patient's MELD score is 35 or higher, UNOS prioritizes the patient to a liver graft from donors in the expanded geographic area in order to increase the probability of an organ offer for that sick patient. It is important to note that the MELD score, which is a powerful predictor of pre-transplant survival, does not predict survival rate after liver transplantation.

In some specific patient groups, the MELD score does not reflect the severity of the liver disease or the patient's actual waiting list mortality risk. Liver function may be normal in patients with HCC, and an allocation system based on "raw" MELD score may not allow a timely transplant prior to cancer progression beyond transplant eligibility. For HCC patients whose outcome after liver transplantation is reasonably good enough to justify the use of deceased-donor organs (a 5-year tumor recurrence-free survival between 60 and 70 %), the current MELD system allows exception points to the patients with HCC meeting one of the following criteria: one lesion ≥ 2 cm and ≤ 5 cm or two or three lesions ≥ 1 cm and ≤ 3 cm. Prior to October 8, 2015, all eligible patients with HCC meeting specific criteria were immediately granted MELD exception points of 22 (independent of the patient's calculated laboratory MELD score), which is equivalent to 15 % risk of 3-month mortality. However, 5 % of all HCC patients still dropped out within 3 months of the listing [24]. Additional MELD points were granted every 3 months as long as the patient remained within Milan criteria. While HCC patients are waiting on the list, various types of locoregional therapies (i.e., transarterial embolization (TACE), microwave ablation, Yttrium 90 radioembolization, radiofrequency ablation) are available to control tumor burden progression [25]. These neoadjuvant therapies have been effective bridge treatments to OLT.

Most recently, a revision to the OPTN/UNOS policy on the timing of exception scores assigned and maximum value of exception scores for candidates with HCC was implemented on October 8, 2015. The revised policy is intended to create a better balance in transplant opportunities between candidates with HCC and those with allocation priority based on their calculated MELD and PELD scores. Under this modification, a new timetable delays assignment of new or extended exception scores. The transplant candidate will be registered with their calculated MELD and PELD scores for at least 6 months and should remain within the HCC criteria prior to receiving a MELD exception score of 28 and PELD score of 34. The revised policy also capped a maximum MELD exception score of 34 for transplant candidates meeting the HCC criteria.

Patients with unresectable, localized hilar cholangiocarcinoma can be considered for liver transplantation after neoadjuvant radio-chemotherapy, and they receive MELD exception points at a UNOS-qualified transplant center. On the other hand, the survival benefit from liver transplantation in patients with intrahepatic cholangiocarcinoma is being debated, and under the current UNOS policy, they do not receive MELD exception points. Other examples of the MELD exception include hepatopulmonary syndrome, portopulmonary hypertension, and neuroendocrine tumor liver metastasis.

Acute liver failure is a rare, lethal, and rapidly progressing type of liver disease. Therefore, UNOS classifies the disease as a special category called "Status 1A." To be listed as Status 1A, an acute liver failure patient must meet at least one the following criteria: ventilator dependence, requirement of dialysis (or continuous hemofiltration), or an international normalized ratio (INR) greater than 2.0. Status 1A patients get top priority for liver organs over all other candidates, regardless of their MELD score. In general, with the exception of Wilson's, acute decompensation of the underlying liver disease is not considered to be a criterion for Status 1A. The immediate failure of liver transplantation (primary nonfunction or hepatic artery thrombosis) is also categorized as Status 1A. All other potential liver transplantation patients receive points based on their MELD score or the MELD exception criteria.

The Key Considerations and Contraindications for Liver Transplantation

Liver transplantation is a spectrum of care including the donor/recipient selection, the surgical procedure, the postoperative management with immunosuppression, education, and rehabilitation. The candidacy should be evaluated from many different angles with the best prediction of short-term and long-term outcomes. The candidate's overall medical history, including the status of the primary liver disease, should be reviewed, and a posttransplant management plan should be established. When the candidate is on the list and eventually receives the organ offer, the quality of the donor and the physical condition of the candidate should be evaluated before the final decision for transplantation is made (Table 36.2).

Careful review of the candidate's medical history is an important initial step. Severe hemodynamic instability is not infrequent during a liver transplantation procedure and the candidate's baseline cardiopulmonary function should be healthy enough to tolerate it. In addition to the risk factor assessment, electrocardiograms and echocardiograms are used to screen candidates for ischemic heart disease, congestive heart failure, valvular heart disease, and arrhythmias. Patients at risk of coronary artery disease, especially those who are elderly or who have diabetes, need a coronary angiogram. Severe coronary artery disease or valvular heart disease, which are not amenable to treatment, preclude liver transplantation. If the echocardiogram result suggests high right ventricular systolic pressure, right heart catheterization is indicated. If the right heart catheterization confirms significant pulmonary hypertension, appropriate medical treatment should be offered to correct it, because the outcome of liver transplantation with persistent severe pulmonary hypertension is dismal. Patients whose pulmonary hypertension responds to medical therapy are considered candidates for transplantation. Patients with fluid overload from acute

Table 36.2 Contraindications to liver transplantation

Cardiopulmonary factors	Other systemic factors
• Severe coronary artery disease or valvular heart disease not amenable to treatment • Persistent severe pulmonary hypertension with medical treatment • Severe respiratory failure with maximum ventilator support • Shock with maximum use of vasopressor agents	• Uncontrolled active infection • A recent history of cancer from nonhepatic origin with high risk of recurrence • Any cancer with distant metastasis • Irreversible severe brain injury • Significant psychosocial issues precluding recovery from transplantation

kidney injury may underestimate the cardiac function and they may require dialysis for an accurate estimation of that function. Some patients have hypoxemia from hepatopulmonary syndrome, and the 5-year mortality rate of those patients reaches 76 % without liver transplantation; however, liver transplantation can decrease the mortality rate to 23 % [26]. UNOS assigns MELD exception points to a patient with significant hepatopulmonary syndrome. After liver transplantation, the hypoxia gradually recovers within a period of 3 months or more. When a suitable donor is available, the cardiopulmonary function of the patient should be re-evaluated. A patient with severe respiratory failure or with shock who requires maximum supportive care cannot tolerate surgical stress from liver transplantation. Uncontrolled active infection, such as pneumonia, is also a known contraindication.

Renal dysfunction is relatively common in patients with liver cirrhosis and ascites. Accurate assessment of renal function is difficult as the Cockcroft-Gault equation overestimates the glomerular filtration rate (GFR) in cirrhotic patients. The Modification of Diet in Renal Disease (MDRD-6) equation with six variables has been suggested as an alternative calculation method for cirrhotic patients [27]. Assessment of renal function in liver transplant candidates is important, because patients with renal impairment frequently develop metabolic acidosis, hyperkalemia, and volume overload during liver transplantation. Planned intraoperative renal replacement therapy can improve the outcome in patients with renal impairment [28]. Hepatorenal syndrome (HRS) is an important cause of acute kidney injury in cirrhotic patients, and the patient's kidney function may return after liver transplantation in 58–94 %. However, 1-year patient survival after liver only transplantation in hepatorenal syndrome was reported low at 66–74 %. Therefore, patients with irreversible acute kidney injury and advanced chronic kidney disease require a combined liver and kidney transplantation. In light of the fact that GFR of liver transplantation recipients drops up to 40 %, consideration for combined liver and kidney transplantation should be individually evaluated. Criteria for combined liver-kidney transplantation based on GFR from MDRD-6 were proposed, but there is a wide disparity in the selection criteria for a simultaneous combined liver and kidney transplantation among transplantation centers [29, 30].

A recent history of cancer from nonhepatic origin is a contraindication of liver transplantation. The decision to perform a liver transplant needs to be informed by carefully considering the type and stage of the cancer and the time period since the last curative treatment. Any evidence of distant metastasis is a contraindication for liver transplantation, but liver metastasis from neuroendocrine tumors is an exception. If the primary neuroendocrine tumor is completely resected and the liver is the only site of the metastasis, liver transplantation can offer a reasonable long-term outcome with a 5-year overall survival rate of 58 % [31]. For patients on the waiting list with primary liver cancer within criteria for liver transplantation, the progression of the disease should be periodically monitored by CT or MRI.

Multiorgan failure, sepsis, and cerebral edema are major causes of death in ALF, and only less than 20 % of all patients can survive without a liver transplant. Because most patients who survive without transplantation can expect a normal life, various prognostic criteria based on age, coagulopathy, causes of the liver injury and encephalopathy have been developed to select patients who do not require liver transplantation. However, all of these criteria have the limitation of low sensitivity, and none of them have been widely accepted in practice because the consequence of false-negative selection for liver transplantation is death which could otherwise have been prevented [32]. The progression of cerebral edema should be carefully monitored in ALF. As noninvasive tests are generally not accurate to predict outcome, invasive monitoring of intracranial pressure can be considered. It has been reported that neurologic recovery is poor when cerebral perfusion pressure is less than 40 mmHg or when intracranial pressure is higher than 40 mmHg. However, bleeding is a known complication and the benefit of this approach has been debated [33]. The progression to irreversible neurologic injury or the development of severe infection precludes liver transplantation as it does in any other indications.

A suitable deceased donor may not be available in a timely manner, and living donor liver transplantation can be an option when it is available. According to a US multicenter study, the median time from listing to first living donor evaluation was 1.5 days and the median time from evaluation to living donor transplantation was only 1 day. Whether or not the potential living donor's decision to donate has been influenced by coercion should be carefully considered even in this time-sensitive situation [34].

Donor Factors

When a deceased donor is available, the risk of transmission of disease from the donor, such as cancer or infection, should be reviewed first. Next, the following factors should be considered when attempting to match a suitable recipient candidate for liver transplantation: ABO blood type, size, and functional capacity. ABO incompatible deceased donor liver transplantation is generally reserved for a desperate situation, such as in acute liver failure, and it is related with poor outcome [32]. In live donor liver transplantation, pretreatment of recipients with plasmaphreresis and rituximab has been shown to improve the outcome of ABO-incompatible liver transplantation [35]. The size match is another important factor. When the capacity of the abdominal cavity in a recipient is small, a relatively large graft implantation may result in impairment of organ perfusion, especially when the abdomen is closed. If a graft, especially a partial graft, is too small for a recipient, it may result in posttransplant graft failure. The third and the most difficult factor to evaluate is the functional capacity of the recipient and the graft. In general, the recipient with a higher metabolic demand (e.g., high MELD score) requires a better quality graft that can support immediate posttransplant recovery. The major factors related to graft "quality" are: age, underlying liver disease (e.g., fatty change and viral infection), and ischemic time. There is no upper limit for the chronological age of a donor. However, when a donor with advanced age is considered, other risk factors should be carefully reviewed. Underlying liver disease of the donor is an important factor to consider. When a donor's blood test result for viral hepatitis C is positive without evidence of significant clinical liver disease, transplantation can still be considered for a patient who already has hepatitis C. In the same manner, a donor with the hepatitis B core antibody without chronic liver disease can donate his or her liver to a patient with hepatitis B. A liver biopsy can aid in making this decision. Significant fatty infiltration of the liver graft (more than 30–60 % of macrovesicular steatosis) assessed by intraoperative visualization and biopsy is related to a higher incidence of primary nonfunction. In general, the assessment of a graft's suitability for transplantation, during organ procurement, to a specific recipient, is based on the direct visualization by experienced transplant surgeons and liver biopsy (if deemed necessary) [36].

During procurement and storage, the liver graft suffers from the interruption of blood flow, and the ischemic time correlates with the incidence of graft dysfunction. To minimize ischemic injury, the timing of the donor's surgery and the recipient's surgery, including transportation time, should be optimally arranged. Ischemic injury is also related to the type of donation.

Liver Graft Options

Liver grafts are donated from either deceased or live donors. For the deceased donor, the organ is procured after brain or circulatory death. Donation after brain death (DBD) donation is the most common type in the US. After a potential donor has been declared to be brain dead, suitable organs are allocated by the local organ procurement organization. All related donor surgery teams work together to procure organs at the designated time. This type of donation is ideal, because the organs receive blood perfusion until the moment when the cold preservation solution is infused into the graft, and ischemic organ injury can be minimized. When an individual has irreversible brain damage but does not meet the brain death criteria and withdrawal of care has been decided by the family, organs from this potential donor can be procured after cardiac arrest and declaration of death. This type of donation is called donation after circulatory (or cardiac) death, DCD [37]. The time between the withdrawal of ventilator support and the time of death is variable, and organs from this donation receive varying degrees of ischemic injury from diminished oxygen supply and blood flow [38]. The additional ischemic injury results in a higher incidence of primary nonfunction and ischemic cholangiopathy, and the impact of these two types of complications is significant [39]. The recipient with primary nonfunction cannot survive without emergency retransplantation; the patient with ischemic cholangiopathy may require multiple biliary interventions, and subsequent retransplantation of the liver.

A healthy live donor can donate a part of his or her liver to a designated recipient. There are a few benefits associated with live donor liver transplantation. It is an elective surgery by directed donation and the graft ischemic duration can be minimized, as it is possible to coordinate the donor's surgery and the recipient's surgery so they can occur simultaneously at the same center. With live donation of partial liver graft, the preservation of the interest and well being of the live donor is a top priority independent of the recipient. As such, a comprehensive evaluation of both the psychosocial and overall health status is an important first step. The surgical approach is planned based on pre-transplant imaging studies. The surgical plan for the liver resection is designed to preserve the vascular inflow and outflow of both the donor and the recipient. Therefore, the amount of liver for donation is determined by the vascular anatomy of the donor's liver. A young and healthy donor can tolerate resection of two-thirds of the liver volume. When the liver volume and quality is sufficient for the immediate postoperative recovery, the liver eventually regenerates to meet the metabolic demand in both the donor and the recipient. When a suitable deceased donor is not presumed to be available in a timely manner, live donor liver transplantation can be considered.

Surgical Procedures in Liver Transplantation

Donor Operation

The deceased donor organ procurement can yield either a whole liver or partial (split) graft. Deceased donor procedure can be variable but typically consists of: (a) evaluation of suitability of the organ for transplantation, (b) cold preservation of the organs through the cannulation into the systemic and portal circulation (e.g., aorta and inferior mesenteric vein), (c) dissection and removal of the organs from the abdominal cavity, and (d) transport of the organ (cold preservation) to the recipient hospital. The organs start to undergo ischemic injury once the blood flow ceases, and this persists until the organ is reperfused with blood flow in the recipient. Even though tissue ischemia terminated at the time of the graft reperfusion, the inflammatory reaction from the reperfusion causes temporary and often severe organ damage. This ischemia-reperfusion injury is the main mechanism of injury in primary nonfunction, and no effective treatment is available to date. As such, shortening the organ ischemic duration is currently the only method to minimize ischemia-reperfusion injury.

The scarcity of organs for transplantation makes any innovation to increase the organ supply extremely important. When the deceased donor liver quality is ideal (e.g., a young donor without risk factors) and the anatomy is favorable, splitting the liver of a deceased donor to yield functional grafts for two recipients have improved the availability of donor organs and lowered mortality on the liver transplant waiting list. Splitting of the liver is an effective approach to expand the donor pool, and when performed by experienced centers, produced long-term survival outcomes comparable to whole organ liver transplantation [3, 40].

Partial liver grafts can also be obtained through live donation. Live donor hepatectomy consists of (a) delicate hilar dissection and liver mobilization and (b) parenchymal division. This procedure requires detailed planning, including the level of vascular division, the need for reconstruction, and the parenchymal volume distribution. All of the blood flow to the graft is kept patent until the recipient is ready for implantation. If there is a need for vascular or biliary reconstruction, the remnant liver (live donor) should remain intact to minimize the complication risk of the live donor while the partial graft intended for the recipient is reconstructed at the back table [41]. The overall complication rate for live donor hepatectomy has been reported to be up to 38 % with an incidence of live donor mortality at 0.2 % [42–45]. Long-term graft and recipient survival in both adults and children for split grafts from deceased and live donors is comparable to whole organ OLT [3].

Recipient Operation

Abdominal exploration is the first step in the recipient procedure. If there is an unexpected cancer spread outside of the liver, the transplantation should be aborted and the graft should be offered to the next candidate on the waiting list. When the intra-abdominal inspection is unremarkable, the hilum is dissected for vascular and biliary reconstruction and the liver is mobilized from the retroperitoneum. Once the native liver is removed (total hepatectomy), the graft liver is implanted in the following manner: the suprahepatic vena cava, infrahepatic vena cava (if caval replacement method is used), followed by the portal vein and hepatic artery.

Once the graft outflow and inflow anastomoses are completed, blood flow in the graft is restored and the graft reperfusion is established. At this time, the outflow of electrolytes and cytokines from the graft may cause temporary hemodynamic instability (reperfusion syndrome), and may cause hemodynamic instability and cardiac arrest in severe cases. The arterial anastomosis is then performed to complete all the vascular anastomoses.

Successful outcomes of liver transplantation are critically dependent on adequate venous outflow and uncompromised inflow to the graft. Hepatic artery and portal vein thrombosis are serious complications after OLT and decrease patient and graft survival [46]. As such, prompt diagnosis for vascular insufficiency and immediate vascular reconstructions (i.e., vascular conduits) are necessary when the portal venous or/and hepatic arterial inflow is/are not optimal for the new graft. Biliary reconstruction is the last step in graft implantation. In most cases, a choledocho-choledochostomy (duct-to-duct anastomosis) is performed. However, a bilio-enteric drainage by Roux-en-Y hepaticojejunostomy is performed in cases when the native bile duct is not suitable for anastomosis, or when there is a risk for native bile duct cancer.

What Is the Success Rate of Liver Transplantation?

OLT is a durable and the definitive lifesaving treatment modality for patients with irreversible liver failure. The current 5-year patient and graft survival rate of primary liver transplantation is 74 % and 67 %, respectively [21]. Recovery after liver transplantation is dependent on overall physical condition, surgical risk, operative factors, and graft function. The graft function is impacted by multiple factors including the age of the donor, the underlying liver condition of the donor (viral liver disease or fatty change), and the duration of time that the liver graft has been outside of the donor's body (ischemic time). After liver transplantation, the recovery can be complicated by vascular thrombosis in the liver graft or primary nonfunction. Other risks in recipients include graft rejection, recurrence of liver disease, and side effects of immunosuppression. Those side effects include infection, increased risk of cancer, hypertension, diabetes, lipid metabolism abnormality, and kidney injury among others.

To date, the balance between serving the "sickest first," as stipulated in the US Department of Health of Human Servises (HHS) "final rule," strikes a delicate balance with avoiding futile transplantation. While patients with MELD scores ≥40 have the highest 3-month waitlist mortality rate (80–100 %), these patients receive the greatest survival benefit from OLT, compared to patients with lower MELD scores. Allocation of organs to the "sickest first" has changed the characteristics of liver transplant recipients during the last decade and has brought new medical and economic challenges to bring these patients through OLT. Patients undergoing OLT today have more severe end-stage liver disease, are older, and have greater comorbidity, compared with the pre-MELD era. The presence of septic shock, cardiac risk, and significant comorbidities are known factors related to diminished survival after liver transplantation. With appropriate patient risk stratification and optimization, the patient with the highest acuity undergoing OLT can achieve a 5-year patient survival rate of 75 % [47].

Despite advances in perioperative management and immunosuppression, up to 22 % of patients suffer hepatic graft failure following primary OLT [48–51]. Causes of early graft failure after OLT include primary graft nonfunction and vascular complications [46, 51]; causes of late graft failure include recurrence of liver disease, chronic rejection, and complex biliary strictures related to a variety of etiologies [49, 52]. Retransplantation of the liver (ReLT) is the only option for survival when the transplanted graft fails. At present, ReLT makes up approximately 10 % of the total number of liver transplants performed in the US [48]. While ReLT is considered a high-risk procedure because of the technical demands of the operation and the severity of illness in the recipient, a 5-year graft failure-free survival rate of 65 % has been demonstrated in a select group of retransplant recipients [53, 54].

Posttransplant Care and Outcome

Immediate posttransplant recovery is related to baseline physical performance status, presence or absence of medical and surgical complications, and graft function. Some degree of multiorgan dysfunction is common, and many of those patients require renal replacement therapy, ventilator support, and frequent blood product transfusions. Severe malnutrition and sarcopenia are common and the risk of infection is high.

The immediate postoperative liver graft function can be assessed by the patient's general condition, such as mental status, requirement of blood transfusion, and overall hemodynamics. Lab values are informative, and trends of lactate dehydrogenase, prothrombin time, aminotransferases, total bilirubin, lactate, and pH are useful ways to monitor the course. If a patient has a T-tube, the amount of output and the color of bile reflect the liver function. Liver Doppler ultrasound can confirm if the blood flow is good in the hepatic artery, the portal vein, and the hepatic vein [55]. The major causes of immediate graft failure that require emergency retransplantation are hepatic artery or portal vein thrombosis, and primary nonfunction. The incidence rate for hepatic artery thrombosis is 5 % while for the portal vein thrombosis is 2 % [46]. Primary nonfunction is a diagnosis of exclusion, and it is a complete failure of liver graft function without any technical factor. The incidence of primary nonfunction has been reported as between 2 and 10 %.

Prevention of rejection is an important part of posttransplant care. During the operation, the patient receives an induction dose of immunosuppression, most commonly with high-dose corticosteroids. The corticosteroid dose can be tapered over varying time periods. In general, the period is shorter in hepatitis C patients, and it is longer or lasts for a lifetime in patients with autoimmune liver diseases. Other induction immunosuppressive agents, i.e. baxiliximab, may be included. Maintenance immunosuppressive agents such as calcineurin inhibitor (CI) (cyclosporine and tacrolimus), mycophenolate mofetil, and mammalian target of rapamycin (mTOR) inhibitors (sirolimus or everolimus) are initiated within a few days after OLT Nephrotoxicity and neurotoxicity are two important side effects of the CI during the early postoperative course. Daily blood levels of the CI are obtained for careful monitoring. Tremor is a common side effect of CI, and it may last for a few months. A single episode of seizure after liver transplantation is not uncommon, and the CI may be the precipitant. Nephrotoxicity needs long-term monitoring, as renal failure is a major cause of longterm morbidity in liver transplantation. Patients on CI should avoid nephrotoxic drugs, such as nonsteroidal anti-inflammatory drugs (NSAIDS), IV contrasts, and aminoglycosides. A third drug, mycophenolate mofetil, is frequently added to support immune suppression especially during the early postoperative period. The side effects of mycophenolate mofetil include gastrointestinal disturbances and neutropenia. These symptoms are common in liver transplantation from other causes, such as other drugs or cytomegalovirus infection, and differentiation is necessary before the dose of mycophenolate mofetil is adjusted. When a patient has significant kidney injury, mTOR inhibitors can be considered to replace or lower the dose of the CI. The mTOR inhibitors do not have nephrotoxicity, but they are associated with pancytopenia and impaired wound healing. Because of their anti-tumor activity, mTOR inhibitors can also be considered in patients whose indication is HCC or other malignancies.

Control of infection is another important issue. Transplantation patients are typically on prophylactic antibiotics including antifungal agents during the perioperative period. Bactrim is typically prescribed for 1 year as a prophylaxis against Pneumocystis jiroveci pneumonia, and dapsone or monthly-inhaled pentamidine are alternative drugs that can be used. Cytomegalovirus is the most common cause of opportunistic infection after solid organ transplantation, and various forms of the prophylactic protocol using intravenous ganciclovir and oral valganciclovir are used for as long as 3–6 months after transplant to prevent it with the recipient and donor baseline CMV status used as a guide. Epstein-Barr virus infection is related to posttransplant lymphoproliferative disease (PTLD), which may progress to malignant lymphoma. No antivirals have yet been proven to have efficacy in treating the

Epstein-Barr virus, and lowering immune suppression is recommended in patients with PTLD.

In practice, long-term posttransplant care is focused on maintaining organ function and controlling the side effects of immune suppression. Medication compliance is important for preventing chronic rejection. Steroid use is not common at this late stage, except in patients with autoimmune liver disease or with combined kidney transplantation. New-onset posttransplant diabetes and hypertension are known side effects of CI, especially in tacrolimus. Hyperlipidemia can be caused by CI, but it is more common in mTOR inhibitors. Proteinuria, pneumonitis, and mouth ulcers are other known side effects of mTOR inhibitors. Women of childbearing potential need counseling, and mycophenolate mofetil has been shown to have teratogenic properties. Cyclosporine has two additional uncommon side effects: gingival hyperplasia and hirsutism. Overall cancer risk is higher with immune suppression and general cancer prevention and monitoring is recommended. Skin cancer is the most common type of posttransplant cancer and the use of sun screen and appropriate surveillance by monitoring are recommended.

Many primary diseases as indications of liver transplantation can recur in the graft liver. Hepatitis B can be effectively controlled by lifelong treatment with antivirals and/or intravenous hepatitis B immunoglobulin. Recurrence of hepatitis C has been almost universal, and treatment has been difficult with traditional interferon-based therapy due to the significant side effects and the increased risk of rejection. Preliminary results of recently introduced direct acting antivirals, with or without combined use of ribavirin, are promising with options now available for almost all of the genotypes [31]. Nonalcoholic steatohepatitis commonly recurs in the graft, and control of metabolic syndrome is a more important issue in this group of patients. In patients with a history of alcoholic liver disease, recurrence of alcohol and other substance abuse should be monitored and patients should receive counseling. Autoimmune hepatitis patients need long-term or lifelong low-dose steroids to prevent recurrence. In rare instances, autoimmune hepatitis can develop in the graft in a patient without a history of the disease; when this occurs it is called de novo autoimmune hepatitis. Other forms of autoimmune liver disease, namely primary biliary cirrhosis and primary sclerosing cholangitis, also can recur. In contrast, metabolic liver diseases, including A_1-antitrypsin deficiency and Wilson's disease, do not recur after liver transplantation. In patients with HCC, the most common site of the recurrence is the liver graft, and appropriate surveillance and early initiation of local control therapy such as transarterial embolization and/or radiofrequency embolization is the mainstay of the treatment. The role of prophylactic adjuvant chemotherapy, including the use of mTOR inhibitors, is being evaluated by multicenter trials.

Overall, the percentage of 5-year patient survival after primary OLT is around 74 %, and more than half of all transplant patients live longer than 20 years [5]. Quality of life and prevention of systemic disease are important issues for those long-term survivors. They need long-term follow up to prevent cardiovascular disease, preserve renal function, and screen for cancer.

Future Trends

The limitation of the donor pool is the biggest challenge in liver transplantation. The high and increasing prevalence of metabolic syndrome and hepatic steatosis in the general population places increasing constraints on this limited donor pool. As such, innovation in organ resuscitation, such as machine perfusion devices that will convert high-risk otherwise discarded organs to transplantable liver, is critical to close the gap between organ demand and supply. Live donor liver transplantation remains a valuable source for expanding the donor pool.

References

1. Agopian VG, Petrowsky H, Kaldas FM, Zarrinpar A, Farmer DG, Yersiz H, et al. The evolution of liver transplantation during 3 decades: analysis of 5347 consecutive liver transplants at a single center. Ann Surg. 2013;258(3):409–21.
2. Farmer DG, Venick RS, McDiarmid SV, Ghobrial RM, Gordon SA, Yersiz H, et al. Predictors of outcomes after pediatric liver transplantation: an analysis of more than 800 cases performed at a single institution. J Am Coll Surg. 2007;204(5):904–14. discussion 14–6.
3. Hong JC, Yersiz H, Farmer DG, Duffy JP, Ghobrial RM, Nonthasoot B, et al. Longterm outcomes for whole and segmental liver grafts in adult and pediatric liver transplant recipients: a 10-year comparative analysis of 2,988 cases. J Am Coll Surg. 2009;208(5):682–9. discussion 9–91.
4. Saab S, Bownik H, Ayoub N, Younossi Z, Durazo F, Han S, et al. Differences in health-related quality of life scores after orthotopic liver transplantation with respect to selected socioeconomic factors. Liver Transpl. 2011;17(5):580–90.
5. Duffy JP, Kao K, Ko CY, Farmer DG, McDiarmid SV, Hong JC, et al. Long-term patient outcome and quality of life after liver transplantation: analysis of 20-year survivors. Ann Surg. 2010;252(4):652–61.
6. Testa G, Crippin JS, Netto GJ, Goldstein RM, Jennings LW, Brkic BS, et al. Liver transplantation for hepatitis C: recurrence and disease progression in 300 patients. Liver Transpl. 2000;6(5):553–61.
7. Gane EJ, Naoumov NV, Qian KP, Mondelli MU, Maertens G, Portmann BC, et al. A longitudinal analysis of hepatitis C virus replication following liver transplantation. Gastroenterology. 1996;110(1):167–77.
8. Recommendations for testing, managing, and treating hepatitis C: the American Association for the Study of Liver Diseases and The Infectious Diseases Society of America. Available from: http://hcvguidelines.org/.
9. Perrillo R, Buti M, Durand F, Charlton M, Gadano A, Cantisani G, et al. Entecavir and hepatitis B immune globulin in patients undergoing liver transplantation for chronic hepatitis B. Liver Transpl. 2013;19(8):887–95.
10. Lee WM, Squires Jr RH, Nyberg SL, Doo E, Hoofnagle JH. Acute liver failure: summary of a workshop. Hepatology. 2008;47(4):1401–15.
11. Forner A, Llovet JM, Bruix J. Hepatocellular carcinoma. Lancet. 2012;379(9822):1245–55.
12. El-Serag HB. Hepatocellular carcinoma. N Engl J Med. 2011;365(12):1118–27.
13. Rahbari NN, Garden OJ, Padbury R, Brooke-Smith M, Crawford M, Adam R, et al. Posthepatectomy liver failure: a definition and grading by the International Study Group of Liver Surgery (ISGLS). Surgery. 2011;149(5):713–24.
14. Mazzaferro V, Bhoori S, Sposito C, Bongini M, Langer M, Miceli R, et al. Milan criteria in liver transplantation for hepatocellular carcinoma: an evidence-based analysis of 15 years of experience. Liver Transpl. 2011;17 Suppl 2:S44–57.

15. Renshaw K. Malignant neoplasms of the extrahepatic biliary ducts. Ann Surg. 1922; 76(2):205–21.
16. Taylor-Robinson SD, Foster GR, Arora S, Hargreaves S, Thomas HC. Increase in primary liver cancer in the UK, 1979-94. Lancet. 1997;350(9085):1142–3.
17. Patel T. Increasing incidence and mortality of primary intrahepatic cholangiocarcinoma in the United States. Hepatology. 2001;33(6):1353–7.
18. Petrowsky H, Hong JC. Current surgical management of hilar and intrahepatic cholangiocarcinoma: the role of resection and orthotopic liver transplantation. Transplant Proc. 2009; 41(10):4023–35.
19. Hong JC, Jones CM, Duffy JP, Petrowsky H, Farmer DG, French S, et al. Comparative analysis of resection and liver transplantation for intrahepatic and hilar cholangiocarcinoma: a 24-year experience in a single center. Arch Surg. 2011;146(6):683–9.
20. Hong JC, Petrowsky H, Kaldas FM, Farmer DG, Durazo FA, Finn RS, et al. Predictive index for tumor recurrence after liver transplantation for locally advanced intrahepatic and hilar cholangiocarcinoma. J Am Coll Surg. 2011;212(4):514–20. discussion 20–1.
21. U.S. Department of Health and Human Services HRaSA, Healthcare Systems Bureau, Division of Transplantation, Rockville, MD. Allocation Calculators. Available from: http://optn.transplant.hrsa.gov/converge/resources/allocationcalculators.asp.
22. Wiesner R, Edwards E, Freeman R, Harper A, Kim R, Kamath P, et al. Model for end-stage liver disease (MELD) and allocation of donor livers. Gastroenterology. 2003;124(1):91–6.
23. Schaubel DE, Guidinger MK, Biggins SW, Kalbfleisch JD, Pomfret EA, Sharma P, et al. Survival benefit-based deceased-donor liver allocation. Am J Transplant. 2009;9(4 Pt 2):970–81.
24. Toso C, Dupuis-Lozeron E, Majno P, Berney T, Kneteman NM, Perneger T, et al. A model for dropout assessment of candidates with or without hepatocellular carcinoma on a common liver transplant waiting list. Hepatology. 2012;56(1):149–56.
25. Llovet JM, Mas X, Aponte JJ, Fuster J, Navasa M, Christensen E, et al. Cost effectiveness of adjuvant therapy for hepatocellular carcinoma during the waiting list for liver transplantation. Gut. 2002;50(1):123–8.
26. Swanson KL, Wiesner RH, Krowka MJ. Natural history of hepatopulmonary syndrome: impact of liver transplantation. Hepatology. 2005;41(5):1122–9.
27. Wong F, Nadim MK, Kellum JA, Salerno F, Bellomo R, Gerbes A, et al. Working Party proposal for a revised classification system of renal dysfunction in patients with cirrhosis. Gut. 2011;60(5):702–9.
28. Agopian VG, Dhillon A, Baber J, Kaldas FM, Zarrinpar A, Farmer DG, et al. Liver transplantation in recipients receiving renal replacement therapy: outcomes analysis and the role of intraoperative hemodialysis. Am J Transplant. 2014;14(7):1638–47.
29. Nadim MK, Sung RS, Davis CL, Andreoni KA, Biggins SW, Danovitch GM, et al. Simultaneous liver-kidney transplantation summit: current state and future directions. Am J Transplant. 2012;12(11):2901–8.
30. Nadim MK, Davis CL, Sung R, Kellum JA, Genyk YS. Simultaneous liver-kidney transplantation: a survey of US transplant centers. Am J Transplant. 2012;12(11):3119–27.
31. Nguyen NT, Harring TR, Goss JA, O'Mahony CA. Neuroendocrine liver metastases and orthotopic liver transplantation: the US experience. Int J Hepatol. 2011;2011:742890.
32. Bernal W, Wendon J. Acute liver failure. N Engl J Med. 2013;369(26):2525–34.
33. Vaquero J, Fontana RJ, Larson AM, Bass NM, Davern TJ, Shakil AO, et al. Complications and use of intracranial pressure monitoring in patients with acute liver failure and severe encephalopathy. Liver Transpl. 2005;11(12):1581–9.
34. Campsen J, Blei AT, Emond JC, Everhart JE, Freise CE, Lok AS, et al. Outcomes of living donor liver transplantation for acute liver failure: the adult-to-adult living donor liver transplantation cohort study. Liver Transpl. 2008;14(9):1273–80.
35. Uchiyama H, Mano Y, Taketomi A, Soejima Y, Yoshizumi T, Ikegami T, et al. Kinetics of anti-blood type isoagglutinin titers and B lymphocytes in ABO-incompatible living donor liver transplantation with rituximab and plasma exchange. Transplantation. 2011;92(10):1134–9.

36. Yersiz H, Lee C, Kaldas FM, Hong JC, Rana A, Schnickel GT, et al. Assessment of hepatic steatosis by transplant surgeon and expert pathologist: a prospective, double-blind evaluation of 201 donor livers. Liver Transpl. 2013;19(4):437–49.
37. Reich DJ, Hong JC. Current status of donation after cardiac death liver transplantation. Curr Opin Organ Transplant. 2010;15(3):316–21.
38. Hong JC, Yersiz H, Kositamongkol P, Xia VW, Kaldas FM, Petrowsky H, et al. Liver transplantation using organ donation after cardiac death: a clinical predictive index for graft failure-free survival. Arch Surg. 2011;146(9):1017–23.
39. Merion RM, Pelletier SJ, Goodrich N, Englesbe MJ, Delmonico FL. Donation after cardiac death as a strategy to increase deceased donor liver availability. Ann Surg. 2006;244(4):555–62.
40. Hong JC, Yersiz H, Busuttil RW. Where are we today in split liver transplantation? Curr Opin Organ Transplant. 2011;16(3):269–73.
41. Kim J, Zimmerman MA. Technical aspects for live-donor organ procurement for liver, kidney, pancreas, and intestine. Curr Opin Organ Transplant. 2015;20(2):133–9.
42. Ghobrial RM, Freise CE, Trotter JF, Tong L, Ojo AO, Fair JH, et al. Donor morbidity after living donation for liver transplantation. Gastroenterology. 2008;135(2):468–76.
43. Abecassis MM, Fisher RA, Olthoff KM, Freise CE, Rodrigo DR, Samstein B, et al. Complications of living donor hepatic lobectomy--a comprehensive report. Am J Transplant. 2012;12(5):1208–17.
44. Chan SC, Fan ST, Lo CM, Liu CL, Wong J. Toward current standards of donor right hepatectomy for adult-to-adult live donor liver transplantation through the experience of 200 cases. Ann Surg. 2007;245(1):110–7.
45. Hashikura Y, Ichida T, Umeshita K, Kawasaki S, Mizokami M, Mochida S, et al. Donor complications associated with living donor liver transplantation in Japan. Transplantation. 2009;88(1):110–4.
46. Duffy JP, Hong JC, Farmer DG, Ghobrial RM, Yersiz H, Hiatt JR, et al. Vascular complications of orthotopic liver transplantation: experience in more than 4,200 patients. J Am Coll Surg. 2009;208(5):896–903. discussion 903–5.
47. Petrowsky H, Rana A, Kaldas FM, Sharma A, Hong JC, Agopian VG, et al. Liver transplantation in highest acuity recipients: identifying factors to avoid futility. Ann Surg. 2014;259(6): 1186–94.
48. Thuluvath PJ, Guidinger MK, Fung JJ, Johnson LB, Rayhill SC, Pelletier SJ. Liver transplantation in the United States, 1999-2008. Am J Transplant. 2010;10(4 Pt 2):1003–19.
49. Jain A, Reyes J, Kashyap R, Dodson SF, Demetris AJ, Ruppert K, et al. Long-term survival after liver transplantation in 4,000 consecutive patients at a single center. Ann Surg. 2000; 232(4):490–500.
50. Busuttil RW, Farmer DG, Yersiz H, Hiatt JR, McDiarmid SV, Goldstein LI, et al. Analysis of long-term outcomes of 3200 liver transplantations over two decades: a single-center experience. Ann Surg. 2005;241(6):905–16. discussion 16–8.
51. Uemura T, Randall HB, Sanchez EQ, Ikegami T, Narasimhan G, McKenna GJ, et al. Liver retransplantation for primary nonfunction: analysis of a 20-year single-center experience. Liver Transpl. 2007;13(2):227–33.
52. Hong JC, Kosari K, Benjamin E, Duffy JP, Ghobrial RM, Farmer DG, et al. Does race influence outcomes after primary liver transplantation? A 23-year experience with 2,700 patients. J Am Coll Surg. 2008;206(5):1009–16. discussion 16–8.
53. Hong JC, Kaldas FM, Kositamongkol P, Petrowsky H, Farmer DG, Markovic D, et al. Predictive index for long-term survival after retransplantation of the liver in adult recipients: analysis of a 26-year experience in a single center. Ann Surg. 2011;254(3):444–8. discussion 8–9.
54. Hong JC. Outcomes predictors in transplantation. In: Busuttil RW, Klintmalm GBG, editors. Transplantation of the liver. 3rd ed. Philadelphia, PA: Elsevier Saunders; 2015. p. 1366–78.
55. Choi EK, Lu DS, Park SH, Hong JC, Raman SS, Ragavendra N. Doppler US for suspicion of hepatic arterial ischemia in orthotopically transplanted livers: role of central versus intrahepatic waveform analysis. Radiology. 2013;267(1):276–84.

Index

A

AASLD. *See* American Association for the Study of Liver Disease (AASLD)

AAT. *See* Alpha-1 antitrypsin (AAT)

AATD. *See* Alpha-1 antitrypsin deficiency (AATD)

AAT ZZ liver disease, 332

Abnormal liver tests, 2
  albumin, 13
  alkaline phosphatase, 8, 10
  aminotransferases, 3–6
  AST/ALT, 2
  bilirubin metabolism, 10, 12
  causes, 1, 2
  histology, 14
  liver function tests, 2
  prothrombin time, 14

ACE. *See* Angiotensin-converting enzyme (ACE)

Acetaminophen (APAP), 2, 17, 24, 95, 107, 121, 182, 390–392, 395, 398, 399, 601

Activities of daily living (ADL), 584

Acute esophageal variceal hemorrhage
  endoscopic therapy, 569
  hemorrhage, 570
  optimal time, 569

Acute fatty liver of pregnancy (AFLP)
  clinical and laboratory findings, 415
  definition, 414
  diagnosis, 415–416
  epidemiology, 414
  management, 416
  maternal and fetal outcomes, 416
  pathogenesis, 415

Acute hepatitis C (AHC), 143, 145

Acute kidney injury (AKI), 108, 109, 536

Acute liver failure (ALF), 23, 102, 415, 486, 601

Acute variceal bleeding
  balloon tamponade, 571
  band ligation, 571
  MELD score, 571
  metal esophageal stents, 570
  mortality rate, 570
  re-bleeding, 571
  stent migration, 570–571
  TIPS, 570

Adefovir, 138, 140, 141

ADL. *See* Activities of daily living (ADL)

ADPKD. *See* Autosomal dominant polycystic kidney disease (ADPKD)

AFP. *See* Alpha fetoprotein (AFP)

AGA. *See* American Gastroenterological Association (AGA)

AH. *See* Alcoholic Hepatitis (AH)

AHC. *See* Acute hepatitis C (AHC)

Akinetic–rigid syndromes, 357

ALAD deficiency porphyria (ADP), 384

Alanine aminotransferase (ALT), 2, 169, 407

Alcoholic hepatitis (AH)
  alcohol withdrawal, 181
  CTP and MELD score, 184
  drug therapy, 187
  fibrosis and cirrhosis, 173
  ICD-9 diagnosis, 175
  Lille score, 185
  liver disease, 182
  liver transplantation, 190
  malnutrition, 177
  mechanisms, 175

© Springer International Publishing Switzerland 2017

K. Saeian, R. Shaker (eds.), *Liver Disorders*,

DOI 10.1007/978-3-319-30103-7

Alcoholic hepatitis (AH) (*cont.*)
   necro-inflammatory process, 183
   nutritional deficiencies, 186
   nutritional intake, 175
   physical exam, 181
   prognostic markers, 174, 184
   symptoms, 180
Alcoholic liver disease (ALD), 600
   cirrhotics, 174
   clinical features
      alcoholic steatosis, 180
      alcohol-induced organ
         injury, 181
      AUDIT, 180
      CAGE questionnaire, 180
      cirrhosis, 180
      laboratory studies, 181
      liver biopsy, 182
      physical exam, 181
   clinical spectrum, 175
   diagnosis, 174, 176
   ER stress, 179
   fibrin/extracellular matrix, 179
   genetic and epigenetic factors, 180
   intestinal barrier dysfunction/microbiota,
      178, 179
   lipid peroxidation, 177
   nutritional abnormalities, 177, 178
   oxidative stress, 177
   prognosis, 183–184, 187–188
   prognostic markers, 174
   steatohepatitis and cirrhosis, 173, 176
   steatosis, 173
   therapies
      corticosteroids and pentoxifylline
         therapy, 188, 189
      drug therapy, 187
      interleukin-1 and inflammasome
         inhibitors, 190
      lifestyle modification, 185
      liver transplantation, 190
      nutrition therapy, 186, 187
   treatment options, 174, 175
Alcohol Use Disorders Identification Test
      (AUDIT), 180
Alcohol withdrawal, 110–111, 181
ALD. *See* Alcoholic liver disease (ALD)
Alkaline phosphatase (ALKP), 169, 171
   causes, 9
   evaluation, 10, 11
   GGT, 8
   isoenzymes, 8
   low serum, clinical significance, 9
   variations, 8

Alpha-1 antitrypsin (AAT)
   definition, 329
   mutations, 331
   NSAIDS, 330
   ZZ liver disease, 332
Alpha-1 antitrypsin deficiency (AATD)
   AAT ZZ liver disease, 332
   carbamazepine and rapamycin, 336
   diagnosis, 330, 333
   liver and lung disease, 329, 330
   lung manifestations, 334
   management, 335
   molecules, 334
Alpha-fetoprotein (AFP), 76, 81, 138, 350
ALT. *See* Alanine aminotransferase (ALT)
American Association for the Study of Live
      Disease (AASLD), 20, 21, 93, 138,
      349, 481
American Gastroenterological Association
      (AGA), 93
American Society of Anesthesiologists (ASA)
      physical status classification
      system, 102, 103
Aminotransferases
   causes, 4, 5
   evaluation, 5–7
   normal values, 3, 4
   SGOT, 3
   SGPT, 3
Angiotensin-converting enzyme (ACE), 431
Antibiotics
   AASLD guidelines, 521
   administration, 523
   blood specimens, 522
   cirrhosis and ascites, 521
   cirrhotics, 567
   neomycin, 492
   norfloxacin group, 568
   patients with liver cirrhosis, 475
   pre and post-procedure, 300
   PMN count, 523
   preliminary findings, 519
   rifaximin, 492
   selection, 523
Antidepressants, 268, 389
Antimitochondrial antibody (AMA), 253, 254,
      256, 258–260, 264, 272–275
Antinuclear antibodies (ANA), 222, 224,
      274, 310
APAP. *See* Acetaminophen (APAP)
Apoceruloplasmin, 357
Ascites
   abdominal distension, 509
   alcohol, 513

blood cultures, 511
causes, 513
chylous, 512
definition, 508
dietary sodium restriction, 514
diuretics, 514, 516
gastrointestinal bleeding, 526
glucose levels, 511
gram stain, 511
hepatic hydrothorax, 513
hypoalbuminemia, 513
incarceration and necrosis, 513
laboratory analysis, 510
liver disease, 519
low salt, 514
malignancy, 509, 512
management, 517
mortality rates, 521
paracentesis, 509, 513, 515
peripheral arterial vasodilation
    hypothesis, 508
peripheral edema, 512
placebo group, 525
portal hypertension, 508, 513
risk factors, 508
SAAG, 510, 511
Terlipressin, 517
TIPS, 516
total protein levels, 511
tuberculous peritonitis, 512
Aspartate aminotransferase (AST), 2, 169
ATP7B gene encoding, 356
Autoantibodies
actin and non-actin components, 222
ANA, 222–224
anti-LKM1, 222
autoimmune hepatitis, 223–224
nonstandard (*see* Nonstandard
    autoantibodies)
Autoimmune hepatitis (AIH), 27, 616
autoantibodies, 222, 224
clinical presentations, 221
codified international criteria, 219
comprehensive scoring systems, 220
concurrent immune diseases, 227
description, 217
drug toxicity, 232–233
extrahepatic malignancies, 234
hepatocellular carcinoma, 233
histological findings, 226
incomplete response, 231
interface hepatitis, 217
nonstandard autoantibodies, 224, 225
progressive fibrosis and cirrhosis, 233
relapse after drug withdrawal,
    234, 235
resolution, 229, 231
salvage therapies, 236–237
simplified scoring systems, 221
suboptimal responses, treatment strategies
    drug toxicity, 238
    incomplete response, 238
    liver transplantation, 239
    relapse after corticosteroid withdrawal,
        238, 239
    treatment failure, 235, 237
symptoms and laboratory tests, 218
treatment
    asymptomatic disease, 227
    azathioprine, 228, 229, 240
    budesonide, 228, 229
    drug intolerance, 218
    monotherapy, 229
    prednisone/prednisolone, 218, 228, 239
Autophagy, 332, 336
Autosomal dominant polycystic kidney
    disease (ADPKD), 64

B

Balloon-occluded retrograde transverse
    obliteration (BRTO), 478, 573, 574
Barcelona Clinic Liver Cancer (BCLC)
    staging system, 76–80
Baxiliximab, 615
BCAAs. *See* Branched chain amino acids
    (BCAAs)
Benign liver lesions
adenomas, 51
cysts, 51
focal nodular hyperplasia (*see* Focal
    nodular hyperplasia)
hemangiomas, 51
hepatic adenoma (*see* Hepatic adenoma)
hepatic cysts (*see* Hepatic cysts)
hepatic hemangioma (*see* Hepatic
    hemangioma)
hormonal therapy, 52
NRH (*see* Nodular regenerative
    hyperplasia (NRH))
polycystic liver disease, 64
Beta oxidation disorders, 372
Bilirubin metabolism
conjugated and unconjugated, 10
causes, 12
evaluation, 13
laboratory assays, 10
normal range, 11

Bilirubinemia, conjugated/unconjugated, 12
Biopsy of liver mass, 43, 44
Bone disease
    low bone density, 93–94
    osteoporosis, 263
    vitamin D deficiency, 92
Branched chain amino acids (BCAAs), 19,
        493, 495
BRTO. *See* Balloon-occluded retrograde
        transverse obliteration (BRTO)
Budd–Chiari syndrome (BCS)
    acute PVT, 418
    cardiac and pericardial diseases, 421
    clinical and laboratory features,
        421–422
    hepatic vein (HV), 421
    histopathology, 423
    inherited and acquired risk factors, 421, 422
    management, 423–424
    outcomes and prognosis, 424
    radiographic findings, 422–423

C
Calcineurin inhibitor (CI), 158, 218, 235, 319,
        425, 615
Carcinoembryonic antigen (CEA), 45, 46, 81
Causality assessment, 394, 396, 398
CBDL. *See* Common bile duct ligation (CBDL)
Ceruloplasmin, 357, 360–362
CFF test. *See* Critical flicker frequency
        (CFF) test
CHE. *See* Covert hepatic encephalopathy
        (CHE)
CHESS. *See* Clinical hepatic encephalopathy
        staging scale (CHESS)
Child-Pugh score, 23, 27, 520, 521, 525
Child-Turcotte-Pugh (CTP) score, 23, 99, 100,
        103–105, 184, 585
Cholangiocarcinoma (CCA), 602
    biliary hilum/hepatic parenchyma, 29
    diagnosis, 81
    dominant strictures, 300
    epidemiology, 80
    liver transplantation, 73
    management, 81
    PSC, 293
    risk factors, 80
    treatment, 301
Cholestasis and AIH
    bile duct injury/loss, 313
    cholangiograms, 313
    corticosteroid response, 321
    liver failure, 320

    outcomes, 320
    prednisone/prednisolone, 320
Cholestatic diseases, 12, 309, 310, 314
Chronic hepatitis C
    liver disease, 147
    liver transplantation, 147, 154
    treatment, 147
Chronic portal vein thrombus
    chronic extrahepatic PVT, 420
    gastrointestinal bleeding, 420
    outcomes, 421
    portal cavernoma, 420
    radiographic findings and diagnosis, 420
    treatment, 420–421
CI. *See* Calcineurin inhibitor (CI)
Ciprofloxacin, 525, 526
Cirrhosis, 14, 233, 251, 252, 329, 331–335,
        343, 350
    alcohol abuse, 110
    ascites, 521
    ASA, 103
    ascites, 109
    baclofen, 186
    cholecystectomy, 104
    coagulopathy, 107
    compensated, 173, 180, 181
    decompensated, 99, 106, 173, 175, 180,
        181, 186
    emergent and elective surgery, 109
    gastrointestinal bleeding, 525
    hepatic encephalopathy, 527
    imaging, 182
    immune/metabolic causes, 182
    kidney function, 108–109
    liver transplantation, 103
    low-sodium diet, 108
    mechanisms, 176
    mesenteric lymph node, 520
    morbidity and mortality, risk of, 99
    mortality rate, 175
    nutritional deficiencies, 186
    paracentesis, 524
    peripheral leukocytosis, 521
    pre- and post-surgery, 110
    probiotic therapy, 189
    prognostic markers, 174, 184
    renal dysfunction, 525
    sarcopenia, 110
    scoring system, 184
Clinical hepatic encephalopathy staging scale
        (CHESS), 488
Clinical Institute Withdrawal Assessment of
        Alcohol Scale, Revised (CIWA-Ar),
        110, 112–114

Common bile duct ligation (CBDL), 547
Coombs-negative hemolytic anemia, 357
Copper
    apoceruloplasmin, 357
    dysfunction, 357
    hepatic, 361–362
    serum free, 362
    transporting P-type ATPase, 356
    urinary copper excretion, 361
Coronary artery bypass grafting procedures
        (CABG), 106
Covert hepatic encephalopathy (CHE), 482,
        485, 488, 489
Critical flicker frequency (CFF)
        test, 490
Crypt cell hypothesis, 342
CTP. *See* Child-Turcotte-Pugh (CTP) score
CYP2E1. *See* Hepatic cytochrome P450 2E1
        (CYP2E1)

D
Deceased-donor liver
    bilirubin, 605
    calculation, 604
    graft, 604
    MELD exception, 605
    mortality rate, 605, 606
    PELD scoring system, 605
    serum bilirubin, 604
Direct acting antivirals (DAA), 144, 149, 152,
        156, 158, 159
Discriminant function (DF), 184, 188
D-Penicillamine, 355, 360, 361, 363, 365
Drug-induced autoimmune hepatitis, 397
Drug-induced liver injury (DILI), 31, 393
    biomarkers and clinical presentation, 390
    cirrhosis/transplantation, 390
    classification, 390
    diagnosis, 389
    idiosyncratic (*see* Idiosyncratic DILI)
    intrinsic, 391, 392
    metabolism and detoxification, 390
    plethora, clinical presentations, 395
    valid methods, 390
Dubin–Johnson syndrome, 13

E
Eastern cooperative oncology group
        (ECOG), 584
Ebola hemorrhagic fever (EHF), 170–171
EHE. *See* Epithelioid hemangioendothelioma
        (EHE)

ELAD. *See* Extracorporeal liver assist device
        (ELAD)
Elective surgery, 102, 104, 106, 109, 611
Emergency surgery, 105
Emphysema, 330, 331, 333, 334
EncephalApp Stroop Test, 489
End stage liver disease, 106–107
Endoscopic band ligation, 561, 563, 565, 572
Endoscopic retrograde cholangio
        pancreatography (ERCP), 587, 588
Endoscopic sclerotherapy, 472–474, 477
Endoscopic ultrasound (EUS), 478, 575
Endoscopic variceal sclerotherapy,
        557, 563
Endoscopy
    GI hemorrhage, 556
    portal hypertension, 556
Entecavir therapy, 134, 139
Epithelioid hemangioendothelioma
        (EHE), 82
Epstein-Barr virus, 168, 616
ERCP. *See* Endoscopic retrograde cholangio
        pancreatography (ERCP)
Erythropoietic protoporphyria (EPP), 382,
        385, 386
Esophageal variceal bleeding, 469, 470,
        472–475, 477
Esophageal varices
    bleeding, 560
    bleeding and re-bleeding, 557
    cirrhotics, 557, 560, 566
    diagnosis, 558
    epidemiology, 557
    GI bleeding, 566
    HVPG, 459
    porto-systemic collaterals, 458
    re-bleeding, 559
    risk factors/natural history, 558
    submucosa, 556
    telangiectasias, 461
    transient elastography (TE), 463
    upper endoscopy, 456, 461
European Association for the Study of Liver
        Disease, 136
European Society for Clinical Nutrition and
        Metabolism (ESPEN), 19, 110
Extracorporeal liver assist device
        (ELAD), 190

F
Familial amyloidotic polyneuropathy (FAP),
        438–440
Familial Mediterranean fever (FMF), 437, 438

Fatty liver
  alcohol consumption, 183
  alcohol-induced liver injury, 176, 181
  clinical spectrum, 175
  endotoxin, 179
  hepatomegaly, 181
  prognosis, 174
Fibrolamellar carcinoma, 80
Florid duct lesion, 259, 308–309, 312
Fluoroquinolones, 567–568
Focal nodular hyperplasia
  diagnosis, 58
  hepatic lesion, 57
  OCPs, 58, 59
Fresh frozen plasma (FFP), 107
Future liver remnant (FLR), 586, 587

G
Galactose elimination capacity (GEC), 586
Gallbladder polyps, 301
Gamma glutamyl transpeptidase (GGT), 8, 10,
      94, 168, 170, 171, 181–183, 310,
      313–315, 407, 410, 431–433
Gastric antral vascular ectasia (GAVE), 556
Gastric varices, 470, 475, 477, 478
  acute bleeding, 573
  primary prophylaxis, 573
  secondary prophylaxis, 574
  types, 573
  web-like arrangement, 573
Glasgow alcoholic hepatitis score (GAHS),
      174, 184
Glasgow coma scale (GCS), 488
Glycogen storage disorders (GSD), 57
  adenomas, 372
  brain damage, 372
  complications, 372
  diagnosis of, 370
  dietary management, 373
  genetic testing, 370
  glucose utilization, 369
  gout, 373
  hyperlipidemia, 373
  hypoglycemia, 370
  liver biopsy, 370
  liver fibrosis, 373
  mortality, 372
  myopathies, 373
  oncotic pressure, 369
  osteoporosis, 373
  renal disease, 373
  skeletal muscle involvement, 370
  types, 370

Granulocyte-macrophage colony-stimulating
      factor (GM-CSF) therapy, 190
Granulomatous liver disease
  autoimmune, 432
  cancer, 435
  causes, 430
  clinical and laboratory findings, 430–431
  definition, 430
  drugs, 435
  foreign body, 435
  idiopathic, 435
  infectious diseases, 433–434
  lipogranuloma, 435
  Q fever, 433–434
  sarcoidosis, 431–432
  types, 430

H
HAV. *See* Hepatitis A virus (HAV)
HBIG. *See* Hepatitis B immune globulin
      (HBIG)
HBV. *See* Hepatitis B virus (HBV)
HCC. *See* Hepatocellular carcinoma (HCC)
HDS. *See* Herbal and dietary supplements
      (HDS)
Heme production, 381, 384
Hemochromatosis, 1, 4, 6, 93, 182, 218
      (*see also* Hereditary
      hemochromatosis (HH))See also
Hepatectomy, 585, 589, 593
Hepatic adenoma, 58, 82
  complications, 55, 56
  management, 56–57
  risk factors, 54
Hepatic amyloidosis
  clinical and laboratory findings, 438
  FAP, 438
  FMF, 438
  histopathology, 439
  management, 439–440
  outcome, 440
  radiographic findings, 438
  systemic amyloidosis, 437
Hepatic angiosarcoma, 82
Hepatic cysts
  biliary cystadenocarcinomas, 64–65
  biliary cystadenomas, 64–65
  diagnosis, 64
  hydatid cysts, 65–68
  simple cysts, 63–64
  types, 63
Hepatic cytochrome P450 2E1 (CYP2E1), 391
Hepatic encephalopathy (HE), 106

brain dysfunction, 481
carbohydrates, 495
causes
    acute confusional states/delirium, 485
    ammonia, 485
    cirrhosis, 486
    diabetes mellitus, 485
    endoplasmic reticulum, 486
    glutamine, 486
    hyponatremia, 485
    inflammatory cytokines, 486
    pathogenesis, 485
    pathophysiology, 485
    portacaval shunt, 486
    portal hypertension, 484
    precipitation, 484, 485
CHE, 482
cirrhosis, 495
classification, 482
CLD, 481
diagnosis
    CHE testing, 488
    classification systems, 488
    clinical evaluation and exclusion, 487
    computerized tests, 489
    grading, OHE, 488
    neurophysiological tests, 490
    paper-and-pencil tests, 489
    strategies, 490
    testing, 487
dietary protein, 495
disease states, 498
driving, 498
electrolyte abnormalities, 496
liver transplantation, 497
malnutrition, 495
MHE treatment, 496, 497
neurocognitive manifestation, 498
neuropsychological testing, 498
neuropsychometric testing, 482
nutrition, 495
OHE, 482
symptoms
    asterixis/disorientation, 483
    dopaminergic neurotransmission, 484
    driving, 483
    extrapyramidal dysfunction, 484
    liver disease and PSS, 484
    mental activities, 483
    MHE, 483
    stages, 483
treatment
    antibiotics, 492, 493
    BCAAs, 493
    intensive care unit, 491
    LOLA, 493
    MARS, 494, 495
    nonabsorbable disaccharides, 491
    PEG, 494
    prebiotics and probiotics, 494
Hepatic encephalopathy scoring algorithm
    (HESA), 488
Hepatic fibrosis, 31, 59, 64, 135, 179, 183, 205,
    206, 227, 233, 310, 348, 399, 465
Hepatic hemangioma
    clinical presentation, 52
    diagnosis, 53
    management, 53–54
Hepatic hydrothorax, 513, 516
Hepatic lymphoma, 84
Hepatic venous pressure gradient (HVPG),
    427, 469, 471–473
    classification, portal hypertension, 459–460
    coagulopathies, 459
    diagnosis, 459
    local anesthesia and conscious sedation, 458
    prognosis, 460
    variceal bleeding, 460, 461
    wedged (WHVP) and free (FHVP), 458
Hepatitis A
    clinical presentation, 126, 127
    diagnosis and treatment, 128
    epidemiology, 122
    pathogenesis, 125
    prevention, 130
    signs and symptoms, 121
    time course, 128
    transmission, 124, 125
    in USA, 123
    vaccine, 90–91, 122
    worldwide prevalence, 123
Hepatitis A virus (HAV), 90, 91, 130
Hepatitis B immune globulin (HBIG), 136
Hepatitis B vaccination, 91, 600, 601, 611, 616
Hepatitis B virus (HBV), 91
Hepatitis C virus (HCV)
    bleeding, 146
    chronic infection, 145
    cirrhosis, 145, 158
    drug–drug interactions, 149–151
    end-stage renal disease (ESRD), 152
    fibrosis/cirrhosis, 156
    HIV, 158, 159
    intravenous drug users, 143
    liver disease, 149, 157
    liver transplantation, 156
    psychiatric effects, 148
    renal impairment, 155

Hepatitis C virus (HCV) (*cont.*)
    side effects, 148, 156, 158
    sofosbuvir/ledipasvir, 149
    symptoms, 143
    T cell response, 144
    testing, 144
    treatment, 153, 158
Hepatitis E virus
    clinical presentation, 127
    diagnosis and treatment, 129
    epidemiology, 124
    pathogenesis, 125
    prevention, 130
    signs and symptoms, 121
    transmission, 125
    vaccine, 122
    worldwide epidemiology, 124
Hepatoblastoma (HB), 73, 83
Hepatocellular carcinoma (HCC), 28, 29, 56,
        95, 137, 233, 252, 269, 302, 349, 602
    Barcelona clinic liver cancer staging
        system, 78
    chemotherapy, 73
    diagnosis, 76
    epidemiology, 74, 75
    fibrolamellar carcinoma, 80
    imaging studies, 72
    incidence of, 75
    liver failure, 208
    liver transplantation, 208
    management, 77–80
    prognosis, 73
    radiographic features, 77
    risk factors, 75, 76
    sorafenib, 73
    staging, 76
Hepatolenticular degeneration, 356
Hepatomegaly, 370, 372
Hepatopulmonary syndrome (HPS)
    cirrhosis, 546
    clinical manifestations and laboratory
        testing, 549–550
    epidemiology and history, 546
    pathophysiology
        animal models, 547
        arterial hypoxemia, 547
        diagnostic criteria, 548
        human disease, 547–548
        IPVD, 548–549
    treatment
        LT, 550–551
        pharmacological therapies, 550
        TIPS, 550
Hepatorenal syndrome (HRS), 109, 609
    ascites and cirrhosis, 535
    cirrhotic cardiomyopathy, 535, 542
    clinical features, 537
    definition, 531, 534
    diagnosis, ICA-AKI criteria, 536
    hypovolemia, 535
    kidney dysfunction, cirrhosis, 533
    liver transplantation, 540–541
    MARS, dialysis, 540
    medical therapy, 538–539
    medications, 532
    neurohumoral vasoconstrictor systems, 535
    portal hypertension, 533
    prevention, 541
    prognosis, 532
    renal biopsy, 536
    RRT, 540
    splanchnic vasodilatation, 534
    subtypes, 537
    symptoms, 531
    TIPS, 539
    treatment, 532, 537–538
Hepatosplenic T-cell lymphoma (HSTCL), 84
Hepatotoxic drugs, 17, 393
Herbal and dietary supplements (HDS), 398
Hereditary hemochromatosis (HH)
    C282Y, 340, 341
    cardiomyopathy, 343
    clinical management
        hepatocellular cancer screening, 349
        phlebotomy, 348, 349
        transplantation, 350
    cysteine substitution, 341
    diagnosis, 339, 344, 345
    epidemiology, 341
    ferritin, 344
    H63D, 340, 341
    homozygotes and compound
        heterozygotes, 351
    liver biopsy, 346–348
    MRI, 340
    mutation analysis, 350
    pathophysiology
        hepcidin, 342
        HFE protein, 343
        increased intestinal iron absorption, 342
        iron-induced liver damage, 343
    primary *vs* secondary iron overload
        syndromes, 341
    prognosis, 340
    progressive iron accumulation, 343
    screening, 351
    superoxide and hydroxyl radicals, 341
    treatment, 340

Herpes viruses
    adenovirus, 168
    cytomegalovirus (CMV), 168
    EHF, 170–171
    epstein-barr virus, 168
    herpes simplex virus, 166–167
    influenza, 169–170
    parvovirus B19 (PV-B19), 169
    VZV, 167
HESA. *See* Hepatic encephalopathy scoring
        algorithm (HESA)
HH. *See* Hereditary hemochromatosis (HH)
Hilar cholangiocarcinoma, 603, 606, 607
HRS. *See* Hepatorenal syndrome (HRS)
HVPG. *See* Hepatic venous pressure gradient
        (HVPG)
Hydatid cysts, 65
Hyperammonemia, 375–378
Hyperbilirubinemia, 12, 13, 167, 168, 385,
        405, 416, 520, 525
Hyperemesis gravidarum
    definition and diagnosis, 408
    etiology, 408–409
    outcomes and recurrence, 409
    pathology, 409
    treatment, 409
Hyperkalemia, 609
Hyperlipidemia, 6, 263, 271, 399,
        509, 616
Hypervascular lesions, 28, 44, 372
Hypoglycemia, 369, 370, 372, 373

I
ICG. *See* Indocyanine green (ICG)
ICT. *See* Inhibitory control test (ICT)
Idiosyncratic DILI
    alcohol consumption, 398
    biochemical pattern, 394
    characterization, 393
    chronic oxidant stress, 398
    diagnosis, 394–397
    drug-induced autoimmune hepatitis, 397
    HDS, 397
    hepatotoxicity, 398
    heterogeneous and rare entity, 393
    LiverTox, 397
    mechanisms, 393
    minor fluctuations, 399
    mitochondrial dysfunction, 398
    plethora, clinical presentations, 394, 395
    PNALD, 399, 400
    treatment, 399
IgG4 cholangiopathy, 296

Incidental hepatic lesions
    benign lesions, 47–48
    CT scan, 43
    history and physical examination, 45
    imaging studies, 46
    investigation, 44–45
    laboratory evaluation, 45
    malignant lesions, 47
    MRI contrast imaging techniques, 48
    MRI of liver, 46–48
    subsequent imaging study, 44–45
Indirect immunofluorescence (IIF), 221,
        222, 225
Indocyanine green (ICG), 586
Infectious mononucleosis (IM), 168
Influenza vaccination, 91
Inhibitory control test (ICT), 489
Interface hepatitis, 217, 222, 226, 234
Interferons, 139, 140, 147, 158
International Autoimmune Hepatits Group
        (IAIHG), 224, 274, 309, 320
International Hepato-Pancreato-Biliary
        Association (IHPBA), 589
International normalized ratio (INR), 585, 607
Intrahepatic cholestasis of pregnancy (ICP)
    clinical manifestations and laboratory
        findings, 410–411
    diagnosis, 411
    maternal and fetal outcomes, 411–412
    medical management, 411
    pathogenesis, 410
    pathology, 411
    pruritus, 409
Intrapulmonary vascular dilatations (IPVD),
        547, 549
Intrauterine fetal demise (IUFD), 411, 412
Intrinsic DILI
    acetaminophen, 391
    APAP, 391
    diagnosis, 392
    hepatic depletion, 391
    hepatotoxicity, 391, 392
    NAFLD, 392
Iron overload syndrome, 341 (*see* Intrauterine
        fetal demise (IUFD))

K
Kayser–Fleischer rings, 357–361, 365
Kendoll histological activity index score, 37
Keratoconjunctivitis, 168
Kidney failure. *See* Hepatorenal syndrome
        (HRS)
King's College Hospital criteria, 23, 24

L
Large volume paracentesis (LVP), 100, 108
Lipogranuloma, 430, 435
Liver adenomatosis, 57
Liver biopsy
    adequate biopsy sampling, 38
    AIH, 28
    complications
        laparoscopic, 35
        percutaneous, 34
        transjugular, 34–35
    diagnosis, 31
    experience of pathologist, 36
    hepatitis C, 28
    liver enzymes, 27, 28
    medication, 32–33
    methods, 33
    pre-biopsy testing, 32
    preparation, 32
    sampling and adequacy, 35
    specimen interpretation, 37–38
    staging, 31
    tissue processing, 35–36
    treatment, 32
    tumor, 28, 29
Liver cancer
    diagnosis and management, 84
    imaging studies, 72
    liver masses, benign/malignant, 72
    prognosis, 73
    treatment options, 72, 73
Liver cirrhosis, 270, 412, 456, 462, 469–471,
        474, 475, 485, 535, 609
Liver cyst, 43, 46, 590
Liver disease
    acetaminophen, 95
    alcoholic and nonalcoholic cirrhosis, 95
    esophageal varices, screening for, 20
    fibrosis progression, 94
    HCC, 20, 95
    hepatitis A vaccination, 90–91
    hepatitis B vaccination, 91
    hepatitis, treatment of, 20, 21
    influenza vaccination, 91
    lifestyle interventions, 19
    liver functions, 17–18
    medication adjustments, 19
    medications, avoidance of
        alcohol consumption, 18
        hepatotoxic drugs, 17
        sodium and fluid, intake of, 18
    NAFLD, 94, 95
    NASH, 95
    NSAIDs and opioids, 95, 96

    nutrition, 19
    opioids, 96
    pneumococcal vaccination, 92
    severity
        CTP score, 23
        imaging, 22
        King's College Hospital criteria, 23
        laboratory tests, 22
        liver biopsy, 22
        MELD score, 23
        portal pressure measurement, 22
        prognostic models, 22
        signs/symptoms, 21
    tramadol, 96
    vaccination, 19
Liver function tests, 2
Liver grafts, 606–608, 611, 612
Liver imaging, 47
Liver metastasis
    cirrhosis, 83
    malignant liver mass, 72
    treatment, 83
Liver panel testing, 1, 2, 14
Liver resection, 81
    chemotherapy and radiation therapy, 596
    classification systems, 585–586
    coagulopathy, 591
    complications and hazards, 595–596
    dynamic liver tests, 586
    imaging modalities, 587–589
    minimally invasive approaches
        conduct of operation, 594–595
        port placement, 594–595
        positioning, 594
    normothermia, 591
    patient positioning, 591
    perioperative preparation, 591
    postoperative analgesia, 591
    postoperative liver volume, 586–587
    preoperative care, 583, 584
    surgical techniques
        biliary tree integrity, 592
        exploration, 592
        incision, 591–592
        mobilization, exposure and
            reassessment, 592
        parenchymal transection, 592
    transplantation and surgical resection, 596
Liver transplantation, 72, 106, 271–272, 379,
        550–551
    bacterial peritonitis, 603
    CCA, 73, 81
    cerebral edema, 610
    diagnosis, 604

donor operation, 612
echocardiogram, 608
EHE, 82
HB, 83
HCC, 79, 80
hepatobiliary malignancy, 601
hepatorenal syndrome, 603
immunosuppression, 608, 614
liver metastasis, 83
MELD exception, 603
MELD scores, 614
neuroendocrine tumor, 609
nonhepatic origin, 609
perioperative management, 614
posttransplant management plan, 608
recipient operation, 613
time-sensitive situation, 610
LiverTox, 17, 397
L-ornithine L-aspartate (LOLA), 493
LT. *See* Liver transplantation (LT)
LVP. *See* Large volume paracentesis (LVP)
Lysophosphatidic acid (LPA), 261

M
Magnetic resonance elastography (MRE),
463, 464
Malignant liver lesions
CCA, 80, 81
HCC, 74–77, 79, 80
metastatic lesions and lymphoma, 83, 84
primary liver tumors, 82, 83
MARS. *See* Molecular adsorbent recirculating
system (MARS)
Mayo PBC risk score, 258
Metabolic bone disease, 252
Metastatic liver lesions, 83–84
Microbubbles, 548
Middle East respiratory syndrome coronavirus
(MERS-CoV), 170
Minimal hepatic encephalopathy (MHE),
106, 107, 483
Mitochondrial trifunctional protein (MTP), 415
Model for end stage liver disease (MELD), 23,
298, 301, 302, 520, 585
allocation system, 607
cholangiocarcinoma, 607
exception points, 607
liver transplantation, 606
MELD/PELD system, 606
mortality, 605
mortality rate, 606
OPTN/UNOS policy, 607
posttransplant mortality, 606
score, 605
types and comorbidities, 605
Model for End-Stage Liver Disease/Pediatric
End-Stage Liver Disease (MELD/
PELD), 604
Modification of Diet in Renal Disease
(MDRD-6), 609
Modified-orientation log (MO-Log), 488
Molecular adsorbent recirculating system
(MARS), 494, 495, 540
MRI cholangiography (MRCP), 10, 587, 589
MTP. *See* Mitochondrial trifunctional protein
(MTP)

N
NAFL. *See* Nonalcoholic fatty liver (NAFL)
NASH. *See* Nonalcoholic steatohepatitis
(NASH)
National Institute on Alcohol Abuse and
Alcoholism, 180
National Institutes of Health (NIH), 601
Nausea and vomiting of pregnancy (NVP), 408
Nephrotoxicity, 159, 267, 391, 492, 615
Neuropathy, 381, 382, 384
Neutropenia, 140, 373, 615
Nodular regenerative hyperplasia (NRH),
59–63, 259
Non-alcoholic fatty liver (NAFL) disease, 94,
392, 600
adiponutrin, 201
antioxidants, 206
bariatric surgery, 205
biopsy, 203, 204
complications, 204, 205
cryptogenic cirrhosis, 201, 208
CVD, 205
diagnosis, 202–203
HCC, 208
hepatic steatosis/steatohepatitis, 202
hepatic triglycerides, 200
insulin resistance, 201
insulin sensitivity, 206
liver tests, 203
macrosteatosis, 200
NASH, 205
obeticholic acid, 207
pioglitazone, 206
statins, 207
steatosis, 199
toxicity, 201
transaminases, 207
type 2 diabetes, 205
vitamin E, 206

Non-alcoholic steatohepatitis (NASH), 95,
        600, 616
    aminotransferases, 201
    cirrhosis, 202, 204
    cryptogenic cirrhosis, 208
    fibrosis, 201
    NAFLD, 199
    *vs.*NAFL, 204
Noncirrhotic liver, 46, 76
Nonselective beta-adrenergic blockers
        (NSBBs), 470–473
Nonselective beta-blockers (NNSB), 560
Nonstandard autoantibodies
    actin (anti-actin), 225
    pANCA, 224–225
Nonsteroidal anti-inflammatory drugs
        (NSAIDs), 95, 615
Norfloxacin, 475, 524, 525, 541, 568
Nucleoside, 134, 138–141
Nucleotide analogues (NAs), 138, 141
NVP. *See* Nausea and vomiting of pregnancy
        (NVP)

O
Occult hepatitis B infection, 135
Octreotide
    acute variceal bleeding, 568
    antibiotics, 557
    somatostain analogues, 568
    vasopressin, 569
Okuda classification, 76
Opiate antagonists, 267–268
Oral contraceptives (OCPs), 54, 59
Organ allocation, 606
Organ Procurement and Transplantation
        Network (OPTN), 606, 607
Ornithine transcarbamylase (OTC) deficiency,
        375–378
Orthodeoxia, 549
Orthotopic liver transplantation (OLT), 135,
        599, 604
Oseltamivir, 170
Osteopenia, 93, 271
Osteoporosis, 93, 263, 271
Overlap syndromes
    autoimmune hepatitis, 309
    cholestatic components, 308, 309
    corticosteroid therapy, 308
    diagnostic features, 311
    frequency, 313
    immune-mediated liver disease, 307
    liver transplantation, 308
    pathogenic possibilities
        antigenic targets, 314
        bile duct injury, 314
        cholestatic disease, 314
        cytotoxic T cells, 315
        immune-mediated diseases, 315
        serum levels, 314
    PBC and PSC, 307, 313
    UDCA, 308, 310
Overt hepatic encephalopathy (OHE), 106, 107

P
Packed red blood cell (PRBC) transfusion
        strategy, 107
pANCA. *See* Perinuclear anti-neutrophil
        cytoplasmic antibodies (pANCA)
Pancreaticoduodenectomy, 602
Paracentesis
    albumin level, 510
    antibiotics, 519
    clinical signs, 522
    coagulation factors, 522
    coagulopathy, 509
    complications, 510
    dietary sodium restriction, 514, 515
    electrolyte abnormalities, 515
    meta-analysis, 526
    SBP, 519
    TIPS, 516
    treatment, 527
Parenteral nutrition-associated liver disease
        (PNALD)
    characterization, 399
    cirrhosis and portal hypertension, 399
    pathogenesis, 399
Parvovirus B19 (PV-B19), 169
PBC. *See* Primary biliary cirrhosis (PBC)
PBC-PSC overlap
    autoimmune cholangitis, 321
    corticosteroids, 322
    liver transplantation, 322
    tumor necrosis, 321
    ursodeoxycholic acid, 321
Percutaneous ablation, 73, 77, 78
Percutaneous transhepatic cholangiography
        (PTC), 294, 587–589
Perinuclear anti-neutrophil cytoplasmic
        antibodies (pANCA), 225
PHES. *See* Psychometric hepatic
        encephalopathy score (PHES)
PHG. *See* Portal hypertensive gastropathy
        (PHG)
PHI. *See* Postoperative hepatic insufficiency
        (PHI)

Phlebotomy
    diagnosis and treatment, 348
    hemochromatosis, 349, 350
    prospective study, 348
    serum ferritin, 349
    vitamin C supplementation, 349
Plasmapheresis, 268, 269
Platypnea, 549
PNALD. *See* Parenteral nutrition-associated
    liver disease (PNALD)
Pneumococcal vaccination, 92
Polycystic liver disease, 64
Porphyrias
    abdominal pain, 382
    abnormal heme production, 381
    acute, 381
    central nervous system, 382
    children, 386
    complexity, 381
    cutaneous presentation, 382
    dietary management, 386
    gastrointestinal symptoms, 385
    genetic testing, 383, 384
    hematological abnormalities, 385
    hepatic changes, 382
    laboratory evaluation, 383
    liver and bone marrow transplant, 386
    medications, 386
    mortality, 384
    neuropathy, 382, 384
    phlebotomy, 386
    photosensitivity, 385
    precipitating drugs, 385
    seizures, 384
    skin protection, 386
    sporadic porphyria cutaena tarda, 381
    symptomatology, 381
    transfusions, 386
Portal hypertension
    abdominal imaging, 462
    ascites (*see* Ascites)
    assessment, 458–464
    bleeding, 469, 470
    causes, 455, 464, 465
    complications, 456, 473–474
    definition, 455
    development, 456
    diagnosis, 456
    endoscopic glue, 477–478
    esophageal varices (*see* Esophageal
      varices)
    fibrosis markers, 462
    gastric variceal bleeding, 475–477
    gastroesophageal varices, 455

    hepatic encephalopathy, 455
    HVPG (*see* Hepatic venous pressure
      gradient (HVPG))
    hyperdynamic circulation, 457
    intrahepatic, 465
    laboratory markers, 462
    liver stiffness, 463
    neoangiogenesis, 458
    nitroprusside, 457
    non-endoscopic approaches, 478
    physical examination, 461
    portal venous flow, 457
    portosystemic collaterals, 458
    posthepatic, 465
    prehepatic, 464–465
    primary prophylaxis, 470–472
    secondary prophylaxis, 473
    spleen stiffness, 463–464
    upper endoscopy, 461
    varices bleed, 474–475
    vasoconstrictors and vasodilators, 457
Portal hypertensive colopathy, 575, 576
Portal hypertensive gastropathy (PHG),
    575, 576
Portal vein embolization (PVE), 587
Portal vein thrombosis (PVT)
    acute, 417
    clinical and laboratory features,
      418–419
    local risk factors, 417, 418
    radiographic features and diagnosis, 419
    treatment, 419–420
Portopulmonary hypertension (PPHTN), 103
Postoperative
    AKI, 108
    ascites, management of, 108
    end stage liver disease, 106–107
    hepatic encephalopathy, 107
    morbidity and mortality, 102, 104
Postoperative hepatic insufficiency
    (PHI), 586
Posttransplant lymphoproliferative disease
    (PTLD), 615
PRBC. *See* Packed red blood cell (PRBC)
    transfusion strategy
Preeclampsia
    clinical presentation, 412–413
    definition, 412
    diagnosis, 413
    epidemiology, 412
    management, 414
    pathogenesis, 412
    pathology, 413
    prognosis, 414

Pregnancy-associated liver disorders
  characteristic timing, 408
  classification, 407–408
  Gadolinium-based contrast, 406
  normal physiological and hormonal
    changes, 406–407
  pregnancy, 405, 406
  ultrasonography, 406
Preoperative checklists, 106
Preoperative Liver Assessment (POLA)
    checklist, 99–101, 106, 114
Pre-primary prophylaxis, 561
Primary biliary cirrhosis (PBC), 27, 93
  AIH, 259, 274, 275, 310, 312, 316, 318
  complications, 252
  diagnosis, 256, 260
  epidemiology, 264, 265
  etiology, 264
  fatigue, 260–261
  food and herbals, 265
  imaging, 260
  liver biochemical tests, 258
  management of symptoms, 266
  natural history, 256
  PBC-specific ANAs, 274
  physical examination, 262
  portal hypertension, 252, 262
  pruritus, 261
  screening, 273
  serum bilirubin, 255
  treatment, 251
  UDCA, 253, 265, 266
  vitamin deficiency, 264
Primary prophylaxis
  band ligation, 563
  carvedilol, 565
  cirrhotics, 565
  endoscopic sclerotherapy, 563
  esophageal variceal bleeding, 564
  high-risk varices, 564
  HVPG, 562
  mortality, 564, 565
  nadolol group, 562
  NSBB, 564
  placebo-controlled trial, 564
  postband ligation, 564
  propranolol group, 562, 564, 565
  surveillance, 566
  treatments, 561, 563
  variceal bleeding, 562, 564
Primary sclerosing cholangitis (PSC)
  AIH, 296, 312, 319, 320
  autoimmune pancreatitis, 296
  bone disease, 290
  cholangiocarcinoma, 291, 293
  cholestatic liver disease
    bone disease, 298
    fat-soluble vitamin deficiency, 298
    portal hypertension, 299
    pruritus, 297–298
  chronic illnesses, 290
  chronic liver disease, 290
  complications
    adenocarcinoma, 301
    biliary stones, 300
    cholangiocarcinoma, 301
    dominant biliary strictures, 300
    inflammatory bowel disease and
      colorectal carcinoma, 299–300
    peristomal varices, 300
  diagnosis
    cholangiography, 294
    histology, 295
    laboratories, 293–294
    onion-skinning, 295
  etiology
    genetics, 292
    immune-mediated, 292
    infectious, 292
    toxin-mediated, 293
    vascular injury, 293
  extrahepatic bile ducts, 291
  IBD, 292
  liver damage, 290
  liver transplantation, 290, 295, 302–303
  onion-skinning, 295
  overactive/abnormal immune system, 290
  small-duct primary sclerosing
    cholangitis, 295
  UDCA, 302
Prophylaxis, 494
  AASLD, 526
  ascitic fluid, 524
  cirrhosis and renal dysfunction, 525
  gastrointestinal bleeding, 525
  hepatorenal syndrome, 525
  hospitalization, 525
  liver transplant, 526
  norfloxacin vs. placebo, 524
  post-sclerotherapy bacteremia, 526
  quinolones, 525
Prothrombin time (PT), 14
Prothrombin time international normalized
    ratio (PT-INR), 606
Pruritus, 261, 267–269
PSC. *See* Primary sclerosing cholangitis (PSC)
Psychometric hepatic encephalopathy score
    (PHES), 489

PTC. *See* Percutaneous transhepatic cholangiography (PTC)
Puncture, aspiration, injection and re-aspiration (PAIR), 65
PVE. *See* Portal vein embolization (PVE)
PVT. *See* Portal vein thrombosis (PVT)

R
Radiation therapy, 78, 81–83
Radiofrequency ablation, 72, 78, 83
Reactive nitrogen species (RNS), 177
Reactive oxygen species (ROS), 177
Renal replacement therapy (RRT), 540
Repeatable battery for the assessment of neuropsychological status (RBANS), 489
Restricted resuscitation, 567
Retransplantation of the liver (ReLT), 614
Ribavirin, 149, 150, 152, 155, 616
Ribonucleoprotein/Sjogren's syndrome A (Ro/SSA), 225
Rifampicin, 267
Rifaximin, 492, 527
Rituximab, 134
Rotor's syndrome, 13
Roussel Uclaf Causality Assessment Method (RUCAM), 394, 397, 398
RRT. *See* Renal replacement therapy (RRT)

S
SAAG. *See* Serum-ascites albumin gradient (SAAG)
Sarcoidosis, 431–432
SARS-CoV. *See* Severe acute respiratory syndrome coronavirus (SARS-CoV)
SBP. *See* Spontaneous bacterial peritonitis (SBP)
Sclerotherapy, 472–474, 477, 526, 557, 563, 569–571, 573
Secondary prophylaxis, 572
Secondary sclerosing cholangitis
    congenital biliary tract disorders, 296
    hepatic artery, 297
Serotonin antagonists, 268
Serum bilirubin, 255
Serum glutamic oxaloacetic transaminase (SGOT), 3
Serum glutamic pyruvic transaminases (SGPT), 3
Serum-ascites albumin gradient (SAAG), 510, 522
Severe acute respiratory syndrome coronavirus (SARS-CoV), 170

Sicca syndrome, 269
Simple cysts, 63–64
Sinusoidal obstruction syndrome (SOS)
    clinical and laboratory findings, 426
    diagnosis, 426–427
    epidemiology and risk factors, 425–426
    HSCT, 425
    medical management, 427–429
    pathogenesis, 425
    prognosis, 429
    prophylactic medical therapy, 428
    TBI, 425
    VOD, 425
Sjogren's Syndrome, 269
Smooth muscle antibodies (SMA), 222, 224
Splenomegaly, 14, 22, 59, 126, 168, 181, 252, 333, 370, 385, 430–431, 461, 462
Spontaneous bacterial peritonitis (SBP), 108, 568
    acid-suppressive therapy, 520
    ascitic fluid analysis, 527
    beta-blockers, 524
    cirrhotic patients, 520
    clinical manifestations, 521
    diagnosis, 522
    diagnostic marker, 526
    Escherichia coli, 520
    immune dysfunction, 521
    intestinal dysmotility, 520
    intraperitoneal infection, 520
    Klebsiella species, 527
    management, 523
    noncirrhotic causes, 521
    paracentesis, 519
    prevention, 519
    prophylaxis, 521
    proton-pump inhibitors, 520
    specimen processing, 526
    treatment, 519, 523, 524
Steroid therapy, 189, 190, 397
Subjective Global Assessment (SGA), 19, 110
Sustained virologic response (SVR), 95, 561

T
TACE. *See* Transarterial embolization (TACE)
Telbivudine, 136, 138–141
Tenofovir, 136, 139–141
Thiopurine methyltransferase (TPMT) activity, 232, 238
Tramadol, 95, 96
Transaminases. *See* Aminotransferases
Transarterial chemoembolization, 73, 78, 79, 83
Transarterial embolization (TACE), 607, 616

Transarterial radioembolization, 78, 79
Transient elastography (TE), 463
Transjugular intrahepatic portosystemic shunt
        (TIPS), 108, 478, 513, 516, 539, 550
Trientine, 355, 363, 364
Trimethoprim-sulfamethoxazole, 525
"Triple-phase" CT scan, 43
Tumor markers, 72
Tumor necrosis factor-alpha (TNF-α), 521

U
United Network for Organ Sharing (UNOS),
        184, 606
Upper limit of normal (ULN), 266
Urea cycle
    brain damage, 378
    children, 379
    complications, 378
    defects, 375, 376
    diagnosis, 376
    dietary management, 378
    genetics, 376
    hyperammonemia, 377
    liver transplant, 379
    mortality, 377
    treatment, 378
Ursodeoxycholic acid (UDCA), 252, 253, 411

V
Variceal bleeding, 109
Varicella zoster (VZV), 167
Varices, esophageal, 19, 20
Vascular endothelial growth factor is observed
        (VEGF), 547
Vasoactive drugs, 568, 569

Viral hepatitis, 599, 600
    chronic infection, 137
    cirrhosis, 137
    HBIG, 136
    HBsAg and anti-HBc IgM, 134
    hepatitis B surface antibody, 133
    intramuscular hepatitis B vaccine, 136
    liver cancer, 137–138
    monotherapy, 140
    occult hepatitis B infection, 135
    risk of reactivation, 133–134
    side effects, HBV medications, 140
    treatment, 138–140
    vaccination, 134–135

W
West Haven criteria (WHC), 482, 487, 488
Wilson's disease (WD), 31
    and children, 355
    background, 356–357
    ceruloplasmin, 360
    clinical manifestations, 357–360
    diagnosis, 360–363
    diet and intake of foods, 355, 356
    genetic testing, 362–363
    hepatocyte transplanted cells, 365
    liver biopsy and hepatic copper, 361–362
    liver transplant, 356
    serum free copper concentration, 362
    treatment, 363–365
    urinary copper excretion, 361

Z
Z allele, 331
Zinc, 355, 356, 363, 364

CPSIA information can be obtained
at www.ICGtesting.com
Printed in the USA
LVOW02s2310280417
532583LV00003B/8/P